I would like to dedicate this handbook to my wife Debbie and to my five sons. This book is also dedicated to all the patients that I have treated over the past 30 years, especially Mr. Roger Rousseau, whose will to live was an example to us all.

—JD

I would like to dedicate this book to my parents, Dr. Ali-Reza Mehran and Dorianne Widmer-Mehran, whose continuous enthusiasm and strength have always been an inspiration.

—RM

Contributors

Jean Bussières, MD, FRCP(C)
Clinical Professor
Anesthesiology
Laval University
Sainte-Foy, Québec, Canada

Jean Deslauriers, MD, FRCS(C)
Professor, Department of Surgery
Laval University Faculty of Medicine
Thoracic Surgery Division
Centre de Pneumologie de L'Hôpital Laval
Sainte-Foy, Québec, Canada

Reza Mehran, MD, FACS, FRCS(C)
Associate Professor, Department of Thoracic and Cardiovascular Surgery
University of Texas M. D. Anderson Cancer Center
Houston, Texas

Mathieu Simon, MD, FRCP(C)
Head, Critical Care
Centre de Pneumologie de L'Hôpital Laval
Sainte-Foy, Québec, Canada

Foreword

I wish to emphasize first some of the comments in the Preface. The practitioner responsible for the management of patients undergoing chest surgery must have knowledge of both the general principles and the practical details of daily care. These principles and practical features of management relate to diagnosis, indications for surgery, complications and their management, practical details of peri- and postoperative care, and any recommended follow-up programs. To quote the authors, "All surgeons who perform chest operations must be familiar and comfortable with general principles of care as well as with practical issues relevant to the daily management of patients.... Such information is often unavailable or difficult to extract from traditional reference textbooks."

I fully acknowledge the difficulty or, sometimes, the impossibility of extracting these practical aspects of management and "daily care" from any of the current reference textbooks on general thoracic surgery. This handbook answers the problem admirably and is a unique contribution, worldwide, for practitioners of general thoracic surgery at any level—student, resident, or clinician.

The senior author, Jean Deslauriers, has directed the preparation of this handbook based on more than 30 years of an intensely busy practice of thoracic surgery. He heads a regional thoracic unit in Quebec City, which is affiliated with Laval University. Dr. Deslauriers is justifiably identified as an internationally recognized leader in his field: an original thinker, a thoughtful and critical observer, and possessed of a knowledge that continues to grow with ongoing experience. He is an able author and speaker who continues to lecture extensively in North and South America, Europe, the Middle East, and Asia. He remains very much abreast of the current "state of the art" in general thoracic surgery.

In addition to his many contributions to the international community, Dr. Deslauriers has spent most of his surgical lifetime mentoring and teaching the surgical residents coming through his program in Quebec City. This handbook is a distillation of his efforts and those of Dr. Reza John Mehran, a former resident of Dr. Deslauriers' who is now a thoracic surgeon with the M. D. Anderson Cancer Center in Houston. Their objective was to define the principles and practical "daily care" issues in thoracic surgery. This labor of love was undertaken because both recognized the complete void that currently exists. The contents are well organized, clearly presented, and liberally illustrated. Each chapter is provided with a relatively small number of carefully selected references. This handbook is an invaluable complement to the current publications in this field.

F. G. Pearson, MD

Preface

Over the past 25 years, interest in the field of general thoracic surgery has increased significantly, not so much as a result of the development of new surgical approaches and techniques but because of the availability of better investigative modalities and more refined perioperative care. Improved tests for early diagnosis and staging of lung cancer, for instance, have resulted in a significant increase in the number of patients with operable disease. The longer life expectancy of the general population observed in large countries such as China has also resulted in an important increase in the absolute number of patients, both men and women.

Although the practice of thoracic surgery is nearly always done within a multidisciplinary system, the thoracic surgeon is the one who directs patient care and who makes final decisions regarding specific issues, such as indications for surgery, operability and resectability of neoplasms, and treatment of perioperative complications. Because of those responsibilities, all surgeons who perform chest operations must be familiar and comfortable with general principles of care as well as with practical issues relevant to the daily management of patients. This handbook was planned because such information is often unavailable or difficult to extract from traditional reference books.

Because Dr. Deslauriers is also an editor of all editions of *Thoracic Surgery* and *Esophageal Surgery*, by Pearson et al., we were able to develop a table of contents in which the topics complement those of the Pearson volumes. We also tried to structure this information in such a way as to allow for easy understanding of the topic at hand. Hence, each chapter is complemented by numerous tables and illustrations. In the text, we have tried to be concise and focus on information that practitioners— whether they are residents or clinicians in the fields of thoracic, cardiac, or general surgery or working in related specialties such as chest medicine, anesthesia, or ear, nose, and throat surgery—must know if they want to be comfortable with the management of thoracic surgical patients.

Although the contents of this handbook reflect the experience and personal approaches of the editors, they also reflect the information contained in peer-reviewed journal articles, review articles, and abstracts published in postgraduate courses. Indeed, the editors have liberally used all types of references to provide the reader with complete and well-structured information on practical aspects of thoracic surgery. To facilitate further reading, the references have been grouped under specific headings at the end of each chapter. Of note, 30% of references are from the years 2000 to 2005, and 80% are from 1990 to 2005.

Finally, we wish to express our gratitude and appreciation to our associates, Maurice Beaulieu, Michel Piraux, Louis F. Jacques, Jocelyn Grégoire, and André Crépeau, who have provided so much insight through daily discussions and constructive criticism, and to F. G. Pearson, who has supported this work and has graciously agreed to write a foreword to this handbook.

Jean Deslauriers, MD
Reza Mehran, MD

Acknowledgments

The editors of this handbook wish to acknowledge the devoted help of
Ann Julien (secretary to Jean Deslauriers) and Josie Martinez (secretary to
Reza Mehran) for typing the entire manuscript, for which we are extremely
grateful. We also wish to thank Jocelyne Bellemare and Hélène Girard
(Medical Library, Centre de Pneumologie de l'Hôpital Laval) for reviewing
all references and doing Medline searches on selected topics. Finally,
we are indebted to Yvonne Wylie Watson (Creative Imagery Inc.,
Albuquerque, New Mexico), who has created most of the artwork included
in this handbook.

In addition, the editors acknowledge the invaluable help of
Drs. Mathieu Simon and Jean Bussières in preparing some of the chapters.
We are also most thankful to all of our residents for their daily discussions
and comments on patient care.

Finally, we wish to extend a special thanks to Maria Lorusso,
Dolores Meloni, and Elyse O'Grady of Elsevier for their expert help and
encouragement during all phases of editing this handbook.

Jean Deslauriers, MD
Reza Mehran, MD

Contents

Multidisciplinary Care of the Thoracic Surgical Patient

Thoracic surgery and especially pulmonary surgery have well-defined indications and operative techniques. Unfortunately, this surgery often involves the removal of lung parenchyma in patients whose cardiopulmonary function is already compromised by comorbidities such as emphysema, coronary artery disease, and other physiologic derangements related to smoking.

In all specialized services that treat thoracic surgical patients on a daily basis, the entire medical team—from nurses to anesthetist, thoracic surgeons, intensive care unit specialists, physiotherapists, chest physicians, and others—knows and understands the indications for surgery as well as how to prepare the patient for the intervention. The medical team also knows how to forecast possible complications, how to prevent them, how to diagnose them early, and, most important, how to treat them efficiently so that a minor event does not progress to a major morbidity.

To be successful, thoracic surgery requires not only good medical knowledge and technical skills from the surgeon but also the involvement of a well-coordinated and well-motivated team of specialists in related fields. Although better knowledge of cardiopulmonary physiology, improvements in anesthesia and postoperative analgesia, and introduction of postoperative monitoring have aided in the management of thoracic surgical patients, the modern approach to this type of work and to these diseases must be multidisciplinary. The primary benefit of this approach is improved care of patients; a non-negligible secondary benefit is that each member of the team can teach colleagues and learn from them.

ROLE OF MULTIDISCIPLINARY TEAM IN SELECTION OF PATIENTS FOR LUNG CANCER SURGERY

Diagnosis and Staging (Table 1-1)

To select the appropriate patients for surgical management, one should try to establish the primary tumor diagnosis by definition of histologic type. One should also try to determine the clinical stage of disease, which includes definition of local extension within the chest and investigation of distant tumor spread.

The *family physician* or *primary care physician* has an important role because he or she is the one who is likely to have seen the patient first, who will have suspected the presence of a thoracic malignant neoplasm, and who will have referred the patient. At present, there is no evidence that lung cancer screening, whether it is done by sputum cytology, tumor markers (monoclonal antibodies for cytologic identification), or low-dose

TABLE 1-1

MULTIDISCIPLINARY CARE OF THE THORACIC SURGICAL PATIENT:
SELECTION FOR SURGERY

Procedure	Collaborators
Diagnosis and staging	Family physician
	Chest physician, internist
	Radiologist, nuclear medicine specialist
	Pathologist, cytopathologist
Technical resectability and induction therapies	Thoracic oncologist
	Multidisciplinary conference
Fitness for surgery	Chest physician
	Consultants: cardiologists, endocrinologists, internists

spiral computed tomographic scan, reduces the number of cancer deaths. None of these techniques is sensitive (when the test result is negative, there is no cancer) or specific (when the test result is positive, there is a cancer) enough to justify its use. Indeed, the majority of nodules identified by spiral computed tomography are either nonmalignant or malignant neoplasms that are unlikely to affect survival (overdiagnosis).

Once the patient has been referred, further investigation is performed by a *chest physician*, *internist*, or *surgeon*. In many centers, diagnostic bronchoscopy is done by *chest physicians*.

The *radiologist* has a crucial role. The radiologist identifies the tumor; defines its local extension to surrounding structures (T status) or to the mediastinum (N status); and rules out distant metastases to common sites such as the musculoskeletal system (bone scanning), liver, and brain. Although computed tomographic scanning is currently the examination of choice, it is possible that in the future, positron emission tomographic scanning *(nuclear medicine specialist)* will provide "one-stop shopping." The radiologist may also be asked to obtain tissue for tumor diagnosis by way of percutaneous needle biopsy.

Preoperatively, the *pathologist* must determine if cancer is present in the biopsy specimens and, if possible, try to establish a correct histologic diagnosis. In the majority of cases, however, the information obtained through biopsy specimens is reliable with regard to the diagnosis of malignancy but less so in terms of tumor classification. If one is involved in the management of patients with early lung cancer, it is important to have good *cytology technicians* as well as *pathologists* who are expert in *cytopathology*. Given that lung tumors show significant heterogeneity, small biopsy specimens should not be overinterpreted, and a diagnosis of non–small cell lung cancer is usually sufficient to distinguish the tumor from small cell lung cancer at this point in the management of the patient.

Technical Resectability and Induction Therapies

The *thoracic surgeon* is the best person to select patients for surgical management and to conduct the surgery safely with minimal mortality and morbidity. The expectation is that approximately 40% of lung cancer patients so treated will survive at least 5 years free of disease. Indeed, the refinements of techniques of pulmonary resection as well as the knowledge that en bloc resection can be performed safely have allowed the *surgeon* some latitude in designing the appropriate treatment for each individual.

Combined modality therapies including induction treatments and chemoprophylaxis have not as yet shown improvement in the patient's survival. Because they are available, however, and because we are currently in an era of multimodality management, some cases should be discussed with a *thoracic oncologist* before surgery.

If an understanding and consensus have been reached by the members of the team as to what should be operated on and by which criteria this decision must be reached (staging protocol), most cases do not need to be discussed in a *multidisciplinary conference (tumor board)*. Cases that should always be discussed at tumor conferences are patients known preoperatively to have advanced disease, patients with tumors who have a low chance of being cured by surgery alone, and patients likely to be eligible to participate in prospective trials of multimodality treatment.

Operability and Fitness for Surgery

Because operative risks are in part related to preexisting pulmonary function, this parameter should be assessed by spirometry. All patients not clearly operable on the basis of spirometry should have complementary testing including estimation of transfer factor (TLco), measurements of gas exchange parameters (Po_2, Pco_2), and quantitative perfusion scans ($\dot{V}/\dot{Q}$), and they should be seen by a *chest physician*. Similarly, cardiac function should be looked at, and if necessary, patients should preoperatively have a *cardiology opinion*. This is most important if the patient has had a myocardial infarction within 6 months or has severe coronary artery disease. Patients with "difficult to control" diabetes mellitus should also be seen preoperatively by an *internist* or *endocrinologist*. Because patients often present with more than one comorbidity and because those factors can interact, the management of some individuals should be discussed at multidisciplinary meetings between *chest physicians*, *surgeons*, and *other specialists* as required.

ROLE OF MULTIDISCIPLINARY TEAM IN PREPARATION FOR SURGERY

All patients being considered for surgery should have adequate preparation; most of the time, this is done on an outpatient basis. All patients are seen by the *thoracic surgery clinical nurse,* who explains the upcoming procedure and may give them a video detailing what has to be done before surgery as well as the different types of procedures. Most important, it explains what will happen during the postoperative period (i.e., epidural, chest tubes). All patients are seen by a *physiotherapist,* who teaches them breathing exercises and exercises designed to improve cough effectiveness. Patients with recent weight loss or poor nutritional status are evaluated by a *dietitian* even though correcting such deficiencies preoperatively does not appear to lower perioperative risks.

It has been shown that aggressive preoperative pulmonary preparation (Table 1-2) and formal preoperative rehabilitation can improve the patient's endurance and decrease pulmonary complications postoperatively. Similarly, smoking cessation for 2 to 4 weeks, bronchodilators, judicious use of corticosteroids, and antibiotics to treat bronchopulmonary infections can decrease postoperative complications by a wide margin. In most centers, preoperative rehabilitation is done under the supervision of a *chest physician*.

It is our habit for all patients taking psychiatric drugs to be seen by a *psychiatrist* preoperatively. Similarly, if the patient is worried about his or her return home after the operation, the patient will be seen by a *social worker*.

Finally, every *surgeon* should spend at least 20 to 30 minutes with the patient and family to explain the indication for surgery as well as the procedure and its risks. In general, the risk is in the range of 2% to 3% for a lobectomy and 5% to 6% for pneumonectomy. Multiple risk factors may yield higher operative mortality rates.

TABLE 1-2

PREOPERATIVE RESPIRATORY CARE REGIMEN: A MULTIDISCIPLINARY EFFORT

Stop smoking (antismoking clinic)
Dilate airways (chest physician)
    Beta$_2$ agonists
    Steroids
    Bronchodilators
Loosen secretions (inhalation therapist)
    Airway humidifier or nebulizer
    Mucolytic and expectorant drugs
    Antibiotics
Remove secretions (physiotherapist)
    Postural drainage
    Coughing
    Chest physiotherapy (percussion and vibration)
Increase education, motivation, and facilitation of postoperative care
    Psychological preparation (surgical nurse, surgeon, social worker)
    Incentive spirometry (inhalation therapist)
    Exercise (rehabilitation specialists)
    Weight gain (dietitian)
    Stabilize the medical problems (consultants)

Modified from Benumof JL, Alfery DD: Anesthesia for thoracic surgery. In Miller RD, ed: Anesthesia, 4th ed. New York, Churchill Livingstone, 1994:1663-1735, with permission.

ROLE OF MULTIDISCIPLINARY TEAM DURING THE OPERATION

Anesthesia

With the ever-increasing number and complexities of thoracic surgical procedures, thoracic anesthesia has evolved into a subspecialty in its own right. Because the *thoracic surgeon* and *anesthetist* share the same operative field (i.e., the airways), it is essential that both communicate preoperatively, intraoperatively, and postoperatively to ensure optimal management of the patient.

Surgical Team

For most cases of lung cancer (Table 1-3), anatomic and complete resection of the primary tumor can be done by one surgeon. On occasion, however, a multidisciplinary approach will be beneficial and will enhance the patient's chances of a complete resection. This is the case, for instance, for Pancoast tumors, for which one must resect the chest wall, often including part of one or more vertebral bodies. In our view, this is best accomplished with the assistance of an *orthopedic surgeon* or a *neurosurgeon* familiar with spinal surgery. Similarly, if a tumor invades the proximal pulmonary artery, aorta, or superior vena cava, it may still be possible to carry out a complete resection; but in such cases, the intraoperative help of a *cardiac or vascular surgeon* is invaluable for the reconstruction.

Another example is that of the reconstruction of the soft tissues of the chest wall after resection of a parietal neoplasm or of other conditions affecting the chest wall. In such cases, *plastic surgeons* are experts in pedicled flap reconstruction, and because the appropriate selection as well as the mobilization of these flaps is important, they should be asked to do this part of the procedure. This is done with the understanding that transposition of any of these flaps requires precise knowledge of its blood supply.

Another area of thoracic surgery in which team work may be useful is that of airway surgery. Subglottic resection and synchronous laryngeal

TABLE 1-3	
IMPORTANCE OF THORACIC SURGEONS WORKING WITHIN A TEAM	
Procedure	**Other Members of the Team**
Pulmonary resection	
Pancoast tumor	Orthopedic surgeon or neurosurgeon
T4 cardiovascular (proximal pulmonary artery, aorta, vena cava)	Cardiovascular surgeon
Vertebral body	Orthopedic surgeon
Chest wall surgery	Plastic surgeon (soft tissue reconstruction)
Tracheal surgery	ENT surgeon (subglottic and glottic resections)
Mediastinal surgery	
Dumbbell tumors	Neurosurgeon

reconstruction are sometimes best managed collaboratively with the *otolaryngologist.*

ROLE OF MULTIDISCIPLINARY TEAM AFTER THE OPERATION

Immediate Postoperative Care

Most of the initial postoperative care is the responsibility of the *thoracic surgeon,* who should be able to prevent, detect early, and treat adequately complications that may arise. It is a matter of controversy as to who should look after postoperative analgesia. In most centers in which postoperative analgesia is provided through epidural administration of opiates, the *anesthetist* is responsible for this part of the postoperative care.

Management of complications such as respiratory failure (1% to 3% of patients), tachyarrhythmias (20% to 40% after pneumonectomy), and renal failure is best done by *chest physicians* or *intensivists, cardiologists,* and *nephrologists,* respectively. Lack or nonavailability of such consultants on a daily basis (including weekends) is certainly a risk factor for catastrophic events. Similarly, it is always desirable to consult with *internists* for the management of patients with diabetes mellitus.

Because life expectancy in developed countries has now increased far beyond 70 years, a large number of elderly patients with lung cancer are presenting as candidates for surgery. In those individuals, postoperative delirium is not uncommon. When this happens, one should consult with a *psychiatrist,* who can adjust the medication on the basis of the patient's age, comorbidities (i.e., renal or liver dysfunction), mental status, and respiratory status.

Hospital Discharge

Because the return home is often a source of anxiety for the patient, it should be prepared. We usually ask the *social worker* to discuss this issue with the patient and the patient's relatives. It is also important that the *surgeon* or a *surgery nurse* spend some time with the patient before he or she leaves the hospital. The patient should understand what he or she can or cannot do during the convalescence as well as which symptoms are an alert to possible late complications.

Adjuvant Therapies

As yet, postoperative adjuvant therapies, with few exceptions, have failed to improve survival of patients with lung cancer. In general, however, the decision to offer lung cancer patients postoperative radiation therapy or chemotherapy is based on whether the patient had pathologic N2 disease and whether there has been a complete resection. The management of individual patients with such diseases should be discussed at *multidisciplinary oncologic conferences* involving *physicians, thoracic surgeons, oncologists,* and *radiation therapists.* These treatments will often be done even if their therapeutic value is uncertain.

Follow-up

Most practitioners are convinced of the value of routine follow-up of patients after surgical therapy for lung cancer, even if its effectiveness has never been measured. Because basic methods of follow-up include history, physical examination, and chest radiograph, these can be done by the *family physician* or preferably by the *thoracic surgeon*. In lung cancer patients, the follow-up must include a proper examination of the supraclavicular region to rule out abnormal adenopathies and a review of chest radiographs with comparison to previous ones.

After resection of lung cancer, most patients generally quit smoking on their own accord. If this proves difficult, they should be referred to an *antismoking clinic*.

CONCLUSION

Although the thoracic surgeon has the responsibility for the individual assessment and the final indication for surgery, the overall management of thoracic surgical patients requires the active interaction of a multidisciplinary team. It is therefore important that major cases of thoracic surgery be done in centers large enough to have the infrastructure, resources, and experience to provide such care.

SUGGESTED READINGS

General Articles

Kay PH, Wells FC, Goldstraw P: A multidisciplinary approach to primary nonseminomatous germ cell tumors of the mediastinum. Ann Thorac Surg 1987;44:578-582.

Patton MD, Schaerf R: Thoracotomy, critical pathway, and clinical outcomes. Cancer Pract 1995;3:286-294.

Gandhi S, Walsh GL, Komaki R, et al: A multidisciplinary surgical approach to superior sulcus tumors with vertebral invasion. Ann Thorac Surg 1999;68:1778-1785.

Sportelli G, Loffredo L, Lupi M, et al: A multidisciplinary approach to the treatment of small-cell lung cancer: the role played by surgery. Eur Rev Med Pharmacol Sci 1999;3:261-263.

Mussi A, Lucchi M, Murri L, et al: Extended thymectomy in myasthenia gravis: a team-work of neurologist, thoracic surgeon and anaesthetist may improve the outcome. Eur J Cardiothorac Surg 2001;19:570-575.

Hulscher JBF, Haringsma J, Benraadt J, et al: Comprehensive Cancer Centre Amsterdam Barrett Advisory Committee: first results. Neth J Med 2001;58:3-8.

Armstrong P, Congleton J, Fountain SW, et al: Guidelines on the selection of patients with lung cancer for surgery. Thorax 2001;56:89-108.

Walsh GL, Davis BM, Swisher SG, et al: A single-institutional, multidisciplinary approach to primary sarcomas involving the chest wall requiring full-thickness resections. J Thorac Cardiovasc Surg 2001;121:48-60.

Ghosh S, Steyn RS, Marzouk JFK, et al: The effectiveness of high dependency unit in the management of high risk thoracic surgical cases. Eur J Cardiothorac Surg 2004;25:123-126.

Multidisciplinary Care of the Thoracic Surgical Patient

Preoperative Assessment

ASSESSMENT OF PULMONARY RESERVE

Chronic obstructive pulmonary disease is probably the most important limiting factor in resectional surgery of the lung not only because it affects the majority of patients with lung cancer but also because it relates directly to postoperative morbidity and mortality. In the "high-risk" patient, resection is not necessarily prohibited, but the type of operation should be carefully selected and prophylactic measures applied to decrease the incidence of complications. As pneumonectomy represents the most extensive type of lung resection feasible, patients should be evaluated predominantly for this procedure.

Although pulmonary function assessment has been studied extensively, *no single parameter* has been shown to predict surgical outcome with accuracy. Risk assessment must therefore include an *in-depth analysis* of a variety of lung function parameters so that a reliable and reproducible profile can be established (low risk, high risk, prohibitive risk) for each individual (Table 2-1). This will ensure that no patient is denied surgery while minimizing the incidence of postoperative complications.

In thoracic surgery, *technical misadventures* do occur but rarely account for significant postoperative morbidity. On the other hand, the majority of postoperative complications and deaths are related to *cardiopulmonary events,* most of which can be identified and prevented preoperatively.

PHYSIOLOGIC EVALUATION OF OVERALL FUNCTION
Evaluation of Pulmonary Status by History—Initial Patient Encounter

The *initial encounter* with the patient is a most important step in the preoperative assessment of pulmonary reserve. It often determines the suitability of the patient to undergo pulmonary resection as well as the need for complementary testing.

A *normally active life,* unimpaired by dyspnea, is generally indicative of sufficient pulmonary reserve. The level of *dyspnea,* however, does not necessarily correlate with results of pulmonary function studies because patients may have adjusted their level of activities according to their limitation. Their actual level of dyspnea should be compared with former abilities. A reasonable assessment of pulmonary function can be obtained by recording the patient's *exercise tolerance* to commonly done manual activities, such as climbing stairs or cutting grass.

TABLE 2-1

PREDICTORS OF POSTOPERATIVE MORTALITY AND MORBIDITY: PATIENT'S PROFILE

	Low Risk	High Risk	Very High Risk or Prohibitive
		Function of Both Lungs	
CLINICAL			
Dyspnea (grade 0-4)	0-1	2-3	3-4
Smoking (current)	0	++	++
Sputum production (1-4)	0	1-2	3-4
SPIROMETRY			
FEV_1	>2.0 L	0.8-2.0 L	<0.8 L
FVC	>3.0 L	1.5-3.0 L	<1.5 L
	>50% predicted	<50% predicted	<30% predicted
FEV_1/FVC	>70%	<70%	<50%
Improvement with bronchodilation	>15%	1%-15%	None
GAS EXCHANGE			
Resting Po_2 (mm Hg)	60-80	45-60	<45
Resting Pco_2 (mm Hg)	<45	45-50	>50
Resting D_{LCO}	>50% predicted	30%-50% predicted	<30% predicted
EXERCISE TESTING			
Submaximal tests			
Stair climbing	>3 flights	≤3 flights	≤1 flight
Exercise oximetry			Resting saturation <90%
			Desaturation of >4% during test
Maximal test			
Exercise oxygen consumption (Vo_2max)	>20 mL/min/kg >75% predicted	11-19 mL/min/kg	<10 mL/min/kg <60% predicted
		Function of Each Lung	
RADIONUCLIDE STUDIES			
Predicted FEV_1	>1.2 L	0.8-1.2 L	<0.8 L
Predicted D_{LCO}			<40% predicted

A *smoking history* is relevant, and patients who have stopped for 3 months or more preoperatively have generally fewer postoperative complications. Similarly, patients who have excessive daily *sputum production* are likely to have a poor outcome from surgical intervention.

Spirometry

Spirometric studies are of value because they provide *objective data on lung function*. They also help to initially *screen the high-risk patient*. For a variety of reasons including medicolegal ones, they should be done routinely before any type of pulmonary resection. A large amount of information can be obtained, for instance, by looking at the relationship between maximal expiratory flow rates and lung volumes. Of these, FEV_1 (quantitative measurement of expiratory volume during the first second of expiration) is the best predictor of pulmonary morbidity after lung resection. FEV_1 values should, however, be adjusted for age, sex, and height, so that it is better to look at percentage of predicted values rather than at absolute values. The ratio FEV_1/FVC (forced vital capacity) is often a better predictor of postoperative complications because it assesses the obstructive pulmonary component more accurately. Abnormal results of these simple spirometric tests as outlined in Table 2-1 give a good profile of the patient's pulmonary reserve and indicate the risk of postoperative complications.

2

Gas Exchange

Preoperative *resting hypoxemia (Po$_2$ < 60 mm Hg)* is not an absolute contraindication to pulmonary resection because the lung to be resected may be a contributing factor. Indeed, arterial partial pressure of oxygen (Pao_2) is not an established predictor of postoperative morbidity. *Resting hypercapnia (Pco$_2$ > 50 mm Hg),* by contrast, indicates advanced lung disease, and such a finding does predict the high likelihood of perioperative morbidity, especially after pneumonectomy.

   Diffusion of carbon monoxide (DLCO) measurements evaluate the ability of the lung to exchange gas. The measurement is based on the principle that diffusion of a gas through the alveolocapillary membrane is equal to the capacity of diffusion of the membrane and the pressure difference between the alveolus and the capillary for this gas. The *coefficient of carbon monoxide diffusion (K_{CO})* is a measurement corrected for the surface of exchange. Several authors have shown that resting DLCO as percentage of predicted is an important predictor of pulmonary morbidity and mortality from all causes after major pulmonary resection (Table 2-1).

   Improvements in flow rates after *bronchodilators* indicate some reversibility of the process, and these patients should be classified by their post-bronchodilator FEV_1. Static lung volumes such as total lung capacity, which is the total amount of air within the lungs at maximal inspiration, and residual volume are indicators of the severity of chronic obstructive pulmonary disease, but they are generally not considered good indicators for perioperative risk in lung resections.

Exercise Testing

Exercise testing measures the ability of the whole organism to perform well because it assesses the interaction of *pulmonary function, hemodynamic performance,* and *peripheral tissue oxygen use.* Since the early 1970s, several authors have demonstrated that exercise testing is the only objective measurement of cardiopulmonary reserve to show a statistically significant difference between groups of patients with benign postoperative courses and groups with cardiac or respiratory complications.

Preoperative Assessment

Submaximal Tests

The available options for such an assessment include self-reporting by patients of their capabilities, stair climbing, and timed walking tests (6- or 12-minute walk) with oximetry.

Although it is not standardized, the *stair climbing* test correlates well with FEV_1 and maximum oxygen consumption (Vo_2max). The ability to pass the test (more than three flights without air hunger or prolonged recovery time) suggests that those patients are likely to tolerate pulmonary resection, including pneumonectomy. The test is also useful in screening patients who may have cardiovascular complaints, such as claudication or angina. One important use of the 6- or 12-minute walk tests is the assessment of severely disabled patients who are capable of only low-intensity exercise.

Exercise oximetry is a cost-effective screening test, and it may be superior to FEV_1 for screening of the high-risk patient. Patients with resting saturation below 90% or those who desaturate above 4% during exercise are in the high-risk category and should have more detailed assessment.

Maximal Tests

The main use of *progressive incremental testing* is the precise measurement of individual response to exercise. In most laboratories, exercise is performed on a calibrated cycle ergometer where the power is increased in equal increments each minute (100 kpm/min or 15 to 20 watts). Observations include arterial blood gases (or oxygen saturation), highest oxygen consumption (Vo_2max), heart rate, blood pressure, and electrocardiogram (ECG). Several studies have shown that a Vo_2max below 10 mL/min/kg is highly predictive of morbidity, whereas few patients with a Vo_2max above 20 mL/min/kg will sustain a pulmonary complication or die postoperatively. Vo_2max expressed as a *percentage of predicted normal* (related to age and body mass) can also be used to discriminate patients, and a Vo_2max value above 75% of predicted is an excellent predictor of uneventful postoperative course irrespective of the extent of resection.

PHYSIOLOGIC EVALUATION OF THE FUNCTION OF EACH LUNG: SPLIT FUNCTION STUDIES

In patients with impaired function, knowledge of the post-resectional function is of importance not only to assess surgical risk but also to predict *long-term chances of disability*. For most patients, a simple calculation based on the preoperative FEV_1 and amount of segments to be resected (5.2% per segment) provides a reasonable estimate of postoperative function. Additional testing includes bronchospirometry, lateral position testing, and quantitative radionuclide scanning.

Bronchospirometry and Lateral Position Test

Bronchospirometry allows the evaluation of one lung compared with the other by insertion of a double-lumen tube in the tracheobronchial tree and measurement of the Vo_2, carbon dioxide elimination, and vital capacity and its subdivisions. Currently, this test is seldom used because it is unpleasant for the patient and requires skilled personnel.

The *lateral position test* estimates the relative function of the right and left lungs by changes in the functional residual capacity when the patient switches from a supine to a left and right decubitus position. Although the accuracy of the test has been challenged, it is technically simple and well tolerated by the patient.

Regional Radionuclide Studies

If preoperative function and extent of planned resection are known, accurate prediction of postoperative pulmonary function can be made by *regional radionuclide studies*. The most popular technique is a split perfusion scan with technetium Tc 99 m–labeled macroaggregate. The formula used for the predicted postoperative (ppo) value is the following:

$$\text{Value ppo} = \text{preoperative value} \times (1 - \text{contribution of parenchyma to be resected})$$

Depending on the author, the lower level of predicted FEV_1 acceptable for operability varies between 0.8 and 1.0 L. These figures are based on medical studies that have shown that once an emphysematous patient has reached an FEV_1 of 0.8 L or less because of disease progression, complications and death from respiratory failure are likely to occur. This situation may, however, be different from the one in which FEV_1 is brought down to similar levels by pulmonary resection and the remaining parenchyma is relatively uninvolved with emphysema. With use of the same formula, other reports have shown that DL_{CO}-ppo and $\dot{V}o_2$max-ppo can also be calculated and used for prediction of perioperative risk.

ALGORITHM FOR THE EVALUATION OF PULMONARY FUNCTION

Despite all of these guidelines, numbers tell only part of the story, and the final preoperative assessment depends on the experience of the assessor. There is no formula for, no absolute criterion of, and, in the case of resectable lung cancer, no absolute contraindication to surgical intervention. One must understand that these parameters predict morbidity, most of which is recoverable; in the case of lung cancer treatment, such recoverable morbidity may be acceptable.

To avoid unnecessary costs, however, it is necessary to take a stepwise approach to the evaluation of the lung cancer patient with presumed resectable disease. The algorithm proposed in this chapter was described by Bolliger et al. It proposes successive steps until the patient is found to be able to tolerate operation or is deemed inoperable (Fig. 2-1).

RISK-REDUCTION STRATEGIES

The identification of pulmonary risk factors allows the institution of *preventive measures* that may permit lung resection in the compromised patient, decrease postoperative complication rates, and ensure acceptable quality of life postoperatively.

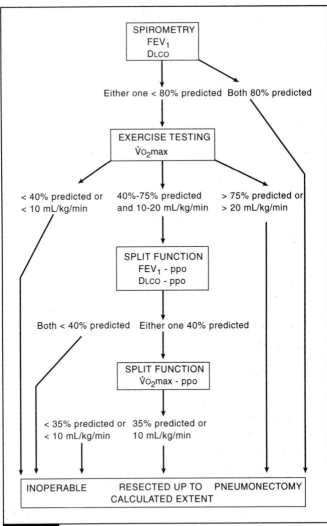

FIG. 2-1

Algorithm for the assessment of lung function before pulmonary resection. ppo, predicted postoperative. *(From Bolliger CT, Perruchoud AP: Functional evaluation of the lung resection candidate. Eur Respir J 1998;11:198-212.)*

TABLE 2-2
RISK-REDUCTION STRATEGIES BEFORE OPERATION
Recognize and estimate severity of chronic obstructive pulmonary disease.
Urge discontinuance of smoking.
Control infection (specific antibiotics).
Control bronchospasm (bronchodilators, corticosteroids).
Discuss care with chest physician and anesthesiologist.
Schedule surgery late in the day for patients with productive cough.
Avoid excessive premedication.
Use formal rehabilitation for 6-8 weeks.
Educate patient about lung expansion maneuvers.

2

Preoperative Assessment

Before Operation (Table 2-2)

Risk-reduction maneuvers that can be used *preoperatively* include cessation of smoking for at least 2 weeks before operation, maintenance of adequate nutrition, and bronchodilation and antibiotic therapy if necessary. If oral corticosteroids are given to improve bronchospasm, as low a dose as possible should be used.

Preoperative teaching of respiratory maneuvers and about the procedure to be done is also most important. This teaching, which is often carried out by physiotherapists, nurses, or other specialized personnel, will improve postoperative cooperation and reduce the incidence of complications. In some individuals, prolonged (up to 8 weeks) and structured preoperative rehabilitation may significantly improve endurance and fitness and thereby allow surgical interventions that otherwise would have been contraindicated.

During Operation (Table 2-3)

For patients undergoing thoracotomy, *standard monitoring requirements* include ECG, direct arterial catheterization, central venous pressure line, pulse oximetry, temperature probe, and urine output measurement. The use of Swan-Ganz catheters is indicated only under specific circumstances.

TABLE 2-3
RISK-REDUCTION STRATEGIES DURING OPERATION
Adequately monitor ECG, arterial blood pressure, temperature, central venous pressure, blood gases, and urine output.
Avoid excessive crystalloids and blood infusion.
Avoid hypotension and hypoxemia.
Regularly suction trachea and main bronchi.
Limit duration of surgery.
Use lung expansion maneuvers when necessary.
Consider use of limited resections (wedges, segmental resections).
Supplement general anesthesia with epidural anesthesia.
Use muscle-sparing incisions or thoracoscopic procedures whenever possible.
Have an anesthetist familiar with thoracic procedures administer anesthesia.
Drain pleural space adequately.

In most patients undergoing pulmonary resection, *one-lung ventilation* is provided by the use of disposable double-lumen endotracheal tubes, and, ideally, anesthesia should be given by an anesthetist *familiar with lung resectional procedures*.

Other important intraoperative risk-reduction strategies include the use of *muscle-sparing incisions or thoracoscopic procedures* whenever possible, the use of *limited resections* if adequate tumor clearance can be achieved, and the use of *surgical lung re-expansion maneuvers* when necessary. These maneuvers include procedures such as pleural tenting and pneumoperitoneum that are designed to decrease the size of the pleural space and therefore lower the incidence of prolonged air leaks.

After Operation (Table 2-4)

After completion of the procedure, it is desirable to have the patient extubated *as soon as possible*. This should not be done, however, until adequate ventilatory ability has been demonstrated.

Because most complications occur in the first 2 to 4 postoperative days, patients should ideally be in an intermediate or intensive care unit where their cardiopulmonary status can be monitored adequately. Indeed, most serious complications can be anticipated and in some cases prevented by early prophylactic treatment. Minimal monitoring, at least during the first 48 hours, includes ECG, blood pressure, urine output, temperature, and oximetry.

Coughing and deep-breathing exercises as well as incentive spirometry have been shown to decrease the risk of atelectasis or of other pulmonary complications by increasing lung volume. If patients are unable to perform deep-breathing exercises adequately, intermittent positive-pressure breathing with saline or a mixture of saline and bronchodilators may be useful. Continuous positive airway pressure (CPAP) can be useful, but it is often poorly tolerated by the postoperative thoracic patient.

TABLE 2-4
RISK-REDUCTION STRATEGIES AFTER OPERATION

Leave endotracheal tube in place until adequate ventilatory ability is demonstrated.
Transfer patient to intermediate or intensive care unit for 24-48 hours postoperatively.
Monitor ECG, blood pressure, urine output, temperature, and oximetry.
Use moist oxygen therapy.
Encourage cough, respiratory physiotherapy, and incentive spirometry.
Carry out fiberoptic bronchoscopy with physical signs or chest radiographic findings of atelectasis.
Carry out intermittent positive-pressure breathing with bronchodilation whenever necessary.
Provide adequate pain control without excessive sedation.
Promote early ambulation.
Avoid excessive fluid infusion.

Epidural analgesia is now the most widespread method of *pain control* for thoracotomy patients. It allows excellent analgesia with relatively minor side effects, such as urinary retention, pruritus, and nausea. Adjuvant therapy with nonsteroidal compounds or intercostal nerve blocks is often added for improved pain control. Adequate pain control is important because pain suppresses cough and deep breathing, thereby increasing the risks of atelectasis and pneumonia.

Patients undergoing pulmonary resection should not receive excessive intravenous fluids because it may lead to higher filtration pressures, transudation into the alveoli, and ultimately pulmonary edema. This is more likely to happen in pneumonectomy patients who have had lymphatic interruption through extensive mediastinal lymphadenectomy.

CONCLUSION

The preoperative assessment of the thoracic surgical patient is of inestimable value in anticipating and preventing postoperative complications. The surgeon should not abrogate the responsibility of this assessment, which requires a complete history and judicious use of pulmonary testing. Ultimately, the incidence of complications can be lowered significantly through the judicious use of risk-reduction strategies.

SUGGESTED READINGS

Review Articles

Miller JI: Preoperative evaluation. Chest Surg Clin North Am 1992;2:701-711.

Marshall MC, Olsen GN: The physiologic evaluation of the lung resection candidate. Clin Chest Med 1993;14:305-320.

Bolliger CT, Perruchoud AP: Functional evaluation of the lung resection candidate. Eur Respir J 1998;11:198-212.

Smetana GW: Preoperative pulmonary evaluation. Current concepts. N Engl J Med 1999;340:937-944.

Reilly JJ: Evidence-based preoperative evaluation of candidates for thoracotomy. Chest 1999;116:474s-476s.

Slinger PD, Johnston MR: Preoperative assessment for pulmonary resection. Anesthesiol Clin North Am 2001;19:411-433.

Schuurmans MM, Diacon AH, Bolliger CT: Functional evaluation before lung resection. Clin Chest Med 2002;23:159-172.

Predicted Function

Bria WF, Kanarek DJ, Kazemi H: Prediction of postoperative pulmonary function following thoracic operations. Value of ventilation-perfusion scanning. J Thorac Cardiovasc Surg 1983;86:186-192.

Kearney DJ, Lee TH, Reilly JJ, et al: Assessment of operative risk in patients undergoing lung resection. Importance of predicted pulmonary function. Chest 1994;105:753-759.

Brunelli A, Monteverde M, Borri A, et al: Predicted versus observed maximum oxygen consumption early after lung resection. Ann Thorac Surg 2003;76:376-380.

Diffusing Capacity

Wang J, Olak J, Ferguson MK: Diffusing capacity predicts operative mortality but not long-term survival after resection for lung cancer. J Thorac Cardiovasc Surg 1999;117:581-587.

Wang JS, Abboud RT, Evans KG, et al: Role of CO diffusing capacity during exercise in the preoperative evaluation for lung resection. Am J Respir Crit Care Med 2000;162:1435-1444.

Exercise Testing

Bolton JWR, Weiman DS, Haynes JL, et al: Stair climbing as an indicator of pulmonary function. Chest 1987;92:783-787.

Bechard D, Wetstein L: Assessment of exercise oxygen consumption as preoperative criterion for lung resection. Ann Thorac Surg 1987;44:344-349.

Gilbreth EM, Weisman IM: Role of exercise stress testing in preoperative evaluation of patients for lung resection. Clin Chest Med 1994;15:389-403.

Bolliger CT, Wyser C, Roser H, et al: Lung scanning and exercise testing for the prediction of postoperative performance in lung resection candidates at increased risk for complications. Chest 1995;108:341-348.

Rao V, Todd TRJ, Kuus A, et al: Exercise oximetry versus spirometry in the assessment of risk prior to lung resection. Ann Thorac Surg 1995;60:603-609.

Bolliger CT, Jordan P, Solèr M, et al: Exercise capacity as a predictor of postoperative complications in lung resection candidates. Am J Respir Crit Care Med 1995;151:1472-1480.

Ninan M, Sommers KE, Landreneau RJ, et al: Standardized exercise oximetry predicts postpneumonectomy outcome. Ann Thorac Surg 1997;64:328-333.

Older P, Hall A, Hader R: Cardiopulmonary exercise testing as a screening test for perioperative management of major surgery in the elderly. Chest 1999;116:355-362.

Brutsche MH, Spiliopoulos A, Bolliger CT, et al: Exercise capacity and extent of resection as predictors of surgical risk in lung cancer. Eur Respir J 2000;15:828-832.

Brunelli A, Monteverde M, Salati M, et al: Stair-climbing test to evaluate maximum aerobic capacity early after lung resection. Ann Thorac Surg 2001;72:1705-1710.

Varela G, Cordovilla R, Jimenez MF, Novoa N: Utility of standardized exercise oximetry to predict cardiopulmonary morbidity after lung resection. Eur J Cardiothorac Surg 2001;19:351-354.

Brunelli A, Al Refai M, Monteverde M, et al: Predictors of exercise oxygen desaturation following major lung resection. Eur J Cardiothorac Surg 2003;24:145-148.

Postoperative Complications and Pulmonary Function

Brunelli A, Al Refai M, Monteverde M, et al: Predictors of early morbidity after major lung resection in patients with and without airflow limitation. Ann Thorac Surg 2002;74:999-1003.

Sekine Y, Iwata T, Chiyo M, et al: Minimal alteration of pulmonary function after lobectomy in lung cancer patients with chronic obstructive pulmonary disease. Ann Thorac Surg 2003;76:356-362.

Solli P, Leo F, Veronesi G, et al: Impact of limited pulmonary function on the management of resectable lung cancer. Lung Cancer 2003;41:71-79.

Jones DR, Stiles BM, Denlinger CE, et al: Pulmonary segmentectomy: results and complications. Ann Thorac Surg 2003;76:343-349.

Pulmonary Function: Cancer and Lung Volume Reduction Surgery

Korst RJ, Ginsberg RJ, Ailawadi M, et al: Lobectomy improves ventilatory function in selected patients with severe COPD. Ann Thorac Surg 1998;66:898-902.

Edwards JG, Duthie DJR, Waller DA: Lobar volume reduction surgery: A method of increasing the lung cancer resection rate in patients with emphysema. Thorax 2001;56:791-795.

Case Series

Ferguson MK, Reeder LB, Mick R: Optimizing selection of patients for major lung resection. J Thorac Cardiovasc Surg 1995;109:275-283.

Wyser C, Stulz P, Solèr M, et al: Prospective evaluation of an algorithm for the functional assessment of lung resection candidates. Am J Respir Crit Care Med 1999;159:1450-1456.

2

Preoperative Assessment

ASSESSMENT OF CARDIAC FUNCTION

Most patients undergoing thoracic operations are current or former smokers and as such are in the age group in which concomitant cardiovascular disease is common. Because both morbidity and mortality from thoracic surgery *increase exponentially* in patients with significant cardiovascular disease, one has to take the appropriate steps to determine potential risks for given individuals. For this evaluation to be successful, *careful teamwork* as well as communication between patients, surgeon, and consultant cardiologist is required. In the end, *clinical judgment* and *experience* remain central to the risk-benefit ratio of the proposed procedure.

OVERALL ESTIMATION OF CARDIOVASCULAR RISKS (TABLE 2-5)

The overall estimation of cardiac risks has been reported by Goldman, who used nine significant preoperative risk factors and assessed point values as determined by multivariate risk analysis (Table 2-6). Although with modern preoperative care it is likely that the actual risks are less than those originally predicted, patients in class 3 or class 4 require additional

TABLE 2-5
CARDIAC RISK PROFILE

	Low Risk	High Risk	Very High Risk or Prohibitive
Overall estimation of cardiovascular risks			
Cardiac risk index (Goldman) (see Table 2-6)	Class 1-2 (0-12 points)	Class 3 (13-25 points)	Class 4 (>25 points)
Cardiopulmonary risk index score (Epstein) (see Table 2-7)	<4 points	>4 points	
Evaluation of the patient with coronary artery disease			
Clinical			
Previous myocardial infarction	None or >6 months	3-6 months	<3 months
Angina (see Table 2-8)	None or class 1	Class 2	Class 3-4 Unstable angina
Exercise testing			
Exercise ECG testing	No changes	Ischemic ECG changes; ST depression >2 mm	
	Ability to reach 85% of age-predicted heart rate maximum	Inability to reach 85% of age-predicted heart rate maximum	
Exercise thallium	Normal or fixed defects	Reversible ischemic defects	
Nonexercise testing			
Nonexercise thallium stress test	Normal or fixed defects	Reversible ischemic defects	
Dobutamine stress echocardiography	Normal	Abnormal; severe wall motion abnormalities	
Coronary angiography	Normal	Lesions amenable to revascularization	Lesions not amenable to revascularization
Evaluation of the patient with congestive heart failure			
New York Heart Association functional class	1	2	3-4

TABLE 2-6			
GOLDMAN CARDIAC RISK INDEX			
Factors			Points
History			
Age >70 years			5
Myocardial infarction <6 months			10
Physical examination			
Congestive failure			11
Aortic stenosis			3
ECG			
Rhythm abnormality			7
Premature ventricular contractions >5/min			7
General			
$Po_2 < 60$ mm Hg; $Pco_2 > 50$ mm Hg; $HCO_3 < 20$ mmol/L			3
↑ Creatinine; liver disease			
↓ Performance status			
Type of operation			
Intraperitoneal or thoracic			3
Emergency surgery			4
Total possible points			53
Class	Points	Severe Morbidity	Cardiac Deaths
1	0-5	0.7%	0.2%
2	6-12	5%	2%
3	13-25	11%	2%
4	>25	22%	56%

From Goldman L, Caldera DL, Nussbaum SR, et al: Multifactorial index of cardiac risk in noncardiac surgical procedures. N Engl J Med 1977;297:848.

investigation as well as intensive perioperative and postoperative monitoring, including pulmonary artery pressure (Swan-Ganz) measurements.

Another method that can be used to estimate cardiac risks is one that is based on a *preoperative risk index* in which points are assigned for various factors including pulmonary and cardiac. These are totaled into a *cardiopulmonary index score* (1 to 10) that is used to predict postoperative risk (Table 2-7). Several authors have shown that this index correlates with values of $\dot{V}o_2max$, which is also an estimate of total physical fitness. A cardiopulmonary risk index score of more than 4 points is highly predictive of complications after lung resection.

THORACIC SURGERY IN THE PATIENT WITH KNOWN OR POSSIBLE CORONARY ARTERY DISEASE

Clinical Evaluation

In most cardiac patients undergoing pulmonary resections, the greatest risks arise from the presence of coronary artery disease. In the general population, the risk of a postoperative myocardial infarction after general anesthesia is in the range of 0.05% to 0.07%. Operations performed within 3 months of a myocardial infarction, however, result in a 27%

TABLE 2-7

CARDIOPULMONARY RISK INDEX

Cardiac Risk Index (CRI)		Pulmonary Risk Index (PRI)	
Variable	Points	Variable	Points
Congestive heart failure	11	Obesity	1
Myocardial infarction during previous 6 months	10	Cigarette smoking (8 weeks)	1
>5 premature ventricular contractions/minute	7	Productive cough (within 5 days of surgery)	1
Rhythm other than sinus rhythm	7	Diffuse rhonchi or wheezing within 5 days of surgery	1
Age > 70 years	5		
Severe aortic valve stenosis	3	$FEV_1/FVC < 70\%$	1
Poor condition	3	$Paco_2 > 45$ mm Hg	1
Total CRI points: 3-46		Total PRI points: 0-6	

CRI score

0-5 points:	1
6-12 points:	2
13-25 points:	3
>25 points:	4

Cardiopulmonary risk index (CPRI) score

CRI + PRI = 1-10 points

From Epstein SK, Faling LJ, Daly BDT, Celli BR: Predicting complications after pulmonary resection. Preoperative exercise testing vs. a multifactorial cardiopulmonary risk index. Chest 1993;104:694-700.

incidence of recurrent infarction. This incidence decreases to about 15% if the myocardial infarction has occurred 4 to 6 months previously and to 6% if the operation is delayed for 6 months or more. Other factors known to be associated with increased reinfarction rates include surgery lasting more than 3 hours, preoperative hypertension, and intraoperative hypotension.

Similar risks have been identified for patients with *angina,* with an increasing risk for each class of the New York Heart Association (NYHA) angina classification (Table 2-8). Patients with unstable or NYHA class 3 or class 4 angina should have further evaluation and potentially be considered for angioplasty or even coronary artery bypass grafting. Increased postoperative morbidity and mortality also correlate with the NYHA functional class that associates dyspnea with congestive heart failure.

For these reasons, *an accurate cardiac history, including documentation of all cardiovascular medication used,* is of utmost importance. Heart auscultation, measurement of blood pressure, and examination for focal

TABLE 2-8
THE NEW YORK HEART ASSOCIATION ANGINA CLASSIFICATION

Class	Description
1	Angina with strenuous exercise
2	Angina with moderate exercise
3	Angina with 1 flight of stairs or 1-2 blocks
4	Angina with any activity

vascular lesions of the carotid, aorta, and femoral vessels should always be done. In addition, a *routine ECG* is valuable to demonstrate asymptomatic arrhythmias, conduction disturbances, or clinically silent coronary artery disease. More specifically, one should look for ST-T wave changes, old Q waves, and bundle branch blocks.

Table 2-9 lists the clinical predictors of *increased perioperative risk* of myocardial infarction, congestive heart failure, and death as established by the American College of Cardiology and American Heart Association Task Force and Practice Guidelines in 1996. Major predictors mandate intensive management; intermediate predictors are well-validated markers of enhanced risk of perioperative cardiac complications. Minor predictors are recognized markers for cardiovascular disease that have not been proved to independently increase perioperative risk.

TABLE 2-9
CLINICAL PREDICTORS OF INCREASED PERIOPERATIVE CARDIOVASCULAR RISK*

MAJOR

Recent myocardial infarction (>7 days but <1 month)
Unstable or severe angina
Decompensated congestive heart failure
High-grade atrioventricular block
Symptomatic ventricular arrhythmias in the presence of underlying heart disease
Supraventricular arrhythmias with uncontrolled ventricular rate

INTERMEDIATE

Mild angina pectoris
Prior myocardial infarction by history or pathologic Q waves
Compensated or prior congestive heart failure
Diabetes mellitus

MINOR

Advanced age
Abnormal ECG
Rhythm other than normal sinus rhythm
Low functional capacity
History of stroke
Uncontrolled systemic hypertension

*Established by the American College of Cardiology and American Heart Association Task Force, 1996. (See reference to ACC/AHA practice guidelines.)

Supplemental Preoperative Evaluation

Exercise Testing

Exercise testing is an objective means of functional assessment and helps identify occult coronary artery disease in presumed healthy patients. It has a sensitivity of 90% in the detection of occult coronary disease. It is recommended that this test be added to routine cardiac assessment for all thoracic surgical patients *older than 45 years* as well as for patients with other risk factors, such as high blood pressure or diabetes. Patients with ischemic responses, with ST segment depression greater than 2 mm, or with hypotension at peak exercise should undergo further testing with a thallium stress test or coronary angiography. The primary limitation of exercise stress testing is often the *patient's inability to complete the test* because of associated peripheral vascular disease, advanced age, deconditioning, or some combination of these factors. Overall, approximately 20% to 25% of patients with a negative cardiac history and normal ECG will have an abnormal exercise ECG.

Nonexercise Testing

In patients unable to exercise adequately, patients with positive exercise test results, and patients with other significant risk factors, *intravenous dipyridamole-thallium imaging is indicated*. In this technique, intravenous administration of thallium causes coronary artery dilatation, which results in increased blood flow to the myocardium supplied by normal vessels but limited perfusion in regions supplied by stenotic vessels. This heterogeneity of flow is reflected in heterogeneous uptake of thallium, which produces a reversible redistribution defect on the immediate images that resolves on delayed images. If a patient has a normal thallium scan or fixed and nonreversible defects, the risk at surgery, especially in relation to postoperative major cardiac events, is minimal. By contrast, several studies have shown a high risk of perioperative cardiac events, including death, for those patients who have *reversible ischemic defects* as documented by thallium testing. Overall, thallium imaging (exercise thallium or nonexercise stress test) is useful to detect asymptomatic coronary artery disease, to assess the functional status of known coronary artery disease, and to show localization of coronary perfusion abnormalities.

Dobutamine stress echocardiography can also be used to document significant coronary artery disease. Although the published experience of dobutamine stress echocardiography is much less than that of thallium imaging, this examination has a negative predictive value that ranges from 93% to 100%.

Algorithm for the Evaluation of Coronary Artery Disease

The algorithm (Fig. 2-2) suggested for investigating the cardiac status of all patients older than 45 years or those with significant risk factors (Table 2-9) is that proposed by Miller. With this approach, one can

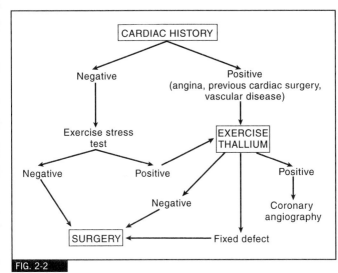

FIG. 2-2

Suggested algorithm for all patients older than 45 years undergoing major thoracic surgery. *(Modified from Miller JI: Thallium imaging in preoperative evaluation of the pulmonary resection candidate. Ann Thorac Surg 1992;54:249-252.)*

identify patients at risk for postoperative cardiac events and quantify this risk in both symptomatic and asymptomatic patients.

In most ambulatory and asymptomatic patients, the test of choice is *exercise ECG testing,* which can both provide an estimate of functional capacity and detect myocardial ischemia. If the result is normal, surgery can be done without further testing. If, on the other hand, the patient has an abnormal result or has a positive cardiac history and is unable to perform the test, a *nonexercise stress test* should be used. The absence of a dipyridamole-thallium–induced reversible defect has a high negative predictive value and indicates low risk for pulmonary resection. As directed by clinical judgment, coronary angiography should be considered in patients with high-risk results during noninvasive testing, patients with unresponsive or unstable angina, and patients with equivocal results of noninvasive testing and other risk factors for cardiac disease. In all of those individuals, a cardiology consultation should be obtained before thoracotomy.

Risk-Reduction Strategies (Table 2-10)

Before Operation

In general, the patient's medication should be continued up to the time of operation and resumed as soon as possible postoperatively. Several studies have shown that prophylactic addition of antiarrhythmic drugs is not useful

TABLE 2-10

RISK-REDUCTION STRATEGIES IN PATIENTS WITH CORONARY ARTERY DISEASE WHO UNDERGO MAJOR THORACIC OPERATIONS

Before operation
Optimization of medical therapy
Coronary angioplasty
Surgical revascularization
During operation
Judicious use of anesthetic agents
Prevention of ischemia
Invasive monitoring
After operation
Intensive monitoring
Adequate pain control

or may even be detrimental. If the patient is taking aspirin, it should be stopped about 1 week preoperatively.

An abnormal thallium scan with reversible ischemia and viable myocardium or a coronary angiogram showing significant coronary artery obstruction should be addressed before thoracotomy. Although no randomized clinical trials have documented whether prophylactic coronary revascularization by angioplasty or bypass operations reduces the incidence of postoperative cardiac complications, several case series suggest that these procedures can indeed be performed safely and help ensure *a low incidence of postoperative cardiac events.* Most people recommend delaying thoracotomy for 10 to 15 days after percutaneous angioplasty and for 4 to 6 weeks after surgical coronary revascularization. We *do not* recommend performing pulmonary resection and coronary artery bypass during the same procedure.

During Operation

In general, the specific type of anesthetic agent being administered does not contribute significantly to the operative cardiac risk since all agents are associated to some degree with depression of myocardial contractility. In the operating room, prevention of ischemia is of paramount importance; clearly, tachycardia, hypotension, and hypoxemia must not be allowed to persist in patients with coronary artery disease. *Invasive hemodynamic monitoring* should be considered in patients with high-risk ischemic heart disease not amenable to revascularization techniques, patients with recent myocardial infarction, and patients with left ventricular failure. This monitoring includes the use of pulmonary artery catheters and of transesophageal echocardiography.

After Operation

Because the majority of cardiac events in thoracic surgical patients will occur during *the first 3 postoperative days,* cardiac monitoring must be maintained during that time. In high-risk patients, it must be supplemented by serial ECG and cardiac-specific enzyme analyses.

Adequate and optimal pain control may be helpful because it releases stress and therefore may lower catecholamine release. As noted before, the preoperative medication should be maintained throughout the postoperative period.

THORACIC SURGERY IN THE PATIENT WITH CONGESTIVE HEART FAILURE

Several studies have shown that patients with congestive heart failure are at risk for *increased operative mortality* during and after thoracic procedures. It is therefore important to identify those individuals with clinical evidence of congestive heart failure so they can be further evaluated and their treatment optimized before surgery. A documented history of prior pulmonary edema or the presence of such physical signs as a third heart sound or jugular vein distention must therefore be sought through careful history and physical examination. Because the operative risk is proportional to the severity of congestive heart failure (Table 2-5), the severity of ventricular dysfunction should be further documented by *two-dimensional echocardiography or radionuclide angiography*. In some cases, it may also be indicated to measure right and left ventricular filling pressures, systemic vascular resistance, pulmonary resistance, and cardiac output.

Currently, there is *no evidence* that cardiac drugs should be given with the sole purpose of preventing perioperative cardiac complications. There is much evidence, however, that risk-reduction strategies (Table 2-11) must include optimization of medical therapy through the use of beta-adrenergic blockers, calcium channel blockers, and nitroglycerin. These drugs can usually be given with a sip of water on the day of surgery, and therapy is continued over the next several days.

Postoperatively, patients should be admitted to the *intensive care unit,* where a Swan-Ganz catheter can be used for hemodynamic monitoring. Continuous recording of wedge pressures (Table 2-12) and of other hemodynamic variables such as arterial blood pressure, central venous pressure, and urine output can guide fluid therapy and use of cardiac inotropic agents. It is well known that mobilization of extravascular fluids coupled to overloading with intravenous fluids can precipitate pulmonary

TABLE 2-11

RISK-REDUCTION STRATEGIES IN PATIENTS WITH CONGESTIVE HEART FAILURE

Before operation
Optimization of medical therapy
During operation
Aggressive hemodynamic monitoring
After operation
Aggressive hemodynamic monitoring
Careful fluid therapy
Use of pressor agents to improve cardiac inotropic action

TABLE 2-12

INTRAOPERATIVE USE OF PULMONARY ARTERY CATHETERS

Class 1	Patients at risk for major hemodynamic disturbances that are most easily detected by a pulmonary artery catheter who are undergoing a procedure that is likely to cause these hemodynamic changes in a setting with experience in interpreting the results
Class 2	Either the patient's condition or the surgical procedure (but not both) places the patient at risk for hemodynamic disturbances
Class 3	No risk of hemodynamic disturbances

From Eagle KA, Brundage BH, Chaitman BR, et al: Guidelines for perioperative cardiovascular evaluation for noncardiac surgery. Report of the American College of Cardiology/American Heart Association Task Force on Practice Guidelines. Circulation 1996;93:1278-1317.

edema in patients with left ventricular dysfunction who have undergone pulmonary resection, especially pneumonectomy. Because of this and because of impaired lymphatic drainage (due to mediastinal lymphadenectomy) associated with pulmonary resection for lung cancer, it is generally recommended that patients not receive excessive fluids.

THORACIC SURGERY IN THE PATIENT WITH DYSRHYTHMIAS AND CARDIAC CONDUCTION ABNORMALITIES

Arrhythmias and conduction disturbances are common preoperative findings in lung cancer patients, who often are 70 years of age or older. Although supraventricular arrhythmias and premature ventricular contractions are known risk factors for postoperative cardiac events, their main significance is that they are likely to reflect the presence of an underlying cardiac disease process, which may need to be investigated and treated. Although these arrhythmias are unlikely to become life-threatening rhythm disturbances, they must be *adequately treated preoperatively*, and this therapy must be maintained postoperatively.

Asymptomatic conduction system disease, such as bundle branch block or bifascicular block, does not presage complete heart block and usually does not require therapy. High-grade cardiac conduction abnormalities, such as complete atrioventricular block, may require preoperative placement of temporary or permanent transvenous pacing. Obviously, all of those patients must have ECG monitoring for at least 48 to 72 hours postoperatively. It is also important to monitor serum electrolytes because both hypokalemia and hypomagnesemia may increase the risk of arrhythmias.

THORACIC SURGERY IN THE PATIENT WITH HYPERTENSION

Although a large number of patients have stable mild or moderate hypertension, this factor alone *is not an independent risk factor* for the occurrence of postoperative cardiovascular events. On the other hand, a severely hypertensive patient, even one whose blood pressure is well controlled with medication, is at risk of high blood pressure variations under anesthesia or postoperatively.

All patients with elevated blood pressure should be evaluated for the severity of the illness and its effect on cardiovascular function and to rule out metabolic abnormalities that may be the cause of the elevated blood pressure. In patients with more severe hypertension (diastolic > 110 mm Hg), antihypertensive medication should be started before surgery, and the blood pressure should be stabilized within normal range before operation.

THORACIC SURGERY IN THE PATIENT WITH CAROTID OCCLUSIVE DISEASE

Carotid occlusive disease in patients undergoing major pulmonary resections raises the question of the perioperative risk of stroke. It also raises the issue of whether asymptomatic carotid artery stenosis should be surgically treated before major thoracic procedures. Although there is no consensus as to what degree of carotid artery stenosis warrants preoperative carotid endarterectomy, some reports have indicated that hemodynamically significant carotid lesions as documented by oculoplethysmography should be repaired before pulmonary resection.

CONCLUSION

Careful attention to cardiac assessment is important because this assessment can demonstrate cardiac conditions (symptomatic or asymptomatic) that should be known and treated before pulmonary resection. Fortunately, available noninvasive testing is likely to identify individuals at risk. In such patients, appropriate management can significantly decrease the risks of cardiac morbidity.

SUGGESTED READINGS

Review Articles

Goldman L, Caldera DL, Nussbaum SR, et al: Multifactorial index of cardiac risk in noncardiac surgical procedures. N Engl J Med 1977;297:845-850.

Wells PH, Kaplan JA: Optimal management of patients with ischemic heart disease for noncardiac surgery by complementary anesthesiologist and cardiologist interaction. Am Heart J 1981;102:1029-1037. Curriculum in Cardiology.

Goldman L: Cardiac risks and complications of noncardiac surgery. Ann Intern Med 1983;98:504-513.

Goldman L: Cardiac risks and complications of noncardiac surgery. Ann Surg 1983;198:780-791.

Jewell ER, Persson AV: Preoperative evaluation of the high-risk patient. Surg Clin North Am 1985;65:3-19.

Freeman WK, Gibbons RJ, Shub C: Preoperative assessment of cardiac patients undergoing noncardiac surgical procedures. Mayo Clin Proc 1989;64:1105-1117.

Mangano DT: Perioperative cardiac morbidity. Anesthesiology 1990;72:153-184.

Mangano DT, Goldman L: Preoperative assessment of patients with known or suspected coronary disease. N Engl J Med 1995;333:1750-1756.

Bronson DL, Halperin AK, Marwick TH: Evaluating cardiac risk in noncardiac surgery patients. Cleve Clin J Med 1995;62:391-400.

Eagle KA, Brundage BH, Chaitman BR, et al: Guidelines for perioperative cardiovascular evaluation for noncardiac surgery. Circulation 1996;93: 1278-1317.

American College of Surgeons: Clinical guideline, Part I. Guidelines for assessing and managing the perioperative risk from coronary artery disease associated with major noncardiac surgery. Ann Intern Med 1997;127:309-328. Position paper.

Joffe II, Morgan JP: Estimation of coronary risk before noncardiac surgery. Up-to-date in Cardiovascular Medicine, October 2002.

ACC/AHA Practice Guidelines: ACC/AHA guideline update for perioperative cardiovascular evaluation for noncardiac surgery—executive summary. J Am Coll Cardiol 2002;39:542-553. (Update of 1996 guidelines.)

Echocardiography

Das MK, Pellikka PA, Mahoney DW, et al: Assessment of cardiac risk before nonvascular surgery. J Am Coll Cardiol 2000;35:1647-1653.

Thallium Imaging

Lette J, Waters D, Lapointe J, et al: Usefulness of the severity and extent of reversible perfusion defects during thallium-dipyridamole imaging for cardiac risk assessment before noncardiac surgery. Am J Cardiol 1989;64:276-281.

Miller JI: Thallium imaging in preoperative evaluation of the pulmonary resection candidate. Ann Thorac Surg 1992;54:249-252.

Brown KA, Rowen M: Extent of jeopardized viable myocardium determined by myocardial perfusion imaging best predicts perioperative cardiac events in patients undergoing noncardiac surgery. J Am Coll Cardiol 1993;21:325-330.

Kontos MC, Brath LK, Akosah KO, Mohanty PK: Cardiac complications in noncardiac surgery: relative value of resting two-dimensional echocardiography and dipyridamole thallium imaging. Am Heart J 1996;132: 559-566.

Stratmann HG, Younis LT, Wittry MD, et al: Dipyridamole technetium 99 m sestamibi myocardial tomography for preoperative cardiac risk stratification before major or minor nonvascular surgery. Am Heart J 1996;132: 536-541.

Predictive Index

Epstein SK, Faling LJ, Daly BDT, Celli BR: Predicting complications after pulmonary resection. Preoperative exercise testing vs. a multifactorial cardiopulmonary risk index. Chest 1993;104:694-700.

Lee TH, Marcantonio ER, Mangione CM, et al: Derivation and prospective validation of a simple index for prediction of cardiac risk of major noncardiac surgery. Circulation 1999;100:1043-1049.

Gilbert K, Larocque BJ, Patrick LT: Prospective evaluation of cardiac risk indices for patients undergoing noncardiac surgery. Ann Intern Med 2000;133:356-359.

Case Series

Steen PA, Tinker JH, Tarhan S: Myocardial reinfarction after anesthesia and surgery. JAMA 1978;239:2566-2570.

Lette J, Waters D, Bernier H, et al: Preoperative and long-term cardiac risk assessment. Predictive value of 23 clinical descriptors, 7 multivariate scoring systems, and quantitative dipyridamole imaging in 360 patients. Ann Surg 1992;216:192-204.

Eagle KA, Rihal CS, Mickel MC, et al: Cardiac risk of noncardiac surgery. Influence of coronary disease and type of surgery in 3368 operations. Circulation 1997;96:1882-1887.

ASSESSMENT OF ESOPHAGEAL FUNCTION

The esophagus extends from the cricopharyngeal muscle to the stomach. Because it is a musculomembranous structure whose *main function is to transport liquids and food,* most benign disorders of the esophagus are related to abnormal function of this transport mechanism.

Before treatment of a patient with esophageal symptoms, it is important to have a full understanding of the underlying disorder and of its pathogenesis. This understanding is necessary not only because preoperative symptoms may not correlate with pathologic changes but also because esophageal symptoms may be nonspecific, may be atypical, or can mimic adjacent organ abnormalities. It is thus important to use the *available esophageal function tests* judiciously because they will provide precise information about diagnosis.

NORMAL ESOPHAGEAL FUNCTION

In general, esophageal motor function is divided into that of the *pharynx and cricopharynx* (upper esophageal sphincter), *body of esophagus*, and *gastroesophageal junction* (lower esophageal sphincter). Motor waves are initiated in the pharynx and move distally through the entire length of the esophagus. These motor waves may vary in duration and amplitude, but they are coordinated and supply a continuous propulsive force.

Upper Esophageal Sphincter

Proximally, the cricopharyngeal muscle acts as an *anatomic sphincter* (upper esophageal sphincter), closing the esophagus and relaxing only in response to swallowing. It is approximately 3 cm in length, and it maintains a constant intraluminal pressure of 10 to 60 cm H_2O. As the pharyngeal motor wave (initiated in the pharynx) passes through the upper

Preoperative Assessment

2

esophageal sphincter, it is preceded by local relaxation, which reduces cricopharyngeal pressure to the resting level of the upper esophagus. After relaxation, the upper esophageal sphincter returns to basal tone, effectively closing off the sphincter and upper end of the esophagus.

Body of Esophagus

Esophageal peristalsis is a continuation of the motor wave initiated in the pharynx, passing through the upper esophageal sphincter and on to the body of the esophagus. Peristaltic waves are *coordinated*. They move rapidly through the upper esophagus but gradually slow down at the lower esophagus.

Lower Esophageal Sphincter

The lower esophagus is demarcated by a *physiologic high-pressure zone* that separates the body of the esophagus from the stomach. It acts as a barrier to reflux of gastric contents into the esophagus. The pressure in the lower esophageal sphincter is 15 to 30 cm H_2O, and the lower esophageal sphincter measures 2 to 4 cm in length. Relaxation of lower esophageal sphincter pressure begins 1.5 to 2.5 seconds after the initiation of swallow and continues for up to 10 seconds. This relaxation neutralizes the pressure barrier and produces a *pressure gradient* from esophagus to stomach. Relaxation terminates with the arrival of the esophageal peristaltic motor wave.

The coordinated wave arrives at the lower esophageal sphincter approximately 10 seconds after the initiation of deglutition. Once it has passed through the lower esophageal sphincter, motor activity in the esophagus ceases until a new motor complex is initiated by swallowing.

ASSESSMENT OF ESOPHAGEAL FUNCTION

Clinical Features

Clinical features are *most important* in the assessment of esophageal function because each symptom may reflect an abnormality in the normal process of swallowing. *Dysphagia,* for instance, relates to the patient's perception of some difficulty in swallowing. The association of *dysphagia and weight loss* is pathognomonic of cancer; a benign stricture may take years to develop, and therefore alterations in weight are less likely.

As stated by Dr. Clement A. Hiebert, deviation from normal may be *subtle* in benign esophageal diseases, and unfortunately, the quality of recorded history depends on the *patient's sensitivity to the dysfunction* as well as the *patient's ability to articulate the matter*. It also depends on the *physician's willingness* to listen and to elicit and arrange the symptoms into a plausible portrait of the illness.

What symptoms should alert the clinician to esophageal dysfunction? Dysphagia is the *most important symptom* indicative of esophageal disease. In motor disorders of the esophagus, dysphagia may be variable in time, and it is often dependent on a specific triggering bolus. In achalasia, for instance, both liquids and solids are delayed at the gastroesophageal junction, but liquids, especially at the extremes of temperature (hot or cold), may profoundly increase the "perception" of the severity of the complaint. Patients with achalasia may also have retrosternal pain associated with obstruction to the passage of food as well as retrosternal fullness and discomfort. Patients with vigorous achalasia complain of spontaneous pain unrelated to eating.

Dysphagia is also the *signature symptom* associated with *pharyngoesophageal disorders*. It may occur with either liquids or solids, but it most commonly occurs with both. The obstruction can be localized by the patient to the cricopharynx, and it is often followed by coughing and choking due to forward spillage of the food bolus to the larynx.

In *gastroesophageal reflux*, typical heartburn with the patient's description of reflux and taste of gastric contents in the mouth is often specific enough to establish the diagnosis. *Regurgitation*, which is characterized by the passive return of swallowed material (undigested food) to the mouth, is typically associated with achalasia or with epiphrenic or Zenker diverticulum.

Chronic aspiration of esophageal contents is also a feature of esophageal dysfunction. Consequences include cough, stridor, bouts of pneumonia, and progressive pulmonary fibrosis.

Although various collagen disorders may involve the esophagus at some stage, *scleroderma* is most frequently associated with esophageal changes. Symptoms described by patients with scleroderma include heartburn and dysphagia, and these symptoms are often indistinguishable from those associated with gastroesophageal reflux.

Diffuse esophageal spasm is a dysfunction of the esophagus in which the lower two thirds loses its normal peristaltic motor coordination and responds to swallowing by segmental spasm. The most common symptoms associated with this condition are pain, dysphagia, regurgitation, and weight loss.

Imaging

Contrast Studies

Barium is the most commonly used contrast agent for examination of the esophagus. It allows a *safe and expedient study* of esophageal mucosa, wall thickness, luminal distensibility, and motility patterns. Videofluoroscopy is used to assess the upper esophageal sphincter, the peristalsis of the body of the esophagus, and the emptying of the esophagus at the gastroesophageal junction.

Despite improved techniques of examination, contrast studies are generally *inefficient* for accurate diagnosis of esophageal dysfunction. Fluoroscopic demonstration of reflux on barium study, for instance, is unreliable. Reflux can be documented in 40% of asymptomatic individuals and in only 20% to 40% of patients with documented reflux esophagitis. Correlation of motor disorders with symptoms and contrast studies remains a challenge.

In achalasia, the esophagus becomes dilated in advanced stages (sigmoid esophagus), whereas it is of normal size in early stages. In both

2

Preoperative Assessment

early and late stages, the esophagus just above the gastroesophageal junction tapers to produce a beak-like appearance. In some cases, the esophagus may show repetitive, simultaneous nonperistaltic contractions (vigorous achalasia).

In diffuse esophageal spasm, the major features are marked nonperistaltic contractions in the lower two thirds of the esophagus (spasm) and an increase in wall thickness to 5 mm or more. In scleroderma, peristalsis is absent in the distal two thirds, and fluoroscopy frequently demonstrates gastroesophageal reflux.

High-speed cinematic or video recording is useful to evaluate the pharyngeal phase of swallowing as well as pharyngoesophageal disorders. Observations suggesting cricopharyngeal dysfunction include the aspiration or misdirection of barium into the larynx, a Zenker diverticulum, and a narrow pharyngoesophageal segment.

Esophageal Transit Scintigraphy

Delayed bolus transit as seen in a variety of esophageal motor disorders can be demonstrated through the *transit of a 10-mL bolus containing* ^{99m}Tc*–sulfur colloid* recorded with a gamma camera. Delayed transit localized in the distal third suggests scleroderma or reflux esophagitis. Incoordinate to-and-fro movements throughout the esophagus are characteristic of diffuse esophageal spasms. Achalasia is characterized by an adynamic esophagus with little motor activity.

Despite these radionuclide signs, the role of this technique in the diagnosis of esophageal dysfunction remains unclear.

Esophageal Function Studies

Esophageal Manometry

Stationary Manometry. Stationary esophageal manometry is an important test in the evaluation of esophageal dysfunction (Table 2-13), gastroesophageal reflux, and pharyngoesophageal disorders. Other possible clinical indications are listed in Table 2-14.

TABLE 2-13

MOST COMMON ESOPHAGEAL MOTILITY DISORDERS

PRIMARY

Achalasia, vigorous achalasia

Diffuse esophageal spasm

Nutcracker esophagus

Hypertensive lower esophageal sphincter

SECONDARY

Gastroesophageal reflux

Collagen vascular diseases (scleroderma)

Neuromuscular diseases and endocrine disorders

Alcoholic neuropathy

TABLE 2-14

CLINICAL APPLICATIONS OF STATIONARY ESOPHAGEAL MANOMETRY

Primary motility disorders

Secondary or nonspecific motility disorders

Pharyngoesophageal disorders

Exclusion of associated esophageal motility disorders when antireflux
   surgery is contemplated

Chest pain of unknown etiology

Failed operation for benign esophageal disease

Manometric studies can be recorded with electronic pressure-sensitive transducers or more commonly through *low-compliance, water-perfused catheters* (Figs. 2-3 and 2-4). Normal manometric values are given in Table 2-15.

Primary Motility Disorders. With the introduction of esophageal manometry, a number of primary esophageal motility disorders have been classified as separate disease entities (Table 2-16). In *achalasia,* there is no peristalsis in the body of the esophagus, and the lower esophageal sphincter does not relax. The classic motility findings in *diffuse esophageal spasm* are the frequent occurrences of simultaneous and repetitive esophageal contractions, which may be of abnormally high amplitude or long duration. *Nutcracker esophagus* is a motor abnormality characterized by peristaltic esophageal contractions of exceedingly high amplitude. *Hypertensive lower esophageal sphincter* is characterized by elevated base pressure of the lower esophageal sphincter with normal relaxation and normal wave progression in the body of the esophagus.

Secondary Motility Disorders. The most common cause of secondary esophageal motility disorders is *gastroesophageal reflux.* The esophagus can also be affected by almost any collagen vascular disease. Typical manometric findings in scleroderma include normal peristalsis in the proximal third of the esophagus (striated muscle), loss or marked diminution of motor activity in the lower two thirds (smooth muscle), and loss of tone in the gastroesophageal junction.

Nonspecific Motility Disorders. Nonspecific motility disorders refer to manometric features that are clearly abnormal but defy classification in one of the previous two groups. Esophageal manometry may show an increased number of multipeaked or repetitive contractions, contractions of prolonged duration, nontransmitted pharyngeal contractions, interrupted contraction waves, or contractions of low amplitude. The significance of those findings is unclear. Fortunately, these problems are uncommon and rarely produce significant symptoms.

Pharyngoesophageal Disorders. Although pharyngoesophageal disorders (Table 2-17) are relatively uncommon, they tend to express themselves through symptoms that are the result of uncoordination of neuromuscular events during swallowing. With this uncoordination,

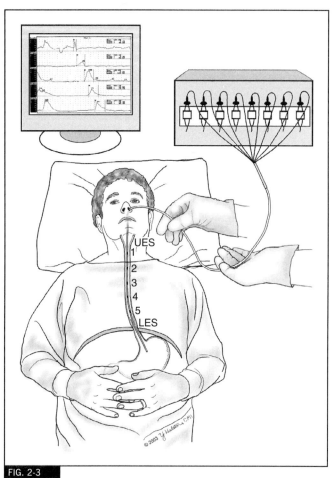

FIG. 2-3

Stationary esophageal manometry with a water-perfused catheter. Note the position
of the five side holes, which are placed at 5-cm intervals along the length of the
catheter. These are necessary to record esophageal peristaltic activity. LES, lower
esophageal sphincter; UES, upper esophageal sphincter.

patients are unable to propel the swallowed material from the oropharynx
into the cervical esophagus. Dysphagia with either liquids or solids or with
both is the most common symptom. Associated symptoms include
regurgitation of food through the nose, choking, coughing, and frank
aspiration. In such cases, carefully performed motility studies may

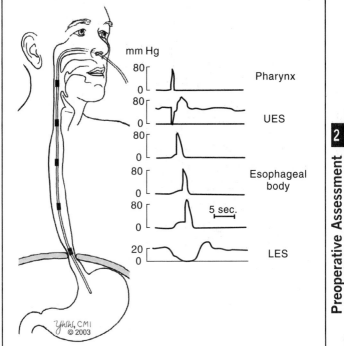

FIG. 2-4

Schematic representation of normal esophageal peristaltism initiated by a pharyngeal swallow and coordinated with relaxation of the upper esophageal sphincter (UES) and the lower esophageal sphincter (LES).

TABLE 2-15

NORMAL MANOMETRIC VALUES

Variable	Normal Value
Esophageal contraction wave	
Amplitude	99 ± 40 cm H_2O
Duration	3.9 ± 0.9 seconds
Lower esophageal sphincter	
Pressure	24 ± 10 mm Hg (mean 14)
Overall length	2.4-5.5 cm (mean 3.7)
Abdominal length	0.8-5.0 cm (mean 2.2)

TABLE 2-16

STATIONARY ESOPHAGEAL MANOMETRY IN PRIMARY ESOPHAGEAL
MOTILITY DISORDERS

Disorder	Diagnostic Criteria	Other Possible Findings
Achalasia	Aperistalsis in body of esophagus Incomplete LES relaxation	Elevated LES pressure
Diffuse esophageal spasm	Spastic motor waves of prolonged duration and high amplitude in lower two thirds of esophagus	Gastroesophageal junction has normal tone Upper third of esophagus is normal
Nutcracker esophagus	Peristalsis of exceedingly high amplitude	Spontaneous contraction
Hypertensive LES	Elevated basal pressure of LES (>40 cm H_2O)	Prolonged contractions >6 sec Normal relaxation Normal wave progression in body of esophagus

LES, lower esophageal sphincter.

demonstrate uncoordination or incomplete relaxation of the upper esophageal sphincter during swallowing.

In patients with pharyngoesophageal disorders, manometric measurements and, most important, *correlation between manometry and radiographic findings* provide an insight as to what disorder is present. A logical basis for therapy is also provided.

Exclusion of Esophageal Motility Disorders When Antireflux Surgery is Contemplated. In general terms, the objectives of investigating gastroesophageal reflux are to establish the source of symptoms, to assess the effects of reflux on the esophagus, and to exclude associated esophageal motility disorders. For instance, it is important to document

TABLE 2-17

MOTOR DISORDERS OF PHARYNGOESOPHAGEAL JUNCTION

Primary	Myogenic: myotonia, thyrotoxic
	Neurogenic
	Congenital: Riley-Day syndrome
	Acquired, central: strokes, bulbar poliomyelitis, post-trauma
	Acquired, peripheral: recurrent nerve palsy
	Myoneurogenic: myasthenia gravis, oculopharyngeal muscular dystrophy
Secondary	Gastroesophageal reflux
Idiopathic	Cricopharyngeal bar, diverticulum
Psychogenic	Globus hystericus

From Henderson RD: Motor Disorders of the Esophagus. Baltimore, Williams & Wilkins, 1976:185.

decreased motor activity in the body of the esophagus before a total fundoplication is performed. If this is not done and the patient has low motor activity, a total fundoplication may lead to severe dysphagia, food retention, and regurgitation. Whether all patients with gastroesophageal reflux should have manometric studies preoperatively remains controversial.

Chest Pain of Unknown Etiology. An estimated 10% to 20% of patients with gastroesophageal reflux or with other motor disorders of the esophagus present with retrosternal distress that is clinically indistinguishable from angina pectoris. The pain, described as "squeezing," "heavy pressure," or "tightness," can be severe and radiate from the retrosternum to the back, jaws, ear, and one or both arms. In such cases, manometric and radiologic studies as well as *perfusion of the esophagus with hydrochloric acid (Bernstein test)* may help distinguish esophageal pain from pain that may arise in adjacent organs. Pain reproduction during an acid "drip test" is a valuable adjunct to diagnosis because it reproduces an important symptom and localizes its origin to the esophagus.

Often, however, patients have more than one type of pain. Each must be clearly defined before proceeding to an operation.

Failed Operation for Benign Esophageal Disease. In any patient in whom an operation has *failed to improve symptoms* or has created a *new set of symptoms,* the investigation should be repeated, and this investigation must include manometric studies. This is especially important if the patient did not have these studies preoperatively. One of the most catastrophic mishaps is that of a patient with primary motor disorder, such as achalasia, who should have a myotomy but instead undergoes fundoplication, thinking that the symptoms are related to gastroesophageal reflux.

Ambulatory Manometry. The intermittent and unpredictable occurrence of motor abnormalities and symptoms in patients with esophageal motility disorders limits the diagnostic value of standard monitoring performed in a laboratory setting during a short period.

Ambulatory 24-hour motility monitoring is done on an outpatient basis. The system allows continuous recording of three esophageal and one pharyngeal pressure channels along with contemporary recording of two pH channels. Approximately 1,000 to 14,000 contractions are recorded by each pressure transducer, and these are transferred to a computer for analysis.

Possible clinical applications of ambulatory 24-hour motility monitoring are listed in Table 2-18. In gastroesophageal reflux, the test is useful to demonstrate disordered motor activity that is secondary to reflux and may affect esophageal clearance after reflux episodes.

24-Hour pH Monitoring

Prolonged esophageal pH monitoring is used to *quantitate* the actual time that the esophageal mucosa is exposed to gastric juice. Possible indications for the test are listed in Table 2-19.

TABLE 2-18

POSSIBLE CLINICAL APPLICATIONS OF AMBULATORY 24-HOUR MOTILITY MONITORING

Diffuse esophageal spasm

Nutcracker esophagus

Nonspecific disorders

    Noncardiac chest pain

    Intermittent dysphagia

    Primary esophagus motor disorders

    Nonobstructive or intermittent dysphagia

    Gastroesophageal reflux disorder

The technique described by Johnson and DeMeester consists of placing a pH electrode 5 cm above the upper border of the lower esophageal sphincter and then continuously recording pH values every 4 seconds during 24 hours. The test is done on an outpatient basis, preferably while the patient is attending normal activities.

Esophageal exposure to gastric juice is best assessed by the following measurements:

1. *Cumulative time* the esophageal pH is below a chosen threshold expressed as the percentage of the total, upright, and supine monitored time.
2. *Frequency of reflux episodes* below a chosen threshold expressed as the number of episodes per 24 hours.
3. *Duration of episodes* expressed as the number of episodes longer than 5 minutes per 24 hours.
4. Time in minutes of the *longest episode* recorded.

To combine the results of the components (Table 2-20) into one expression of the overall esophageal acid exposure below a pH threshold, a pH score can be calculated, and this score can discriminate between physiologic and pathologic reflux. Limitations of the study include possible intolerance of the patient, electrode malfunction or displacement, and modification of daily routine by the patient.

CONCLUSION

Careful and orderly assessment of esophageal function must be done in most patients with esophageal symptoms or complaints. This assessment includes good history taking as well as more sophisticated testing, such as

TABLE 2-19

POSSIBLE INDICATIONS FOR 24-HOUR pH MONITORING

Gastroesophageal reflux nonresponsive to medication

Atypical symptoms like chest pain

Pulmonary problems like adult-onset asthma

Preoperative and postoperative evaluation of antireflux surgery

TABLE 2-20	

NORMAL VALUES FOR THE COMPONENTS OF 24-HOUR pH MONITORING

24-Hour Component	Normal
% total time with pH < 4	<4.2%
% upright time with pH < 4	<6.3%
% supine time with pH < 4	<1.2%
Number of episodes	<50
Number of episodes ≥ 5 min	3 or less
Longest episode	<9.2 min

$$\text{Composite score} = \frac{\text{patient value} - \text{mean}}{\text{standard deviation}} + 1$$

From Johnson LF, DeMeester TR: Development of the 24-hour intraesophageal pH monitoring composite scoring system. J Clin Gastroenterol 1986;8:52-58.

ambulatory manometric recording. The results of this investigation should provide an answer to three questions: Is there something wrong with the esophagus? If the answer is yes, what is it? And finally, what should be done about it?

SUGGESTED READINGS

Review Articles

Henderson RD: Motor Disorders of the Esophagus. Baltimore, Williams & Wilkins, 1976.

Stein HJ, DeMeester TR, Hinder RA: Outpatient physiologic testing and surgical management of foregut motility disorders. Curr Probl Surg 1992;34:415-555.

Kahrilas PJ, Clouse RE, Hogan WJ: American Gastroenterological Association technical review of the clinical use of esophageal manometry. Gastroenterology 1994;107:1865-1884.

Stewart ET, Dot WJ: Radiology of the esophagus. In Freeny PC, Stevenson GW, eds: Margulis and Burhennes' Alimentary Tract Radiology, 5th ed. St. Louis, Mosby, 1994:192.

Eslami MH, Richards WG, Sugarbaker DJ: Esophageal physiology. Chest Surg Clin North Am 1994;4:635-652.

Dent J, Holloway RH: Esophageal motility and reflux testing. State-of-the-art and clinical role in the twenty-first century. Gastroenterol Clin North Am 1996;25:51-73.

Adhami T, Shay SS: Esophageal motility in the assessment of esophageal function. Semin Thorac Cardiovasc Surg 2001;13:234-240.

Zuccaro G: Esophagoscopy and endoscopic esophageal ultrasound in the assessment of esophageal function. Semin Thorac Cardiovasc Surg 2001;13:226-233.

DeMeester TR, Constantin M: Function tests. In Pearson FG, Cooper JD, Deslauriers J, et al: Esophageal Surgery, 2nd ed. Philadelphia, Churchill Livingstone, 2002:158-191.

Nonspecific Motor Disorders

Benjamin SB, Richter JE, Cordova M, et al: Prospective manometric evaluation with pharmacologic provocation of patients with suspected esophageal motility dysfunction. Gastroenterology 1983;84:893-901.

Hsu JJ, O'Connor MK, Kang YW, Kim CH: Nonspecific motor disorder of the esophagus: a real disorder or a manometric curiosity? Gastroenterology 1993;104:1281-1284.

Leite LP, Johnston BT, Barrett J, et al: Ineffective esophageal motility (IEM). The primary finding in patients with nonspecific esophageal motility disorder. Dig Dis Sci 1997;42:1859-1865.

Achalasia

Magovern CJ, Altorki NK: Achalasia of the esophagus. Chest Surg Clin North Am 1994;4:721-739.

Van Dam J, Falk GW, Sivak MV, et al: Endosonographic evaluation of the patient with achalasia. Appearance of the esophagus using the echoendoscope. Endoscopy 1995;27:185-190.

Kostic SV, Rice TW, Baker ME, et al: Timed barium esophagogram: a simple physiologic assessment for achalasia. J Thorac Cardiovasc Surg 2000;120:935-946.

Chest Pain and Esophagus

Katz PO, Dalton CB, Richter JE, et al: Esophageal testing of patients with noncardiac chest pain or dysphagia. Results of three years' experience with 1161 patients. Ann Intern Med 1987;106:593-597.

Diffuse Esophageal Spasm

Allen ML, Dimarino AJ: Manometric diagnosis of diffuse esophageal spasm. Dig Dis Sci 1996;41:1346-1349.

Intraesophageal pH Monitoring

Johnson LF, DeMeester TR: Development of the 24-hour intraesophageal pH monitoring composite scoring system. J Clin Gastroenterol 1986;8(suppl):52-58.

Reflux Disease

Dent J, Holloway RH, Toouli J, Dodds WH: Mechanisms of lower esophageal sphincter incompetence in patients with symptomatic gastroesophageal reflux. Gut 1988;29:1020-1028.

Bremner RM, DeMeester TR, Crookes PF, et al: The effect of symptoms and nonspecific motility abnormalities on outcomes of surgical therapy for gastroesophageal reflux disease. J Thorac Cardiovasc Surg 1994;107:1244-1250.

Waring JP, Hunter JG, Oddsdottir M, et al: The preoperative evaluation of patients considered for laparoscopic antireflux surgery. Am J Gastroenterol 1995;90:35-38.

McLauchlan G: Oesophageal function testing and antireflux surgery. Br J Surg 1996;83:1684-1688.

Fibbe C, Layer P, Keller J, et al: Esophageal motility in reflux disease before and after fundoplication: a prospective, randomized, clinical, and manometric study. Gastroenterology 2001;121:5-14.

Others

Russell COH, Whelan G: Oesophageal manometry: how well does it predict oesophageal function. Gut 1987;28:940-945.

Foglia RP: Esophageal disease in the pediatric age group. Chest Surg Clin North Am 1994;4:785-809.

Fuller L, Huprich JE, Theisen J, et al: Abnormal esophageal body function: radiographic-manometric correlation. Am Surg 1999;65:911-914.

Specific Preoperative Assessment

ASSESSMENT OF TECHNICAL RESECTABILITY OF LUNG CANCER

Lung cancer is a *significant health problem*, with more than 170,000 new cases being diagnosed annually in the United States. Of these, approximately 45% are *limited to the thorax*, where surgery is the most effective method of controlling the disease. Recognizing this concept, surgeons want an operation to be performed when it has been clearly determined that cancer resection is the *most appropriate* course of management.

The necessity for a compulsive attitude toward preoperative assessment is therefore to be emphasized because rational treatment and ultimately prognosis depend largely on the clinical stage of disease. The techniques used to determine the clinical stage should define the patients *most likely* to benefit from pulmonary resection while ensuring that *no individual is denied the chance of curative resection* on the basis of radiologic or clinical findings alone. If proper pretreatment staging is accomplished, the rate of exploratory thoracotomy or incomplete resection should not exceed 8% to 10%.

Patients with T1N0 and T2N0 disease have early lung cancers, and for most of them, technical resectability of the tumor is not an issue. For higher stage tumors, however, the surgeon must have the knowledge that "en bloc" resection *might need to be carried out* and that it can be performed *safely*. This includes the resection of T3 tumors that involve the chest wall, the superior sulcus, the mediastinal pleura, or the pericardium and endobronchial tumors located within 2 cm of the carina. It also includes the resection of selected T4 tumors that may invade the heart, the mediastinum, or the vertebral bodies.

In all of those cases, the local extent of disease must be *carefully assessed*. Ultimately, the results of this evaluation will determine whether a given tumor is technically resectable.

GENERAL GUIDELINES FOR THE SELECTION OF PATIENTS FOR SURGERY: RESECTABILITY AND OPERABILITY

The selection of patients for resection of non–small cell lung cancer must take into account not only the *technical resectability* of the tumor but also *the operability* of the disease. The ability to accomplish a complete resection is the technical consideration, and with new refinements in techniques and operative support, the limits of resectability have been expanded. For instance, localized invasion of the trachea does not contraindicate operation, although involvement of the lower trachea for more than 3 cm does not allow complete resection.

Operability implies that surgical resection is the *best management option* for the patient; its definition includes consideration of age, pulmonary function, cardiovascular fitness, and nutritional and performance status. Most important, the definition of operability must take into account the *clinical nodal status*. Five-year survival rates for completely resected T3N0M0 tumors is, for instance, in the range of 35% to 40%. However, once N1 disease is present, the 5-year survival decreases to 15% to 20%, and most often surgery is not recommended if N2-3 disease is documented preoperatively. Patients with T4N1-2 lesions are virtually *incurable* by surgery.

Because the presence of N1-3 disease is such an ominous prognostic sign, *invasive techniques* of mediastinal staging should be used before embarking on the resection of higher stage tumors.

EVALUATION OF TECHNICAL RESECTABILITY OF PATIENTS WITH SUSPECTED CHEST WALL INVOLVEMENT

Rib (T3) Involvement (Table 3-1)

About 5% of resected lung cancers involve the ribs. In such cases, *preoperative determination* of the need for chest wall resection is important for the planning of the operation.

Chest wall invasion must be first suspected in patients complaining of severe *chest wall pain* at a site adjacent to a peripheral lung tumor. Indeed, localized or increasingly severe chest wall pain is one of the best predictors of the need for chest wall resection. Obvious *bone destruction* as seen on standard chest radiographs is always indicative of chest wall invasion.

Computed tomography (CT) has an accuracy up to 90% in predicting chest wall invasion. Positive signs include rib destruction, extension of the tumor into the muscles overlying the rib cage, and obliteration of the extrapleural fat plane. The combination of *chest wall pain* and *abnormal bone scan* nearly always indicates the need for chest wall resection.

On occasion, chest wall involvement will only be identified at thoracotomy. If this is the case, it is reasonable to first attempt to develop

TABLE 3-1
SIGNS OF PROBABLE RIB INVOLVEMENT
Localized chest wall pain
Abnormal isotope bone scan
Imaging
Rib destruction
Extension to muscles of the rib cage
Obliteration of extrapleural fat plane
At surgery
Resistance to extrapleural dissection plane

an extrapleural (between parietal pleura and endothoracic fascia) dissection plane. However, if any resistance is encountered or if frozen section analysis reveals malignant invasion of the parietal pleura, an en bloc resection of the chest wall must be carried out.

Tumors Adherent to (T3) or Invading (T4) the Vertebral Body

Overall, *little success* has been obtained after resection of non–small cell lung cancer abutting or invading vertebral bodies, although tumors closely related to the paravertebral fascia but without destruction of the vertebral body can be resected.

Involvement of a vertebra can be anticipated when the patient complains of persistent pain over the appropriate portion of the spine. This can be further documented by demonstrating erosion of a vertebral body on chest radiographs. Magnetic resonance imaging (MRI) is, however, the *best imaging technique* to document the extent of vertebral body invasion. It will show if the tumor is only adherent to the prevertebral fascia, if it involves the transverse process of the vertebra, or if there is invasion of the vertebral body itself with or without extension into the intervertebral foramina.

In general, tumors adjacent to the paravertebral plane or those involving the transverse process or the lateral part of the vertebral body can be resected. However, direct and frank invasion of the vertebral body or tumor extension in the spinal canal remains for most surgeons an absolute contraindication to surgery.

If one is attempting to resect such tumors, the operation must be carefully planned. It is important to carry out the procedure with the help of a neurosurgeon or an orthopedic surgeon. Incomplete resections *do not improve survival,* and their ability to palliate is questionable.

Pancoast Tumors (T3-4)

Pancoast tumors refer to primary lung cancers that are located at the *apex of the lung,* usually posteriorly (the pulmonary sulcus is located paravertebrally). They often invade the upper two or three ribs (T3), vertebral bodies (T4), lower part of the brachial plexus (T4), and stellate ganglion, causing a clinical syndrome characterized by pain, neurologic deficit in the territory of the ulnar nerve, and Horner syndrome.

To adequately select patients with Pancoast tumors for surgery, the surgeon must have *clear knowledge of the tumor's anatomy* in the lower neck and thoracic inlet. Although CT is helpful in evaluating vertebral and rib involvement, it is not nearly as accurate as MRI, which is also useful to assess vascular involvement (subclavian artery or vein), invasion of nerve roots, or tumor extension into the intervertebral foramina. On occasion, subclavian artery angiography will be useful to demonstrate subclavian arterial involvement and, most important, that of *the vertebral artery.* As part of clinical staging of patients with Pancoast tumors, we also recommend *cervical ultrasonography* because such tumors can metastasize transpleurally to the ipsilateral cervical nodes (Table 3-2).

TABLE 3-2

CLINICAL STAGING OF PATIENTS WITH PANCOAST TUMORS

Patients often have chest wall and shoulder pain, Horner syndrome, and
  ulnar nerve deficit
MRI is the best imaging technique
Subclavian artery angiography sometimes recommended
Ultrasonographic examination of ipsilateral neck

With modern surgical techniques and a multidisciplinary approach, it is
possible to *completely resect* tumors that locally invade part of the
vertebral body, subclavian artery, and C8-T1 nerve roots. If the subclavian
artery needs to be resected en bloc with the tumor, it can be reconstructed
usually by end-to-end anastomosis but on occasion with the use of a
prosthesis. If the *vertebral artery* is also involved, surgery can be
hazardous because major intraoperative bleeding can occur.

EVALUATION OF TECHNICAL RESECTABILITY OF PATIENTS WITH SUSPECTED AIRWAY INVOLVEMENT (TABLE 3-3)

Proximal Airway (T3) Involvement

Tumors within 2 cm of the carina are T3 tumors that can be resected by
sleeve resection, thus avoiding the need for pneumonectomy, which
carries a significantly *higher rate* of operative morbidity and mortality.
Sleeve resections are applicable to any lobe or segment on either side.

The only preoperative finding that identifies a possible candidate for
sleeve resection is the *bronchoscopic appearance of the tumor*, which
may extend to a lobar orifice or into the adjacent main bronchus (Fig. 3-1).
Bronchoscopy is also useful to determine the endobronchial extent of
tumor and to plan the resection accordingly. In some cases, CT scanning
or pulmonary angiography may also be used to determine the technical
feasibility of a sleeve resection.

The final decision to carry out a sleeve resection is generally based
on operative findings, such as evidence (microscopic or macroscopic)
of residual cancer along the resection line of the lobectomy, extraluminal
extension of the carcinoma, or sometimes presence of N1 disease.
Ultimately, the technical feasibility of a sleeve resection can be determined
only by *frozen section* biopsies of the involved bronchi and adjacent
lymph nodes.

TABLE 3-3

TECHNICAL RESECTABILITY OF PATIENTS WITH AIRWAY INVOLVEMENT

Usually suspected during bronchoscopic examination
Importance of operative findings including frozen section biopsies
Final decision made at surgery
For sleeve pneumonectomy, tension-free anastomosis unlikely to be possible if length
  of resection is more than 4 cm

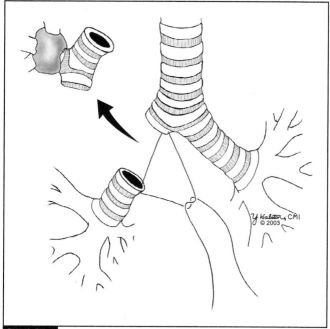

FIG. 3-1

Schematic representation of a right upper lobectomy with sleeve resection of the main bronchus. Note the location of the neoplasm at the origin of the right upper lobe bronchus.

In planning to carry out a sleeve resection, it is therefore important to have *frozen section capabilities* and *pathologic expertise*.

Carina (T4) Involvement

Most lung cancers involving the carina or lower trachea are so extensive that *complete resection is not possible*. This involvement is usually due to metastatic subcarinal nodes growing through the airway and into the tracheal lumen. On occasion, however, tumors arising in upper lobes or in the origin of either main bronchus may be *sufficiently localized* to be amenable to complete resection and reconstruction.

Tracheal sleeve pneumonectomy (Fig. 3-2) is a demanding operation with a high risk of complications. Selection of patients is therefore important, and it is mostly done during the preoperative bronchoscopic examination. When this possibility is suspected, random biopsy specimens should be taken of the tracheal mucosa and submucosa *at least 2 cm proximal to the tumor*; a tension-free or tumor-free reconstruction is

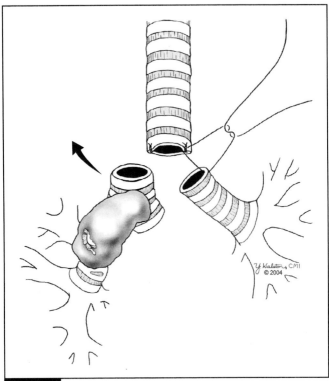

FIG. 3-2

Schematic representation of a right pneumonectomy with sleeve resection of the carina. The neoplasm is in the right upper lobe but extends to the lower end of the trachea.

unlikely to be possible if the tumor extends more than 3 cm or four cartilaginous rings above the carina or beyond 1.5 cm in the contralateral bronchus. If sleeve pneumonectomy is contemplated, *transesophageal echocardiography* must be done to evaluate the degree of tumor extension to organs of the posterior mediastinum, such as the esophagus, or extension into the superior vena cava.

The final decision to perform a sleeve pneumonectomy is made at surgery. For a tension-free anastomosis to be accomplished, the safe length between the distal end of the lower trachea and the contralateral main bronchus *should not surpass 4 cm*. Preoperative or intraoperative documentation of superior vena cava invasion and limited spread to the muscular wall of the esophagus are *additional difficulties*, but they are not considered to be absolute contraindications to tracheal sleeve pneumonectomy.

EVALUATION OF TECHNICAL RESECTABILITY OF PATIENTS WITH SUSPECTED MEDIASTINAL INVOLVEMENT

Mediastinal Pleura, Mediastinal Fat, Pericardium (T3)

Invasion of the mediastinal pleura, pericardium, or mediastinal fat constitutes T3 disease, for which a *complete resection is possible* most of the time. Determination of technical resectability before operation is difficult, however. CT scanning is of little value in detecting direct mediastinal invasion by lung cancer.

At operation, localized attachments to the mediastinal pleura can often be easily mobilized. Invasion of the pericardium in the vicinity of pulmonary blood vessels may mandate *intrapericardial division* of these vessels.

Main Stem of Pulmonary Arteries (T4)

Intrapericardial involvement of right or left main pulmonary arteries constitutes T4 disease. This type of involvement is difficult to document preoperatively, although CT scan may suggest that these vessels are invaded. It is important, however, that *no patient be denied operation strictly on the basis of CT scanning* because it is often relatively easy to resect intrapericardially the involved portion of the artery.

Heart and Great Vessels (T4)

Direct invasion of the heart, whether it is the atria or ventricle, is considered to be *unresectable disease*. This type of invasion can be predicted preoperatively through the combined results of CT, MRI, and transesophageal echocardiography.

In selected cases, small localized areas of the left atrium may be resected; this usually applies to tumors that have tracked down the pulmonary vein. Similarly, infiltration of the aorta is usually a contraindication to surgery, although in some cases one might be able to peel off the tumor when only the adventitia is involved. Again, this is difficult to document preoperatively; often, the decision will have to be made only after full mobilization of the lung and involved cardiovascular structure.

In patients in whom cardiac or aortic invasion is suspected preoperatively, the *planning of operation* must be done with great care. Cardiac surgeons must be involved in the decision-making process; for most of these lesions, cardiac invasion is due to metastatic local nodes rather than the primary tumor. In general, more aggressive maneuvers, such as cardiopulmonary bypass, are *not indicated*.

Superior Vena Cava (T4)

Local invasion of the superior vena cava by tumors in the anterior segment of the right upper lobe is sometimes amenable to resection. This can be done by tangential lateral clamping of the superior vena cava and partial resection of its wall or by complete proximal and distal clamping, resection, and reconstruction. These techniques apply, however, to *highly selected patients* in whom the point of caval attachment is the only limiting factor to a curative resection. Indeed, most of the time, the superior vena cava is involved by metastatic nodes rather than by the primary tumor.

The preoperative documentation of superior vena cava invasion is usually made by contrast-enhanced CT scanning and by vena cava angiography. The presence of a superior vena cava syndrome is an *absolute contraindication* to surgery.

Esophagus (T4)

The esophagus is rarely the sole point of attachment of T4 tumors, although paraesophageal tissues can occasionally be mobilized to the extent that the esophagus is the remaining point of fixation. If the tumor has not penetrated into the esophageal mucosa, a *superficial resection of the esophageal musculature* can be performed. Full-thickness invasion of the esophagus is an absolute contraindication to resection.

Preoperatively, esophageal invasion is best demonstrated by contrast esophageal studies and esophagoscopy.

Recurrent Nerve and Phrenic Nerve (T4)

Recurrent nerve palsy is easy to document preoperatively because patients present with hoarseness. In all cases, it is important to document vocal cord paralysis by direct examination because, on occasion, hoarseness may be due to other causes, such as synchronous laryngeal cancer. As a rule, recurrent nerve palsy is due to N2 disease, and most of these patients *should not have an operation*.

Phrenic nerve palsy can be suspected by the identification of a high diaphragm on the side of the tumor. Documentation is done by fluoroscopic studies, which demonstrate an immobile diaphragm or a diaphragm with paradoxical movements. Once again, this must be documented; several patients will have an elevated hemidiaphragm only because of loss of volume or atelectasis of the involved lung rather than from phrenic nerve palsy.

As a general rule, phrenic nerve involvement through upper lobe tumors is considered to be a contraindication to surgery because in nearly all cases it relates to N2 disease. By contrast, phrenic nerve involvement more caudally (over the pericardium) may be related to *direct invasion* by lower lobe or middle lobe tumors, and in such cases, complete resection may be possible.

EVALUATION OF TECHNICAL RESECTABILITY OF PATIENTS WITH SUSPECTED INVOLVEMENT OF OTHER STRUCTURES

Diaphragm (T3)

Most patients with *direct extension of lung cancer into the diaphragm* also have invasion of the cardiophrenic angle or chest wall or subdiaphragmatic extension into the liver or abdominal lymph nodes, which precludes resection. An occasional patient, however, may present with localized disease that can be managed by full-thickness resection of a portion of the hemidiaphragm.

If such a case is suspected preoperatively, careful examination of the area should be carried out through CT scanning and upper abdominal ultrasonography.

Pleural Effusion

Malignant effusions should be considered an *absolute contraindication to surgery* when these are confirmed cytologically or pathologically. However, a few patients will have a cytologically negative effusion due to atelectasis or obstructive pneumonitis or due to a condition unrelated to their primary tumor. These patients should not be denied surgery even if the presence of an effusion by itself (even if it is negative) is a predictor of unresectability and a poor prognostic sign.

All pleural effusions associated with lung cancer should be investigated at least by thoracentesis and cytologic analysis. If the effusion is significant

TABLE 3-4			
TECHNICAL RESECTABILITY OF LUNG CANCER			
Structure Involved	Resectable	Doubtful[1]	Not Resectable
CHEST WALL			
Ribs[2]	✓		
Spine			
Prevertebral fascia, transverse process	✓		
Lateral portion of vertebra		✓	
Vertebral body			✓
Pancoast tumors			
Lower trunk of brachial plexus (C8-T1)	✓		
Subclavian artery	✓		
PROXIMAL AIRWAYS			
Less than 2 cm of trachea	✓		
More than 3 cm of trachea			✓
More than 1.5 cm of contralateral bronchus			✓
MEDIASTINUM			
Mediastinal pleura and fat, pericardium	✓		
Main stem of pulmonary arteries	✓		
Heart and great vessels			✓
Superior vena cava		✓	
Esophagus			
Superficial muscular	✓		
Full thickness			✓
Recurrent nerve			✓
Phrenic nerve			✓
Diaphragm	✓		
PLEURAL EFFUSION			
Malignant			✓
Reactional	✓		

[1]Doubtful indicates that it can be done in highly selected cases.

[2]Any number of ribs can be resected. A defect of 5 cm anterolaterally or of 10 cm posteriorly needs prosthetic reconstruction.

or associated with higher stage tumors, patients should also undergo *videothoracoscopy* with pleural biopsy.

As a rule, every attempt should be made to rule out malignant neoplasia as the cause of pleural effusion in patients with primary lung cancer.

CONCLUSION (TABLE 3-4)

Resectability of lung cancer was traditionally considered a state of mind because almost any tumor could be resected. Currently, however, the decision to resect a particular neoplasm must depend on objective and reliable information obtained preoperatively as well as on the potential for complete resection, keeping in mind that *incomplete resection consistently fails to cure*. Because penetration of other thoracic structures will often necessitate their removal, proper planning of surgery is essential, as is consultation with other surgical specialists such as cardiovascular, orthopedic, and plastic surgeons. Above all, these cases must have proper clinical nodal staging, and they should be discussed at tumor conferences. As stated by Dr. D. Weissberg, these considerations are important if one is to avoid surgical decisions based on the surgeon's philosophy rather than on objective facts.

SUGGESTED READINGS

Review Articles

Martini N: Surgery for T3 disease. Proceedings of the American College of Surgeons Postgraduate Course in Thoracic Surgery. New Orleans, October 1986.

Luketich JD, Van Raemdonck DE, Ginsberg RJ: Extended resection for higher-stage non–small-cell lung cancer. World J Surg 1993;17:719-728.

Armstrong P, Congleton J, Fountain SW, et al: Guidelines on the selection of patients with lung cancer for surgery. British Thoracic Society and Society of Cardiothoracic Surgeons of Great Britain and Ireland Working Party. Thorax 2001;56:89-108.

Orlowski TM, Szczesny TJ: Surgical treatment of stage III non–small cell lung cancer. Lung Cancer 2001;34(suppl 2):S137-S143.

Deslauriers J: Current surgical treatment of nonsmall cell lung cancer 2001. Eur Respir J 2002;19(suppl):61s-70s.

Rice TW, Blackstone EH: Radical resections for T4 lung cancer. Surg Clin North Am 2002;82:573-587.

CT Scanning

Rendina EA, Bognolo DA, Mineo TC, et al: Computed tomography for the evaluation of intrathoracic invasion by lung cancer. J Thorac Cardiovasc Surg 1987;94:57-63.

Webb WR, Gatsonis C, Zerhouni EA, et al: CT and MR imaging in staging for non–small cell bronchogenic carcinoma: report of the radiologic diagnostic oncology group. Radiology 1991;178:705-713.

VATS Evaluation

Roviaro G, Varoli F, Rebuffat C, et al: Videothoracoscopic staging and treatment of lung cancer. Ann Thorac Surg 1995;59:971-974.

Technical Resectability of Pancoast Tumors

McLoud TC, Filion RB, Edelman RR, Shepard JAO: MR imaging of superior sulcus carcinoma. J Comput Assist Tomogr 1989;13: 233-239.

Heelan RT, Demas BE, Caravelli JF, et al: Superior sulcus tumors: CT and MR imaging. Radiology 1989;170:637-641.

Laissy JP, Soyer P, Sekkal SR, et al: Assessment of vascular involvement with magnetic resonance angiography (MRA) in Pancoast syndrome. Magn Reson Imaging 1995;13:523-530.

Rusch VW, Parekh KR, Leon L, et al: Factors determining outcome after surgical resection of T3 and T4 lung cancers of the superior sulcus. J Thorac Cardiovasc Surg 2000;119:1147-1153.

Jett JR: Superior sulcus tumors and Pancoast's syndrome. Lung Cancer 2003;42:s17-s21.

Kent MS, Bilsky MH, Rusch VW: Resection of superior sulcus tumors (posterior approach). Thorac Surg Clin 2004;14:217-228.

Technical Resectability of Chest Wall Invasion

Ratto GB, Piacenza G, Frola C, et al: Chest wall involvement by lung cancer: computed tomographic detection and results of operation. Ann Thorac Surg 1991;51:182-188.

Allen MS: Chest wall resection and reconstruction for lung cancer. Thorac Surg Clin 2004;14:211-216.

Technical Resectability of Tumors Invading the Airway

Deslauriers J, Grégoire J, Jacques LF, Piraux M: Sleeve pneumonectomy. Thorac Surg Clin 2004;14:183-190.

Rendina EA, Venuta F, De Giacomo T, et al: Sleeve resection after induction therapy. Thorac Surg Clin 2004;14:191-197.

Technical Resectability of Vertebral Body Invasion

Grunenwald DH, Mazel C, Girard P, et al: Radical en bloc resection for lung cancer invading the spine. J Thorac Cardiovasc Surg 2002;123:271-279.

Fadel E, Missenard G, Chapelier A, et al: En bloc resection of non–small cell lung cancer invading the thoracic inlet and intervertebral foramina. J Thorac Cardiovasc Surg 2002;123:676-685.

Martin LW, Walsh GL: Vertebral body resection. Thorac Surg Clin 2004;14:241-254.

Technical Resectability of Mediastinal Invasion

Fukuse T, Wada H, Hitomi S: Extended operation for non–small cell lung cancer invading great vessels and left atrium. Eur J Cardiothorac Surg 1997;11:664-669.

3

Specific Preoperative Assessment

Spaggiari L, Regnard JF, Magdeleinat P, et al: Extended resections for bronchogenic carcinoma invading the superior vena cava system. Ann Thorac Surg 2000;69:233-236.

Grunenwald DH: Resection of lung carcinomas invading the mediastinum including the superior vena cava. Thorac Surg Clin 2004;14:255-263.

Surgery

Shirakusa T, Kawahara K, Iwasaki A, et al: Extended operation for T4 lung carcinoma. Ann Thorac Cardiovasc Surg 1998;4:110-118.

Grunenwald DH: Surgery for advanced stage lung cancer. Semin Surg Oncol 2000;18:137-142.

ASSESSMENT OF THE PATIENT WITH A MEDIASTINAL MASS

True mediastinal tumors and masses are lesions arising from *structures normally located* in the mediastinum or from structures that are transiting through it. Lesions arising from structures outside the mediastinum and anomalies of vascular origin are considered false mediastinal tumors.

To provide optimal care, one should establish *a clear diagnosis* in every case. Although this diagnosis will, on occasion, be obtained through simple methods, often a more complex and integrated investigation will be necessary. To be successful, this investigation involves a close collaboration between thoracic surgeons, radiologists, and pathologists as well as a structured and cost-effective framework.

ANATOMIC DIVISIONS OF THE MEDIASTINUM

Because specific lesions have a predilection for certain sites, dividing the mediastinum into different compartments is helpful.

Classically, the mediastinum is divided into *superior and inferior compartments* by an imaginary line extending from the sternal angle to the fourth intervertebral disk (Fig. 3-3). The inferior compartment is further subdivided into anterior, middle, and posterior compartments (Fig. 3-4). The *anterior mediastinum* extends from the back of the sternum to the front of the ascending aorta and pericardium; the *posterior mediastinum* is situated between the posterior pericardium and spine. The *middle mediastinum*, located between the anterior and posterior mediastinum, contains the heart and great vessels as well as trachea and main stem bronchi.

In 1972, Shields proposed a more simple anteroposterior division of the mediastinum. In his schema, there are two true mediastinal compartments (anterior and visceral) and *bilateral paravertebral sulci* that lie alongside the spine (Fig. 3-5).

TRUE AND FALSE MEDIASTINAL TUMORS

The differential diagnosis of a mediastinal mass is highly dependent on *its location*.

Thymic lesions, germ cell tumors, lymphomas, and connective tissue tumors including lipomas (sarcomas) and hemangiomas are more commonly located in the *anterior mediastinum* (Table 3-5). In the majority

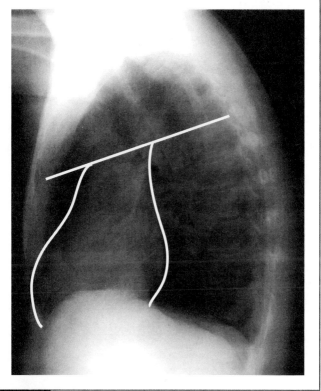

FIG. 3-3

Classic mediastinal compartments. The mediastinum is divided into a superior and an inferior compartment by a line drawn from the sternal angle to the fourth intervertebral disk.

of cases, substernal goiters are also located in the anterior mediastinum, although they are downward extensions from the neck and as such maintain their cervical vascular supply. Other anterior mediastinal shadows that may simulate primary mediastinal masses include sternal tumors, abnormalities of the vascular system, and lung cancer of upper lobes invading directly through the mediastinal pleura.

Lesions of lymphoid origin (enlarged lymph nodes) are largely found in the *middle mediastinum* (Table 3-6). These include benign diseases such as sarcoidosis and granulomatous disease as well as malignant enlargement such as that seen in lymphomas or metastatic carcinomas. Bronchogenic cysts are also commonly located in the middle mediastinum

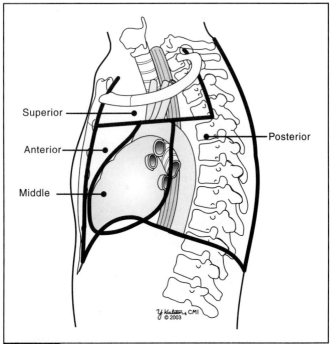

FIG. 3-4

Diagram showing the classic mediastinal compartments: superior, anterior, middle, posterior.

near the carina. A variety of cardiovascular shadows may simulate middle mediastinal masses; primary tracheal tumors seldom present as mediastinal masses.

Neurogenic tumors (benign or malignant) are usually found in the *posterior mediastinum* (Table 3-7) or paravertebral sulci. Lesions originating from the esophagus and aneurysms of the descending thoracic aorta are also considered in the differential diagnosis of false posterior mediastinal masses. Contents of diaphragmatic hernias, specifically Morgagni hernia, paraesophageal hernia, and posterolateral hernia of Bochdalek, may also present as mediastinal masses.

METHODS OF INVESTIGATION

If the tumor is clearly mediastinal, a *likely presumptive diagnosis* should be entertained before management is considered. Of equal importance, pretreatment evaluation must provide a *clear understanding* of possible difficulties that may be encountered should surgery be required.

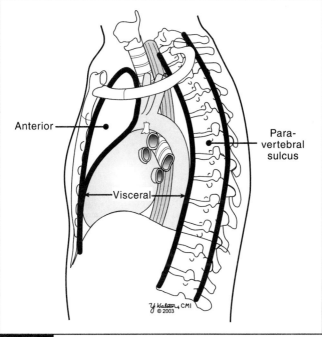

Anterior

Para-
vertebral
sulcus

Visceral

Y. Walton, CMI
© 2003

FIG. 3-5

Proposed anatomic subdivision of the mediastinum by Shields. *(From Shields TW: Mediastinal Surgery. Philadelphia, Lea & Febiger, 1991.)*

TABLE 3-5

COMMON ANTERIOR MEDIASTINAL MASSES

True Masses	False Masses
Thymic tumors	Substernal goiters (extension from neck)
Germ cell tumors	Sternal and costochondral tumors
Lymphomas	Lymphangiomas
Mesenchymal tumors	Aneurysms of ascending aorta, innominate artery, subclavian artery
	Abnormal dilatation of superior vena cava or azygos vein
	Lung cancer invading through mediastinal pleura

TABLE 3-6

COMMON MIDDLE MEDIASTINAL MASSES

True Masses	False Masses
Enlarged lymph nodes (benign, malignant)	Aneurysm (or dilatation) of heart cavities or aortic arch
Foregut cysts (bronchogenic)	Aneurysm of pulmonary artery
Pericardial cysts	Mediastinitis, pericarditis

TABLE 3-7	
COMMON POSTERIOR MEDIASTINAL MASSES	
True Masses	**False Masses**
Neurogenic tumors (benign, malignant)	Esophageal shadows: megaesophagus (achalasia), tumors
Foregut cysts (bronchogenic, enterogenic)	Diaphragmatic hernias
Meningocele	Aneurysms of descending aorta
	Pott abscesses
	Extramedullary hematopoiesis

Noninvasive Methods

Clinical Considerations

The mediastinal location of masses is *age dependent* (Table 3-8). In children, posterior mediastinal localization is more common because of the predominance of neurogenic tumors. In adults, the anterior mediastinum is more commonly involved because of the high incidence of thymomas and lymphomas, which are rarely observed in children. In the anterior mediastinum, a distinct pediatric-adult differentiation is indeed due to the high incidence of thymomas in the adult (Table 3-9). Overall, 92% of mediastinal tumors occur in the adult population (age 15 years or older) and only 8% in children.

Approximately *25% of all mediastinal tumors* are malignant, in both adults and children. Roughly two thirds of children are symptomatic at presentation, whereas only one third of adults have symptoms. Tumors in the upper half of the mediastinum are more likely to be symptomatic because in that area, several organs are distributed in a narrow and rigid anteroposterior space. The presence or absence of symptoms also depends on whether the mass is *benign or malignant* and on the *size of the tumor*. In general, malignant and bigger lesions *are more likely* to be symptomatic than are benign and smaller lesions.

Most symptoms relate to mediastinal structures that are either *compressed* or *invaded*. Respiratory symptoms, such as cough, stridor, and dyspnea, are the most common, followed by chest pain, which may mimic that of angina. Other possible symptoms and signs include dysphagia, superior vena cava syndrome, cardiac tamponade, hoarseness, and Horner syndrome. In 80% to 90% of cases, the presence of chest pain associated with a mediastinal mass *is indicative of malignancy*.

TABLE 3-8		
LOCALIZATION OF MEDIASTINAL TUMORS BASED ON AGE		
	Pediatric (≤15 yr)	Adult (>15 yr)
Anterior	38%	65%
Middle	10%	10%
Posterior	52%	25%

TABLE 3-9		
ANTERIOR MEDIASTINAL TUMORS ACCORDING TO AGE		
	Pediatric	Adult
Thymic	17%	47%
Germ cell	24%	15%
Lymphoma	45%	28%
Mesenchymatous	15%	—
Others	—	16%

Systemic manifestations may include fever, weight loss, anemia, and myasthenia gravis seen in association with thymomas.

Imaging

Plain chest radiography continues to be a *highly satisfactory examination* for the initial evaluation of mediastinal masses. On the posteroanterior view, one can determine if the mass is *superior or inferior* and if it is unilateral or bilateral. On the lateral film, the site of the mass can be assessed, thereby starting a differential diagnosis based on location. Several clues about the nature of the mass can also be discerned from its borders and density. Other simple techniques that may be useful include fluoroscopic examination and barium swallow study. Under fluoroscopy, one can assess the *volume, contours,* and *transparency* of the mass. Barium examination is an excellent method to document signs of *esophageal compression* as well as intrinsic lesions of the esophagus that may indeed be responsible for the mass.

CT is now the *examination of choice* in virtually all cases of mediastinal masses. It is accurate in defining the *density of the mass* in relation to the density of adjacent structures such as the lungs (air), soft tissues, and bones. Masses with low attenuation are consistent with fat; cystic lesions have attenuation values close to or higher than that of water. Solid masses have attenuation values higher than that of water, and if the mass is malignant (versus benign), it often has irregular margins with suggestions of infiltration into adjacent tissues. Contrast-enhanced CT has a more than 90% accuracy rate in distinguishing vascular from nonvascular etiology. CT is also useful to determine the *most suitable* approach for the biopsy of the lesion under investigation.

MRI is *not routinely* used in the investigation of mediastinal masses, although the lack of ionizing radiation, the availability of cross-sectional images in multiple imaging planes, and the ability to distinguish vascular structures without intravenous administration of contrast agents have made MRI a *potentially valuable alternative* to CT (Table 3-10). Neurogenic tumors involving the intervertebral foramen or with intraspinal extension are best assessed by MRI. Similarly, invasion or encasement of major vascular structures may also be best demonstrated by MRI. Myelography is no longer performed because CT and MRI can provide a clearer definition of the neural foramina. A potential use of angiography is the localization of

3

Specific Preoperative Assessment

TABLE 3-10

CT AND MRI IN THE EVALUATION OF MEDIASTINAL MASSES

CT Superior	MRI Superior	CT and MRI Equal
Spatial resolution	Multiplanar imaging capability and no contrast material needed	Detection of pure fluid collections
Detection of bone destruction	Identification of complex fluid collection	Detection of chest wall invasion
Detection of calcification	Soft tissue differentiation	Evaluation of vascular obstruction (contrast CT)
Detection of lung nodules	Tumor vs. fibrosis	
Evaluation of lung parenchyma	Tumor vs. obstructive pneumonitis	
Screening for lung, liver, adrenals	Evaluation of brachial plexus, neural foramina, diaphragm, bone marrow	
	Mediastinal tissue invasion	

From Moore EH: Radiologic evaluation of mediastinal masses. Chest Surg Clin North Am 1992;2:1.

parathyroid adenomas or possible involvement of the artery of Adamkiewicz by neurogenic tumors.

Ultrasonography is *not routinely used* to evaluate mediastinal masses because ultrasound beams cannot significantly transmit through lung or bone. On occasion, ultrasound examination can be used to distinguish between cystic and solid masses that are located at the cardiophrenic angle. The use of gallium scans has been recommended by some authors to evaluate anterior mediastinal masses such as lymphomas or any other pathologic process involving active inflammation. Gallium uptake by germ cell tumors is unpredictable, and thymomas rarely take up gallium.

Tumor Markers

Tumor markers are *measurable biologic substances* that indicate the presence of a neoplasm. They include anti–acetylcholine receptor (anti-AChR) antibodies, useful to diagnose thymomas and myasthenia gravis, and tumor markers such as human chorionic gonadotropin β (β-hCG) and alpha-fetoprotein, useful in the diagnosis of non-seminomatous germ cell tumors. About 90% of patients with non-seminomatous germ cell tumors have elevation of at least one of these markers. Changes in the titer of markers roughly parallel the *tumor activity*, and these are invaluable for *estimating prognosis* as well as for *selecting therapy* and following its effect.

Needle Biopsy

Biopsy of mediastinal tumors can be performed when the diagnosis remains *unclear* after extensive imaging. Indeed, *it is mandatory* when primary treatment is likely to be nonsurgical, such as in lymphomas or germ cell tumors. Unfortunately, fine-needle aspiration biopsy often does not provide enough material to diagnose or subclassify lymphomas or germ cell tumors or to differentiate between lymphoma and thymoma. If larger cutting needles are used, the biopsy route must be planned carefully to *avoid potential vascular injury*. In all cases in which biopsy has been performed, specimens must be submitted for immunohistochemical staining and electronic microscopy.

Invasive Methods

Open Biopsy

A variety of techniques are available for open biopsy of mediastinal masses. *Cervical mediastinoscopy* allows access to masses in the paratracheal or subcarinal spaces and occasionally to masses extending from the anterior mediastinum to the middle compartment. *Mediastinotomy* is carried out through a short transverse incision over the second cartilage and affords access for adequate biopsy of all anterior mediastinal masses. Both of these procedures are associated with few complications, and when they are combined, nearly all tumors in the anterior or middle mediastinum are accessible to biopsy.

Thoracoscopic biopsy (VATS) is minimally invasive, and nearly all areas of the mediastinum can be approached with equal safety and efficacy. One additional advantage of VATS is that certain benign lesions, such as cystic masses, can be completely excised during the procedure.

Anesthesia for Open Biopsy

Large mediastinal tumors can be associated with significant impairment of cardiopulmonary dynamic, which may in turn lead to *catastrophic complications during general anesthesia*. These issues need to be addressed preoperatively, and adequate evaluation and preparation of the patient are of foremost importance. In general, the degree of airway compression or narrowing documented by CT scan or flexible bronchoscopy is a good predictor of whether anesthetic difficulties with the airway will be encountered. If the patient has severe airway compromise or cannot tolerate general anesthesia because of vascular compression (pulmonary artery, superior vena cava), empirical therapy can be based on the presumed diagnosis of the mediastinal tumor, or an open biopsy can be performed under local anesthesia.

DIAGNOSTIC STRATEGIES

Anterior Mediastinal Tumors

Common causes of anterior mediastinal masses are thymic neoplasms, germ cell tumors, lymphomas, mesenchymal tumors, and substernal goiter.

Thymomas are the *most common anterior mediastinal tumors* in adults. Their peak incidence is between 40 and 60 years of age, and there is no sex predilection. Approximately 50% of patients are asymptomatic, and 30% of patients with a known thymoma have associated myasthenia gravis. In addition to myasthenia gravis, another 5% to 10% of patients will have other "parathymic" syndromes, such as red cell aplasia, hypogammaglobulinemia, systemic lupus, Cushing syndrome, and inappropriate antidiuretic hormone secretion.

TABLE 3-11
CLASSIFICATION OF PRIMARY THYMIC NEOPLASMS
Thymomas
Noninvasive (stage I, Masaoka staging system)
Minimally invasive (stages IIa-b)
Invasive (stage III)
Thymic carcinomas
Squamous or lymphoepithelioma-like
Thymic carcinoids
Thymolipomas
Thymic cysts
Congenital or acquired
Thymic lymphomas

Chest radiographs and CT scan usually show a *rounded or lobulated soft tissue mass* in the anterior mediastinum near the junction of the heart and great vessels. On occasion, there are areas of cystic degeneration or hemorrhage. Calcifications are present in about 20% of cases and *do not* indicate benignancy. Contrast-enhanced CT is best to demonstrate local invasion into mediastinal fat, pleura and lung, pericardium, and great vessels. The diagnosis and stage of a thymoma are usually based on the CT scan appearance. Well-circumscribed thymic masses are almost always benign, whereas vascular or pericardial invasion or encasement suggests an invasive thymoma. This distinction is significant because patients with invasive tumors may not be suitable candidates for immediate surgery and may therefore require preoperative biopsy, best done through a limited anterior mediastinotomy on the side over which the tumor projects. In most patients with suspected thymoma, however, surgical excision should be performed *without preoperative biopsy*. A classification of other primary thymic neoplasms is given in Table 3-11.

Germ cell tumors of the mediastinum (Table 3-12) are rare but still account for most primary extragonadal germ cell tumors. Benign teratomas

TABLE 3-12
CLASSIFICATION OF PRIMARY GERM CELL TUMORS OF THE MEDIASTINUM
BENIGN
Mature teratoma
Dermoid or epidermoid cysts
MALIGNANT
Teratocarcinoma
Seminomas (dysgerminomas)
Non-seminomatous germ cell tumors
Yolk sac tumors (endodermal sinus)
Choriocarcinomas
Embryonal cell carcinomas

occur more frequently in young adults and are equally distributed between men and women. CT is highly suggestive with a well-demonstrated fatty and cystic lesion, often with calcifications. Cough productive of hair or sebum is a *pathognomonic sign* of rupture in the tracheobronchial tree. When a benign teratoma is suspected, *surgical excision is recommended without biopsy*.

Mediastinal seminomas occur in men in their third decade, and most are symptomatic. Although 10% of patients may have an elevated β-hCG level, they almost never have elevated alpha-fetoprotein levels. On CT scan, seminomas present as bulky lobulated homogeneous anterior mediastinal masses. Because most of these tumors are infiltrative and their treatment is primarily nonsurgical, a *biopsy should be performed* and the patient referred for chemoradiotherapy. In some cases, an open biopsy is necessary to distinguish between pure and mixed seminomas. This distinction is *important* because pure seminomas are highly radiosensitive and have a good prognosis (cure rates of 50% to 100%), whereas mixed (seminoma and non-seminoma) tumors have a much poorer prognosis.

Non-seminomatous germ cell tumors are *rapidly growing neoplasms*, and approximately 80% have at least one site of metastatic disease at the time of diagnosis. Almost all patients are young men younger than 30 years, and most are symptomatic at the time of presentation. On CT, the tumor presents as a large and irregular anterior mediastinal mass with extensive areas of necrosis and hemorrhage. Measurements of serum levels of β-hCG and alpha-fetoprotein are indispensable in the diagnosis and management of these tumors, and *one or both markers are elevated in about 90% of cases*. It is generally agreed that despite positive tumor markers, all patients should have *tissue confirmation* before treatment.

The majority of patients with lymphomas in the mediastinum also have *systemic disease*. However, 5% to 10% of patients will present with primary mediastinal disease, usually *enlarged nodes* located in the anterior and superior mediastinum. They often produce symptoms related to respiratory compression, pleuropericardial involvement, or superior vena cava compression. The surgeon's role in suspected lymphomas of the mediastinum is primarily diagnostic, and one must ensure that enough material is obtained not only to establish the diagnosis but also to *subtype the tumor*.

Connective tissue tumors such as lipomas, hemangiomas, fibromas, and lymphangiomas and their malignant counterparts are *uncommon*, and most are found in the anterior mediastinum. Resection is usually indicated and is often the best way to confirm the diagnosis. Mediastinal lymphangioma (cystic hygroma) is a benign proliferation of lymphatic vessels and sacs that may grow in an infiltrative fashion. Typically, they are tumors of *very young children* and involve primarily the neck. In about 10% of cases, they will extend in the superior mediastinum, where they present as rounded, multicystic, and infiltrative lesions. Complete surgical excision may be difficult, and postoperative recurrences are common.

The vast majority of intrathoracic goiters are *continuous* with an enlarged cervical thyroid gland and have a typical CT appearance. They are usually located in the anterosuperior mediastinum, where they present with smooth borders and multinodularity; they may also have coarse calcifications and low-density cystic areas. Most are asymptomatic and discovered during chest radiography. All symptomatic substernal goiters should be removed without preoperative biopsy.

Tumors of the Middle Mediastinum

Common lesions located in the middle mediastinum include pericardial and foregut cysts and *lesions arising from lymph nodes*. Several arterial abnormalities are also located in this compartment, and they can be recognized by contrast-enhanced CT. A list of the most common mediastinal cysts by location is given in Table 3-13.

Pleuropericardial cysts are characteristically located at the right cardiophrenic angle (60%), where they present as smooth, round, and homogeneous soft tissue masses contiguous with the hemidiaphragm. CT shows a mass with an attenuation coefficient consistent with a cystic lesion. If fine-needle aspiration biopsy is carried out, it yields clear and watery fluid.

Most bronchogenic cysts are in sites *adjacent to the tracheobronchial tree*. Many are asymptomatic. On standard radiography, they present as rounded, sharply demarcated homogeneous masses in close association with the trachea and carina. On CT, they usually have low Hounsfield units indicating clear fluid, but they may be infected or contain sufficient mucus to give a high CT number. They can be readily recognized by VATS, and occasionally complete cyst excision can be carried out during the procedure.

TABLE 3-13

COMMON CYSTS BY LOCATION OF THE MEDIASTINUM

ANTERIOR MEDIASTINUM

Lymphangiomas (cystic hygroma)

Thymic cysts
    Congenital
    Acquired

MIDDLE MEDIASTINUM

Pleuropericardial cysts

Foregut cysts—bronchogenic

POSTERIOR MEDIASTINUM

Foregut cysts
    Enteric
    Neuroenteric

Thoracic duct cysts

By far, the most common masses in the middle mediastinum are in relation to enlarged lymph nodes distributed around the tracheobronchial tree. The differential diagnoses of these nodes include sarcoidosis, lymphoma, and metastatic disease from the lung. Cervical mediastinoscopy is useful in biopsy of mediastinal nodes and for correct diagnosis of the underlying process.

Tumors of the Posterior Mediastinum

Mediastinal masses in the posterior mediastinum include *neurogenic tumors* and some *foregut cysts,* such as enteric (esophageal duplications) and neuroenteric cysts.

Neurogenic tumors arise from the peripheral nerves or sympathetic ganglion. In adults, the majority (90%) are benign, slow growing, and asymptomatic. In this population, the most common neurogenic tumors are of nerve sheath origin (Table 3-14), and these include schwannomas and neurofibromas. About 40% of mediastinal neurogenic tumors derive from the autonomic nervous system, and these include ganglioneuromas (young adult), neuroblastomas (children), and ganglioneuroblastomas (children). On radiographic examination, neurogenic tumors present as *rounded masses* arising in the *paravertebral sulcus.* Erosion, destruction, or spreading of the ribs may occur, as may vertebral abnormalities and intraspinal extension (dumbbell tumors). These features are best examined by MRI, which accurately describes the existence and longitudinal extension of the spinal component of the tumor. Preoperative biopsy of neurogenic tumors is unnecessary.

CONCLUSION

Mediastinal masses must be investigated in depth not only to establish diagnosis but also to document the degree of local invasiveness before surgery. Fortunately, modern imaging techniques facilitate this investigation.

For most tumors for which primary treatment is likely to be nonsurgical, a biopsy specimen should be obtained.

TABLE 3-14
CLASSIFICATION OF COMMON NEUROGENIC TUMORS OF THE MEDIASTINUM
TUMORS OF THE SYMPATHETIC NERVOUS SYSTEM
Most common in patients <10 years
Neuroblastoma
Ganglioneuroblastoma
Ganglioneuroma (most common variety)
TUMORS OF THE PERIPHERAL NERVES
Most common in patients >20 years
Schwannoma
Neurofibroma
Malignant peripheral nerve sheath tumor (most commonly seen in the context of Recklinghausen disease, also known as malignant neurofibroma)

SUGGESTED READINGS

Review Articles

Mullen B, Richardson JD: Primary anterior mediastinal tumors in children and adults [collective review]. Ann Thorac Surg 1986;42:338-345.

Kohman LJ: Approach to the diagnosis and staging of mediastinal masses. Chest 1993;100:328s-330s.

Strollo DC, Rosado de Christenson ML, Jett JR: Primary mediastinal tumors. Part 1. Tumors of the anterior mediastinum. Chest 1997;112:511-522.

Wright CD: Surgical management of mediastinal tumors and fibrosis. Semin Respir Crit Care Med 1999;20:473-481.

Yoneda KY, Louie S, Shelton DK: Mediastinal tumors. Curr Opin Pulm Med 2001;7:226-233.

False Tumors

Kelley MJ, Mannes EJ, Ravin CE: Mediastinal masses of vascular origin. A review. J Thorac Cardiovasc Surg 1978;76:559-572.

Imaging

Graeber GM, Shriver CD, Albus RA, et al: The use of computed tomography in the evaluation of mediastinal masses. J Thorac Cardiovasc Surg 1986;91:662-666.

Glazer HS, Siegel MJ, Sagel SS: Low-attenuation mediastinal masses on CT. AJR Am J Roentgenol 1989;152:1173-1177.

Brown K, Aberle DR, Batra P, Steckel RJ: Current use of imaging in the evaluation of primary mediastinal masses. Chest 1990;98:466-473.

Moore EH: Radiologic evaluation of mediastinal masses. Chest Surg Clin North Am 1992;2:1-22.

Markers

Minton JP, Chevinsky A: Present status of serum markers. Semin Surg Oncol 1989;5:426-435.

Needle Biopsy

Herman SJ, Holub RV, Weisbrod GL, Chamberlain DW: Anterior mediastinal masses: utility of transthoracic needle biopsy. Radiology 1991;180:167-170.

Morrissey B, Adams H, Gibbs AR, Crane MD: Percutaneous needle biopsy of the mediastinum: review of 94 procedures. Thorax 1993;48:632-637.

Hsu WH, Chiang CD, Hsu JY, et al: Ultrasonically guided needle biopsy of anterior mediastinal masses: comparison of carcinomatous and non-carcinomatous masses. J Clin Ultrasound 1995;23:349-356.

Surgical Biopsy

Kern JA, Daniel TM, Tribble CG, et al: Thoracoscopic diagnosis and treatment of mediastinal masses. Ann Thorac Surg 1993;56:92-96.

Rendina EA, Venuta F, De Giacomo T, et al: Comparative merits of thoracoscopy, mediastinoscopy, and mediastinotomy for mediastinal biopsy. Ann Thorac Surg 1994;57:992-995.

Gossot D, Toledo L, Fritsch S, Celerier M: Mediastinoscopy vs. thoracoscopy for mediastinal biopsy. Results of a prospective nonrandomized study. Chest 1996;110:1328-1331.

Solaini L, Bagioni P, Campanini A, Poddie BD: Diagnostic role of videothoracoscopy in mediastinal diseases. Eur J Cardiothorac Surg 1998;13:491-493.

Demmy TL, Krasna MJ, Detterbeck FC, et al: Multicenter VATS experience with mediastinal tumors. Ann Thorac Surg 1998;66:187-192.

de Montpréville VT, Dulmet EM, Nashashibi N: Frozen section diagnosis and surgical biopsy of lymph nodes, tumors, and pseudotumors of the mediastinum. Eur J Cardiothorac Surg 1998;13:190-195.

Hutter J, Junger W, Miller K, Moritz E: Subxiphoidal videomediastinoscopy for diagnostic access to the anterior mediastinum. Ann Thorac Surg 1998;66:1427-1428.

Rendina EA, Venuta F, De Giacomo T, et al: Biopsy of anterior mediastinal masses under local anesthesia. Ann Thorac Surg 2002;74:1720-1723.

Case Series

Ferguson MK, Lee E, Skinner DB, Little AG: Selective operative approach for diagnosis and treatment of anterior mediastinal masses. Ann Thorac Surg 1987;44:583-586.

Fradet G, Evans KG, Nelems B, et al: Primary anterior mediastinal tumours: "an investigational algorithm." Can J Surg 1989;32:139-143.

Cohen AJ, Thompson L, Edwards FH, Bellamy RF: Primary cysts and tumors of the mediastinum. Ann Thorac Surg 1991;51:378-386.

Azarow KS, Pearl RH, Zurcher R, et al: Primary mediastinal masses. A comparison of adult and pediatric populations. J Thorac Cardiovasc Surg 1993;106:67-72.

Temes R, Chavez T, Mapel D, et al: Primary mediastinal malignancies: findings in 219 patients. West J Med 1999;170:161-166.

Hoerbelt R, Keunecke L, Grimm H, et al: The value of a noninvasive diagnostic approach to mediastinal masses. Ann Thorac Surg 2003;75:1086-1090.

ASSESSMENT OF THE PATIENT WITH A CHEST WALL MASS

Patients with chest wall masses present diagnostic problems that are often unique to that region of the body. Primary neoplasms, for instance, include a wide spectrum of tumors that may originate from soft tissues, cartilage, or bone. Such lesions can be asymptomatic or more commonly present as *painful masses*. In many cases, the pain was initially misinterpreted as being a nonspecific musculoskeletal complaint, only to be associated with a mass after months or even years of observation.

A multitude of nontumoral abnormalities can also mimic tumors of the chest wall both clinically and radiologically, and these must be included in the differential diagnosis. Among them are anatomic variants or *congenital deformities, sequelae of thoracic trauma,* and *soft tissue infections*.

In all cases of chest wall tumor, the assessment should be aimed at determining the *site, size, and histology of the tumor* as well as the degree of involvement of adjacent structures. It should also be aimed at planning adequate resection and establishing a reliable method for reconstruction.

CLASSIFICATION OF CHEST WALL MASSES

Neoplastic

Primary tumors of the chest wall are rare (Table 3-15) and can arise from any of the structures of the chest wall. They account for approximately 0.04% of all new tumors diagnosed annually in the United States. Fifty percent to 60% of these tumors are *malignant,* and these are almost always sarcomas. The average age at presentation for benign tumors (26 years) is approximately *15 years younger* than for their malignant counterparts (40 years). The male-to-female ratio is 2:1 except for desmoid tumors, for which there is a preponderance of females (1:2). Chest wall tumors affect the *ribs more than the sternum,* and they originate more often from the soft tissues (two thirds of cases) than from the bone or cartilage (one third of cases).

Primary Benign Tumors (Table 3-16)

Chondromas are the most common tumors of the chest wall. They usually arise in the region of the costochondral junction, anteriorly in young adults. The patient will often present with a painful mass that has been growing slowly for a period of years. On radiologic examination, the lesion may have a small lytic area in the rib associated with a sclerotic border. Typically, chondromas have calcifications that may be diffuse or focal with a stippled pattern. On *histologic evaluation,* there is mature hyaline cartilage with foci of myxoid degeneration and calcifications, and it is sometimes difficult to differentiate them from low-grade chondrosarcomas.

Osteochondromas, which typically occur in the first and second decades of life, originate from the bony cortex of a rib and are most often asymptomatic.

TABLE 3-15

GENERAL FEATURES OF PRIMARY CHEST WALL TUMORS

Incidence is low (0.04% of all new tumors diagnosed in the United States).

Fifty percent to 60% are malignant.

Age at presentation for benign tumors is 26 years.

Age at presentation for malignant tumors is 40 years.

Male-to-female ratio is 2:1 (except for desmoid tumors).

Ribs are affected more than sternum.

Tumors originate more often from soft tissues (two thirds) than from bone or cartilage (one third).

TABLE 3-16
COMMON PRIMARY BENIGN TUMORS OF THE CHEST WALL
Bone and cartilage
Chondromas, osteochondromas
Fibrous dysplasia
Osteoblastomas, giant cell tumors, aneurysmal bone cysts
Soft tissues
Desmoid tumors
Lipomas, fibromas, lymphangiomas, hemangiomas, neurofibromas

Patients with osteochondromatosis (multiple lesions) have a higher propensity for sarcomatous degeneration.

Fibrous dysplasia occurs in young adults and presents as a *painless chest wall mass*, most commonly over the posterior ribs. The lesion shows a central, fusiform, expanded mass radiologically with thinning of the cortex and *absence of calcifications*. On occasion, it is necessary to excise the lesion to differentiate it from a malignant tumor.

Desmoid tumors are rare tumors that some consider to be *low-grade fibrosarcomas*. They occur more commonly in women and have a high rate of local recurrences. On histologic evaluation, they contain sheets of fibroblasts with well-differentiated abundant collagen fibers.

Primary Malignant Tumors (Table 3-17)

Chondrosarcomas and osteogenic sarcomas are the most common primary malignant tumors arising in the chest wall.

The majority of chondrosarcomas arise in the anterior costochondral junction or sternochondral junction, and they usually present as slow-growing painful masses. Most are seen in the third or fourth decade of life. Conventional radiologic findings are those of a lobulated mass originating in the medullary portion of the rib or sternum, often with stippled calcification pattern and cortical bone destruction. CT scan may demonstrate involvement of adjacent structures (mediastinum, lung), which distinguishes it from benign chondromas. The natural history of these tumors is one of slow growth with frequent local recurrences.

TABLE 3-17
COMMON PRIMARY MALIGNANT TUMORS OF THE CHEST WALL
Bone and cartilage
Chondrosarcomas
Osteogenic sarcomas (osteosarcomas)
Ewing sarcomas, Askin tumors
Solitary plasmacytomas
Soft tissues
Soft tissue sarcomas, fibrosarcomas, rhabdomyosarcomas, synovial sarcomas, malignant fibrous histiocytomas

Osteogenic sarcomas are *rapidly growing tumors* that typically occur in teens and young adults. They appear radiologically as osteosclerotic or osteolytic masses with calcifications and new periosteum bone formation (sunburst appearance). These tumors have a much worse prognosis than chondrosarcomas.

Ewing sarcomas of the thorax are rare and mostly seen in *adolescent boys*. Most patients present with progressive chest wall pain with or without the presence of a mass. The typical radiographic picture is the onion-peel appearance produced by multiple layers of periosteal new bone formation. Ewing sarcomas are thought to be of *neural cell origin.* Another closely related and highly malignant lesion is the primitive neuroectodermal tumor described by Askin and colleagues. About half of patients with Ewing sarcomas or Askin tumors have metastatic disease at the time of their presentation.

Plasma cell myelomas occurring in the solitary form are not uncommon tumors, especially in older men. They usually present with pain or with a mass, and radiographically they project as *well-defined "punched-out" lytic lesions of the ribs*. The diagnosis of a solitary plasmacytoma should be made only if the results of all studies for multiple myeloma are negative.

Direct Extension from Lung or Breast Carcinomas

Involvement of soft tissues or bony structures of the chest wall by contiguous spread from lung cancer is common, but these patients usually *do not present with a chest wall mass*. The mode of presentation is often that of insidious chest pain in a patient who has a peripherally located neoplasm. On occasion, breast cancer recurring after mastectomy will have chest wall involvement and present with a chest wall mass.

Ribs and sternum are not uncommon sites of metastatic disease from a primary in other systems, but again, most of these patients do not present with chest wall masses.

Non-neoplastic (Table 3-18)

A variety of non-neoplastic disorders can mimic chest wall tumors and present with chest wall masses. These include *anatomic variants*, such as prominent xiphoids, and *congenital deformities* of the anterior chest wall, such as unilateral costochondral prominences. This latter deformity is usually seen in adolescent girls, and because of the superimposed breast, it can be difficult to differentiate from a true chest wall tumor. Traumatic *fractures of ribs or sternum* can also present with chest wall masses. This is the case, for instance, with sternal fractures where proximal and distal fragments overlap.

In developed countries, better control of tuberculosis with systemic antibiotics has virtually eliminated tuberculous cold abscesses of the chest wall. By contrast, these are not uncommon in underdeveloped countries where hygiene is poor and bacteria have become resistant. These cold abscesses present as fluctuating masses over the anterior chest wall with or without sinus track formation. CT typically shows obvious bone destruction and calcifications.

TABLE 3-18

NON-NEOPLASTIC CHEST WALL MASSES

Anatomic variants
    Hypertrophy of costal cartilages, prominence of xiphoid
Congenital anomalies
    Pectus carinatum
    Unilateral costochondral prominence
Trauma
    Fractures (rib, sternum) with exuberant callus
    Costochondral separation
Infectious lesions
    Tuberculosis (cold abscesses), actinomycosis, pyogenic osteomyelitis
Inflammatory lesions
    Nonspecific costochondritis (Tietze syndrome)
    Osteoarthritis

Tietze syndrome is characterized by tender swelling of one or more costal cartilages, usually the second or third.

DIAGNOSTIC MODALITIES IN THE INVESTIGATION OF PATIENTS WITH CHEST WALL MASSES

Noninvasive evaluation of patients with chest wall masses should include careful history, physical and laboratory examinations, and imaging through conventional chest radiography and CT scanning.

Clinical Features

Although history and physical examination are important, common clinical features such as *pain* and the presence of a *palpable mass* are often unreliable in distinguishing between benign and malignant tumors of the chest wall. The *age of the patient* at presentation, for instance, is not a useful criterion because the age ranges for patients with benign and malignant tumors overlap considerably. The same applies to the *duration of symptoms*.

In some instances, however, age is important. Plasmacytomas, for example, always occur in people who are older. Ewing sarcomas and Askin tumors are fast-growing tumors seen exclusively in young patients.

The clinical features that suggest that a tumor of the chest wall is or has become malignant are *recent rapid increase in size* and *invasion of adjacent organs*. Less common symptoms that may also suggest malignancy include weight loss, fever, and brachial plexus neuropathy.

On physical examination, the texture and mobility of the mass can provide clues to its diagnosis. A fluctuating mass with no evidence of cutaneous inflammation can be a cold abscess (tuberculosis), especially if it is localized over costal cartilages. A mobile lesion probably originates from the soft tissues; an immobile mass originates from the bony chest wall.

3

Specific Preoperative Assessment

Imaging

Conventional chest radiographs are still of value, especially if new and old radiographs can be compared to detect the *tumor growth rate*. They can also be useful in distinguishing neoplastic from non-neoplastic chest wall lesions.

CT and MRI have complementary roles in the evaluation of patients with chest wall masses. CT is useful to delineate the extent of bone, soft tissue, and mediastinal involvement, and this information is helpful to plan surgical resection. CT also readily shows small calcifications as well as areas of bone destruction. CT signs that suggest malignancy include *rapid increase in tumor size, cortical bone destruction,* and *involvement of surrounding structures*.

MRI is helpful in defining compression or invasion of major vascular structures. It is also the best imaging technique to demonstrate *invasion of the spine*.

Radiologic characteristics of the most common chest wall tumors are given in Table 3-19. Additional useful diagnostic techniques include *ultrasonography,* to document the tumor's relationship to the pleura and lung, and *bone scans,* which are not specific but may help identify other sites of disease or distant metastases.

Biopsy Techniques

A definitive diagnosis can be achieved only by histologic confirmation. Biopsy options include *fine-needle aspiration* (poor diagnostic yield),

TABLE 3-19
RADIOLOGIC CHARACTERISTICS OF MOST COMMON CHEST WALL TUMORS

	Age	Usual Site	Characteristics
BENIGN TUMORS			
Chondromas	10-30 yr	Anterior chest wall	Well-defined small, oval area of bone lysis Focal (stippled) calcifications
Fibrous dysplasia	Young adults	Posterior chest wall	Fusiform lytic lesion that erodes cortical bone
MALIGNANT TUMORS			
Chondrosarcomas	>40 yr	Anterior chest wall	Large, lobulated, destruction of cortical bone Mottled calcifications
Ewing sarcomas	<30 yr	—	Bone destruction and sclerosis Onion-peel appearance
Osteosarcoma	Teens and young adults	—	Sunburst pattern
Plasmacytoma	>60 yr	Upper ribs	Well-defined punched-out lytic lesion

core needle biopsy (diagnostic accuracy of more than 95%, and histologic grading is possible), *incisional biopsy* (excellent diagnostic yield), and *excisional biopsy* (definitive diagnosis). Evaluation of biopsy specimens with optical microscopy, electron microscopy, and immunohistochemical techniques including the use of monoclonal antibodies can usually provide a definitive diagnosis.

Excisional biopsy is appropriate for small lesions (<2 to 4 cm) or for lesions that are radiographically benign in appearance. *Less invasive biopsy procedures* are preferable for larger tumors or for tumors for which treatment is unlikely to be primarily surgical. These include Ewing sarcomas, plasmacytomas, metastasis to the chest wall from a primary elsewhere, and tumors likely to require major chest wall resection or multimodality therapies.

In some cases, an incisional biopsy is done under general anesthesia, and this can be converted to wide resection if necessary. One of the problems associated with this approach is that clinical decisions will occasionally be based on the wrong diagnosis. This applies to chondromas and chondrosarcomas, in which some tumor areas may appear to be histologically benign while frank malignancy is present in other areas. This may also apply to other types of sarcomas that have spindle-shaped appearances.

In general, the selection of a particular biopsy technique *must be individualized*. With few exceptions, tumor implantation at the site of biopsy and increased local recurrence rates have not been a problem.

Other Investigations

In malignant tumors, additional investigation must include appropriate testing for distant metastases. Pretreatment consultation with a medical oncologist is also appropriate, particularly for multimodality treatment of tumors such as Ewing sarcomas or solitary plasmacytomas.

If surgery is contemplated, chest wall reconstruction may warrant a consultation with the plastic surgeon. Similarly, a neurosurgical consultation may be required if the tumor encroaches the spine.

MODALITIES IN PREPARING THE PATIENT FOR CHEST WALL RESECTION

What Type of Resection Is Required?

Surgical treatment of benign tumors consists of resecting the involved structures with a *2-cm free margin of normal tissue*. The resulting defects are usually small and easily reconstructed without the use of prosthesis or muscle flaps.

When surgical resection of a primary malignant tumor is warranted, the resection should be wide and complete. In most institutions, this type of surgery involves a *4-cm or greater lateral margin* as well as the removal of one rib above and one below the tumor. Attached structures such as lung and pericardium should be resected in continuity.

3

The repair of these full-thickness chest wall defects often requires *skeletal reconstruction* to ensure chest wall stability as well as *re-creation of soft tissue coverage.* These must be planned before surgery, and indeed no chest wall resection should be undertaken without a plan for closure of the defect and at least one backup plan should the initial strategy not prove to be feasible.

Skeletal Reconstruction

Although skeletal reconstruction may not be necessary for small or posteriorly placed defects (under the scapula), patients generally do better after reconstruction if the defect is larger than two adjacent ribs or about 5 cm in diameter. The most commonly used prostheses are the Marlex mesh alone,[*] the composite Marlex mesh–methyl methacrylate "sandwich," the 2-mm-thick Gore-Tex (polytetrafluoroethylene) soft tissue patch,[†] and the Prolene mesh.[‡] The Marlex sandwich type of prosthesis is particularly useful because it *can be shaped according to the patient's anatomy,* and this may be more cosmetically acceptable. It is composed of two layers of Marlex mesh and the methyl methacrylate. A 1- to 2-cm cuff of Marlex is left around the methyl methacrylate to secure the sandwich to the adjacent ribs. Other advantages of the Marlex sandwich include *its light weight, versatility, radiolucency,* and *firm bonding to surrounding chest wall*. Reconstruction with autogenous tissue, such as fascia lata or bone grafts, is less satisfactory and requires experienced operators.

Soft Tissue Coverage

Soft tissue coverage can be attained with muscle flaps, pedicled myocutaneous flaps, and omental flaps. These flaps are used in association with a prosthesis, and they *are readily available to fill almost any size defect* in the chest wall.

Myocutaneous flaps are particularly useful because they offer large amounts of skin and soft tissues. These flaps have an axial blood supply that permits elevation and rotation for a significant distance with or without transposition of the overlying skin. Because of their thickness, myocutaneous flaps also provide *added chest wall stability* and have *a low incidence of complications*. The most commonly used muscle flaps are listed in Table 3-20.

In assessing the preoperative state of these flaps, one must be aware of any previous surgery that may have compromised the blood supply of the flap or of previous irradiation. This evaluation should be done by the plastic surgeon, who can best follow the basic principles of flap design and plan for a flap of choice to be used for the reconstruction.

---

[*]La Med Gmbh, D-82041, Deisenhofen, Germany.
[†]W. L. Gore and Associates, Inc., Elkton, Md.
[‡]Ethicon, Inc., Somerville, NJ.

TABLE 3-20		
CHOICES OF MUSCLE FLAPS FOR THORACIC RECONSTRUCTION		
Flap	Blood Supply	Uses
Pectoralis major	Dual: thoracoacromial vessels and internal mammary (perforators)	Mostly for sternal reconstruction
Latissimus dorsi	Predominantly from thoracodorsal artery	Full-thickness reconstruction of anterior lateral defects
Rectus abdominis	Dual: superior and inferior epigastrics	Across anterior chest wall
Omentum	Gastroepiploic arteries	Useful in exposed, contaminated, necrotic chest wall

3

CONCLUSION

Pathologic processes that involve the chest wall include a variety of congenital anomalies, inflammatory diseases, and neoplastic conditions. In this context, each patient warrants individual evaluation including careful imaging and selection of biopsy technique. Operative selections should be based primarily on tumor diagnosis as well as on technical feasibility of complete resection.

SUGGESTED READINGS

Review Articles

Chicarilli ZN, Ariyan S, Stahl RS: Costochondritis: pathogenesis, diagnosis, and management considerations. Plast Reconstr Surg 1986;77:50-59.

Anderson BO, Burt ME: Chest wall neoplasms and their management [current review]. Ann Thorac Surg 1994;58:1774-1781.

Shamberger RC, Grier WS: Chest wall tumors in infants and children. Semin Pediatr Surg 1994;3:267-276.

Faber LP, Somers J, Templeton AC: Chest wall tumors. Curr Probl Surg 1995;32:665-747.

Urschel JD, Takita H, Antkowiak JG: Necrotizing soft tissue infections of the chest wall. Ann Thorac Surg 1997;64:276-279.

Nesbitt JC: Primary tumors of the chest wall. Proceedings of the Refresher Course in Thoracic Surgery, Washington University, St. Louis, October 1998:2-5.

Somers J, Faber LP: Chondroma and chondrosarcoma. Semin Thorac Cardiovasc Surg 1999;11:270-277.

Allen MS, Miller DL, Deschamps C, et al: Chest wall tumors (key references). Ann Thorac Surg 1999;67:889-890.

Imaging

Saito T, Kobayashi H, Kitamura S: Ultrasonographic approach to diagnosing chest wall tumors. Chest 1988;94:1271-1275.

Specific Preoperative Assessment

Schaefer PS, Burton BS: Radiographic evaluation of chest-wall lesions. Surg Clin North Am 1989;69:911-945.

Sharif HS, Clark DC, Aabed MY, et al: MR imaging of thoracic and abdominal wall infections: comparison with other imaging procedures. AJR Am J Roentgenol 1990;154:989-995.

Swischuk LE, Stransberry SD: Radiographic manifestations of anomalies of the chest wall. Radiol Clin North Am 1991;29:271-278.

Kuhlman JE, Bouchardy L, Fishman EK, Zerbouni EA: CT and MR imaging evaluation of chest wall disorders. Radiographics 1994;14:571-595.

Fortier M, Mayo JR, Swensen SJ, et al: MR imaging of chest wall lesions. Radiographics 1994;14:597-606.

Jeung MY, Gangi A, Gasser B, et al: Imaging of chest wall disorders. Radiographics 1999;19:617-637.

Gladish GW, Sabloff BM, Munden RF, et al: Primary thoracic sarcomas. Radiographics 2002;22:621-637.

Case Series

Sabanathan S, Salama FD, Morgan WE, Harvey JA: Primary chest wall tumors. Ann Thorac Surg 1985;39:4-15.

King RM, Pairolero PC, Trastek VF, et al: Primary chest wall tumors: factors affecting survival. Ann Thorac Surg 1986;41:597-601.

Eng J, Sabanathan S, Pradhan GN, Mearns AJ: Primary bony chest wall tumors. J R Coll Surg Edinb 1990;35:44-47.

Burkhart HM, Deschamps C, Allen MS, et al: Surgical management of sternoclavicular joint infections. J Thorac Cardiovasc Surg 2003;125:945-949.

ASSESSMENT OF THE PATIENT WITH AN ELEVATED HEMIDIAPHRAGM

True eventration of the diaphragm is a *congenital condition* in which all or a portion of one hemidiaphragm is permanently elevated yet retains its continuity and normal attachments to the costal margin. It is differentiated from a diaphragmatic hernia by the *unbroken continuity* of the diaphragm.

By contrast, diaphragmatic paralysis is an *acquired condition* generally related to pathologic involvement of the phrenic nerve. Although different from true eventration, it often produces the same radiographic appearance and leads to the same physiologic disturbances.

TERMINOLOGY (TABLE 3-21)

True eventrations are developmental abnormalities characterized by *failure of proper muscularization of the diaphragm*. They can be partial or involve the entire central part of one or both hemidiaphragms. The eventrated diaphragm is thin with a membranous appearance, whereas the more peripheral portion is still muscular with normal bone attachments.

Acquired elevation of the diaphragm (often inappropriately termed eventration) can be associated with an intact or an abnormal phrenic nerve.

TABLE 3-21

CLASSIFICATION OF CAUSES OF ELEVATED DIAPHRAGM

True eventration
    Partial or total
Acquired elevation
    Intact phrenic nerve
    Abnormal phrenic nerve

If the phrenic nerve is involved and the diaphragm is paralyzed, the loss of contractility will progressively lead to muscular atrophy and distention of the dome.

The main differences between eventration and elevation of the diaphragm are given in Table 3-22.

Most cases of diaphragmatic elevation with an intact phrenic nerve are related to *mechanical factors* (Table 3-23), and the condition is reversible. A classic example is that of an elevated diaphragm associated with atelectasis and due to high negative pleural pressure. Another example is an elevated hemidiaphragm secondary to an intra-abdominal condition. The only situation in which diaphragmatic function may not return to

TABLE 3-22

DIFFERENCES BETWEEN CONGENITAL EVENTRATION AND ACQUIRED ELEVATION OF THE DIAPHRAGM

Feature	Eventration	Elevation
Incidence	Rare	Common
Etiology	Congenital	Acquired
Associated anomalies	Yes	No
Phrenic nerve	Intact	Often abnormal
Appearance of the diaphragm	Marked decrease in muscular fibers; membranous appearance	Atrophic but still muscular
Side predominance	Left	No predominance
Type	Total or partial	Always total
Sniff test	Weak motion	Paradoxic motion

TABLE 3-23

DIAPHRAGMATIC ELEVATION WITH INTACT PHRENIC NERVE

Intrapleural process
    Atelectasis, loss of volume of lung
    Postpneumonectomy
    Reflex diaphragmatic paralysis: empyema, postoperative
    Pulmonary fibrosis
    Restrictive pleural disease
Intra-abdominal process
    Any intra-abdominal collection or mass
    Reflex paralysis–subphrenic abscess
    Hepatomegaly, splenomegaly
Trauma to the diaphragm
Idiopathic

3

Specific Preoperative Assessment

TABLE 3-24
ETIOLOGY OF PHRENIC NERVE PALSY
CERVICAL
Birth injury
Blunt or penetrating trauma to spine or soft tissue
Operative injury
Neck surgery: thyroid, neck dissection, scalenotomy
Jugular vein cannulation
THORACIC
Trauma (rare)
Operative injury
Thymectomy, mediastinal tumor
Pulmonary resection
Cardiovascular operations
Coronary artery bypass grafting: pericardial traction, topical hypothermia, internal mammary artery harvest
Tumors
Lung cancer with N2 disease
Malignant mediastinal tumor, lymphoma
Infectious
Typhoid, measles, polio, herpes
Idiopathic

normal is in the case of blunt trauma where the muscle is torn but yet the pleuroperitoneal membrane is intact, preventing herniation.

Diaphragmatic elevation related to involvement of the phrenic nerve can be classified as post-traumatic, secondary to neuromuscular or infectious diseases, neoplastic, or idiopathic (Table 3-24). Injuries to the phrenic nerve can occur after any type of operation in the thorax or in the neck, but they are more commonly reported after *surgery for congenital cardiac anomalies*. Injury to the phrenic nerve can also occur with breech or difficult and prolonged deliveries. These injuries are usually the result of a pull on the C3-5 nerve roots. A number of neuromuscular or infectious disorders affecting the phrenic nerve (or diaphragm) can also be associated with an elevated diaphragm (Table 3-24).

INVESTIGATION OF THE PATIENT WITH AN ELEVATED HEMIDIAPHRAGM

Physiologic Consequences of Elevated Diaphragm

The most significant physiologic derangements associated with a high hemidiaphragm relate to the *respiratory system*. Patients are dyspneic, and one is usually able to demonstrate a restrictive pattern characterized by a reduction in lung volumes and mild hypoxemia. These changes will often be worse when measurements are obtained with the patient in the supine position. These findings are due to the inability of the paralyzed diaphragm to resist the push of abdominal contents into the chest on lying down.

Elevation of the diaphragm can also be the cause of *digestive symptoms* related to the rotation of the gastric fundus underneath the diaphragm.

Clinical Considerations

The symptoms associated with an elevated diaphragm are different if the problem occurs in children or in adults.

In children, the symptoms are *mostly respiratory*; the spectrum ranges from mild respiratory difficulties or cyanosis during feedings to frank respiratory failure necessitating intubation and mechanical ventilation. Often, difficulty in feeding, repeated bouts of pneumonitis, and dyspnea are the prominent symptoms. Interestingly, the clinical course of elevated diaphragm (eventration or phrenic nerve paralysis) in infants and children *does not always correlate* with involvement; patients are sometimes asymptomatic with large or complete eventration. Diminished breath sounds, contralateral shift, and depression of the abdomen on the involved side can be found on clinical examination.

The Hoover sign of accentuated outward excursion of the costal margin on inspiration is due to the failure of the diaphragmatic action to oppose that of the intercostals.

In the adult population, symptoms associated with an elevated diaphragm are *also predominantly respiratory*. Most patients complain of dyspnea, cough, and retrosternal pain. A variety of gastrointestinal symptoms can also be present. These include gas bloat, nausea and vomiting, heartburn, uncontrollable belching, and loud and abnormal noises originating from air moving along the gastrointestinal tract. These digestive symptoms are usually associated with left-sided elevated diaphragms.

Imaging

On chest radiographs, the superior margin of each hemidiaphragm forms a *dome-shaped interface* between lung and soft tissues of the abdomen. On the full-inspiration posteroanterior chest radiograph, the right hemidiaphragm is normally 1 to 2 cm higher than the left. It usually projects at about the level of the sixth rib anteriorly and tenth rib posteriorly. The left hemidiaphragm is positioned one rib interspace below (1 to 3 cm).

On fluoroscopy, the diaphragm moves down with inspiration and up with expiration, with an average excursion of 3 to 5 cm. These diaphragmatic movements can be observed only if there is spontaneous respiratory motion without mechanical ventilation. For most patients, this examination is done in the upright position; the patient is asked to perform deep inspiration and expiration, forced inspiration and expiration, and sniffing. A paralyzed hemidiaphragm will have a *paradoxical movement* (i.e., upward motion on inspiration). In infants and young children, the examination is best carried out while the patient is crying. As part of standard chest radiographs and fluoroscopic examination, the lungs and mediastinum should be examined for possible causes of phrenic nerve palsy.

On CT scan, the diaphragm is seen as a curved soft tissue density with fat below and aerated lung above. It is best depicted when it is separated from liver and spleen by lower attenuation fat. The direct multiplanar imaging capability of MRI technology can improve depiction of normal or abnormal diaphragm anatomy. These examinations can also help define *pulmonary, pleural, or mediastinal anomalies* not seen on chest radiographs.

Ultrasonography can be used to assess diaphragmatic motion and thickness. It can also be useful to differentiate between an eventration (thin but intact diaphragm) and a hernia. Finally, it can help identify the context of the eventration.

Imaging in Infants and Children with Elevated Diaphragm

The diagnosis of congenital diaphragmatic eventration is usually suggested on chest radiographs. The classic appearance of total eventration is that of an *elevated diaphragm* often associated with *loss of volume of the ipsilateral lung* and *displacement of the mediastinum* toward the contralateral side. On fluoroscopy, it results in smooth elevation of the hemidiaphragm with little or only slightly paradoxical movement during forced inspiration or crying. Focal areas of partial eventration appear as upward bulges in otherwise normally shaped diaphragms. On fluoroscopy, the partially eventrated diaphragm moves downward in synchronicity with the contralateral diaphragm. Differentiating a complete eventration from a paralyzed diaphragm may be difficult, although a paralyzed hemidiaphragm is likely to have paradoxical motion.

Imaging in Adults with Elevated Diaphragm

The diagnosis of acquired elevation can usually be made on a standard chest radiograph. The diaphragm is clearly elevated and forms a *round, unbroken line* arching from the mediastinum to the costal arch. The stomach is drawn up into the chest; it may be normally positioned with a high fundus, or it may be inverted with a partial or complete volvulus. Fluoroscopy is the simplest and most efficient and reliable means of assessing for diaphragmatic paralysis. The paralyzed hemidiaphragm paradoxically moves upward on inspiration and downward on expiration, passively following changes in intrapleural and intra-abdominal pressure. The *sniff test* is usually necessary to confirm that abnormal hemidiaphragm excursion is due to paralysis.

Electromyography and Phrenic Nerve Stimulation

Because of major complexities, diaphragm electromyography and phrenic nerve stimulation *have not found extensive clinical utility*. Electrical stimulation of the phrenic nerve is performed by needle electrodes positioned at the posterior border of the sternocleidomastoid muscle. The response to stimulation reflects nerve conduction velocity, and it is recorded by electrodes that can be implanted subcostally near the diaphragm or by surface electrodes placed between the seventh or eighth intercostal space. The response to nerve stimulation can also be recorded by fluoroscopic examination.

Diagnostic Pneumoperitoneum

Diagnostic pneumoperitoneum might be useful *to distinguish between an elevated diaphragm and frank herniation*, although in chronic hernias, adhesions may prevent air from reaching the pleural space. The technique involves the introduction of air into the peritoneal cavity followed by an upright chest radiograph to outline the diaphragmatic continuity.

Differentiating an Elevated Diaphragm from a Diaphragmatic Hernia

On occasion, it can be difficult to differentiate between an intact but elevated or eventrated diaphragm and a diaphragm with broken continuity and true herniation of abdominal contents in the pleural space. In newborns, Bochdalek hernia results from failure of the pleuroperitoneal membrane to close the pleuroperitoneal canal; visceral herniation involves the stomach, spleen, colon, or small bowel. Most are left sided, and they are seen on the chest radiograph as a soft tissue mass bulging upward through the posterior aspect of the diaphragm. There is contralateral shift of the mediastinum, and as air is swallowed, bowel loops in the chest become filled with gas. In adults, CT and MRI studies can demonstrate the diaphragmatic defect.

Diaphragmatic ruptures due to blunt trauma are usually associated with large defects that produce herniation of hollow viscera in the chest. The identification of a *nasogastric tube in the intrathoracic stomach* is a specific sign. In cases of late diagnosis or in right-sided ruptures, an apparent elevation of the diaphragm can be the only radiographic sign. In such cases, CT, spiral CT, and direct coronal or sagittal imaging with MRI may be indicated for definitive diagnosis. Diagnostic pneumoperitoneum can also be useful in such cases.

INVESTIGATION OF THE PATIENT BEING CONSIDERED FOR SURGERY

In all newborns or infants with severe respiratory difficulties, initial treatment must aim at supporting oxygenation and achieving gastric decompression. Once the patient is stabilized, the diagnosis is confirmed and surgical plication, often a lifesaving procedure, is carried out in a timely fashion. Before proceeding with operation, it is particularly important to ensure that the respiratory symptoms are *due to the eventration and not to associated cardiopulmonary malformations*. If the eventration is only partial, if the child is asymptomatic, or if he or she responds well to conservative management, most surgeons agree that operation can be delayed or even totally avoided. In infants with phrenic nerve paralysis secondary to difficult delivery or open heart surgery, aggressive treatment by plication of the diaphragm is recommended if the child is symptomatic or cannot be weaned off the respirator.

Most cases of eventration or phrenic nerve palsy diagnosed in the adult should be treated conservatively unless severe dyspnea interferes with normal activities or gastrointestinal symptoms are clearly related to the high position of the diaphragm. Indications for surgery are *uncommon*, and the

3

Specific Preoperative Assessment

clinician must be careful before recommending plication for respiratory or digestive symptoms thought to be related to elevation of the diaphragm. Typically, patients with respiratory symptoms due to the elevated diaphragm are moderately hypoxic; the total lung capacity, vital capacity, and expiratory reserve volume are lower than predicted with the patient seated, falling farther from predicted volumes with the patient in the supine position.

CONCLUSION

Eventration of the diaphragm denotes an abnormally high position of the diaphragm due to developmental malformation of diaphragmatic musculature; acquired elevation of the diaphragm is usually due to phrenic nerve paralysis. These are distinct entities, although the distinction is of little importance in the decision for surgical repair. The correct diagnosis can be made by standard chest radiography and fluoroscopy, which show *paradoxical movement* during forced inspiration. CT and MRI are useful to outline the contours of the diaphragm and to rule out a diaphragmatic hernia.

SUGGESTED READINGS

Review Articles

Christensen P: Eventration of the diaphragm. Thorax 1959;14:311-319.

McNamara JJ, Paulson DL, Urschel HC, Razzuk MA: Eventration of the diaphragm. Surgery 1968;64:1013-1021.

Thomas TV: Congenital eventration of the diaphragm [collective review]. Ann Thorac Surg 1970;10:180-192.

Panicek DM, Benson CB, Gottlieb RH, Heitzman ER: The diaphragm: anatomic, pathologic, and radiologic considerations. Radiographics 1988;8:385-425.

Imaging

Shackleton KL, Stewart ET, Taylor AJ: Traumatic diaphragmatic injuries: spectrum of radiographic findings. Radiographics 1988;18:49-59.

Tarver RD, Conces DJ, Cory DA, Vix VA: Imaging the diaphragm and its disorders. J Thorac Imaging 1989;4:1-18.

Brink JA, Heiken JP, Semenkovich J, et al: Abnormalities of the diaphragm and adjacent structures: findings on multiplanar spiral CT scans. AJR Am J Roentgenol 1994;163:307-310.

Houston JG, Fleet M, Cowan MD, McMillan NC: Comparison of ultrasound with fluoroscopy in the assessment of suspected hemidiaphragmatic movement abnormality. Clin Radiol 1995;50:95-98.

Israel RS, Mayberry JC, Primack SL: Diaphragmatic rupture: use of helical CT scanning with multiplanar reformations. AJR Am J Roentgenol 1996;167:1201-1203.

Gottesman E, McCool FD: Ultrasound evaluation of the paralyzed diaphragm. Am J Respir Crit Care Med 1997;155:1570-1574.

Gierada DS, Curtin JJ, Erickson SJ, et al: Fast gradient echo magnetic resonance imaging of the normal diaphragm. J Thorac Imaging 1997;12:70-74.

Gierada DS, Slone RM, Fleishman MJ: Imaging evaluation of the diaphragm. Chest Surg Clin North Am 1998;8:237-280.

Physiology

Clague HW, Hall DR: Effect of posture on lung volume: airway closure and gas exchange in hemidiaphragmatic paralysis. Thorax 1979;34: 523-526.

Pacia EB, Aldrich TK: Assessment of diaphragm function. Chest Surg Clin North Am 1998;8:225-237.

Surgery for Elevated Diaphragm

Wright CD, Williams JG, Ogilvie CM, Donnelly RJ: Results of diaphragmatic plication for unilateral diaphragmatic paralysis. J Thorac Cardiovasc Surg 1985;90:195-198.

Graham DR, Kaplan D, Evans CC, et al: Diaphragmatic plication for unilateral diaphragmatic paralysis: a 10-year experience. Ann Thorac Surg 1990; 49:248-252.

Ribet M, Linden JL: Plication of the diaphragm for unilateral eventration or paralysis. Eur J Cardiothorac Surg 1992;6:357-360.

Ciccolella DE, Daly BDT, Celli BR: Improved diaphragmatic function after surgical plication for unilateral diaphragmatic paralysis. Am Rev Respir Dis 1992;146:797-799.

Case Series

Piehler JM, Pairolero PC, Gracey DR, Bernatz PE: Unexplained diaphragmatic paralysis: a harbinger of malignant disease? J Thorac Cardiovasc Surg 1982;84:861-864.

Guth AA, Pachter HL, Kim U: Pitfalls in the diagnosis of blunt diaphragmatic injury. Am J Surg 1995;170:5-9.

ASSESSMENT OF THE PATIENT WITH POSSIBLE AIRWAY OBSTRUCTION

A number of diseases can cause obstruction of major airways. These include laryngeal abnormalities, benign or malignant tumors, benign strictures, and diseases causing extrinsic compression. Patients may be asymptomatic or may present with nonspecific symptoms such as cough or dyspnea. Often, they will have stridor or wheezing, and these symptoms may be interpreted as being due to asthma. The obstruction can be fixed or variable, and the symptoms can be experienced during inspiration, expiration, or both phases of the respiratory cycle. Symptoms can be present at rest or be felt only during exercise. The obstruction can affect the extrathoracic trachea or the intrathoracic trachea or main bronchi. Overall, this is a heterogeneous population of patients with wide variations in the etiology and severity of the underlying conditions.

Successful management depends on *careful assessment* of the clinical status of the patient; precise determination of the location, length, and extent of airway compromise; and determination of the pathologic condition causing the obstruction.

CAUSES OF AIRWAY OBSTRUCTION

Non-neoplastic Conditions (Table 3-25)

A variety of benign conditions can be associated with airway obstruction. This obstruction can be located at any level from the larynx and subglottis to the trachea or main bronchi.

Subglottic strictures are defined as a *narrowing of the airway immediately below the vocal cords*. These strictures are often the result of *cervical trauma* in which the patient sustains an injury to the anterior neck with fracture of the cricoid cartilage. Typically, these occur in motor vehicle accidents, where the hyperextended neck of the driver hits the steering wheel, or in motorcycle mishaps, where the driver hits an unseen rope or chain. If the initial impact is survived, the patient may present with symptoms and signs of acute airway obstruction, or a late subglottic stricture may develop. *Postintubation or post-tracheotomy injuries* are the

---

TABLE 3-25

NON-NEOPLASTIC CONDITIONS ASSOCIATED WITH AIRWAY OBSTRUCTION

Supraglottic or glottic lesions
Subglottic lesions
    Congenital
    Acquired
        External trauma
        Postintubation or post-tracheotomy
        Postoperative
        Systemic lesions
        Idiopathic
Tracheal lesions
    Congenital stenosis, webs; congenital vascular anomalies
    Acquired
        External trauma
        Postintubation or post-tracheotomy
        Postoperative
        Systemic lesions
        Postinfectious: tuberculosis, histoplasmosis
Bronchial lesions
    Post-traumatic
    Postoperative
    Postinfectious: tuberculosis, histoplasmosis
Foreign bodies
Tracheobronchomalacia

most common causes of subglottic strictures, however. Risk factors include large size of endotracheal tubes, prolonged duration of intubation, cuff pressure, and high location (near the cricoid cartilage) of the tracheotomy tube. The stenosis is the result of full-thickness fibrous scarring of the subglottic region. *Idiopathic subglottic strictures* usually occur in women younger than 40 years, and they can progress to severe airway obstruction.

Most tracheal stenoses are also the result of *prolonged endotracheal intubation*, or they occur as a *complication of tracheotomy*. They are characterized by chronic scarring of the trachea, which can occur at the site of the tracheotomy (stomal stricture) or at the site of the cuff of the endotracheal tube (cuff stricture). These patients will often have a combination of intrinsic scarring and tracheomalacia, both of which can create airway obstruction. Systemic lesions that may occasionally be associated with subglottic or tracheal obstruction include amyloidosis and *Wegener granulomatosis*. Endotracheal tuberculosis is uncommon, but it may produce narrowing of the airway, usually at several levels (tracheal and bronchial). Mediastinal fibrosis secondary to histoplasmosis is rare but, when present, often associated with diffuse tracheobronchial narrowing.

Most acquired benign obstructive lesions of main bronchi are secondary to *blunt chest trauma*. They usually occur within 2 cm of the carina, and 80% of them will affect the right main bronchus. When these injuries are not immediately recognized and treated, they will almost inevitably progress to a bronchial stenosis or complete obstruction. Nontraumatic bronchial inflammatory strictures are rare.

Foreign body inhalation is especially prevalent in young children, and pieces of toy or of any small object can be aspirated and produce airway obstruction. Foreign bodies can be located in the distal trachea or more commonly *in the right lung* (right main bronchus, bronchus intermedius, right lower lobe bronchus); their presence should be suspected in young children presenting with lobar pneumonia.

Tracheobronchomalacia is characterized by a weakening or destruction of the airway cartilage. Patients usually present clinically with symptoms of airway obstruction. It can be localized, such as in association with chronic extrinsic airway compression, or diffuse, as often seen in patients with severe end-stage emphysema (soft trachea).

Neoplastic Conditions (Table 3-26)

Respiratory obstruction may be the presenting sign of *airway neoplasms*. Although tracheal neoplasms are relatively rare, lung cancers originating in the upper lobes and infiltrating the main bronchi and carina or laryngeal carcinomas extending to the subglottic region are not uncommon.

Primary malignant neoplasms of the trachea are rare, accounting for less than 0.1% of all malignant neoplasms. Squamous cell carcinoma is the most frequent, and adenoid cystic carcinoma arising from mucous glands in the tracheal wall is next in frequency. Carcinoids are low-grade

---

TABLE 3-26

NEOPLASTIC CONDITIONS ASSOCIATED WITH AIRWAY OBSTRUCTION

Primary tumors of the airway
    Benign
        Carcinoids
        Adenomas
        Papillomas
        Schwannomas
    Malignant
        Squamous cell carcinomas
        Adenoid cystic carcinomas
        Mucoepidermoid carcinomas
        Lung cancer invading main bronchi and trachea
Metastatic endotracheal or endobronchial tumors
Tumors of the mediastinum invading or compressing the airway
    Mesenchymal tumors of anterior mediastinum
    Germ cell tumors
    Lymphomas
    Metastatic lung cancer to mediastinal nodes
Tumors of adjacent organs invading the airway
    Tumors of the thyroid
    Tumors of the esophagus

---

malignant neoplasms that arise in the central airways (including lobar bronchi) in approximately 80% of cases.

Malignant neoplasms of the mediastinum or those arising in the thyroid gland or esophagus can be responsible for airway obstruction either through *direct invasion of the subglottic region or trachea* or through *extrinsic compression*. Malignant tumors of the upper or middle third of the esophagus will often encase and invade the trachea. Hematogenous metastases to the endotracheal mucosa are exceedingly rare; the most common originate from breast carcinomas, melanomas, and genitourinary tract carcinomas.

INVESTIGATION OF THE PATIENT WITH POSSIBLE AIRWAY OBSTRUCTION

Clinical Considerations

The clinical presentation of patients with upper respiratory tract obstruction can be variable, but it is usually characterized by inspiratory dyspnea with stridor as the air flows through the restricted airway. Wheezing occurs when the airway diameter is *less than 8 mm*, and stridor occurs when the airway diameter is *less than 5 mm*.

Often, 50% of the tracheal lumen will be compromised without undue symptoms, particularly in sedentary patients. It is the next 20% narrowing that will produce the severe symptoms of dyspnea and an audible stridor that often gets *louder during exercise* because of the increased resistance to airflow. It is therefore reasonable to assume that a major obstruction of the airway has occurred when stridor is present. It is also reasonable to assume that relief of a small fraction of that obstruction may improve airflow enough to remove the urgency of the situation. In addition to the stridor, the increased effort necessary to pull the air in may cause indrawing of the suprasternal notch and intercostal spaces.

Other nonspecific symptoms of airway obstruction include cough, hoarseness, and hemoptysis. A *recent history of predisposing factors*, such as previous intubation, thoracotomy, or trauma, should also alert the physician to the possibility of airway obstruction.

Auscultation of the patient over the neck area may detect coarse low-pitched sounds of turbulence in the trachea. These sounds are different from the wheeze related to asthma or chronic obstructive pulmonary disease that is best heard over the lung fields and is predominant during the expiratory phase of inspiration. In spite of those differences, the clinical recognition of upper airway obstruction *can be difficult*, and the clinical features are often misinterpreted as being due to asthma, especially if the obstruction is intrathoracic and variable.

Noninvasive Testing
Imaging

Imaging of a known or suspected abnormality of central airways causing obstruction *should always be done before bronchoscopic examination* because modern imaging techniques can characterize the location and length of the stenotic segment, identify external compression causes, and qualify the degree of airway obstruction. All of this information allows safer bronchoscopic examination, tracheobronchial dilatation, or surgical intervention if necessary.

The usual initial radiologic examinations are standard chest radiographs. These are useful even if it is recognized that airway abnormalities *are often missed* because of the considerable overlap of the trachea and main bronchi with the spine and other mediastinal structures. Indeed, only two thirds of abnormalities involving the trachea and main bronchi can be detected on chest radiographs as opposed to CT scanning, which allows detection in approximately 95% of cases. Standard posteroanterior and lateral radiographs are nevertheless important to screen associated mediastinal, pulmonary, pleural, or cardiac abnormalities.

In the past, multidirectional planar tomography with or without contrast (air tomography) was the examination of choice, and it produced images of good spatial resolution. The technique had the advantage of *including the entire trachea and main bronchi in one image*. Unfortunately, this type of equipment and expertise are now found in a limited number of centers.

Conventional thin-section CT scanning is currently the imaging technique of choice to evaluate the airways. Several studies have documented its usefulness to depict both the morphology and anatomy of obstructing lesions of the tracheobronchial tree. Because the trachea

3

Specific Preoperative Assessment

lies perpendicular to the plane of the CT scan, it is readily studied by cross-sectional imaging. CT scan also provides *accurate localization of the site of obstruction* as well as determination of the intraluminal versus extraluminal component of the abnormality. This latter finding, not easily shown on planar tomography, may potentially be significant should the patient become a candidate for surgical resection. CT scan will also demonstrate if the narrowing is diffuse or if the abnormality is localized (stricture, neoplasm). Precise knowledge of these characteristics allows *safer bronchoscopic evaluation* and dilatation and better planning of surgical intervention.

More recently, the use of *helical CT with multiplanar reconstruction* has been described in the evaluation of central airways. This technique provides better anatomic details and on occasion will show lesions not evident or seen on conventional axial imaging. Perhaps more important, it may demonstrate with greater accuracy the site, length, and degree of severity of the obstruction (Fig. 3-6). Potential drawbacks of helical CT include the need for a longer breath-hold (15 to 45 seconds), increased complexity of data, and difficulties in correctly classifying the lesion into benign or malignant.

Although MRI can section and study the central airways in both coronal and sagittal planes, it does not provide more information than conventional or helical CT scanning does.

Flow-Volume Curves

Flow-volume curves provide a *graphic recording of maximum airflow* for the vital capacity during forced inspiration and expiration (Fig. 3-7A). They can be useful to detect even mild airway obstruction, and they can help differentiate between extrathoracic and intrathoracic obstruction.

Although this type of information is not helpful to categorize specific lesions, flow-volume curves are *easy to perform,* and to the trained eye, they allow immediate recognition of the severity and localization of the obstruction. They are very helpful in differentiating between a wheeze due to asthma or chronic bronchitis and stridor due to mechanical large airway obstruction.

If the obstruction is fixed, there is flow limitation during *both phases of respiration* as shown in Figure 3-7B. If the obstruction is extrathoracic and variable (Fig. 3-7C), the narrowing is worse during inspiration because intraluminal pressure is subatmospheric while extraluminal pressure is approximately atmospheric. During expiration, intraluminal pressure becomes positive relative to extraluminal pressure, which tends to dilate the airway and obscure the presence of the lesion.

The situation is reversed when the variable lesion is intrathoracic (Fig. 3-7D). During expiration, intraluminal pressure is less relative to extraluminal intrathoracic pressure, which tends to reduce the airway at the site of the lesion.

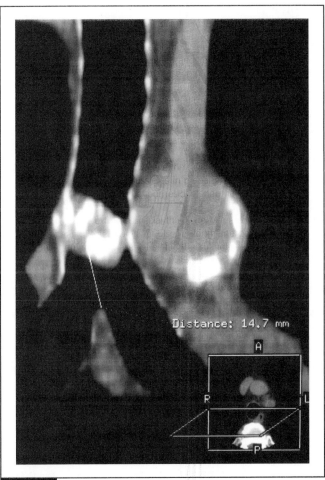

Distance: 14.7 mm

FIG. 3-6

Helical CT demonstrating an obstructive lesion of the distal trachea (1 cm above the carina). The tumor was a hamartoma.

Invasive Testing

Bronchoscopy provides *both assessment and therapy*. If the patient has severe airway obstruction, the examination should be performed in a controlled environment with all options available. It is thus reasonable to bring the patient to the operating room, and it is also advisable to have

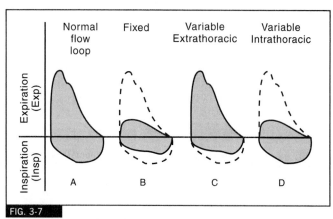

FIG. 3-7

Flow-volume curves to detect airway obstruction. **A,** Normal flow-volume curve.
B, Obstruction is fixed (equal flattening of maximal peak inspiratory and expiratory
flow rates) during both inspiration and expiration; it is unable to change cross-
sectional area in response to transmural pressure differences. **C,** Obstruction is
variable and extrathoracic (cervical trachea, larynx, supraglottic). The narrowing
is worse during inspiration, producing a typical flow-volume curve where airflow is
limited during inspiration. **D,** Obstruction is variable and intrathoracic. Because of
pressure differences between intraluminal and extraluminal pressure, the narrowing
is worse during expiration.

available a *flexible bronchoscope, a complete set of rigid bronchoscopes,*
and a *tracheostomy tray.*

The procedure is usually performed with the patient breathing
spontaneously. Sedation is extremely important and narcoleptic anesthesia
provides excellent support. Careful *local anesthesia* to the oropharynx and
larynx is accomplished by having the patient gargle with 4% aqueous
lidocaine (Xylocaine) before insertion of the bronchoscope or with
additional topical lidocaine spray. Lidocaine 2% is then injected through the
bronchoscope to anesthetize the larynx, vocal cords, and tracheobronchial
tree in progressive downward fashion. If sedation and topical anesthesia
have been appropriately used, the glottis should be readily visualized,
and the bronchoscope can be advanced through the vocal cords.

Flexible Bronchoscopy

If an obstruction is found, flexible bronchoscopy can be used to appreciate
the lesion in terms of its *location, macroscopic appearance,* and, most
important, *severity of the narrowing.* Secretions (or blood) can be aspirated,
and if the obstruction is not too severe or hemorrhagic, biopsy specimens
can be taken and the airways distal to the obstruction can be evaluated.
A *video of the procedure* is useful for further management discussion.

Rigid Bronchoscopy

If the obstruction is severe, it is best managed with the *rigid bronchoscope*. This is again done under local anesthesia, carefully explaining the procedure to the patient as you progress. Benign inflammatory strictures can almost always be dilated, and initial attempts should be made with the patient still breathing spontaneously. To do so, one has to insert the bevel of the bronchoscope into the stricture and, with pressure on the scope, *rotate or corkscrew the instrument through* it. It is important to have available rigid bronchoscopes of graded sizes 3.5 to 9 mm because a small pediatric rigid bronchoscope may be the only bronchoscope that can be inserted through very tight strictures. Should the obstruction encountered be neoplastic, the bronchoscopist must evaluate the vascularity of the tumor and the potential for significant bleeding should biopsy be performed; even minor hemorrhage in a compromised airway may lead to total obstruction or loss of visibility. A *useful means of appreciating the reversibility of the obstruction* is to pass a flexible bronchoscope down the rigid instrument to examine the length of the tumor and ensure the patency of the distal airway beyond the apparent obstruction.

In all of those cases, it is clear that prior imaging allows safer evaluation and avoidance of life-threatening airway obstructions. Indeed, prior knowledge of the pathologic process being examined is desirable so that one can be prepared for urgent surgical intervention, should it be required.

If bronchoscopy is done by medical doctors or if general anesthesia is required, the surgeon must be in attendance so that if sudden compromise of the airway occurs, rigid bronchoscopy can be carried out.

Once the exact nature of the obstruction is known, a decision about management can be made. At this point, general anesthesia may be used if the stricture has been dilated or if it has been decided that débridement of a tumor will be done either with laser or with biopsy forceps and rigid bronchoscope. The airway can also be stented if required.

CONCLUSION

Airway obstruction is a significant and challenging clinical problem for the thoracic surgeon. Its presentation varies from asymptomatic to life-threatening situation, depending on the severity of obstruction and cardiopulmonary reserve.

Basic principles of investigation include judicious use of modern imaging techniques allowing safe bronchoscopy, dilatation, or surgical intervention.

SUGGESTED READINGS

Review Articles

Miller RD, Hyatt RE: Obstructing lesions of the larynx and trachea: clinical and physiologic characteristics. Mayo Clin Proc 1969;44:145-161.

Courey MS: Airway obstruction. The problem and its causes. Otolaryngol Clin North Am 1995;28:673-684.

Evaluation

Shepard JAO, McLoud TC: Imaging the airways. Computed tomography and magnetic resonance imaging. Clin Chest Med 1991;12:151-168.

Kwong JS, Adler BD, Padley SPG, Müller NL: Diagnosis of diseases of the trachea and main bronchi: chest radiography vs. CT. AJR Am J Roentgenol 1993;161:519-522.

Quint LE, Whyte RI, Kazerooni EA, et al: Stenosis of the central airways: evaluation by using helical CT with multiplanar reconstructions. Radiology 1995;194:871-877.

Ferretti GR, Knoplioch J, Bricault I, et al: Central airway stenoses: preliminary results of spiral-CT–generated virtual bronchoscopy simulations in 29 patients. Eur Radiol 1997;7:854-859.

Burke AJ, Vining DJ, McGuirt WF, et al: Evaluation of airway obstruction using virtual endoscopy. Laryngoscope 2000;110:23-29.

Management

Lorch DG, Sahn SA: Post-extubation pulmonary edema following anesthesia induced by upper airway obstruction. Are certain patients at increased risk? Chest 1986;90:802-805.

DeLaurier GA, Hawkins ML, Treat RC, Mansberger AR: Acute airway management. Role of cricothyroidotomy. Am Surg 1990;56:12-15.

Mehta AC, Harris RJ, De Boer GE: Endoscopic management of benign airway stenosis. Clin Chest Med 1995;16:401-413.

Horak J, Weiss S: Managing the airway in the critically ill patient. Crit Care Clin 2000;16:1-15.

Case Series

Mathisen DJ, Grillo HC: Endoscopic relief of malignant airway obstruction. Ann Thorac Surg 1989;48:469-475.

Stephens KE, Wood DE: Bronchoscopic management of central airway obstruction. J Thorac Cardiovasc Surg 2000;119:289-296.

ASSESSMENT OF THE PATIENT WITH A PLEURAL DISORDER

Although pleural disorders are common in the practice of thoracic surgery, their assessment can be problematic. Pleural effusions, for instance, can be secondary to a variety of thoracic, abdominal, or systemic diseases. For those patients, clinical history, physical examination, and imaging of the pleural space represent first-line investigation. If required, more invasive techniques, such as thoracentesis or percutaneous pleural biopsies, can be used and a diagnosis be firmly established in 80% of cases. Recent advances in thoracoscopy (VATS) have further improved the diagnostic accuracy of investigational procedures.

ANATOMY OF THE PLEURAL SPACE

The pleura is made of two serosal membranes, one covering the lung (the visceral pleura) and one covering the inner chest wall and mediastinum (the parietal pleura). The transition between parietal and visceral pleura *is at the hilum;* the reflection covers all constituents of the hilum except inferiorly, where the reflection extends down to the diaphragm (inferior pulmonary ligament).

The visceral pleura *covers the surface of the lung and extends into the fissures*. It is thin, transparent, and tightly adherent to the underlying lung. The parietal pleura can be divided into costal, mediastinal, and diaphragmatic pleura. At the level of the thoracic wall, it is attached to the bony chest wall by a fibrous layer known as the endothoracic fascia. This fascia is a cleavage layer within which the parietal pleura can be separated from the chest wall. The transition between each segment of the parietal pleural is at the level of *the pleural sinuses* (Table 3-27).

The blood supply of the parietal pleura comes exclusively from systemic arteries (intercostals, internal mammary, bronchial, subclavian); for the most part, venous blood drains into the venae cavae through intercostal veins. The visceral pleura is vascularized by both the systemic (bronchial arteries) and the pulmonary circulation.

The visceral pleura is devoid of somatic innervation. The parietal pleura is innervated through a rich network of somatic, sympathetic, and parasympathetic fibers. At the level of the costal pleura, these fibers travel through intercostal nerves; stimuli of the diaphragmatic pleura are transmitted through the phrenic nerve.

PHYSIOLOGY OF THE PLEURAL SPACE

Pleural Pressure

The pleural pressure is proportional to the pressure developed within the lung. When the lung volume is at its functional residual capacity (end-expiration), the elastic forces of the lung and thorax are in equilibrium, and the pleural pressure equals -2 to -5 cm H_2O. In any condition in which the elastic recoil of the lung is increased (e.g., interstitial fibrosis, atelectasis), the pleural pressure becomes *more subatmospheric*. The pleural pressure is not uniform around the surface of the lung, being more negative at the apex (-7 to -9 cm H_2O) than at the base (0 to -2 cm H_2O).

Pleural Fluid

Pleural fluid is *constantly secreted*, mostly by filtration from the microvessels in the parietal pleura. The composition of the normal pleural

TABLE 3-27
PLEURAL SINUSES
Costomediastinal sinuses: anterior, posterior
Costophrenic sinus
Mediastinophrenic sinus

TABLE 3-28

COMPOSITION OF NORMAL PLEURAL FLUID

Volume: 0.1-0.2 mL/kg
Protein: 10-20 g/L
Albumin: 50% to 70%
Glucose: as in plasma
Lactate dehydrogenase: <50% of plasma level
Cells/mm³: 4500
    Mesothelial cells: 3%
    Monocytes: 54%
    Lymphocytes: 10%
    Granulocytes: 4%
    Unclassified: 29%
pH: 7.38 (mixed venous blood + 0.02)
Partial pressure of carbon dioxide: 45 mm Hg (= mixed venous blood)
Bicarbonate: 25 mmol/L (= mixed venous blood)

fluid is shown in Table 3-28. The mechanisms of pleural fluid exchanges (formation and reabsorption) have traditionally been explained by the *balance of hydrostatic and osmotic pressures* (Fig. 3-8). The flow of fluid depends on the permeability coefficient of the pleura, difference of hydrostatic pressures, and difference of osmotic pressures across the pleura. Studies in large mammals have recently shown, however, that resorption of pleural fluid may be *through lymphatic stomata* in the parietal pleura rather than through the visceral pleura.

ASSESSMENT OF THE PATIENT WITH A PNEUMOTHORAX

Terminology

Pneumothorax is a condition characterized by the *presence of air in the pleural space*. It is generally classified as being spontaneous, post-traumatic, or iatrogenic (Table 3-29). Whereas primary spontaneous pneumothoraces occur in young people without lung disease, secondary spontaneous pneumothoraces occur in patients with clinical or radiologic evidence of underlying lung disease, most often chronic obstructive pulmonary disease (Table 3-30).

Assessment and Diagnosis

Primary Spontaneous Pneumothorax

Almost all patients present with sudden onset of sharp chest pain, and about 60% will also be dyspneic (Table 3-31). The symptoms usually *correlate* with the degree of lung collapse. The diagnosis is best confirmed by erect chest radiograph, although *expiratory films* may on occasion be useful to demonstrate a small pneumothorax that may have been missed on a standard film. Quantification of the size of a pneumothorax may be useful for making a therapeutic decision. Unfortunately, the methods used for this quantification vary greatly and lack standardization (Fig. 3-9). CT scanning can better estimate the size of the pneumothorax as well as delineate the distribution of bullae and blebs.

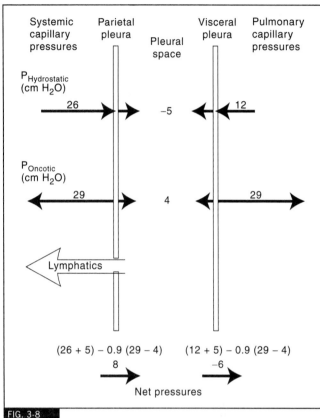

FIG. 3-8

Mechanisms of pleural fluid transportation across the pleural space. The arrows indicate the direction of the flow. The balance of pressures (Starling equation) favors the filtration of fluid through the pleural space, from the parietal pleura to the visceral pleura, where it is reabsorbed.

Secondary Spontaneous Pneumothorax

Most patients with secondary pneumothoraces are male, are older than 45 years, and have documented or clinically apparent pulmonary disease (Table 3-30). Clinically, nearly all patients will present with *acute shortness of breath,* often associated with hypoxia, hypercapnia, and acidosis. Because of their limited pulmonary reserve, these patients often show little tolerance to even a small pneumothorax.

TABLE 3-29

CLASSIFICATION OF PNEUMOTHORAX

SPONTANEOUS

Primary (healthy individuals and normal lung)
Secondary (underlying pulmonary disease)
    Chronic obstructive pulmonary disease
    Infection
    Neoplasm
    Catamenial
    Miscellaneous

TRAUMATIC

Blunt chest trauma
Penetrating chest trauma

IATROGENIC

Diagnostic
Inadvertent

The correct diagnosis is made by chest radiograph, which on occasion will be difficult to interpret because of the increased radiolucency of the diseased lung. In those cases, CT scan may be helpful to confirm the diagnosis and sometimes to distinguish between a large bulla and a pneumothorax.

TABLE 3-30

POSSIBLE CAUSES OF SECONDARY SPONTANEOUS PNEUMOTHORAX

Airway and pulmonary disease
    Chronic obstructive pulmonary disease
    Asthma
    Cystic fibrosis
Interstitial lung disease
    Pulmonary fibrosis
    Sarcoidosis
Infectious disease
    Tuberculosis and other mycobacterial infections
    Bacterial infections
    Pneumocystis carinii infections
    Parasitic infections
    Mycotic infections
    AIDS
Neoplastic
    Bronchogenic carcinoma
    Metastatic (lymphoma, sarcoma)
Catamenial (endometriosis)
Miscellaneous
    Marfan syndrome
    Ehlers-Danlos syndrome
    Histiocytosis X
    Scleroderma
    Lymphangiomyomatosis
    Collagen diseases

TABLE 3-31		
MAIN DIFFERENCES BETWEEN PRIMARY AND SECONDARY SPONTANEOUS PNEUMOTHORACES		
	Primary	Secondary
Age	<30 yr	>45 yr
Sex	Predominantly male	Predominantly male
Underlying disease (clinical, radiologic)	No	Yes
Body type	Tall and healthy young man	—
Symptoms	Dominated by pain	Dominated by shortness of breath
Histopathology	Apical blebs	Diffuse lung disease
Chances of recurrence	10%-15%	>50%

Pneumothorax and Acquired Immunodeficiency Syndrome

Several reports have now described the association of spontaneous pneumothorax, pneumomediastinum, and acquired immunodeficiency syndrome (AIDS). In those patients, the high incidence of pneumothoraces is the result of *cystic lesions that are most common at lung apices*. These lesions consist of subpleural air spaces filled with eosinophilic exudate, *Pneumocystis carinii* organisms, fibrous material, and macrophages.

Catamenial Pneumothorax

Pneumothoraces occurring *within 48 to 72 hours of the onset of menstruation* are called catamenial pneumothoraces. Most occur on the right side, and they may be recurrent for several years before being diagnosed. They are usually small, and patients present with chest pain and dyspnea.

The pathogenesis of catamenial pneumothorax in unclear, although it is likely that air reaches the pleural space through congenital diaphragmatic defects. It is also possible that there are focal endometrial implants on the visceral pleura or in the lung, with air leakage occurring during menstruation.

ASSESSMENT OF THE PATIENT WITH A PLEURAL EFFUSION

Pathophysiology of Pleural Effusions

Pleural effusions develop because of a *disturbance* in the mechanisms that normally move 5 to 10 L of fluid across the pleural space every day. Increased capillary permeability (inflammation, tumor implants), increased hydrostatic pressure (heart failure), reduced oncotic pressure (hypoalbuminemia), increased negative intrapleural pressure (atelectasis), and decreased lymphatic drainage (lymphatic obstruction by tumor or radiation-induced fibrosis) can all cause a pleural effusion (Tables 3-32 and 3-33).

Assessment and Diagnosis

The typical symptoms associated with pleural effusion are *dyspnea*, cough, and chest discomfort. Physical findings include decreased breath sounds and dullness to percussion.

3

Specific Preoperative Assessment

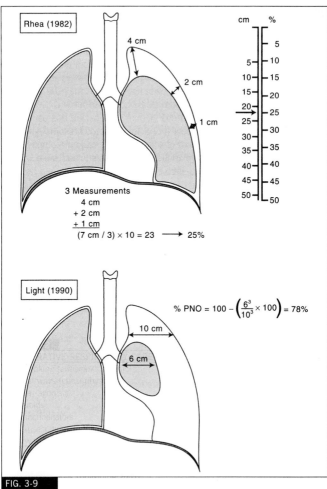

FIG. 3-9

Quantification of the size of a pneumothorax. With the method described by Rhea et al, one must first find the average interpleural distance at the apex and at the midpoints of both upper and lower lungs. The average interpleural distance is then calculated and the number reported on a nomogram, which gives an estimate of the size of the pneumothorax (PNO). *(From Rhea JT, DeLuca SA, Greene RE: Determining the size of pneumothorax in the upright patient. Radiology 1982;144:733-736.)* Another method is that described by Light, in which the amount of collapse can be estimated by measuring an average diameter of the lung and the thorax, cubing these two diameters, and finding the ratios between them. *(From Light RW: Management of spontaneous pneumothorax. Am Rev Respir Dis 1993;148:245-248.)*

TABLE 3-32

HOW DOES THE EXIT OF PLEURAL FLUID EXCEED ITS RATE OF ENTRY?

Increased vascular hydrostatic pressure (usually pulmonary venous pressure)

Reduced vascular oncotic pressure due to hypoalbuminemia

Increased microvascular permeability due to inflammation

Impaired lymphatic drainage due to malignant lymphatic infiltration or
  interruption of the thoracic duct

More negative pressure in the pleural space due to atelectasis of the adjacent lung

Transdiaphragmatic passage of fluid from the peritoneal cavity

From Sahn SA: State of the art. The pleura. Am Rev Respir Dis 1988;138:184-234.

Conventional imaging is the mainstay of the evaluation of these patients. Small effusions cause *blunting of the costophrenic angle* (200 to 500 mL required); larger effusions produce the classic *meniscus sign*. Massive effusions cause a complete opacification of the hemithorax. Loculated effusions may be difficult to diagnose on standard radiographs because they present as densities that can be difficult to distinguish from a pulmonary parenchymal process. A lateral decubitus view may be useful to determine if the fluid is mobile. *Subpulmonic effusion* refers to an accumulation of pleural fluid between the diaphragm and the lung. An upright radiograph will show an apparent elevation of the diaphragm.

CT scanning facilitates detection of small amounts of pleural fluid; it is also helpful to detect loculated collections or to distinguish pleural lesions

---

TABLE 3-33

INTERACTION AMONG PATHOGENETIC MECHANISMS AND CONTRIBUTING FACTORS FAVORING THE ACCUMULATION OF PLEURAL FLUID IN PATIENTS WITH CANCER

Pathogenetic Mechanisms	Impaired Lymphatic Drainage	Increased Pleural Osmotic Pressure	Increased Capillary Permeability	Increased Venous Pressure
Pleural implants	+	+	+	−
Lymphatic metastases				
Mediastinal nodes	+	+	−	−
Lymphangitis	+	+	−	−
Tumor cell suspension	+	+	+	−
Contributing syndromes				
Superior vena cava	+	+	−	+
Congestive heart failure	+	+	−	+
Pericardial effusion	+	+	−	−
Infection	+	+	+	−
Mediastinal irradiation	+	+	−	−
Hypoalbuminemia	−	+	−	−

+, contributes; −, does not contribute.

From Roth JA, Ruckdeschel JC, Weisenberger TH, eds: Thoracic Oncology. Philadelphia, WB Saunders, 1989:596; and Harper GR: Pleural effusion in cancer. Clin Cancer Briefs 1979;1:1.

TABLE 3-34

MOST COMMON CAUSES OF PLEURAL EFFUSIONS

TRANSUDATES

Congestive heart failure, myxedema

Cirrhosis

Nephrotic syndrome, glomerulonephritis, peritoneal dialysis

Pulmonary emboli, sarcoidosis

EXUDATES

Neoplastic: primary or secondary

Infection: bacterial (parapneumonic effusion), tuberculosis, viral, fungal (rare)

Gastrointestinal: pancreatitis, subphrenic abscess, esophageal rupture

Collagen diseases: rheumatoid, systemic lupus erythematosus, Sjögren, Wegener

Miscellaneous: trauma, radiation injury, postoperative, drugs

from parenchymal processes. Ultrasonography is complementary to CT in detecting small amounts of pleural fluid (it can detect 3 to 5 mL). It is also useful to *characterize* the effusion. Indeed, the demonstration of septa may indicate an infectious cause. MRI is of little clinical relevance at present.

As described by Valerie W. Rusch, the *clinical setting* in which an effusion occurs is important and often influences the approach to diagnosis. A patient who develops a small effusion in conjunction with pneumonia is likely to have a parapneumonic effusion. The same is true of a patient with known congestive heart failure who develops a right-sided effusion. In contrast, a woman who develops a new pleural effusion after having been treated for breast cancer is likely to have metastatic pleuritis.

Knowledge of the most common causes of pleural effusion is helpful in defining its cause (Table 3-34). The four most common causes of pleural effusions in North America are *congestive heart failure, bacterial pneumonia, malignant neoplasm,* and *pulmonary emboli*. The most common causes of malignant pleural effusions are lung cancer, breast cancer, and lymphoma.

Biopsy Procedures

If the diagnosis is not clinically obvious, thoracentesis (Table 3-35) should be performed under ultrasound guidance. It is diagnostic in 50% to 60% of cases, and higher yields can be obtained for diseases such as empyemas

TABLE 3-35

ANALYSIS OF PLEURAL FLUID OBTAINED BY THORACENTESIS

Character of fluid: bloody, turbid, purulent, milky

Cytologic examination

Cell count (white blood cells)

Culture and sensitivity

Biochemistry

    pH, glucose, protein, lactate dehydrogenase

    Amylase (elevated in pancreatitis, esophageal perforation)

    Triglyceride (elevated [>110 mg/dL]) in chylothorax

TABLE 3-36	
EXAMINATION OF PLEURAL FLUID	
Color of Fluid	Suggested Diagnosis
Red (bloody)	Malignant neoplasm, pulmonary embolism, trauma, tuberculosis, ruptured aneurysm
Yellow (straw color)	Not diagnostic
Yellow (greenish color)	Rheumatoid
White (milky)	Chylothorax
Brown (chocolate sauce)	Anaerobic liver abscess
Black	*Aspergillus*
Character of fluid	
Viscous	Malignant mesothelioma (hyaluronic acid) or long-standing pyothorax
Pus	Empyema
Turbid	Many leukocytes or lipid effusion
Debris	Rheumatoid

From Al-Jahdali H, Menzies RI: How to diagnose pleural effusions. Can J Diagn 1996;13:105-113.

(turbid or purulent fluid), hemothoraces (bloody fluid), and chylothoraces (clear milky fluid) (Table 3-36). The pleural fluid (approximately 50 mL in routine cases) should be sent for cytologic examination, culture, and cell count. Approximately *60% to 80% of patients with metastatic pleuritis* will have positive cytology.

Simultaneous pleural fluid and serum glucose, protein, and lactate dehydrogenase (LDH) levels should be obtained. Normal pleural fluid is clear; it has low protein concentration (1.0 to 1.5 g/dL), fewer than 1500 nucleated cells/mm³, glucose and LDH concentrations equal to those of serum, and pH higher than 7.62. Effusions are classified as exudates or transudates on the basis of the protein and LDH levels. An effusion is considered an *exudate* if the pleural fluid–to–serum ratio is greater than 0.5 for protein and greater than 0.6 for LDH. The pleural fluid concentration of glucose is also helpful because a level below 60 mg/dL (or less than 50% of serum glucose concentration) is seen only in malignant or tuberculous effusions, parapneumonic effusions, and effusions associated with rheumatoid arthritis. Several authors have also reported that a pH of less than 7.00 in conjunction with a glucose level below 60 mg/dL is indicative that a parapneumonic effusion is likely to progress to frank empyema.

Patients whose effusions remain undiagnosed after a thoracentesis may have a percutaneous needle biopsy. Unfortunately, percutaneous pleural biopsy has a *low yield in malignant neoplasia* because of the patchy distribution of disease.

If the cause of the effusion is still unclear after thoracentesis and needle biopsy, the patient should undergo a bronchoscopy and *videothoracoscopy* (Table 3-37). Bronchoscopy is useful to diagnose endobronchial tumors

TABLE 3-37

INDICATIONS FOR DIAGNOSTIC THORACOSCOPY IN PLEURAL DISORDERS

Unexplained pleural effusion
Biopsy of a pleural mass
Thoracic malignant neoplasm and associated pleural effusion
Mesothelioma
    Diagnosis
    Need for additional biopsy specimens to confirm the diagnosis
    Enlarged mediastinal nodes
    Confirm the T status of the tumor
Other metastatic effusions or lesions
    Need for additional biopsy specimens for pathologic studies
Unexplained pericardial effusion
Pneumothorax
    To evaluate at first occurrence
Traumatic hemothorax
Evacuation of intrapleural foreign body

that may be responsible for the effusion; thoracoscopy allows direct access to 90% to 100% of the surfaces of both the visceral and parietal pleura. Often, the examination will clarify whether the effusion is due to a malignant process, and a pleurodesis can also be done should it be necessary. Several large series report a diagnostic accuracy of 90% to 100% for thoracoscopy, depending on the reasons for which thoracoscopy was performed. In experienced hands, *diagnostic thoracoscopy*, particularly when it is limited to inspection and biopsy, is *a safe procedure* with few complications (Table 3-38).

With the development of thoracoscopy techniques, few circumstances occur in which open thoracotomy is necessary. It may be indicated when the pleural space is obliterated or when one wishes to proceed immediately with a surgical procedure, such as decortication or pulmonary resection.

ASSESSMENT OF THE PATIENT WITH POSSIBLE EMPYEMA

Terminology

The American Thoracic Society divides the evolution of an empyema into three distinct stages *indicative of disease progression* in the pleural space (Table 3-39). During the *exudative phase (stage I),* the pleural membranes

TABLE 3-38

POSSIBLE COMPLICATIONS ASSOCIATED WITH DIAGNOSTIC THORACOSCOPY

Prolonged air leak
Subcutaneous emphysema
Bleeding (entry site, adhesions, biopsy site)
Inadequate lung re-expansion
Empyema
Arrhythmias
Entry-track implant or metastasis

TABLE 3-39		
PATHOLOGIC FINDINGS OF EMPYEMA		
Stage	Phase	Characteristics
Stage I	Exudative (acute phase)	Swelling of pleura
		Pleural fluid with low viscosity and cellular contents
Stage II	Fibrinopurulent (transitional phase)	Heavy fibrin deposits with turbid or purulent fluid
Stage III	Organizing (chronic phase)	Ingrowth of fibroblasts and capillaries with lung trapping by collagen

swell considerably and discharge a thin exudative fluid. Fibrin is deposited over all pleural surfaces, but the peel is not thickened enough to prevent complete lung re-expansion. During the *fibrinopurulent phase (stage II),* there are heavy fibrin deposits over all pleural surfaces, and the pleural fluid is turbid or frankly purulent. Loculations form during that stage. Within 3 to 4 weeks, *organization (stage III)* begins with massive ingrowth of fibroblasts and formation of collagen fibers over both parietal and visceral surfaces. The pus is thick, and the lung that is imprisoned within a thick peel can no longer re-expand. Although complications can occur at any time during the formation of an empyema, they are *more likely* to develop during the chronic stage of disease (Table 3-40).

Patients with bacterial pneumonia may have an associated pleural effusion, which is called a *parapneumonic or a postpneumonia effusion.* Uncomplicated effusions are nonpurulent, have a negative Gram stain result and culture, and do not loculate in the pleural space. They resolve spontaneously with antibiotic treatment of the underlying pneumonia. Complicated effusions are either empyemas or loculated parapneumonic effusions that *require surgical drainage* for adequate resolution.

Assessment and Diagnosis

An empyema should be suspected in patients with acute respiratory illnesses and associated pleural effusion. Typical symptoms such as pleuritic chest pain, high fever, cough, tachypnea, tachycardia, toxicity, and local tenderness are often present. These symptoms can occur acutely

TABLE 3-40
COMPLICATIONS OF EMPYEMA
Pulmonary fibrosis
Contraction of the chest wall
Empyema necessitatis: spontaneous drainage through the skin
Bronchopleural fistula: spontaneous drainage through the bronchus
Osteomyelitis (rib, spine)
Pericarditis
Mediastinal abscess
Subphrenic abscess

or develop insidiously during a period of a few days or even weeks. Physical examination nearly always shows diminished mobility of the involved hemithorax, decreased breath sounds, and dullness to percussion.

Chest radiographs show a pleural effusion with or without underlying pneumonia or lung abscess. On lateral radiographs, the empyemas are *nearly always posterior,* and most extend to the diaphragm. The classic image is that of a posteriorly located, inverted D–shaped density (pregnant lady sign) as seen in the lateral chest film. Decubitus views are useful to determine if the collection is free flowing (stage I) or loculated (stage II). CT scan is useful to ascertain the underlying lung as well as to stage the empyema as determined by the presence of loculations, thickness of the pleura, and presence or absence of a trapped lung. In recent years, *ultrasonography* has become the *best imaging technique* to document the presence of fluid, to demonstrate loculations, and to guide thoracentesis.

Once the presence of fluid has been confirmed, diagnostic thoracentesis should be done; the aspirate should be sent for cytologic study, biochemical analysis, Gram stain, and aerobic and anaerobic studies (Table 3-41). The gross appearance and odor of pleural fluid are among the most significant items of information obtainable by thoracentesis. Thin fluid, even with positive bacteriologic findings, may respond to selective antibiotherapy and thoracentesis; thick pus requires formal surgical drainage. Anaerobic pus is usually foul; aerobic pus has no offensive odor.

The relevance of pleural fluid biochemistry to diagnosis of empyema is controversial. Most authors believe that pleural effusions with low fluid pH (<7.0), low glucose concentration (<50 mg/dL), and high LDH contents (>1000 U/L) should be drained because these parameters indicate a *complicated effusion or impending empyema.*

During the investigation of patients with empyema, one should also look for the causative process, such as decayed teeth or endobronchial obstructive processes.

TABLE 3-41

ANALYSIS OF PLEURAL EFFUSIONS AND EMPYEMA

Specimen	Simple Parapneumonic Effusion	Complicated Parapneumonic Effusion	Empyema
Pleura	Thin, leaky	Fibrin deposition, loculi	Thick granulation tissue
Fluid appearance	Clear	Opalescent	Pus
White blood cell count	PMN +	PMN ++	PMN ++
Bacteria	–/sterile	±/–	+/+
pH	>7.3	<7.1	<7.1
Lactate dehydrogenase (U/L)	<500	>1000	>1000
Glucose (mg/dL)	>60	<40	<40
Fluid/serum glucose	>0.5	<0.5	<0.5

PMN, polymorphonuclear cells; +, positive; ++, more positive; –, negative.
From Muers MF: Streptokinase for empyema. Lancet 1997;349:1491.

ASSESSMENT OF THE PATIENT WITH A POSSIBLE CHYLOTHORAX

Clinical Features and Imaging

Initially, the clinical manifestations of a chylothorax are the result of *mechanical compression* of the mediastinum (superior vena cava, inferior vena cava, heart) and ipsilateral lung causing dyspnea, fatigue, and heaviness. If there is rapid accumulation of lymph, the patient may become tachypneic, tachycardic, and hypotensive, and frank cardiovascular instability can occur if fluids are not replaced. After a few days, the patient will start to lose weight (protein), fat-soluble vitamins, and antibodies, making the patient more susceptible to infection.

Unfortunately, there is *no valid radiologic finding* that allows one to differentiate between a chylothorax and pleural effusions due to other causes. Bipedal lymphangiograms and radionuclide imaging with technetium Tc 99m antimony sulfide colloid can demonstrate obstruction to lymph flow, but they are limited in localizing the site of chyle leakage.

Fluid Analysis

Chylothorax is suggested by the presence of *nonclotting milky fluid* obtained from the pleural space at thoracentesis. The characteristics of chyle are listed in Table 3-42. The diagnosis is confirmed by finding free microscopic fat, a fat content that is higher than that of plasma, and a protein content that is less than half the plasma level. The fat globules

TABLE 3-42

NORMAL CHARACTERISTICS AND COMPOSITION OF CHYLE

CHARACTERISTICS

Milky appearance with a creamy layer that clears when fat is extracted
    by alkali or ether
pH: 7.4-7.8 (alkaline)
Odorless
Specific gravity: 1.012-1.015
Sterile and bacteriostatic
Fat globules staining with Sudan III
Lymphocytes: 400-6800 × 10^6/L
Erythrocytes: 0.050-0.6 × 10^9/L

COMPOSITION

Chyle	Normal Plasma Concentration
Total protein: 21-59 g/L	65-80 g/L
Albumin: 12-41.6 g/L	40-50 g/L
Globulin: 11-30.8 g/L	25-35 g/L
Fibrinogen: 0.16-0.24 g/L	1.5-3.5 g/L
Total fat: 14-210 mmol/L	
Triglycerides: above plasma value	0.84-2.0 mmol/L
Cholesterol: plasma values or lower	4.4-6.5 mmol/L
Glucose: 2.7-11.1 mmol/L	2.5-4.2 mmol/L
Urea: 1.4-3.0 mmol/L	3.0-7.0 mmol/L

clear with alkali or ether and stain with Sudan III. Chyle is milky white only when the patient is eating (i.e., when fat is being transported from the gut). A chylous leak in the fasting state yields blood-stained fluid or clear and serous fluid. Lymphocytes are the predominant cells in chyle, and a 90% lymphocyte count is virtually diagnostic.

CONCLUSION

In the investigation of a pleural disorder, it is important to have a methodical and structured approach. One must begin with simple methods, such as careful history taking, standard chest radiographs, and thoracentesis, rather than proceed immediately with more invasive techniques such as thoracoscopy. This approach not only reduces the cost of investigation but also minimizes the patient's morbidity.

SUGGESTED READINGS

Review Articles

Black LF: The pleural space and pleural fluid. Mayo Clin Proc 1972;47:493-506.

Sahn SA: Pleural fluid analysis: narrowing the differential diagnosis. Semin Respir Med 1987;9:22-29.

Lorch DG, Sahn SA: Pleural effusions due to diseases below the diaphragm. Semin Respir Med 1987;9:75-85.

Sahn SA: State of the art. The pleura. Am Rev Respir Dis 1988;138:184-234.

Morris V, Wiggins J: Current management of pleural disease. Br J Hosp Med 1992;47:753-758.

Kennedy L, Sahn SA: Noninvasive evaluation of the patient with a pleural effusion. Chest Surg Clin North Am 1994;4:451-465.

Hammar SP: The pathology of benign and malignant pleural disease. Chest Surg Clin North Am 1994:4:405-430.

Sahn SA: The diagnostic value of pleural fluid analysis. Semin Respir Crit Care Med 1995;16:269-278.

Radiology

Rosenberg ER: Ultrasound in the assessment of pleural densities. Chest 1983;84:283-285.

Leung AN, Müller NL, Miller RR: CT in differential diagnosis of diffuse pleural disease. AJR Am J Roentgenol 1990;154:487-492.

McLoud TC, Flower CDR: Imaging the pleura: sonography, CT, and MR imaging. AJR Am J Roentgenol 1991;156:1145-1153.

Carretta A, Landoni C, Melloni G, et al: 18-FDG positron emission tomography in the evaluation of malignant pleural disease—a pilot study. Eur J Cardiothorac Surg 2000;17:377-383.

Pleural Biopsy

Prakash UBS: Comparison of needle biopsy with cytologic analysis for the evaluation of pleural effusion: analysis of 414 cases. Mayo Clin Proc 1985;60:158-164.

Tomlinson JR, Sahn SA: Invasive procedures in the diagnosis of pleural disease. Semin Respir Med 1987;9:30-36.

Metintaş M, Özdemir N, Işiksoy S, et al: CT-guided pleural needle biopsy in the diagnosis of malignant mesothelioma. J Comput Assist Tomogr 1995;19:370-374.

Thoracoscopy

Rusch VW, Mountain C: Thoracoscopy under regional anesthesia for the diagnosis and management of pleural disease. Am J Surg 1987;154:274-278.

Menzies R, Charbonneau M: Thoracoscopy for the diagnosis of pleural disease. Ann Intern Med 1991;114:271-276.

Daniel TM: Diagnostic thoracoscopy for pleural disease. Ann Thorac Surg 1993;56:639-640.

Kohman LJ: Thoracoscopy for the evaluation and treatment of pleural space disease. Chest Surg Clin North Am 1994;4:467-479.

Harris RJ, Kavuru MS, Rice TW, Kirby TJ: The diagnostic and therapeutic utility of thoracoscopy. A review. Chest 1995;108:828-841.

Malthaner RA, Inculet RI: Minithoracoscopy for pleural effusions. Can Respir J 1998;5:253-254.

Investigation of Pneumothorax

Rhea JT, DeLuca SA, Greene RE: Determining the size of pneumothorax in the upright patient. Radiology 1982;144:733-736.

Light RW: Management of spontaneous pneumothorax. Am Rev Respir Dis 1993;148:245-248.

Investigation of Pleural Effusion

Collins TR, Sahn SA: Thoracentesis. Clinical value, complications, technical problems and patient experience. Chest 1987;91:817-822.

Smyrnios NA, Jederlinic PJ, Irwin RS: Pleural effusion in an asymptomatic patient: spectrum and frequency of causes and management considerations. Chest 1990;97:192-196.

Bartter T, Santarelli R, Akers SM, Pratter MR: The evaluation of pleural effusion. Chest 1994;106:1209-1214.

Al-Jahdali H, Menzies RI: How to diagnose pleural effusions. Can J Diagn 1996;13:105-113.

ASSESSMENT OF TECHNICAL RESECTABILITY OF ESOPHAGEAL CANCER

In oncologic surgery, resectability addresses the issue of whether the removal of a neoplasm is *technically feasible*, a decision generally based on accurate preoperative definition of the tumor (T) factor (clinical staging). In patients with esophageal cancer, precise assessment of locoregional tumor extension is even more important because attempted resection of advanced tumors not only offers *no hope for cure* but also carries *high operative mortality* as well as *significant morbidity*. Evidence of airway invasion, for instance, precludes safe resection and is considered an absolute contraindication to esophagectomy.

The judicious use of preresection investigative techniques thus facilitates the allocation of patients to surgical treatment when it is likely that this treatment will provide the most benefits. Fortunately, advances in CT scanning techniques, MRI, and more recently endoscopic ultrasonography have markedly improved the accuracy of clinical staging (accuracy of more than 90%). Similarly, thoracoscopic exploration (VATS) may help avoid unnecessary operations when it is known that the tumor has spread to neighboring structures such as the aorta, pericardium, or left atrium.

STAGING TECHNIQUES

In general, tumor invasion into *neighboring mediastinal structures* such as airway, pericardium, aorta, azygos vein, or recurrent nerve indicates unresectable disease. Limited extension to mediastinal fat, mediastinal pleura, or lung is considered a *relative contraindication* to resection. Patients with more localized tumors can usually have complete resection of their neoplasm.

Preoperatively, this information is obtained through a variety of imaging and endoscopic techniques.

Imaging

Plain Chest Radiographs and Barium Swallow Study

Plain chest radiographs are seldom useful to predict invasion of vital neighboring structures. By contrast, upper gastrointestinal tract contrast studies are useful to determine tumor length as well as severity of tumor obstruction. For many surgeons, a lesion longer than 10 cm is *unlikely to be resectable*, whereas a lesion shorter than 5 cm is an *accurate predictor* of resectability. As nicely demonstrated by Dr. K. Sugimachi, other abnormal findings that may suggest marked extraluminal extension, thus unresectability, include deformities of the esophageal axis, deep ulcerations of the esophageal wall, and clear demonstration of a tracheobronchial fistula.

CT Scan and MRI

CT scanning is useful to demonstrate the depth of tumor infiltration into or through the esophageal wall. Wall thickness of 5 to 10 mm is a sign of limited disease. Wall thickness *of more than 10 mm*, tumor infiltration into periesophageal fat, disappearance of fat planes between esophagus and surrounding tissues, and abnormal contacts with other mediastinal structures are usually considered accurate signs of nonresectability.

CT scan can identify *airway invasion*, whether it is direct tumor extension into the tracheobronchial lumen or tracheoesophageal fistula. *Aortic invasion* can also be predicted from CT findings. An interface arc of contact between aorta and esophageal cancer of less than 45 degrees suggests absence of aortic invasion, whereas an interface arc of more than 90 degrees strongly suggests aortic invasion. Extension to the pericardium is characterized by pericardial thickening and effusion; invasion of diaphragmatic crura by distal esophageal carcinomas can also be demonstrated by CT. For an optimal CT examination, oral contrast agents (barium, water soluble) as well as intravenous contrast material should be administered.

Although MRI can better differentiate invasion from abutment of surrounding structures, it is *seldom used* for the clinical staging of esophageal carcinomas.

Endoscopic Ultrasonography

Endoscopic ultrasonography is accurate in assessment of the depth of tumor invasion and is indeed the *procedure of choice* to determine the clinical tumor status (cT). Endoscopic ultrasonography is also useful to evaluate *interfaces between primary tumor and neighboring structures.* Unfortunately, echoendoscopes cannot be passed in patients with significant narrowing of the esophageal lumen (15% to 20% of all patients). In such cases, the tumor can be dilated before endoscopic ultrasonography or the examination can be performed with small ultrasonic probes. Accurate interpretation of endoscopic ultrasonography images may be difficult and is often dependent on the *experience of the operator.*

Fluorodeoxyglucose–positron emission tomography does not provide definitions of the esophageal wall or paraesophageal tissues. It thus has little value in determining the clinical T status.

In the past, azygos venography was used to demonstrate vein compression and obstruction because these were considered strong indicators of extraluminal extension. Currently, the same information can be obtained from CT scans with intravenous contrast material administered by the dynamic bolus technique.

Endoscopic

Bronchoscopy

Bronchoscopy is still the best technique to evaluate esophageal carcinomas with *possible airway invasion*. Bronchoscopic findings suggestive of invasion include indentations of the normally flat membranous wall of the trachea or main bronchi, actual permeation of tumor into the airway, and presence of a tracheoesophageal fistula. Bronchoscopy should be done under local anesthesia so that vocal cord mobility can also be assessed during the examination.

Thoracoscopy

Videothoracoscopy can exclude a cT4 unresectable tumor, but this determination requires *dissection of the primary tumor* from the adjacent structure presumed to be invaded. For visualization of the entire intrathoracic esophagus, the examination should nearly always be done on the right side, and if necessary, the azygos vein can be divided and the mediastinal pleura incised.

In addition to tumor staging, preresection nodal staging (cN) can also be accomplished during thoracoscopy.

Operative Staging

Ultimately, the decision as to whether an esophageal carcinoma is or is not resectable may have to be made *at operation*. This is an important consideration because imaging modalities are sometimes imperfect or their interpretation is incorrect. Because complete resection is an important prognostic factor, patients should not be denied surgery if tumor resectability is still doubtful after clinical investigation. Patients should be excluded from operation only when unresectability has been clearly documented.

TECHNICAL RESECTABILITY OF ESOPHAGEAL CANCER

General Principles of Surgery

Although resection is still the mainstay for the treatment of esophageal carcinoma, there are still controversies about the resectability of some tumors. These controversies have become even more important in this era of induction treatment modalities.

All surgeons agree, however, that *incomplete resections* negate the primary purpose of the operation and that they should be avoided. This is the reason why every surgeon must adopt a compulsive attitude toward accurate clinical staging of the T factor with the understanding that, sometimes, precise determination of technical resectability can be defined only at operation.

Unresectable Tumors (Tables 3-43 and 3-44)

All tumors with clear evidence of mediastinal invasion are considered technically unresectable. This includes tumors that invade the tracheobronchial tree, the aorta, the pericardium, or the left atrium. This type of direct invasion is not uncommon because the esophagus is located in a *confined area (mediastinum)* and has *no adventitia*.

Patients with airway invasion documented by bronchoscopy or biopsy have unresectable disease. Obviously, this includes patients with tracheoesophageal fistulas. Because bronchoscopic findings may have such an impact on treatment strategies, this examination is recommended for every patient with esophageal carcinomas in the neck as well as those in the upper or middle third of the thorax. During open surgery, airway invasion may present as tight adhesions between tumor and membranous airway. *Fixity of the carcinoma to the carina or lower trachea* documented during transhiatal esophagectomy is an indication to abort the procedure.

Invasion of the aorta is also an absolute contraindication to surgery, and this is best documented by CT scan or at operation (dense fibrosis, fixed tumor to aorta). In addition to an interface arc of contact between tumor and aorta greater than 90 degrees, other CT signs that suggest

TABLE 3-43

TECHNICAL RESECTABILITY OF ESOPHAGEAL CARCINOMA

Factor (best test)	Resectable	Relative Contraindication	Absolute Contraindication
Length of carcinoma (upper gastrointestinal tract series)			
>10 cm		✓	
<5 cm	✓		
Tumor diameter (CT scan)			
>4 cm		✓	
<4 cm	✓		
Abnormal axis of esophagus (upper gastrointestinal tract series)		✓	
Deformity (upper gastrointestinal tract series)		✓	
Deep ulceration (upper gastrointestinal tract series)		✓	
Wall thickness (endoscopic ultrasonography)			
<10 mm	✓		
>10 mm		✓	
Fat planes (CT, endoscopic ultrasonography)			
Infiltration of periesophageal fat		✓	
Preservation of fat planes	✓		
Disappearance of fat planes		✓	
Abnormal contacts with other structures		✓	
Invasion of neighboring structures			
Respiratory			
Abnormal contact with airway (CT scan)		✓	
Extension into airway lumen (bronchoscopy)			✓
Tracheobronchial fistula (upper gastrointestinal tract series, bronchoscopy)			✓
Lung (CT scan)		✓	
Pulmonary artery or veins (CT, MRI)			✓
Cardiovascular			
Aorta (CT)			
Interface arc of contact <45 degrees on CT	✓		
Interface arc of contact >90 degrees on CT		✓	
Pericardium, atrium (CT, cardiac ultrasonography)			✓
Azygos vein compression or obstruction (CT)			✓
Diaphragm (crura) (CT)		✓	
Recurrent nerve (endoscopy)			✓

3

Specific Preoperative Assessment

TABLE 3-44
ABSOLUTE CONTRAINDICATIONS TO SURGERY
Documented invasion of
Trachea, main bronchi
Aorta
Pericardium, left atrium
Pulmonary blood vessels
Recurrent nerve

invasion include marked deformity of the aorta and tumor invasion of the space between aorta and spine. Simple absence of the fat plane between cancer and aorta does not necessarily indicate unresectability.

Pericardial invasion (pericardial thickening, pericardial effusion), invasion of the left atrium, invasion of pulmonary blood vessels (artery or veins), and recurrent nerve paralysis are other *absolute contraindications* to esophagectomy.

Relative Contraindications to Surgery (Table 3-45; see also Table 3-43)

Patients are considered to have relative contraindications to surgical resection if they have tumors whose length is greater than 10 cm or tumors with a diameter greater than 4 cm. *Full-thickness invasion of the esophageal wall* documented by endoscopic ultrasonography, mediastinal fat invasion (CT scan), deformity of the esophageal axis (upper gastrointestinal tract series), deep ulcerations, and disappearance of fat planes on CT are all relative contraindications to surgical treatment. In all of those cases, the tumor has a clinical T4 designation without actually invading neighboring organs.

Although uncommon, invasion of the lung or invasion of the diaphragmatic crura by distal esophageal tumors does not preclude curative resection.

When any of these findings is combined with significant weight loss, N1 disease, or other comorbidities, surgery should *probably be avoided* because the benefits (survival) versus the risks (morbidity and mortality) are not in favor of the patient.

Resectable Tumors

Resectable tumors are those with lengths less than 5 cm, diameters smaller than 3 cm, and no evidence of mediastinal involvement by

TABLE 3-45
RELATIVE CONTRAINDICATIONS TO SURGERY
Tumors measuring > 10 cm in length
Tumors with a diameter > 4 cm
Full-thickness invasion of esophageal wall
Deformity of esophageal axis
Deep ulcerations
Disappearance of fat planes
Invasion of lung, diaphragmatic crura

endoscopic ultrasonography (wall thickness of 5 to 10 mm). These represent a small subgroup of patients in whom surgery has an excellent chance of being uncomplicated, and the patient has a good chance of prolonged survival.

CONCLUSION

Because it is important preoperatively to identify which patients might benefit from esophagectomy, and because surgery offers *the best hope for cure,* every effort should be made to predict the extent of local invasion of esophageal carcinomas before operation. It is also important to understand that each test can by itself be inaccurate but that all modalities are complementary to each other. CT scanning and endoscopic ultrasonography remain, however, the *mainstays* of determining the resectability of esophageal carcinomas.

SUGGESTED READINGS

Review Articles

Krasna MJ: Advances in staging of esophageal carcinoma. Chest 1998;113:107s-111s.

Buenaventura P, Luketich JD: Surgical staging of esophageal cancer. Chest Surg Clin North Am 2000;10:487-497.

Ultrasonography

Dittler HJ, Siewert JR: Role of endoscopic ultrasonography in esophageal carcinoma. Endoscopy 1993;25:156-161.

Rösch T: Endosonographic staging of esophageal cancer: a review of literature results. Gastrointest Endosc Clin North Am 1995;5:537-547.

Zuccaro G, Rice TW, Goldblum J, et al: Endoscopic ultrasound cannot determine suitability for esophagectomy after aggressive chemoradiotherapy for esophageal cancer. Am J Gastroenterol 1999;94:906-912.

Heidemann J, Schilling MK, Schmassmann A, et al: Accuracy of endoscopic ultrasonography in preoperative staging of esophageal carcinoma. Dig Surg 2000;17:219-224.

Mariette C, Balon JM, Maunoury V, et al: Value of endoscopic ultrasonography as a predictor of long-term survival in oesophageal carcinoma. Br J Surg 2003;90:1367-1372.

Airway Involvement

Altorki NK, Migliore M, Skinner DB: Esophageal carcinoma with airway invasion. Evolution and choices of therapy. Chest 1994;106:742-745.

Riedel M, Hauck RW, Stein HJ, et al: Preoperative bronchoscopic assessment of airway invasion by esophageal cancer. A prospective study. Chest 1998;113:687-695.

Radiology

Picus D, Balfe DM, Koehler RE, et al: Computed tomography in the staging of esophageal carcinoma. Radiology 1983;146:433-438.

3

Specific Preoperative Assessment

Takashima S, Takeuchi N, Shiozaki H, et al: Carcinoma of the esophagus: CT vs MR imaging in determining resectability. AJR Am J Roentgenol 1991;156:297-302.

Sugimachi K, Watanabe M, Sadanaga N, et al: Preoperative estimation of complete resection for patients with oesophageal carcinoma. Surg Oncol 1994;3:327-334.

Saunders HS, Wolfman NT, Ott DJ: Esophageal cancer. Radiologic staging. Radiol Clin North Am 1997;35:281-294.

Rankin SC, Taylor H, Cook GJR, Mason R: Computed tomography and positron emission tomography in the preoperative staging of oesophageal carcinoma. Clin Radiol 1998;53:659-665.

Thoracoscopy

Krasna MJ: Minimally invasive staging for esophageal cancer. Chest 1997;112:191s-194s.

Surgery

Kato H, Tachimori Y, Watanabe H, Itabashi M: Surgical treatment of thoracic esophageal carcinoma directly invading the lung. Cancer 1992;70:1457-1461.

Sariego J, Mosher S, Byrd M, et al: Prediction of outcome in "resectable" esophageal carcinoma. J Surg Oncol 1993;54:223-225.

Matsubara T, Ueda M, Kokudo N, et al: Role of esophagectomy in treatment of esophageal carcinoma with clinical evidence of adjacent organ invasion. World J Surg 2001;25:279-284.

Mariette C, Finzi L, Fabre S, et al: Factors predictive of complete resection of operable esophageal cancer: a prospective study. Ann Thorac Surg 2003;75:1720-1726.

Positron Emission Tomography

Block MI, Patterson GA, Sundaresan RS, et al: Improvement in staging of esophageal cancer with the addition of position emission tomography. Ann Thorac Surg 1997;64:770-777.

Kobori O, Kirihara Y, Kosaka N, Hara T: Positron emission tomography of esophageal carcinoma using [11]c-choline and ^{18}F-fluorodeoxyglucose. A novel method of preoperative lymph node staging. Cancer 1999; 86:1638-1648.

Flamen P, Lerut A, Van Cutsem E, et al: Utility of positron emission tomography for the staging of patients with potentially operable esophageal carcinoma. J Clin Oncol 2000;18:3202-3210.

ASSESSMENT OF THE PATIENT WITH A SOLITARY PULMONARY NODULE

The solitary pulmonary nodule is a single, usually sharply defined spherical lesion that is fairly well circumscribed. There are approximately 150,000 of these nodules detected every year in the United States, and about 40% to 50% of resected lesions will be malignant. With improvements in the technology of CT scanning, it is likely that more and more nodules will be detected, but unfortunately, they will be *more difficult to diagnose* because of their smaller size.

As stated by Dr. E. Spratt, the correct management of solitary pulmonary nodules often remains elusive despite the multiplicity of diagnostic tests available. At one end of the spectrum, there are people who think that *all nodules should be excised,* therefore subjecting patients with benign lesions to unnecessary operations. At the other end of the spectrum are those who think that only *patients with tissue-proven malignant neoplasms* should undergo surgery. In this group, obviously, many malignant lesions will be allowed to grow and spread when a curative resection could have been performed earlier.

Short of subjecting every patient with a solitary pulmonary nodule to thoracotomy, there are unfortunately no 100% reliable tests for the definitive diagnosis of these abnormalities. It is thus important to have a clear understanding of all possible causes of pulmonary nodules. It is also important to have complete knowledge of the diagnostic methods available, beginning with the least invasive, such as accurate recording of clinical history. It is finally important to have a *safe, cost-effective, and cohesive investigative approach* so that either a positive diagnosis is reached or there is a strong likelihood that the nodule is benign.

DEFINITION AND INCIDENCE

Although there are many definitions of solitary pulmonary nodules (Table 3-46), most agree that these are *well-defined lung opacities* that measure less than 4 to 5 cm in diameter. They may have smooth, lobulated, or umbilicated contours and any shape. They are completely surrounded on all sides by aerated lung, and they are free of the mediastinum or pleura. They are not associated with atelectasis or adenopathies. They may contain calcifications or be cavitary, but these characteristics are not necessarily obvious on a standard chest radiograph.

Most solitary pulmonary nodules are *asymptomatic;* they are usually picked up coincidentally on chest radiography. Radiographic surveys of adults have demonstrated nodules in 0.1% to 0.2% of the population; but in high-risk patients recently screened for lung cancer by low-dose spiral CT, pulmonary nodules have been found in up to 20% of individuals.

ETIOLOGY OF PULMONARY NODULES (TABLE 3-47)

Among malignant lesions, *primary bronchogenic carcinoma* is the most common entity. Breakdown by cell type shows that tumors often presenting

TABLE 3-46

THE SOLITARY PULMONARY NODULE

Must be 4-5 cm or less in diameter

Must be solitary

Must be in lung parenchyma and surrounded by aerated lung

May have any contour or shape

No obvious calcification on standard chest radiograph

Specific Preoperative Assessment

3

TABLE 3-47	
COMMON CAUSES OF PULMONARY NODULES	
MALIGNANT	
Bronchogenic carcinomas (adenocarcinomas)	
Pulmonary metastasis (sarcomas, kidney, colorectal, breast)	
Lymphomas	
NONMALIGNANT	
Infectious granulomas: tuberculosis, histoplasmosis, coccidioidomycosis	
Noninfectious granulomas: sarcoidosis, rheumatoid arthritis, Wegener	
Benign lung tumors: hamartomas	
Congenital: bronchogenic cysts, arteriovenous malformations	
Others: pneumoconiosis, scar tissue, chronic pneumonitis	

in the form of solitary pulmonary nodules are *adenocarcinomas* including bronchoalveolar cell carcinomas. Pulmonary metastases from extrathoracic tumors are also common. On occasion, peripheral carcinoids or low-grade lymphomas may also present as solitary nodules.

In virtually every series of solitary pulmonary nodules, *granulomas*— whether they are tuberculomas or histoplasmomas—account for the bulk of the benign nodules. These granulomatous foci are usually negative for bacteria both on culture and histologically, especially when the nodule is old and partly calcified. Other benign lesions that may present as solitary nodules include hamartomas, bronchogenic cysts, and areas of chronic pneumonitis. Hamartomas are not uncommon; the majority present as *well-circumscribed nodules* usually less than 4 cm in diameter. *"Popcorn"* calcifications are virtually diagnostic. Bronchogenic cysts are foregut developmental anomalies that can also assume the appearance of a nodule when distended with mucus. They have a predilection for lower lobe locations.

Noninfectious granulomatous conditions such as sarcoidosis, rheumatoid arthritis, and Wegener granulomatosis usually present with multiple pulmonary nodules.

ASSESSMENT OF THE PATIENT WITH A SOLITARY PULMONARY NODULE

The most relevant question posed by the presence of a solitary pulmonary nodule is whether the lesion is malignant. This is important because small (<3 cm) solitary primary lung cancers have a better prognosis with surgical resection than do larger tumors. Indeed, the 5-year survival rate for T1N0M0 resected lung cancers is 75% to 80%, whereas it is 55% to 60% for T2N0M0 tumors.

The probability that a nodule is malignant relates to clinical factors, such as age of the patient and smoking history, and radiologic characteristics, such as presence or absence of occult calcifications and nature of the contours. Ultimately, definitive diagnosis is based on histologic documentation of the exact nature of the nodule.

TABLE 3-48
CLINICAL FACTORS IN FAVOR OF MALIGNANT DISEASE

Age > 40 years
History of cigarette smoking for >20-25 years
Previous history of malignant disease
Family history of lung cancer
Presence of local symptoms: cough, hemoptysis
Presence of systemic symptoms: weight loss, osteoarthropathy

Noninvasive Methods

Clinical Assessment

The clinical history of a patient with a solitary pulmonary nodule may provide important clues in arriving at the actual diagnosis. Because these clues may be vague, they should not, however, affect subsequent diagnostic procedures.

If the patient, for instance, is younger than 40 years and is a nonsmoker, the risk of malignancy is less than 1%. By contrast, a solitary pulmonary nodule in a patient with a previous history of malignant disease has a 50% chance of being malignant (Table 3-48). If the previous malignant neoplasm was a sarcoma or a melanoma, this probability is increased by 10-fold; and if the tumor was from the head and neck region (squamous cell carcinoma), it is increased by 2-fold.

The *presence of symptoms* also favors a diagnosis of malignancy. Symptoms such as cough and hemoptysis may be due to local encroachment on surrounding intraparenchymatous airways by a malignant tumor. Systemic symptoms such as weight loss and pulmonary hypertrophic osteoarthropathy are also significant risk factors for malignancy.

Clinical factors favoring a nonmalignant diagnosis (Table 3-49) are present in only *a few patients* with solitary pulmonary nodules. These include previous history of tuberculosis or close contact with individuals known to have active tuberculosis or a history of other nonmalignant disease, such as sarcoidosis, rheumatoid arthritis, or Wegener granulomatosis. Telangiectasis may suggest arteriovenous malformations. Living in regions endemic for

TABLE 3-49
CLINICAL FACTORS IN FAVOR OF BENIGN LESION

Age < 40 years
Patient is a nonsmoker
No previous history of malignant disease
No symptoms
Previous personal history of tuberculosis or contact with tuberculous patient
Personal history of rheumatoid arthritis, Wegener granulomatosis
Patient lives in endemic region for histoplasmosis
Patient is immunosuppressed

3

Specific Preoperative Assessment

histoplasmosis is a risk factor for a granulomatous lesion; *immunosuppressed patients* may develop solitary mycotic foci.

Radiographic Assessment

The purpose of the radiographic assessment is to determine which lesion will require further work-up and which lesion can be confidently called benign and therefore not require any additional diagnostic procedure.

Is There a Lung Nodule or Not? The first item to be addressed when a solitary pulmonary nodule is discovered is *whether the nodule is indeed in the lung* or originates from an adjacent structure. The differential diagnosis includes lesions from the pleura (benign pleural fibromas), from the subpleural area (lipomas, schwannomas), and from the chest wall. It also includes intrapleural fibrin deposits and localized pleural effusions within lung fissures (pseudotumors). On occasion, mediastinal lesions or diaphragmatic tumors may also be mistaken for solitary pulmonary nodules.

Comparison with Previous Films. *Radiographic stability* provides substantial evidence of a benign origin, and the absence of any detectable growth of a nodule for a prolonged time is the *single most reliable way* of establishing that the nodule is benign. A review of old radiographs can therefore be extremely useful because if there has been no growth for a 2-year period, the nodule is probably benign (average doubling time for malignant neoplasms is 120 days).

Appearance of the Lesion. Although the radiologic appearance of the nodule cannot reliably separate malignant and benign lesions, radiologic "benignancy" can be established with some confidence if specific patterns are identified. For individual cases, however, these patterns offer no absolute guidance as to the etiology of the nodule.

In general, nodules of benign origin (Table 3-50) are smaller (<3 cm), have *better defined borders,* and have a heavier radiologic density. For instance, nodules smaller than 2 cm and dense are usually granulomas. By contrast, malignant nodules are more likely to be larger and have irregular contours, with ill-defined or irregular margins. Umbilication of the border of a solitary pulmonary nodule is usually interpreted as a sign of malignancy (Fig. 3-10).

TABLE 3-50

RADIOLOGIC FEATURES IN FAVOR OF BENIGN LESION

Stability for 2 years
Size smaller than 3 cm in diameter
Well-defined borders
Heavier density
Specific patterns of calcifications

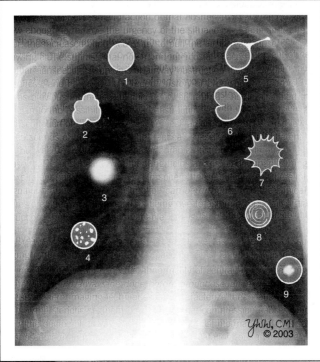

FIG. 3-10

Radiographic characteristics of different pathologic processes that may present as solitary pulmonary nodules: 1, round and well-defined nodule in granuloma; 2, lobulated with well-defined margin in hamartoma; 3, ill-defined margin with pneumonia; 4, round with speckled calcifications in hamartoma; 5, pleural tail with cancer; 6, umbilicated at the entrance of a feeding vessel in cancer; 7, stellate margin in cancer; 8, concentric calcifications in granuloma; 9, central calcifications, nonspecific.

Calcifications within a pulmonary nodule are best seen on CT scan and generally *are a reliable sign that the lesion is benign,* especially if specific patterns of calcium deposition are manifest. These include a dense central core of calcification, a laminated pattern with calcium in concentric layers (granuloma), and a popcorn type of calcification that is associated with hamartomas. The mere presence of calcifications, however, is inadequate evidence that the lesion is benign because microcalcifications are present in 15% to 25% of resected carcinomas. These calcifications may occur in necrotic areas of the tumor, or it may be a previous calcific focus that is incorporated by the tumor.

Growth Rate (Doubling Time). The use of growth rate is much less reliable in a prospective manner than retrospectively (comparison with old films). The doubling time of a lesion can be appreciated by *comparing two radiographs taken at an interval of 3 to 4 months,* and this measurement can be used to determine if the nodule is benign or malignant. The calculation analyzes doubling of tumor volume rather than doubling of its diameter. It uses the formulation of a sphere, and the results are entered in a tumor volume–time graph (Fig. 3-11). In practice, these measurements are difficult to interpret because the volume of a given tumor may double while its diameter only increases by 25%. In general, the doubling in the volume of a malignant tumor varies from 1 month to 18 months (Table 3-51). If a nodule shows rapid growth in a period of less than 1 month, it is usually infectious; those growing very slowly during a period of several years are often benign.

Use of CT Scan. Computed tomography is the *imaging technique of choice* to evaluate a solitary nodule not clearly calcified on plain radiography. Because it is 10 to 20 times more sensitive to density differences than standard radiographs, CT can demonstrate benign calcifications not seen otherwise.

Nodule densitometry can also be performed, and the determination of Hounsfield numbers depends on the density of the lesion. A high Hounsfield number (>600) is generally a reliable indicator of benign disease, whereas those nodules with numbers 50 to 150 are viewed to be the most suspicious for malignancy.

CT scan can also identify satellite nodules not seen on conventional radiographs. Unfortunately, satellite lesions can be found in both carcinomas and infectious granulomatous diseases.

Skin Testing

The PPD tuberculin test and fungal serology tests are essentially *unreliable* because a positive test result only indicates previous exposure rather than actual disease. It does not in any way exclude the possibility of malignancy in the lesion.

Histologic Analysis

When clinical and radiologic clues remain vague, histologic analysis becomes important.

Sputum Cytology and Culture. Sputum cytology is *not particularly useful* in the diagnosis of solitary pulmonary nodules. A diagnostic yield of less than 1% can be expected because the lesion is peripheral and does not exfoliate cells into the bronchial tree. Sputum cultures might be more reliable if fungal or acid-fast bacilli are recovered.

Fiberoptic Bronchoscopy and Transbronchial Biopsy. In solitary pulmonary nodules, the yield of fluoroscopy-guided transbronchial biopsy is in the range of 40% to 60%, but *specific benign diagnoses are established in only 10% of nodules examined*. One advantage of fiberoptic bronchoscopy

3

Specific Preoperative Assessment

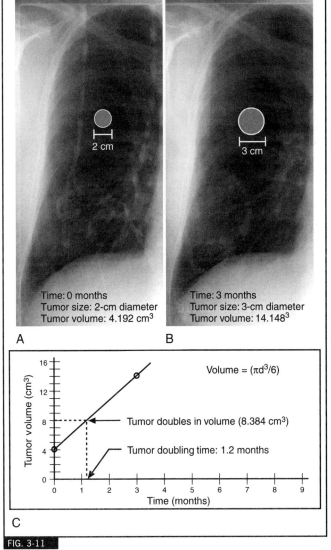

Time: 0 months
Tumor size: 2-cm diameter
Tumor volume: 4.192 cm³

A

Time: 3 months
Tumor size: 3-cm diameter
Tumor volume: 14.148³

B

Volume = (πd³/6)

Tumor doubles in volume (8.384 cm³)

Tumor doubling time: 1.2 months

C

FIG. 3-11

The calculation of the tumor doubling time. Serial measurements of the volume of the tumor (**A** and **B**) are entered in a tumor volume–time graph (**C**). The doubling time is calculated by measuring the time to double the volume of the tumor.

TABLE 3-51

RADIOLOGIC FEATURES IN FAVOR OF MALIGNANT LESION

Evidence of growth of the lesion within 2 years or less
Volume doubling time of 1-18 months
Size larger than 3 cm in diameter
Irregular contours and margins
Umbilication of border

---

is that it permits visual inspection of the bronchial tree. Samples are obtained by washing and brushing the affected segment, followed by transbronchial biopsy under biplane fluoroscopic guidance. Results are dependent on the *size of the nodule,* its *proximity to central airways,* and *skills of the operator.* If the lesion is less than 2 cm in diameter, a specific diagnosis will be obtained in 10% of cases; if the nodule is 2 to 4 cm, the technique will be diagnostic in 40% to 50% of cases. Fiberoptic bronchoscopy is a safe procedure; significant hemorrhage occurs in less than 1% of cases and pneumothorax in less than 10% of cases.

Transthoracic Needle Biopsy. Transthoracic needle biopsy (fine-needle aspiration) is performed under fluoroscopic or CT guidance. It is a safe procedure, with less than 10% of patients requiring tube drainage because of a pneumothorax.

In malignant lesions, a positive diagnosis can be established in up to 95% of cases, provided the material is handled by experienced pathologists. Limiting factors are the visibility and location of the lesion and the experience of the operator. With CT guidance, however, nodules as small as 7 to 8 mm in diameter can be safely sampled, with yields of positive diagnosis in the presence of malignancy in the range of 50% to 60%.

Specific benign lesions (e.g., granulomas, hamartomas, active infection, infarct) are diagnosed in only 10% of cases, mostly because benign lesions are difficult to penetrate as they tend to be pushed away by the needle. These benign diagnoses are often reported as *nonspecific inflammatory changes or fibrosis.* A negative biopsy finding without a specific benign diagnosis therefore provides *insufficient evidence* of a nonmalignant origin of the nodule, and further diagnostic procedures may be indicated.

Invasive Methods

By the time initial investigations are completed, the nodule is either a known malignant neoplasm requiring surgical resection or a nodule in which no malignant cells have been found and no definitive diagnosis has been established. This uncertainty of a benign diagnosis is thus the most compelling argument for thoracoscopic excision of these nodules. VATS has a sensitivity and specificity of 100%, and it can be done with no mortality and minimal morbidity. In benign lesions, it becomes a therapeutic procedure.

CT scan is used to *localize the nodule,* and at operation, the nodule is either visualized or palpated. A wedge excision is then carried out including surrounding normal lung parenchyma with an endoscopic stapler. Other techniques, such as hook wire localization with CT or fluoroscopic imaging, can be used if the nodule is located away from the pleural surface. If a primary lung cancer is identified, formal thoracotomy and anatomic resection can be carried out.

Open Thoracotomy

Thoracoscopic resection may be difficult for small nodules (<1.5 cm) or for centrally located lesions that are close to hilar structures and unsuitable for thoracoscopic wedge excision. In those cases, standard limited thoracotomy is the definitive procedure to establish the diagnosis of the nodule. The mortality is low, but the morbidity is higher than that of thoracoscopy.

OVERALL APPROACH TO THE DIAGNOSIS OF A PULMONARY NODULE (FIG. 3-12)

The most appropriate approach for the diagnosis of indeterminate pulmonary nodules is still controversial, although everyone agrees that these nodules should be investigated until a *diagnosis is reached* or until there is *a strong likelihood* that the nodule is benign.

An observation-only approach is recommended (Table 3-52) if the patient is *young* (<35 years), is a *nonsmoker,* and has *no previous history of malignant disease.* On chest radiographs, the nodule must have been present and unchanged in size or contours for at least 2 years, and it must be small (<1.0 cm) or have a benign pattern of calcifications. A definitive diagnosis of benign disease obtained by transthoracic needle biopsy or transbronchial bronchoscopic biopsy is also a criterion that justifies observation. The follow-up of these nodules must include serial CT scans for at least 2 years (every 4 to 6 months), keeping in mind the possibility that granulomas can undergo malignant changes at any time.

In most other clinical settings, a biopsy procedure must be carried out, and there are basically two different approaches to obtaining tissue from the lesion. The first one is to use noninvasive biopsy techniques such as transthoracic needle biopsy. This approach is justified because technologic advances in the field of CT-guided needle aspiration biopsy as well as skills in cytologic interpretation of small specimens have increased the diagnostic yield of the technique to 95% or better in cases of malignant neoplasms. In most cases, transthoracic needle biopsy can be rapidly performed, is low cost, and has few complications. The real advantage is that both patient and surgeon know the diagnosis before surgery. That knowledge not only allows better planning of the operative procedure but also avoids relying on intraoperative diagnostic maneuvers before definitive therapy.

The second approach is to use invasive biopsy techniques such as thoracoscopy or open thoracotomy without prior transthoracic needle

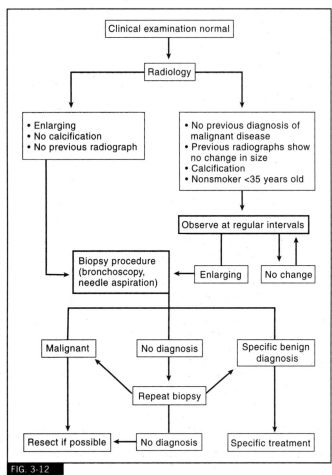

FIG. 3-12

Suggested approach to the diagnosis of a pulmonary nodule. *(Modified from Stubbing DG: Pulmonary nodules. Med Clin North Am 1985;24:3224-3228.)*

TABLE 3-52

CHARACTERISTICS OF BENIGN NODULES

Patient <30-35 years old and nonsmoker
No previous history of malignant disease
Nodule unchanged in size or contours for 2 years or more
Nodule is small (<1.0 cm)
Benign pattern of calcifications
Definitive diagnosis of benign disease by transthoracic needle biopsy

aspiration biopsy. This approach is justified by the fact that transthoracic needle biopsy may have a false-negative rate in the presence of malignancy as high as 5% to 7%. In addition, there may be significant difficulties in making a specific benign diagnosis. The final and most quoted argument in favor of this approach is that transthoracic needle biopsy adds another diagnostic step in a situation where *operation will be warranted anyway*. For those surgeons who prefer this approach, transthoracic needle aspiration biopsy is reserved for patients who are not surgical candidates and those who have unresectable malignant neoplasms and in which a tissue diagnosis is needed.

APPROACH TO THE PATIENT WITH MULTIPLE PULMONARY NODULES

Although most patients with multiple pulmonary nodules have metastatic disease, it is important to obtain histologic confirmation. Alveolar cell carcinoma and multifocal adenocarcinomas are primary lung tumors that may regularly present with multiple nodules. On occasion, noninfectious granulomatous conditions may also present with multiple pulmonary nodules.

CONCLUSION

Because the 5-year survival for malignant solitary pulmonary nodules is high, it is important that these are *diagnosed early* and resected. On the other hand, thoracotomy and even thoracoscopy carry some morbidity and mortality, and these should be avoided whenever possible for benign lesions. Although multiple techniques can be used to diagnose these nodules, it is still better to resect a benign lesion than to delay the excision of a malignant tumor until there is metastatic spread.

SUGGESTED READINGS

Historical Reference

Davis EW, Peabody JW, Katz S: The solitary pulmonary nodule. A ten-year study based on 215 cases. J Thorac Surg 1956;32:728-770.

Review Articles

Spratt EH: Management of the solitary pulmonary nodule. Proceedings of the University of Toronto Thoracic Surgery Postgraduate Course, June 1984.

Stubbing DG: Pulmonary nodules. Med North Am 1985;24:3224-3228.

Khouri NF, Meziane MA, Zerhouni EA, et al: The solitary pulmonary nodule. Assessment, diagnosis, and management. Chest 1987;91:128-133.

Caskey CI, Templeton PA, Zerhouni EA: Current evaluation of the solitary pulmonary nodule. Radiol Clin North Am 1990;28:511-520.

Swensen SJ, Jett JR, Payne WS, et al: An integrated approach to the evaluation of the solitary pulmonary nodule. Mayo Clin Proc 1990;65:173-186.

Lillington GA: Management of solitary pulmonary nodules. Dis Mon 1991;37:271-318.

Midthun DE, Swensen SJ, Jett JR: Clinical strategies for solitary pulmonary nodule. Annu Rev Med 1992;43:195-208.

Shulkin AN: Management of the indeterminate solitary pulmonary nodule: a pulmonologist's view. Ann Thorac Surg 1993;56:743-744.

Lillington GA, Caskey CI: Evaluation and management of solitary and multiple pulmonary nodules. Clin Chest Med 1993;14:111-119.

Leef JL, Klein JS: The solitary pulmonary nodule. Radiol Clin North Am 2002;40:123-143.

Imaging

Edwards FH, Schaefer PS, Callahan S, et al: Bayesian statistical theory in the preoperative diagnosis of pulmonary lesions. Chest 1987;92: 888-891.

Jones FA, Wiedemann HP, O'Donovan PB, Stoller JK: Computerized tomographic densitometry of the solitary pulmonary nodule using a nodule phantom. Chest 1989;96:779-783.

Webb WR: Radiologic evaluation of the solitary pulmonary nodule. AJR Am J Roentgenol 1990;154:701-708.

Erasmus JJ, Connolly JE, McAdams HP, Roggli VL: Solitary pulmonary nodules: Part I. Morphologic evaluation for differentiation of benign and malignant lesions. Radiographics 2000;20:43-58.

Erasmus JJ, McAdams HP, Connolly JE: Solitary pulmonary nodules: Part II. Evaluation of the indeterminate nodule. Radiographics 2000;20:59-66.

Gould MK, Maclean CC, Kuschner WG, et al: Accuracy of positron emission tomography for diagnosis of pulmonary nodules and mass lesions: a meta-analysis. JAMA 2001;285:914-924.

Ohtsuka T, Nomori H, Horio H, et al: Radiological examination for peripheral lung cancers and benign nodules less than 10 mm. Lung Cancer 2001;42:291-296.

Needle Biopsy

Khouri NF, Stitik FP, Erozan YS, et al: Transthoracic needle aspiration biopsy of benign and malignant lung lesions. AJR Am J Roentgenol 1985;144:281-288.

Calhoun P, Feldman PS, Amstrong P, et al: The clinical outcome of needle aspirations of the lung when cancer is not diagnosed. Ann Thorac Surg 1986;41:592-596.

Mitruka S, Landreneau RJ, Mack MJ, et al: Diagnosing the indeterminate pulmonary nodule: percutaneous biopsy versus thoracoscopy. Surgery 1995;118:676-684.

Murphy JM, Gleeson FV, Flower CDR: Percutaneous needle biopsy of the lung and its impact on patient management. World J Surg 2001; 25:373-380.

Baldwin DR, Eaton T, Kolbe J, et al: Management of solitary pulmonary nodules: how do thoracic computed tomography and guided fine needle biopsy influence clinical decisions? Thorax 2002;57:817-822.

Thoracoscopy

Shennib H: Intraoperative localization techniques for pulmonary nodules. Ann Thorac Surg 1993;56:745-748.

Mack MJ, Hazelrigg SR, Landreneau RJ, Acuff TE: Thoracoscopy for the diagnosis of the indeterminate solitary pulmonary nodule. Ann Thorac Surg 1993;56:825-832.

Suzuki K, Nagai K, Yoshida J, et al: Video-assisted thoracoscopic surgery for small indeterminate pulmonary nodules. Indications for preoperative marking. Chest 1999;115:563-568.

Jiménez MF, The Spanish Video-Assisted Thoracic Surgery Study Group: Prospective study on video-assisted thoracoscopic surgery in the resection of pulmonary nodules: 209 cases from the Spanish Video-Assisted Thoracic Surgery Study Group. Eur J Cardiothorac Surg 2001;19:562-565.

Okumura T, Kondo H, Suzuki K, et al: Fluoroscopy-assisted thoracoscopic surgery after computed tomography–guided bronchoscopic barium marking. Ann Thorac Surg 2001;71:439-442.

Saito H, Minamiya Y, Matsuzaki I, et al: Indication for preoperative localization of small peripheral pulmonary nodules in thoracoscopic surgery. J Thorac Cardiovasc Surg 2002;124:1198-1202.

Yamada S, Kohno T: Video-assisted thoracic surgery for pure ground-glass opacities 2 cm or less in diameter. Ann Thorac Surg 2004;77:1911-1915.

Daniel TM, Altes TA, Rehm PK, et al: A novel technique for localization and excisional biopsy of small or ill-defined pulmonary lesions. Ann Thorac Surg 2004;77:1756-1762.

Others

Goldberg-Kahn B, Healy JC, Bishop JW: The cost of diagnosis. A comparison of four different strategies in the work-up of solitary radiographic lung lesions. Chest 1997;111:870-876.

Andrea S, Paolo C, Ascanelli S, et al: Significance of a single pulmonary nodule in patients with previous history of malignancy. Eur J Cardiothorac Surg 2001;20:1101-1105.

3

Specific Preoperative Assessment

ASSESSMENT OF THE PATIENT WITH PULMONARY METASTASES

For patients with metastatic neoplasms, the lung is one of the *most common sites* of involvement. Approximately 30% of patients with malignant disease will eventually develop pulmonary metastases; for melanomas or sarcomas, the incidence may be as high as 80%. This propensity of malignant tumors to metastasize to the lungs is related to the *venous drainage of most organs,* which is through the caval system into the heart, and then to the lungs. Another reason is the ease of detection of pulmonary metastases through conventional radiographic studies.

In the past, the diagnosis of pulmonary metastases was regarded as evidence of uncontrolled disseminated malignant disease. Autopsy reports have shown, however, that many patients who die of metastatic disease have *no other foci* than those within the lung. For these individuals, the use of local surgical treatment may be appropriate, remembering that of all patients with metastatic disease to the lung, few will be candidates for surgical resection, and even *fewer will be cured* by this modality.

In general, therapeutic success depends on early diagnosis of pulmonary metastases, appropriate selection of patients for operation, complete resection of all metastatic tissue, and above all favorable tumor-host relationship. It also depends on such risk factors as histology of the primary tumor; disease-free interval; and number, size, and location of metastases. When all of these considerations have been looked at and rigid selection criteria have been applied, surgical resection of pulmonary metastases *may have* an impact on survival.

SELECTION CRITERIA FOR RESECTION OF PULMONARY METASTASES

Most institutions have developed guidelines (Table 3-53) for considering patients with malignant neoplasms and pulmonary metastases for resection. The first and foremost criterion is that the *primary tumor must be controlled* (usually by surgical resection), and there must be no evidence of local recurrence. The second is that *complete excision* of all intrathoracic disease is considered feasible by CT scanning. This includes patients likely to require pneumonectomy or extended resections (i.e., pulmonary resection en bloc with chest wall or other intrathoracic structure) and patients who will require bilateral thoracotomies. Third, the patient must have *adequate pulmonary reserve* to allow complete resection of all metastases and a general medical condition that permits thoracotomy. Fourth, no more effective systemic therapy must be available.

Traditionally, the only patients with pulmonary metastasis thought to be resectable were the patients with solitary metastasis. It is now accepted that no single number of lung metastasis excludes patients from metastasectomy as long as a *complete resection* is possible. If present, synchronous extrapulmonary metastasis can also be resected, usually

---

TABLE 3-53

SELECTION CRITERIA FOR RESECTION OF PULMONARY METASTASES

Primary lesion must be controlled locally.

All metastases are presumed resectable.

Adequate pulmonary reserve.

?Metastatic lesions must be limited to the lung without evidence of other sites of distant metastatic disease.

before lung metastasectomy. This is the case, for instance, of patients with synchronous liver and lung metastases from colorectal cancer. One should understand, however, that these aggressive surgeries are only done under *unusual and rare circumstances*.

INVESTIGATION OF THE PATIENT WITH PULMONARY METASTASES

Clinical Assessment

Detection of pulmonary metastases is usually made through imaging techniques because less than 15% of patients will present with symptoms such as cough, hemoptysis, chest pain, or fever. However, a number of other clinical considerations are important in the judicious selection of patients for thoracotomy. Among the most important are the documentation of the *presence or absence of significant weight loss,* of clinical symptoms suggesting *extrapulmonary disease,* and of symptoms relating to a *possible recurrence* of the primary tumor. The surgeon must also look for lymph node or liver enlargement. Indeed, supraclavicular or axillary nodes may be involved in such malignant neoplasms as those from the head and neck region, breast carcinomas, colorectal carcinomas, or renal cell tumors. It is also essential to obtain all possible information about the histology and stage of the primary tumor and about the nature of its treatment before the occurrence of pulmonary metastases.

Imaging Studies

Of the chest radiologic techniques available, conventional radiographs are the least sensitive with a limiting resolution of 5 to 9 mm. CT scanning is currently the *"gold standard"* for the evaluation of pulmonary metastases, with high-resolution and helical CTs able to detect millimetric lung nodules. Unfortunately, CT scanning is not specific because it cannot differentiate benign from malignant processes. It also has some limitations in detecting nodules smaller than 5 to 6 mm.

In patients who have had standard chest radiographs and conventional CT, the overall risk of *underestimating* the number of metastases is 35% to 40%, and the risk of *overestimating* them is in the range of 25% to 30%. Thus, these techniques provide accurate information in only about 70% to 75% of patients.

Biopsy Techniques

When a new lesion develops in the lung of a patient previously treated for a malignant tumor, it *cannot be assumed* that it is automatically a metastasis. Indeed, it is important to differentiate between a metastasis and a primary lung cancer because techniques for staging, operation, and adjuvant treatments are likely to differ substantially. In general, a solitary pulmonary nodule is likely to be a metastasis in 60% to 80% of patients with prior sarcoma or melanoma, in 50% of patients with prior adenocarcinoma, and in less than 20% of patients with prior squamous cell or prostatic carcinoma.

In recent years, transthoracic needle biopsy has been relied on for diagnosis because it provides an accurate and specific means of determining histology. Bronchoscopy, even with transbronchial biopsy, is much less useful, demonstrating diagnostic capabilities in less than 10% of patients. In all cases where an adequate specimen has been obtained by one of these techniques, it is pertinent to *compare it with that of the primary tumor* to determine with maximum accuracy if it is the same neoplasm.

Staging Techniques

The value of mediastinoscopy for assigning stage in patients with lung metastasis is unclear. It appears to be appropriate in patients with large or central metastases; in patients with enlarged mediastinal nodes on CT scan; in patients with multiple metastases; and in patients with primary breast, colorectal, or kidney tumors.

Before recommending surgery, it is also important to restage the primary tumor with appropriate examinations to *rule out* local recurrence. It is also important to determine by the most complete possible work-up if the patient has evidence of other visceral metastatic disease.

ASSESSMENT OF OTHER CONSIDERATIONS FOR OUTCOME AFTER SURGERY

Numerous studies have tried to evaluate prognostic factors (Table 3-54) for patients with metastatic pulmonary disease. Factors such as number of metastases, disease-free interval, tumor doubling time, and tumor histology have been reported by some as important determinants of survival, but none of these factors has been shown to be consistently related to good outcome after surgery.

Histology of the Primary Tumor (Table 3-55)

The histology of the primary tumor is an important consideration. As discussed by Dr. E. C. Holmes, *bone and soft tissue sarcomas* as well as germ cell tumors (testicular) are particularly suitable for resection. Presumably, it is because these tumors tend to preferably metastasize to the lung rather than to other viscera early in the course of disease. By contrast, the role of lung metastasectomy is less clear in tumors such as breast carcinomas and malignant melanomas because these tumors tend to metastasize to other viscera before invading the lung.

Tumor-Host Relationship

Clearly one of the most important factors influencing long-term survival in patients with metastatic cancer to the lung is the *tumor-host relationship* or biologic behavior of the tumor. This tumor-host relationship explains the marked variability in aggressiveness of particular tumor types. Two recognized indexes of specific tumor aggressiveness are the calculated *tumor doubling time* and the *disease-free interval*. Surgery should not be denied on the basis of those criteria alone, especially if the patient is an otherwise good candidate for operation.

TABLE 3-54

RISK FACTORS IN RELATION TO OUTCOME AFTER SURGERY

Risk Factor	Outcome		
	Good	Moderate	Poor
Histology of primary tumor			
Sarcomas, germ cell (testicular)	✓		
Epithelial (colorectal), kidney		✓	
Melanoma, breast			✓
Tumor-host relationship			
Tumor doubling time			
>40 days	✓		
<20 days			✓
Disease-free interval			
>2 years	✓		
6-24 months		✓	
<6 months			✓
Extent of disease			
Number of metastases			
1	✓		
>4			✓
Size of metastases			
<3 cm in diameter	✓		
>3 cm in diameter		✓	
Bilaterality of lesions	✓		
Presence of regional or mediastinal lymph nodes			✓
Availability of effective chemotherapy	✓		

Calculated Tumor Doubling Time

Several authors have shown a *constant rate of growth* for each tumor and an *excellent correlation* between the tumor doubling time of a metastatic tumor and the survival after resection of the pulmonary metastases. Earlier studies have indicated that patients with a tumor doubling time of less than 20 days have a median survival of less than 1 year, whereas patients with a tumor doubling time of more than 40 days have a 65% 5-year survival.

For most patients, however, prospective tumor doubling time measurements are *not particularly useful* not only because it is difficult to

TABLE 3-55

RESULTS OF RESECTION OF PULMONARY METASTASES

	5-Year Survival
Soft tissue sarcoma	30%-60%
Colorectal sarcoma	25%-30%
Renal cell carcinoma	20%-50%
Testicular carcinoma	60%-80%
Melanoma	Very poor
Head and neck squamous cell carcinoma	20%-30%
Breast carcinoma	Very poor

assess the doubling time of small metastases (<1 cm) but also because not all metastases in the same patient may have a similar doubling time.

Disease-Free Interval

The disease-free interval is defined as the time interval *between control of the primary tumor and first observed pulmonary metastases*. In general, most observations have shown that survival rate increases as the disease-free interval becomes longer. This is because longer disease-free intervals are good indicators that the host has been strong enough to contain the disease. Patients who have a disease-free interval of less than 6 months generally do not do well after pulmonary resection of lung metastases, whereas those with an average disease-free interval longer than 2 years fare much better.

Extent of Disease

The extent of disease includes the *number* of pathologically proven metastases, *their sizes*, whether they are *unilateral or bilateral,* and finally whether there is spread to *regional or mediastinal* lymph nodes.

Several studies have shown comparable 5-year survival rates after excision of solitary or multiple metastases. Although there is no threshold number above which pulmonary resection is contraindicated, most studies show *lower survival rates* in patients with four or more metastases. This is particularly true for osteogenic and soft tissue sarcomas.

The size of lung metastases as a predictive value is seldom discussed in the literature. Some authors do, however, report a correlation between a significant drop in 5-year survival rate and metastases that were more than 3 cm in diameter.

Although bilaterality of the lesions does not appear to be detrimental as long as complete resection of the deposits is achievable, the presence of regional or mediastinal lymph nodes is associated with *worse prognosis*. The role of lung metastasectomy is at best doubtful under those circumstances.

Availability of Effective Chemotherapy

The availability of chemotherapy that is *effective* against that particular neoplasm is critical. The excellent chemotherapy available for non-seminomatous testicular tumors, for instance, has permitted the resection of pulmonary metastasis with tumor doubling time of less than 40 days. A trial of chemotherapy will often be an indication that the pulmonary metastases are sensitive to the regimen, and in those cases, surgical resection of the metastases can be carried out. Patients are then continued on postoperative chemotherapy.

PULMONARY METASTASES IN CHILDREN

In children, pulmonary metastases are the most common lung malignancy that is likely to require surgical treatment, and in many cases, surgical excision of lung metastases in association with chemoradiotherapy is beneficial. This strategy applies particularly to children with *Wilms tumors* or those with *osteogenic sarcomas*. In both cases, survival is increased significantly with pulmonary resection regardless of the disease-free interval or bilaterality of the lesions.

CHOICE OF SURGICAL APPROACH

The operative approach in patients with pulmonary metastases varies from institution to institution. In patients with unilateral metastases, some advocate unilateral thoracotomy whereas others support median sternotomy or transverse sternotomy so that both lungs can be examined. This last approach assumes that even the best scanning techniques will have missed 15% to 25% of metastatic nodules.

Patients with initial bilateral disease can be approached by bilateral staged thoracotomies or by median or transverse sternotomy. Resection can also be done through bilateral axillary or anterior thoracotomies.

The role of *video-assisted thoracoscopic surgery* (VATS) has not been fully evaluated and therefore cannot be recommended at this time. The obvious drawback of VATS techniques is that they do not allow adequate palpation of the lungs, and therefore resection is likely to be incomplete.

RESULTS OF SURGICAL RESECTION

The results of surgical resection for the most common primary solid malignant tumors for which pulmonary metastasectomy may be done are listed in Table 3-55.

Osteosarcomas and germ cell tumors are initially treated by chemotherapy before consideration of pulmonary metastasectomy. For patients with renal cell carcinomas, head and neck squamous cell carcinomas, soft tissue sarcomas, and colorectal carcinomas, the initial treatment for pulmonary metastases is resection.

CONCLUSION

Although surgeons have become more aggressive and liberal in their indications for resection of pulmonary metastases, the two prognostic factors that are most important are the tumor-host relationship and the likelihood of resecting all metastatic lung tissue. Increased possibilities of effective chemotherapy may be important in the future.

SUGGESTED READINGS

Review Articles

Holmes EC: The surgical management of pulmonary metastases. Proceedings of the University of Toronto Thoracic Surgery refresher course, Toronto, June 1979.

Harvey JC, Lee K, Beattie EJ: Surgical management of pulmonary metastases. Chest Surg Clin North Am 1994;4:55-66.

Downey RJ: Surgical treatment of pulmonary metastases. Surg Oncol Clin North Am 1999;8:341-354.

3

Specific Preoperative Assessment

Åberg T: Selection mechanisms as major determinants of survival after pulmonary metastasectomy [editorial]. Ann Thorac Surg 1997;63: 611-612.

Putnam JB Jr.: New and evolving treatment methods for pulmonary metastases. Semin Thorac Cardiovasc Surg 2002;14:49-56.

Evaluation

Margaritora S, Porziella V, D'Andrilli A, et al: Pulmonary metastases: can accurate radiological evaluation avoid thoracotomic approach? Eur J Cardiothorac Surg 2002;21:1111-1114.

Pastorino U, Veronesi G, Landoni C, et al: Fluorodeoxyglucose positron emission tomography improves preoperative staging of resectable lung metastases. J Thorac Cardiovasc Surg 2003;126:1906-1910.

Endobronchial Metastases

Katsimbri PP, Bamias AT, Froudarakis ME, et al: Endobronchial metastases secondary to solid tumors: report of eight cases and review of the literature. Lung Cancer 2000;28:163-170.

Thoracoscopy and Pulmonary Metastases

McCormack PM, Ginsberg KB, Bains MS, et al: Accuracy of lung imaging in metastases with implications for the role of thoracoscopy. Ann Thorac Surg 1993;56:863-866.

McCormack PM, Bains MS, Begg CB, et al: Role of video-assisted thoracic surgery in the treatment of pulmonary metastases: results of a prospective trial. Ann Thorac Surg 1996;62:213-217.

Sonett JR: VATS and thoracic oncology: anathema or opportunity [editorial]. Ann Thorac Surg 1999;68:795-796.

Landreneau RJ, De Giacomo T, Mack MJ, et al: Therapeutic video-assisted thoracoscopic surgical resection of colorectal pulmonary metastases. Eur J Cardiothorac Surg 2000;18:671-677.

Laser Surgery

Rolle A, Koch R, Alpard SK, Zwischenberger JB: Lobe-sparing resection of multiple pulmonary metastases with a new 1318-nm Nd:YAG laser—first 100 patients. Ann Thorac Surg 2002;74: 865-869.

Results of Pulmonary Metastasectomy

Wright JO, Brandt B, Ehrenhaft JL: Results of pulmonary resection for metastatic lesions. J Thorac Cardiovasc Surg 1982;83:94-99.

Mountain CF, McMurtrey MJ, Hermes KE: Surgery for pulmonary metastasis: a 20-year experience. Ann Thorac Surg 1984;38:323-330.

Ris HB, Vorburger T, Noce R, et al: Surgery and chemotherapy for pulmonary metastases: long-term results from a combined modality approach. Thorac Cardiovasc Surg 1991;39:224-227.

Putman JB, Swell DM, Natarajan G, Roth JA: Extended resection of pulmonary metastases: is the risk justified? Ann Thorac Surg 1993;55:1440-1446.

Pastorino U, Buyse M, Friedel G, et al: Long-term results of lung metasta-sectomy: prognostic analyses based on 5206 cases. The International Registry of Lung Metastases. J Thorac Cardiovasc Surg 1997;113:37-49.

Robert JH, Ambrogi V, Mermillod B, et al: Factors influencing long-term survival after lung metastasectomy. Ann Thorac Surg 1997;63:777-784.

Spaggiari L, Grunenwald DH, Girard P, et al: Pneumonectomy for lung metastases: indications, risks and outcome. Ann Thorac Surg 1998;66:1930-1933.

Kandioler D, Krömer E, Tüchler H, et al: Long-term results after repeated surgical removal of pulmonary metastases. Ann Thorac Surg 1998;65:909-912.

Jaklitsch MT, Mery CM, Lukanich JM, et al: Sequential thoracic metastasectomy prolongs survival by re-establishing local control within the chest. J Thorac Cardiovasc Surg 2001;121:657-667.

Loehe F, Kobinger S, Hatz RA, et al: Value of systematic mediastinal lymph node dissection during pulmonary metastasectomy. Ann Thorac Surg 2001;72:225-229.

Metastases from Specific Primaries

Okumura S, Kondo H, Tsuboi M, et al: Pulmonary resection for metastatic colorectal cancer: experiences with 159 patients. J Thorac Cardiovasc Surg 1996;112:867-874.

Regnard JF, Grunenwald D, Spaggiari L, et al: Surgical treatment of hepatic and pulmonary metastases from colorectal cancers. Ann Thorac Surg 1998;66:214-219.

Temple LKE, Brennan MF: The role of pulmonary metastasectomy in soft tissue sarcoma. Semin Thorac Cardiovasc Surg 2002;14:35-44.

Friedel G, Pastorino U, Ginsberg RJ, et al: Results of lung metastasectomy from breast cancer: prognostic criteria on the basis of 467 cases of the International Registry of Lung Metastases. Eur J Cardiothorac Surg 2002;22:335-344.

Rena O, Casadio C, Viano F, et al: Pulmonary resection for metastases from colorectal cancer: factors influencing prognosis. Twenty-year experience. Eur J Cardiothorac Surg 2002;21:906-912.

Pfannschmidt J, Muley T, Hoffmann H, Dienemann H: Prognostic factors and survival after complete resection of pulmonary metastases from colorectal carcinoma: experience in 167 patients. J Thorac Cardiovasc Surg 2003;126:732-738.

Monteiro A, Arce N, Bernardo J, et al: Surgical resection of lung metastases from epithelial tumors. Ann Thorac Surg 2004;77:431-437.

Inoue M, Ohta M, Iuchi K, et al: Benefits of surgery for patients with pulmonary metastases from colorectal carcinoma. Ann Thorac Surg 2004;78:238-244.

Metastases in Children

Torre W, Rodriguez-Spiteri N, Sierrasesumaga L: Current role for resection of thoracic metastases in children and young adults. Do we need different strategies for this population? Thorac Cardiovasc Surg 2004;52:90-95.

Others

Joseph WL, Morton DL, Adkins PC: Variation in tumor doubling time in patients with pulmonary metastatic disease. J Surg Oncol 1971;3:143-149.

Rehabilitation and Preparation for a General Thoracic Surgical Procedure

In the 1960s, many centers across North America and Europe began to include rehabilitation as an integral part of the management of patients with chronic obstructive pulmonary disease (COPD). Striking improvements were noted after exercise training, and it soon became clear that *exercise tolerance* and *quality of life* could be optimized through formal rehabilitation. In addition, rehabilitation programs could integrate a comprehensive approach to management that included patient education, energy conservation, relaxation, nutrition, and psychological counseling.

As a result, patients undergoing surgery for emphysema, whether it is lung volume reduction surgery (LVRS) or lung transplantation, have also been asked to participate in formal rehabilitation programs. Indeed, several institutions will not operate on a patient without the patient's active participation in programs in which the focus is on the teaching of proper *breathing exercises, pulmonary toilet, upper body strengthening,* and *nutritional repletion*. In most of these centers, formal rehabilitation is continued postoperatively to improve exercise tolerance and chest wall mechanics.

Rehabilitation of patients with COPD who are to undergo pulmonary resection for lung cancer is based on similar objectives but is currently done in few centers across North America. The ultimate goal of these programs is to improve the patient's endurance and likelihood of normal postoperative recovery.

In addition to pulmonary rehabilitation, preparation for a general thoracic surgical procedure must include optimization of the medical management of comorbidities, education of the patient and psychological support, and correction of nutritional deficiencies if necessary.

PULMONARY REHABILITATION

Objectives

The goals of pulmonary rehabilitation (Table 4-1), according to the American Thoracic Society, are to lessen airflow limitation, to prevent and treat secondary medical complications such as hypoxemia and infections, to decrease respiratory symptoms, and to improve quality of life. Its goal before thoracic surgical intervention is to improve the *patient's endurance* and general health in the hope that these improvements will translate into greater likelihood of a *normal postoperative period*. Stated differently, the assumption is that if the patient is in better physical condition preoperatively, it is less likely that she or he will suffer from major postoperative complications.

TABLE 4-1

GOALS OF PULMONARY REHABILITATION
(AMERICAN THORACIC SOCIETY, 1981)

To lessen airflow limitation
To prevent and treat secondary medical complications
To decrease respiratory symptoms
To improve quality of life
To improve patient's endurance and emotional health

Rehabilitation Before Lung Cancer Surgery

Background

Lung cancer is currently the most common malignant neoplasm in men and women, and approximately 175,000 new cases are diagnosed in the United States each year. Since most of these patients are smokers, it is estimated that 80% to 90% of them have COPD and that 20% to 30% have severe disease. In numerous studies, patients with COPD have been found to be at *higher risk* for postoperative morbidity and death.

Approaching the High-Risk Patient

In approaching the high-risk patient, judgment and experience are paramount in assessing the risks of operation versus its benefits. A carefully obtained clinical history with particular detail to the patient's overall activity level, stamina, and motivation is often *as important* as the FEV_1 or the arterial Po_2.

Over the years, many combinations of parameters, such as forced expiratory volume in 1 second (FEV_1), forced vital capacity (FVC), and diffusion capacity ($DLco$), have been used to assess patients. Unfortunately, these traditionally used criteria have only a modest ability to predict risk. In addition, there has *never been unanimity* in regard to which of these values are absolute contraindications to resection. In some situations, for instance, when the tumor is in an emphysematous lobe, a combination of cancer resection and lung volume reduction (LVRS) may result in an appropriate cancer operation and improved pulmonary function.

Exercise testing has also become increasingly popular to assess risk. Because the results of the test generally correlate with postoperative morbidity, the risk of complications is likely to be reduced if *exercise tolerance is maximized* before operation. In one early report, patients who could not tolerate climbing one flight of stairs without severe dyspnea had a postoperative mortality of 50% versus 10% of those with better tolerance. Other studies have since positively correlated the ability to climb two or three flights of stairs to reduced postoperative morbidity rates. More formalized exercise tests have now been shown to provide *better insight* into the outcome after resection. These include the measurements of oxygen consumption (MVo_2), maximal oxygen uptake ($\dot{V}o_2max$), and exercise oximetry.

Rationale and Goals of Rehabilitation

The main goal of rehabilitation (Table 4-2) is to improve the patient's endurance and exercise performance in the hope that this improvement will result in *more effective cough, increased respiratory muscle strength,* and *lower incidence of major postoperative events.* Another component of preoperative rehabilitation of lung cancer patients is to optimize pharmacologic therapy for COPD. If the patient is a current smoker, immediate cessation of smoking and delay of surgery for at least 3 to 4 weeks is worthwhile, understanding that this delay is *unlikely* to significantly reduce chances for a long-term cure.

Components of Rehabilitation

Most rehabilitation programs for patients awaiting lung cancer surgery are *home based.* The duration and intensity of exercise training depend on the severity of COPD and the patient's prior conditioning and motivation. The form of exercise is directed toward activities that involve large muscles or that mimic activities the patient does every day. For instance, patients are instructed to *walk rather than cycle,* and activities involving upper extremities, such as lifting, are considered less important. Patients are provided with a log book in which they can record dates of exercise, distances walked, and heart rate.

Rehabilitation Before Surgery for End-Stage Emphysema

Background

Historically, plication of giant bullae was the *first operation* advocated for the relief of dyspnea in patients with COPD. Patients were improved if the bulla occupied at least one third of the volume of the hemithorax and was compressive of adjacent lung. Better results were also obtained if the *underlying emphysema was not too severe* and if the compressed lung had potential for function as documented by adequate perfusion and dynamic ventilation. Although a number of authors have reported improvements in expiring flow rates, dyspnea, and exercise tolerance postoperatively, indications for bullectomy are infrequent, mostly because the ideal candidate is seldom seen.

On the contrary, generalized nonbullous emphysema is a progressive, disabling disease that affects almost 2 million people in the United States. Its prevalence is rising, especially among women, whose tobacco use has

---

TABLE 4-2

GOALS OF REHABILITATION IN LUNG CANCER PATIENTS

To increase patient's endurance and exercise performance
To have more effective cough
To have increased respiratory muscle strength
To optimize medical and pharmacologic management
To stop smoking

4

Rehabilitation and Preparation

steadily increased since World War II. The prognosis of patients with COPD is related to a number of factors including decreasing FEV_1 on serial testing. In patients with severe disease characterized by an FEV_1 less than 30% of predicted, the 1-year and 5-year survival rates are 90% and 40%, respectively. In addition to poor survival, the consequent need for repeated admissions to the hospital with ongoing supervision has resulted in a major impact on the use of health care resources.

In 1957, Brantigan and Mueller reported the procedure of LVRS as an innovative surgical approach for the management of emphysema. The operation was aimed at reducing lung volume by resection of functionless tissue. The objective was for the *improved elastic recoil* of the remaining smaller lung to enhance ventilation by placing the muscles of respiration, such as the diaphragm and intercostals, at an improved mechanical advantage. Since then and particularly since 1995, numerous studies have shown that LVRS improves lung function and quality of life at least in the short term. Lung transplantation has also become a viable option for some patients with COPD, with 2-year survival rates exceeding 75%.

Rationale and Goals of Rehabilitation

Preoperative rehabilitation is considered by many the most important component of the entire program of LVRS. The rationale for the use of rehabilitation before LVRS is summarized in Table 4-3.

In general, the primary goal of preoperative rehabilitation is to improve the *strength and aerobic conditioning* of patients, making surgery less traumatic and postoperative recovery faster. Some patients might improve with exercise to such a degree that they no longer need or desire surgery. Similarly, patients not motivated enough for rehabilitation or not compliant with the program are likely to struggle throughout the recovery period, and those patients should not have surgery.

It is understood that *conditioning of the patient* as measured by the 6-minute walk test does improve significantly with rehabilitation. The level of dyspnea and measured pulmonary function do not.

Components of Rehabilitation

In most centers, the targeted goals of rehabilitation are 30 consecutive minutes on a bicycle at 1.5 mph and 30 consecutive minutes on a treadmill at 1.0 mph. These objectives are carried out within a supervised structured rehabilitation program for an average of 8 to 10 weeks before surgery.

TABLE 4-3	
RATIONALE FOR REHABILITATION BEFORE LVRS	
Potential Result of Rehabilitation	Outcome
Improvement in symptoms	May eliminate need for surgery
Noncompliance, poor motivation, inability to exercise	Eliminates poor candidates for LVRS
Improvement in exercise tolerance	Decreases risk of postoperative morbidity

Modified from Kesten S: Pulmonary rehabilitation and surgery for end-stage lung disease. Clin Chest Med 1997;18:173-181.

During exercise, the patient's pulse and oxygen saturation are monitored, and supplemental oxygen is given as necessary to maintain saturation at more than 90%. An evaluation is sent regularly to the physician so that progress can be monitored. Patients may also be asked to do exercise arm ergometry to improve the strength of their upper extremities.

In motivated patients, *home training is effective* and allows the training of patients in regions where supervised programs are unavailable.

Pharmacologic Therapy

Before surgery, all attempts must be undertaken *to optimize pharmacologic therapy* for COPD. The therapy goals are to induce bronchodilation, to decrease bronchial inflammatory reaction, and to facilitate expectorations (Table 4-4). Obviously, such measures will help decrease postoperative morbidity.

Maximum bronchodilation is achieved through the use of beta$_2$ agonists, anticholinergic agents, and theophylline. In dyspneic patients, one can initiate bronchodilation with metered-dose inhalation of a beta$_2$ agonist such as albuterol (Ventolin) or terbutaline (Bricanyl) taken three or four times a day (1 or 2 puffs). Topical administration of an anticholinergic aerosol such as ipratropium (Atrovent), 2 to 6 puffs every 6 to 8 hours, may also be effective, possibly with less troublesome side effects than with albuterol. Theophylline given at a dose of 200 to 400 mg twice a day is of particular value in less compliant or less capable patients, but it has *greater potential for toxicity*. Theophylline may have positive cardiac effects, such as improving cardiac output and reducing pulmonary vascular resistance.

The role of anti-inflammatory drugs like corticosteroids in the preoperative setting is less clear because their use can lead to *postoperative morbidities* related to poor tissue healing (prolonged air leaks, bronchopleural fistula) and infection (pulmonary, empyemas). If they are given, it should be in low doses (40 mg/day) and for a short time (2 to 3 weeks). Patients should be weaned quickly so that steroids have been completely discontinued at the time of operation. In some cases, it is possible to use aerosol steroids such as budesonide (Pulmicort) instead of oral steroids.

Antibiotics should be given if there is pulmonary infection as evidenced by fever, purulent sputum, or radiologic infiltrates. The choice of antibiotic

TABLE 4-4	
PHARMACOTHERAPY FOR COPD	
Objectives	**Drugs**
Bronchodilation	Albuterol (Ventolin), terbutaline (Bricanyl): 1-2 puffs 3-4 times/day
	Ipratropium (Atrovent): 2-6 puffs q 6-8 h
	Theophylline: 200-400 mg bid (orally)
Anti-inflammatory	Corticosteroids, orally: 40 mg/day × 10-14 days
	Budesonide (Pulmicort 400): 2 puffs bid
Drugs affecting mucus	Antibiotics (choice based on sputum culture)

TABLE 4-5
PHYSICAL THERAPY

Objective	Technique
Improved mobilization and clearance of secretions	Chest percussion
	Vibrations, postural drainage
	Cough training
Improved ventilation and cough efficiency	Breathing exercises
Improved deep breathing and lung expansion	Intermittent positive-pressure breathing
	Incentive spirometry

is based on sputum cultures; the major bacteria to be considered are *Streptococcus pneumoniae* and *Haemophilus influenzae*.

Physical Therapy

The objective of aggressive physical therapy (Table 4-5) given preoperatively is to prevent or at least to *minimize* factors that might promote postoperative alveolar collapse and lobar atelectasis. These factors include decreased tidal volume (V_T), decreased functional residual capacity (FRC), absence of sighs, and decreased force of cough. All of these factors are aggravated through the use of sedation, narcotics, and immobility.

Pulmonary physiotherapy includes techniques of *chest percussion, vibration,* and *postural drainage* and teaching of techniques for improved efficiency of cough (chest physiotherapy). The rationale for such measures is based on the belief that additional mechanical and gravitational forces will assist in the mobilization and clearance of airway secretions. Chest physiotherapy is particularly important, and it is our policy that *all patients*, even those with minimal sputum production, must be seen by the physiotherapist before major thoracic surgical procedures.

Breathing training includes the teaching of breathing exercises such as pursed-lip breathing, respiratory muscle training, and exercise training. Collectively, these techniques are designed to improve *diaphragmatic action* and therefore efficiency of ventilation and cough.

More recently, the use of *intermittent positive-pressure breathing* and *incentive spirometry* has been advocated to induce deep breathing and regional expansion of the lung. The presence of an experienced physiotherapist enhances the effectiveness of these mechanical devices, and again, these measures are more useful if they have been taught preoperatively.

OTHER COMPONENTS OF PREPARATION FOR A GENERAL THORACIC PROCEDURE

Optimal Treatment of Comorbidities

One of the goals that must be achieved in preparing a patient for a major thoracic surgical procedure, whether it is for lung or esophageal disease, is the optimization of medical management of comorbidities. If the patient is diabetic (usually type II), for instance, the patient must be seen by an internist (or endocrinologist) to make certain that *medication is well adjusted*.

This is even more important if the patient has borderline renal failure with elevated creatinine. Indeed, the consultant might be invaluable in observing the patient postoperatively and making *necessary readjustments* in both medication and fluid intake.

Cardiovascular therapy may also need to be reviewed, and this is best done by a cardiologist. Diuretics, angiotensin-converting enzyme inhibitors, and calcium channel blockers are useful drugs, but they must be given cautiously to avoid electrolyte imbalance, hypotension, and arrhythmias.

Patients who undergo surgical resection of lung or esophageal cancers are at *increased risk for supraventricular arrhythmias*, the incidence being in the range of 15% to 20%. Unfortunately, this incidence has never been shown to decrease significantly with prophylactic drug management. Over the years, several drugs including digoxin, calcium channel blockers, and beta blockers have been tried, usually in small trials, and have never proved useful. In fact, drugs such as amiodarone have been found to be associated with pulmonary toxicity, and digoxin has the potential to cause or aggravate arrhythmias. Other drugs, such as propranolol, may be associated with such adverse events as hypotension and bradycardia. Currently, the consensus is that because the efficacy of prophylactic drug management has never been clearly documented in the setting of general thoracic procedures, these drugs *should not be given*.

Nutrition

Nutritional deficiencies are commonly associated with COPD, lung cancer, and esophageal cancer. Clinically, these may translate into a significant weight loss or abnormalities of serum nutritional indexes such as albumin, total protein, transferrin, and cholesterol. A deficient nutritional status can also be identified by determination of body mass index. Ultimately, malnutrition will be associated with *impaired respiratory muscle strength, decrease in ventilatory drive,* and *impairment of immune responses*. All of these effects are detrimental to the thoracic surgical patient, who may be more susceptible to postoperative respiratory failure.

Even if common sense dictates that correction of these deficiencies may reduce postoperative morbidity, there is little scientific evidence that this is the case other than for patients with esophageal cancer awaiting esophagectomy.

Patient Education and Psychological Support

On the basis of the premise that better knowledge will translate into improvements in behavior, compliance, and emotional stability, *preoperative education* of patients and their immediate family becomes important. Several studies have shown that patients instructed about the nature of their disease and possible implications of surgery will cooperate better during the postoperative period. This education is done not only by physicians but also by nurses, respiratory therapists, and physical therapists.

Psychosocial support and other similar interventions are also considered essential aspects of a comprehensive approach to general

TABLE 4-6

TOPICS TO BE COVERED DURING PREOPERATIVE INTERVIEW

Results of investigation
Nature of the disease
Treatment options
Indications for surgery
Risks and benefits of surgery
Surgical procedure to be done
Results of surgery

thoracic surgical procedures. In some cases, emotional disorders such as depression or anxiety may become so disabling that patients must be seen by a psychologist or psychiatrist and have some kind of medication introduced before surgery.

Informed Consent and Medicolegal Issues

Before any thoracic surgical procedure, the surgeon must take the time *to meet privately with the patient and the patient's close family* (Table 4-6). During that interview, the surgeon must discuss the results of the investigation, the nature of the disease, the treatment options, the indication for surgery and its risks and benefits, and the surgical procedure to be done. Specific risks, such as recurrent nerve palsy after left upper lobectomy, must be explained. The main causes of postoperative death, usually cardiorespiratory, as well as the possible results of the intervention must also be addressed. This interview usually takes about 20 to 25 minutes or longer if the patient and the family have specific questions that they want to discuss.

At the end of the interview, a *contemporary note (in legible characters)* should be left in the chart, and the patient must sign a consent form for operation. An informed consent does not automatically prevent medicolegal difficulties, but should they arise, this informed consent and the contemporary note will be extremely useful to the surgeon and the defense team.

CONCLUSION

Preparing a patient for a thoracic surgical procedure is complex; most of the time, it requires a *multidisciplinary* and *comprehensive approach*. Exercise training programs are important because they increase strength and endurance of the patient. Other interventions might improve the patient's understanding of the operation and reduce the level of anxiety.

Although scientific evidence that these interventions make a difference is often lacking, a review of clinical endpoints including reduced operative mortality, decreased length of hospital stay, and facilitated hospital discharge suggests that *rehabilitation* and *compulsive preparation* for surgery are useful to the patient.

SUGGESTED READINGS

Review Articles

Peters RM, Turnier E: Physical therapy: indications for and effects in surgical patients. Am Rev Respir Dis 1980;122:147-154.

Rochester DF, Goldberg SK: Techniques of respiratory physical therapy. Am Rev Respir Dis 1980;122:133-146.

Hodgkin JE, Farrell MJ, Gibson SR, et al: American Thoracic Society. Medical Section of the American Lung Association. Pulmonary rehabilitation. Am Rev Respir Dis 1981;124:663-666.

Ries AL: Position paper of the American Association of Cardiovascular and Pulmonary Rehabilitation. Scientific basis of pulmonary rehabilitation. J Cardiopulm Rehab 1990;10:418-441.

Kesten S: Pulmonary rehabilitation and surgery for end-stage lung disease. Clin Chest Med 1997;18:173-181.

Chronic Obstructive Pulmonary Disease and Rehabilitation

Howland J, Nelson EC, Barlow PB, et al: Chronic obstructive airway disease. Impact of health education. Chest 1986;90:233-238.

American Thoracic Society: Comprehensive outpatient management of COPD. Am J Respir Crit Care Med 1995;152:s84-s96.

Celli BR: Pulmonary rehabilitation in patients with COPD [clinical commentary]. Am J Respir Crit Care Med 1995;152:861-864.

O'Donnell DE, Aaron S, Bourbeau J, et al: Canadian Thoracic Society recommendations for management of chronic obstructive pulmonary disease—2003. Can Respir J 2003;10(suppl A):11a-33a.

Nutrition

Wilson DO, Rogers RM, Hoffman RM: Nutrition and chronic lung disease. Am Rev Respir Dis 1985;132:1347-1365.

Schols AMWJ, Soeters PB, Dingemans AMC, et al: Prevalence and characteristics of nutritional depletion in patients with stable COPD eligible for pulmonary rehabilitation. Am Rev Respir Dis 1993;147:1151-1156.

Mazolewski P, Turner JF, Baker M, et al: The impact of nutritional status on the outcome of lung volume reduction surgery. A prospective study. Chest 1999;116:693-696.

Arrhythmias

Bayliff CD, Massel DR, Inculet RI, et al: Propranolol for the prevention of postoperative arrhythmias in general thoracic surgery. Ann Thorac Surg 1999;67:182-186.

Rehabilitation and Lung Volume Reduction

Brantigan OC, Mueller E: Surgical treatment of pulmonary emphysema. Am Surg 1957;23:789-804.

Cooper JC, Patterson GA, Sundoresan RS, et al: Results of 150 consecutive bilateral lung volume reduction procedures in patients with severe emphysema. J Thorac Cardiovasc Surg 1996;112:1319-1330.

Exercise Capacity and Postoperative Complications

Bolliger CT, Jordan P, Solèr M, et al: Exercise capacity as a predictor of postoperative complications in lung resection candidates. Am J Respir Crit Care Med 1995;151:1472-1480.

Others

Lheureux M, Raherison C, Vernejoux JM, et al: Quality of life in lung cancer: does disclosure of the diagnosis have an impact? Lung Cancer 2004;43:175-182.

Intraoperative Care

BRONCHOSCOPY BY SURGEONS

Bronchoscopy is invaluable to all physicians dealing with diseases of the respiratory system. It permits clear visualization of the tracheo-bronchial tree with little risk and discomfort to the patient. It is an *essential diagnostic modality*, and it may also have therapeutic implications in many situations.

The rigid bronchoscope became popular in the 1950s, and it is still the optimal instrument for control of hemoptysis or management of severe airway obstruction. The flexible bronchoscope, which was introduced in the 1970s, has its greatest use in *diagnostic procedures*. Both should be considered complementary to each other in their indications and applications.

Bronchoscopy is currently performed by a variety of physicians including pneumologists, thoracic surgeons, anesthetists, intensivists, and otolaryngologists. In several institutions throughout the United States, all diagnostic bronchoscopies are performed by *chest physicians* who have become familiar and experienced with the technique. This should not, however, be considered a reversal of roles, and the thoracic surgeon must still have a *clear understanding* of all aspects of flexible and rigid bronchoscopy, including indications, anesthetic techniques, instrumentation, and possible complications. The thoracic surgeon must also be familiar with the basic techniques of airway examination, such as biopsy, washing, and brushing.

PREBRONCHOSCOPIC EVALUATION AND POSSIBLE CONTRAINDICATIONS

Clinical history and review of available radiographs and computed tomographic (CT) scans form the basis of the prebronchoscopic evaluation. This information allows the physician to *determine the indication* and to *formulate a plan of examination*, including techniques of anesthesia, instrumentation, and specimens to be obtained.

Platelet count, bleeding time, and prothrombin time should be obtained. Any abnormality must be corrected before bronchoscopy.

One of the most important aspects of prebronchoscopic evaluation is to *inform the patient* about the upcoming procedure and possible discomforts. If the endoscopist takes the appropriate time to do this interview properly, few patients will be unable to cooperate during the examination.

Possible contraindications are all relative, and they do not necessarily preclude a carefully performed bronchoscopy. These include bleeding disorders (whether they are pathologic or due to anticoagulants), severe hypoxemia, cardiovascular instability, and severe asthma. In some cases, severe cervical arthritis may prevent neck extension, which is necessary for rigid bronchoscopy, or maxillofacial abnormalities may prevent the safe passage of the flexible bronchoscope.

FLEXIBLE BRONCHOSCOPY

The flexible bronchoscope has revolutionized the procedure of bronchoscopy because of *extended visual range* into the bronchial tree, *ease of insertion*, and *minimal discomfort*. The procedure is relatively easy to learn and can be used with topical anesthesia and minimal sedation. It is relatively *low risk* to the patient.

Indications

Diagnostic Bronchoscopy (Table 5-1)

The most common indication for diagnostic flexible bronchoscopy is an *abnormal finding on chest radiography*, such as a lung mass, atelectasis, diffuse pulmonary infiltrates, or unresolving pleural effusions. The exact location of the lesion can be identified, and biopsy of the mass can be performed. If the lesion is in an intermediate or peripheral location, it can be brushed under biplane fluoroscopic control. In cases of diffuse infiltrates, bronchoalveolar lavage with or without transbronchial lung biopsy frequently helps determine the cause of the infiltrates. These techniques are particularly useful in debilitated or immunosuppressed individuals.

Symptoms of bronchopulmonary disease sometimes suggest a bronchial lesion even in the absence of chest radiographic abnormalities. These include a *persistent cough, hemoptysis,* and *pulmonary osteoarthropathy.* Hemoptysis associated with a wheeze may be caused by bronchial obstruction whether it is malignant or not.

Flexible bronchoscopy can also be useful to localize a bronchogenic carcinoma in a patient with positive sputum but normal radiographs and in the planning of lung cancer operations. Indeed, no patient should have lung cancer surgery without prior bronchoscopy because the decision to perform specific types of resection is often based on the determination of the exact location of the tumor. In all cases of central tumors that may require sleeve resection, or if it is unclear whether a lobectomy or a pneumonectomy will be required, the surgeon must assess the location

TABLE 5-1

POSSIBLE INDICATIONS FOR DIAGNOSTIC FLEXIBLE BRONCHOSCOPY

Abnormal radiographic finding: lung mass, diffuse infiltrates, atelectasis, pleural effusion
Abnormal symptom: cough, hemoptysis, stridor, wheeze (localized)
Lung cancer: diagnosis, localization of occult cancer, planning of resection,
   transbronchial needle aspiration of lymph nodes
Significant hemoptysis (≤400 mL/24 h)
Follow-up of patients after lung transplantation
Diagnosis and follow-up with bronchoalveolar lavage of sarcoidosis, fibrosing alveolitis
Others: possible airway obstruction, lung abscess, possible laryngeal abnormality
   (vocal and paralysis), thoracic trauma

of the tumor. Mediastinal lymph nodes can be sampled by the technique of transbronchial needle aspiration.

Significant ($\leq$400 mL/24 h) but not life-threatening (>150 mL/1 h) hemoptysis is also an indication for diagnostic fiberoptic bronchoscopy. The purpose of the examination is to locate the *site of hemoptysis* and *its cause*. The flexible bronchoscope is also used extensively in the management of the lung transplant recipient. The diagnosis of infection or rejection, for instance, is heavily dependent on bronchoscopy. The patient may undergo transbronchial lung biopsy for diagnosis of rejection, and bronchoalveolar lavage is used to diagnose pulmonary infections.

Other possible indications are listed in Table 5-1. In lung abscesses, bronchoscopy is used not only to determine if there is bronchial obstruction (cancer, foreign body) but also to try to *enter the cavity endobronchially* and *initiate drainage*. In thoracic trauma, all patients with possible airway injury should have bronchoscopy.

Therapeutic Bronchoscopy (Table 5-2)

One of the most common indications for therapeutic flexible bronchoscopy is pulmonary toilet through aspiration of retained secretions or mucous plugs. This is used in patients unable to clear their secretions, whether they have had a thoracic operation or not. If the patient is intubated, the bronchofiberscope can also be used to check and reposition the endotracheal tube if necessary. In this setting, fiberoptic bronchoscopy should be used liberally, and it is always done at bedside.

The flexible bronchoscope can be used for difficult intubations. In such cases, the bronchoscope is advanced in the airway and used as a guide to introduce the endotracheal tube. It is also used by anesthetists to check that a *disposable double-lumen tube is properly positioned.* This is done after insertion of the tube, after the patient has been placed in the lateral decubitus (posterolateral thoracotomy) position, and at any other time that the tube may have been displaced during the operation.

The fiberoptic bronchoscope can be helpful in the management of postoperative bronchopleural fistulas. It can be used to help position long endotracheal tubes for single-lung ventilation or for fistula occlusion with tissue glues or glutaraldehyde glues. These glues are delivered to the fistula site through the operating channel of the bronchoscope or more often through a catheter passed alongside the bronchoscope.

TABLE 5-2
POSSIBLE INDICATIONS FOR THERAPEUTIC FLEXIBLE BRONCHOSCOPY
Bronchial toilet (aspiration of bronchial secretions)
Difficult endotracheal intubation and placement of double-lumen endotracheal tube
Treatment of bronchopleural fistula
Removal of foreign bodies
Laser therapy, brachytherapy

TABLE 5-3	
TECHNIQUE OF FIBEROPTIC BRONCHOSCOPY	
Most are done on an outpatient basis	
Nothing by mouth for 12 hours before procedure	
Premedication	
Atropine, 0.3-0.6 mg	
Midazolam (Versed), 2-4 mg; or fentanyl, 100-200 µg	
Topical anesthesia with lidocaine 2%	
Oxygen therapy and monitoring of oxygen saturation	
Nothing by mouth for 2-4 hours after bronchoscopy	

On occasion, the flexible bronchoscope can be used to identify or even to remove small foreign bodies. For larger foreign bodies, however, the rigid bronchoscope is the instrument of choice.

The development of lasers has permitted the treatment of a wide variety of lesions through the flexible bronchoscope. Similarly, the flexible bronchoscope is necessary to institute brachytherapy, in which catheters containing radioactive materials are placed close to endobronchial malignant tumors.

Technique and Instrumentation (Table 5-3)

Flexible bronchoscopy is a safe and reliable technique that is usually done in an outpatient facility. Ideally, the patient has had nothing by mouth for at least 12 hours before the procedure.

Most patients are premedicated with an anticholinergic drug (atropine, 0.3 to 0.6 mg) to reduce secretions and to inhibit vasovagal responses. They also receive an intravenous sedative (midazolam [Versed], 2 to 4 mg; fentanyl, 100 to 200 µg) for comfort. Local topical anesthetics are then applied to the airway with the purpose of blunting laryngeal and cough reflexes. These agents, such as lidocaine 2%, are applied to nasal, posterior pharyngeal, and proximal airway and are administered by spray or gargle. Additional lidocaine may be administered by direct spray through the suction port of the bronchoscope under direct vision. The flexible bronchoscope is then introduced nasally or orally by use of a mouth guard, or it can be inserted through an endotracheal tube under general anesthesia. To prevent aspiration, the patient should have nothing by mouth for 2 to 4 hours after bronchoscopy.

Fiberoptic bronchoscopes are *classified* according to the *diameter of their distal ends.* Standard adult scopes are 5 or 6 mm in outside diameter with a 2.2- to 2.8-mm working channel. Pediatric scopes are typically 3.5 or 3.6 mm with a smaller working channel. Light is transmitted through fiberoptic bundles, and the field of vision is usually 80 degrees.

Advantages (Table 5-4)

There are several advantages of fiberoptic bronchoscopy over rigid bronchoscopy. First and foremost, there is *minimal discomfort for the patient* during or after the procedure. The small-diameter flexible scope

TABLE 5-4

ADVANTAGES OF FLEXIBLE BRONCHOSCOPY

Minimal discomfort for the patient
Extended visual range to subsegments
Specimens obtained by various methods
Low risk to patient
Done as outpatient procedure and at bedside
Complications are infrequent and mild

offers *extended visual range*, even into subsegmental levels, allowing more precise cytologic and histologic diagnosis. Specimens are obtained by direct forceps biopsy, washings, needle biopsies, or transbronchial biopsies, all at relatively low risk to the patient. It can be done at bedside in an outpatient facility.

Limitations and Complications

The most important limitation relates to the size of the fiberoptic bronchoscope. Smaller scopes do not allow easy clearing of secretions, mucus, or blood (smaller suction channels).

Flexible bronchoscopy performed by experienced endoscopists is a *safe procedure.* The risk of mortality is less than 1%, and major complications occur in less than 2% of patients. These include respiratory depression, hypercapnia, bronchospasm (which can be severe), hypoxia, arrhythmias, aspiration, pneumothorax, and significant hemorrhage. It is uncommon, however, that bleeding significant enough to warrant thoracotomy is initiated.

RIGID BRONCHOSCOPY

Rigid bronchoscopy is preferable in cases of airway obstruction, with massive hemoptysis, and for the removal of foreign bodies. With the introduction of rigid telescopes with high-quality optics, large biopsy specimens can be obtained, and visualization of segmental bronchi is now possible.

Indications (Diagnostic and Therapeutic) (Table 5-5)

One of the most important indications of rigid bronchoscopy is the *evaluation and management* of patients with massive (>600 mL/24 h) or life-threatening (>150 mL/1 h) hemoptysis. In such cases, the rigid

TABLE 5-5

INDICATIONS FOR RIGID BRONCHOSCOPY (DIAGNOSTIC AND THERAPEUTIC)

Massive (>600 mL/24 h) or life-threatening (>150 mL/1 h) hemoptysis
Control of airway obstruction
    Benign disease: dilatation, diagnosis, evaluation of resectability
    Malignant disease: diagnosis, debulking to provide early treatment, evaluation of
       resectability, stenting, laser
Removal of foreign body
Pediatric bronchoscopy

5

Intraoperative Care

bronchoscope provides the operator with *immediate control of the airway.* In addition, it permits the use of large-bore suction equipment to keep the airway clear of blood and clots.

The rigid bronchoscope is also the instrument of choice and safest modality for diagnosis of conditions that produce significant airway obstruction. These include benign processes, such as *tracheal strictures* after intubation or after tracheotomy, and *malignant diseases* of the airway. On occasion, the bronchoscope can be used to débride the tumor directly with biopsy forceps or electrocautery and re-establish airway control. If the tumor is unresectable, additional intervention that can be done with the rigid bronchoscope includes airway stenting or laser therapy. If the obstruction is due to a benign stricture, it can be dilated with sequential passage of bronchoscopes of increasing diameters. In both cases (malignant and benign obstruction), the rigid bronchoscope allows an *accurate assessment* of the location, caliber, length, and rigidity of the stricture as well as the status of the distal airway.

In general, large foreign bodies in proximal bronchi are much easier to remove with the rigid bronchoscope than with the flexible scope. In children with small airways, often the only available option to inspect the airway is the use of a pediatric rigid bronchoscope.

Technique and Instrumentation (Table 5-6)

Although rigid bronchoscopy can be carried out at bedside and under topical anesthesia, it is usually done under *general anesthesia* and in *an operating room.* Intravenous or inhalation general anesthesia can be used for induction. During bronchoscopy, various techniques of ventilation are available; these include intermittent insufflation, continuous insufflation, and jet ventilation. The most common form of ventilation is the *Venturi technique or jet ventilation.* Through the side port or the open proximal end of the scope, a high-pressure jet of oxygen entrains surrounding air, thus ventilating the patient throughout the procedure (Fig. 5-1).

The rigid, open-tube bronchoscopes commonly used in adults have an internal diameter of 6, 7, or 8 mm and are 40 cm in length. A ventilating side port (ventilating bronchoscope) permits assisted ventilation (Fig. 5-1). Visualization can be enhanced with 0-, 30-, and 90-degree telescopes.

Advantages

There are several advantages to rigid bronchoscopy over flexible bronchoscopy in dealing with significant airway obstruction. In such cases, the rigid bronchoscope allows dilatation of the lesion, maintenance of adequate control of the airway, and evacuation of clots and secretions if necessary.

TABLE 5-6

TECHNIQUE OF RIGID BRONCHOSCOPY

Generally done under general anesthesia in operating room

Extensive cervical fusion may prevent adequate positioning

Induction with intravenous drugs or inhalation general anesthesia

Jet ventilation during the procedure (Venturi technique) through ventilating side port

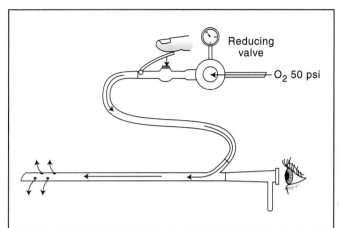

FIG. 5-1

Schematic illustration of the modified Sanders jet ventilation technique for ventilation through a rigid bronchoscope. The side port of the bronchoscope is used as the Venturi injector site, and the open end can be used for continuous viewing by the endoscopist. *(From Ehrennerth J, Brull S: Anesthesia for thoracic diagnostic procedures. In Kaplan JA, ed: Anesthesia, 2nd ed. New York, Churchill Livingstone, 1991.)*

The rigid bronchoscope is also necessary when the airway has to be stented. The other significant usefulness of rigid bronchoscopy is the investigation of life-threatening hemoptysis. In such cases, bleeding is profuse, and complete removal of blood may be difficult to achieve with a flexible bronchoscope. Rigid bronchoscopy provides the operator with *immediate and safe control* of the airway.

Limitations and Complications (Table 5-7)

Two major disadvantages of rigid bronchoscopy are, first, that it must be done under general anesthesia and, second, that it must be done by an

TABLE 5-7

LIMITATIONS AND COMPLICATIONS OF RIGID BRONCHOSCOPY

Must be done under general anesthesia
Must be done by an operator familiar with the technique
Inability of the patient to extend the neck is a contraindication
Visualization of only major lobar orifices
Biopsy not possible at segmental level
Possible complications
    Complications related to general anesthesia
    Major hemorrhage
    Subcutaneous emphysema or pneumothorax from the use of Venturi ventilation

operator who is *familiar with the technique.* Unfortunately, most people currently doing bronchoscopic examinations are unfamiliar with the technique of rigid bronchoscopy. Indeed, most young chest physicians or thoracic surgeons have never seen let alone done a single rigid bronchoscopy. Another limitation of rigid bronchoscopy is that the patient must be able to extend the neck, and that may be prevented by extensive cervical fusion or ankylosing spondylitis. From a visual point of view, the limitation of rigid bronchoscopy is that it goes only as far as major lobar orifices, so that brushing and biopsy *cannot easily* be accomplished at the segmental level.

There are many potential complications of rigid bronchoscopy, but most can be avoided with careful technique. Major hemorrhage can occur when excessive or ill-advised biopsy specimens are taken. Major anesthetic complication can occur with misuse of the Venturi technique. High-pressure jet ventilation can produce surgical emphysema or rupture of pulmonary bullae with secondary pneumothorax.

VIRTUAL BRONCHOSCOPY (TABLE 5-8)

During recent years, thin-section spiral CT and three-dimensional image data-processing techniques have become important diagnostic methods for depicting endoluminal airway diseases. Most commonly, these radiologic techniques use spiral CT data that are reconstructed into a large number of axial images for diagnostic interpretation. The advantage of virtual bronchoscopy over flexible bronchoscopy is that it is *less invasive* and *better tolerated by patients*. Another advantage is that it allows simultaneous visualization of airways and adjacent mediastinal structures such as blood vessels, therefore enabling a more accurate assessment of the surgical implication of the lesion being studied. It is also useful in the planning of palliative treatments, such as laser therapy and application of stents.

The main disadvantage of virtual bronchoscopy is that biopsy specimens *cannot be obtained.* Other potential disadvantages are that it may not be accurate in all cases, especially if the lesion is in more peripheral airways, and that it is unable to provide reliable information about mucosal

TABLE 5-8
ADVANTAGES AND DISADVANTAGES OF VIRTUAL BRONCHOSCOPY
ADVANTAGES
Better tolerated by patients
Simultaneous visualization of airway and adjacent mediastinal structures
More accurate assessment of surgical implications
Planning of palliative procedures
DISADVANTAGES
Biopsy not possible
Not 100% accurate
Underestimation of mucosal involvement
Radiation exposure

abnormalities proximal or distal to the lesion. Finally, a significant disadvantage is the radiation exposure that is necessary to scan the patient.

CONCLUSION

Although the introduction of the fiberoptic bronchoscope has led to its widespread use mostly by medical specialists (nonsurgeons), every thoracic surgeon should be familiar with the technique, and *proper training* should be an integral part of every thoracic surgery residency program. Every resident should be comfortable with the use of both the rigid and flexible bronchoscope under local or general anesthesia. The current availability of computerized training models may help achieve these goals.

SUGGESTED READINGS

Review Articles

Sokolowski JW, Burgher LW, Jones FL, et al: American Thoracic Society Guidelines for fiberoptic bronchoscopy in adults. Am Rev Respir Dis 1987;136:1066.

Dellinger RP: Fiberoptic bronchoscopy in adult airway management. Crit Care Med 1990;18:882-887.

Arroliga AC, Matthay RA: The role of bronchoscopy in lung cancer. Clin Chest Med 1993;14:87-98.

Ahmad M, Dweik RA: Future of flexible bronchoscopy. Clin Chest Med 1999;20:1-17.

Karmy-Jones R, Cuschieri J, Vallières E: Role of bronchoscopy in massive hemoptysis. Chest Surg Clin North Am 2001;11:873-906.

Raoof S, Mehrishi S, Prakash UB: Role of bronchoscopy in modern medical intensive care unit. Clin Chest Med 2001;22:241-261.

Becker HD: Bronchoscopy. Year 2001 and beyond. Clin Chest Med 2001;22:225-239.

Wain JC: Rigid bronchoscopy: the value of a venerable procedure. Chest Surg Clin North Am 2001;11:691-699.

Wood DE: Management of malignant tracheobronchial obstruction. Surg Clin North Am 2002;82:621-642.

Anesthesia for Flexible and Rigid Bronchoscopy

Perrin G, Colt HG, Martin C, et al: Safety of interventional rigid bronchoscopy using intravenous anesthesia and spontaneous assisted ventilation. A prospective study. Chest 1992;102:1526-1530.

Dich-Nielsen JO, Nagel P: Flexible fiberoptic bronchoscopy via the laryngeal mask. Acta Anaesthesiol Scand 1993;37:17-19.

Sivarajan M, Stoler E, Kil HK, Bishop MJ: Jet ventilation using fiberoptic bronchoscopes. Anesth Analg 1995;80:384-387.

Ferson DZ, Nesbitt JC, Nesbitt KK, et al: The laryngeal mask airway: a new standard for airway evaluation in thoracic surgery. Ann Thorac Surg 1997;63:768-772.

Natalini G, Cavaliere S, Seramondi V, et al: Negative pressure ventilation vs. external high-frequency oscillation during rigid bronchoscopy. A controlled randomized trial. Chest 2000;118:18-23.

Okada S, Ishimori S, Sato M, et al: Endoscopic surgery with use of a laryngeal mask and a fiberoptic flexible bronchoscope. J Thorac Cardiovasc Surg 2001;121:1196-1197.

High-Risk Bronchoscopy

Snow N, Lucas AE: Bronchoscopy in the critically ill surgical patient. Am Surg 1984;50:441-445.

Flores RM, Sugarbaker DJ: High-risk bronchoscopy. Ann Thorac Surg 2000;69:1604-1605.

Virtual Bronchoscopy

Seemann MD, Claussen CD: Hybrid 3D visualization of the chest and virtual endoscopy of the tracheobronchial system: possibilities and limitations of clinical application. Lung Cancer 2001;32:237-246.

Lacasse Y, Martel S, Hébert A, et al: Accuracy of virtual bronchoscopy to detect endobronchial lesions. Ann Thorac Surg 2004;77:1774-1780.

Bronchoscopy Training

Hilmi OJ, White PS, McGurty DW, Oluwole M: Bronchoscopy training: is simulated surgery effective? Clin Otolaryngol 2002;27:267-269.

Blum MG, Powers TW, Sundaresan S: Bronchoscopy simulator effectively prepares junior residents to competently perform basic clinical bronchoscopy. Ann Thorac Surg 2004;78:287-291.

Others

Slinger P, Robinson R, Shennib H, et al: Alternative technique for laser resection of a carinal obstruction. J Cardiothorac Vasc Anesth 1992;6:749-755.

Hollaus PH, Lax F, Janakiev D, et al: Endoscopic treatment of postoperative bronchopleural fistula: experience with 45 cases. Ann Thorac Surg 1998;66:923-927.

Zerella JT, Dimler M, McGill LC, Pippus KJ: Foreign body aspiration in children: value of radiography and complications of bronchoscopy. J Pediatr Surg 1998;33:1651-1654.

McLean AN, Semple PD, Franklin DH, et al: The Scottish multi-center prospective study of bronchoscopy for bronchial carcinoma and suggested audit standards. Respir Med 1998;92:1110-1115.

Dasgupta A, Mehta AC: Transbronchial needle aspiration. An underused diagnostic technique. Clin Chest Med 1999;20:39-51.

Duhamel DR, Harrell JH: Laser bronchoscopy. Chest Surg Clin North Am 2001;11:769-789.

PRINCIPLES OF ANESTHESIA FOR PULMONARY RESECTION

During the past 20 years, anesthesia for noncardiac thoracic surgical procedures has evolved substantially. The *"disposable" double-lumen tube* introduced in the early 1980s, for instance, is a good example of new technology that has made "one-lung anesthesia" much safer. Similarly, the introduction of *epidural catheters* in the mid-1980s not only changed the conduct of postoperative analgesia but also allowed the anesthetist to reduce the "depth" of anesthesia during lung resectional procedures. During the 1990s, potent new "short-acting" drugs allowed a more controlled anesthesia with rapid emergence.

To be safe and reliable, thoracic anesthesia must be administered by anesthetists who are well trained and have gained experience in this field. They also must have good knowledge of the anatomy and physiology of the respiratory system, and, most important, they must be able to work in conjunction with a surgeon with whom they share the airway.

PREANESTHETIC EVALUATION

Most patients are evaluated on an outpatient basis a few days or weeks before the actual surgery (Table 5-9). During this visit, the anesthetist evaluates the upper airway and makes sure that there are no problems that could preclude the introduction of a double-lumen tube. For instance, the anesthetist approximates the tracheal diameter so that he or she can select the proper size of the double-lumen tube. Similarly, he or she documents significant tracheal deviation or compression that could have important implications during intubation.

The anesthetist reviews the results of routine laboratory tests and, most important, of the *pulmonary function studies*. The results of cardiac evaluation are looked at carefully, as are those related to other significant comorbidities that may possibly affect the conduct of general anesthesia.

The anesthetist is interested in musculoskeletal disorders, such as osteoarthritis of the spine, which may complicate the insertion of an epidural catheter, or frozen shoulders, which may complicate lateral positioning. The anesthetist finally wants to document the presence of *neuromuscular abnormalities*, such as myasthenia gravis, which are sometimes associated with intrathoracic tumors.

5

Intraoperative Care

TABLE 5-9
OBJECTIVES OF PREANESTHETIC VISIT
Evaluation of upper airway
Assessment of pulmonary function
Assessment of cardiac function
Recording of significant comorbidities
Recording of musculoskeletal or neuromuscular disorders

At the end of the visit, the anesthetist *discusses the anesthetic plan* and postoperative analgesic program with the patient and prescribes the premedication.

IMMEDIATE PREOPERATIVE CARE

On the day of surgery, the patient is requested to take *his or her regular cardiovascular and pulmonary medication;* other drugs are given on a per case basis. A few hours before the operation, the patient receives a premedication, which is usually a benzodiazepine. At that time, the attending anesthetist may further review the results of the preoperative evaluation and look again at standard radiographs and CT scans just to make sure that there will be no problems inserting the double-lumen tube.

Before arterial cannulation and before insertion of the epidural catheter, the patient's sedation is further readjusted with intravenous benzodiazepine and narcotics.

CONDUCT OF ANESTHESIA

Monitoring

In addition to basic and standard monitoring (Table 5-10), peripheral arterial cannulation is an important consideration for patients undergoing pulmonary resection. It allows for monitoring of arterial (systemic) blood pressure, recording of possible hemodynamic perturbations likely to occur during mediastinal compression, and serial blood gas determinations, which are essential during one-lung anesthesia. Standard requirements also include electrocardiography and urine output, which is usually quantified every 15 to 30 minutes.

Central venous pressure monitoring can be added, although most centers use this modality only when *fluid management is a critical issue,* such as in the patient with known heart failure or the patient undergoing pneumonectomy. Although central venous pressure values are not completely reliable when the patient is in the lateral position and has the chest and pleural space opened, a trend can be recorded, and this trend is usually helpful for fluid administration. To avoid iatrogenic pneumothoraces while inserting the central venous pressure line, some anesthetists use the

---

TABLE 5-10

MONITORING DURING PULMONARY RESECTION

Hemodynamic monitoring
    Essential: electrocardiography, arterial line, urinary catheter
    By indication: central venous line, Swan-Ganz catheter
Respiratory monitoring
    Essential: FIO_2, $ETCO_2$, pulse oxymetry, arterial blood gases (arterial line)
    By indication: sidestream spirometry
Others
    Essential: monitoring of central temperature
    By indication: transesophageal echocardiography

internal or external jugular vein. When a patient has superior vena cava obstruction, one must install an intravenous line in the lower extremity so that fluids, blood, or drugs can reach the systemic circulation.

Pulmonary artery catheterization is *seldom used* during lung resection because most patients with severe cardiac failure are not candidates for this type of surgery. If a Swan-Ganz catheter has been used and is positioned on the side of surgery, it must always be *withdrawn* before vascular stapling just to make sure it is not included in the stapling line or transected. On occasion, *transesophageal echocardiography* will be used to monitor cardiac function.

Standard respiratory monitoring includes measurements of *fraction of inspired oxygen (FIO_2)*, end-tidal carbon dioxide ($ETCO_2$), *pulse oxymetry (SpO_2)*, and *arterial blood gases.* This monitoring is extremely valuable during one-lung ventilation, when respiratory parameters are likely to fluctuate. An oxygen saturation of 97% to 100% as documented by SpO_2 can, for instance, reflect large variations in PaO_2 (89 to 400 mm Hg), and, because of such variations, continuous online monitoring of PaO_2 is still considered unreliable.

During one-lung ventilation, additional respiratory monitoring can include sidestream spirometry, which provides continuous monitoring of volume, pressure, and flow within the respiratory circuit. Plotted in pressure-volume and flow-volume loops, these measurements are helpful to evaluate the airtightness or displacement of endobronchial tubes, the presence of auto-positive end-expiratory pressure (auto-PEEP), and the effect of ventilatory pattern on pulmonary mechanics and air leaks after reinstitution of bilateral ventilation.

Central body temperature is finally monitored, and efforts must be made to prevent intraoperative hypothermia.

Position of the Patient

Most patients undergoing pulmonary resection are placed in the lateral decubitus position. During positioning, the anesthetist must make sure that neurologic and vascular structures of the shoulder *are protected* from pressure or traction injuries. A pillow placed in the axilla is often enough protection against compression of the brachial plexus.

Despite these precautions, it is not unusual that the shoulder is painful for one or more days postoperatively. Possible explanations for this phenomenon include stretching of the brachial plexus due to hyperextension of the shoulder, stretching of the shoulder capsule due to inadequate support of the arm, compression of nerve roots as they exit the spine (often related to a poor alignment of the cervical spine), or irritation of the brachial plexus from the chest tube, or the pain can originate from the diaphragm and be referred to the shoulder.

During positioning, it is nearly impossible to prevent some displacement of the double-lumen tube. It is therefore important to *reassess endoscopically* where the tube is located once the patient has been turned on the side.

5

Intraoperative Care

Induction and Maintenance of Anesthesia

For most patients, general anesthesia is induced by an intravenous agent and maintained throughout the procedure by volatile anesthetics and intravenous narcotics. Although volatile anesthetics inhibit hypoxic pulmonary vasoconstriction, a phenomenon that may interfere with oxygenation during one-lung ventilation, this effect is dose and agent dependent. General anesthesia can also be maintained through the continuous infusion of short-acting agents, such as propofol, and of narcotics, which do not interfere with hypoxic pulmonary vasoconstriction.

Deep muscle relaxation (curarization) is important to prevent diaphragmatic movements because such movements may interfere with the conduct of the operation. Inadequate muscle relaxation may also compromise ventilation of the down lung.

Intraoperative Analgesia

Although it is still controversial, most anesthetists agree that the use of "preincisional" analgesia drugs or of regional anesthesia techniques helps decrease the "depth" of general anesthesia required during surgery. It may also promote earlier awakening during the immediate postoperative period as well as decrease the intensity of immediate post-thoracotomy pain.

These are some of the reasons why epidural catheters are inserted before the induction of anesthesia while the patient is still awake and in the lateral decubitus position (or sitting down). The catheter is introduced at the level of the *thoracic or lumbar spine*, and nervous stimulation confirms its proper location. Some centers also use fluoroscopic imaging to make sure that the epidural catheter is indeed at the right place. During the operation, bupivacaine in combination with fentanyl citrate or less frequently with morphine sulfate is used.

Because there is a risk of intraspinal hematoma associated with spinal puncture, the administration of subcutaneous heparin should be postponed for at least 1 hour after an atraumatic peridural catheterization.

Other analgesic medications can be administered in association with peridural analgesia; these include acetaminophen, given at a dose of 650 to 1300 mg intrarectally, and other nonsteroidal anti-inflammatory drugs.

Lung Separation

One-lung ventilation is used in nearly all cases of pulmonary resection because it improves surgical exposure while preventing excessive retraction of the lung, which may cause parenchymal hemorrhage and contusion. One-lung ventilation also *prevents potential soiling* of the contralateral lung by purulent bronchial secretions (absolute indication for double-lumen tube). Most often, one-lung ventilation is carried out through a double-lumen tube (Fig. 5-2). Alternatively, endobronchial blockers can be used (Fig. 5-3).

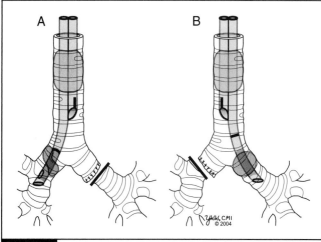

FIG. 5-2

Schematic diagrams depicting the use of right-sided **(A)** and left-sided **(B)** double-lumen tubes. When surgery is performed on the left lung, a right-sided double-lumen tube is used **(A)**. When surgery is performed on the right lung, a left-sided tube is used **(B)**.

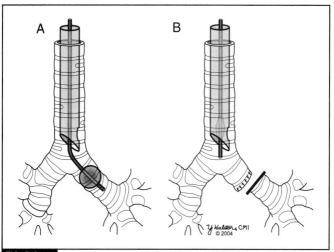

FIG. 5-3

Schematic diagrams depicting the use of an endobronchial blocker for left lung blockade. Once the tip of the catheter has been directed into the appropriate location, the balloon is inflated, producing total bronchial occlusion **(A)**. The bronchial blocker is pulled back in the endotracheal tube to allow safe stapling of the left main bronchus **(B)**.

TABLE 5-11

ONE-LUNG VENTILATION: LUNG SEPARATION

	Advantages	Disadvantages
Double-lumen tubes	Ease of placement	Need to be changed for postoperative ventilation
	Ease of continuous positive airway pressure to the nonventilated lung	
	Rapid switch from one-lung to two-lung ventilation	Risk of right upper lobe obstruction
	Suction of two lungs	
Endobronchial blockers	Ease with difficult airways	Frequent failure of separation
	Selective lobar blockade	
	Ease of postoperative ventilation	Risk of contamination from one lung to the other

Double-lumen tubes consist of *two catheters bonded together* so that one lumen is long enough to reach a main stem bronchus and the second lumen ends with an opening in the distal trachea (Fig. 5-2). A proximal tracheal cuff and a distal endobronchial cuff in the main stem bronchus allow separation of the lungs when these cuffs are inflated. Left disposable double-lumen tubes are relatively easy to insert, but right double-lumen tubes are more difficult to position. Both have different cuff arrangements that minimize lobar obstruction. Advantages of double-lumen tubes (Table 5-11) include *ease of placement, easy and rapid conversion* from two-lung ventilation to one-lung ventilation at any time during surgery, suctioning of secretions from *both lungs*, and provision of continuous positive airway pressure to the nonventilated lung.

Endobronchial blockers usually consist of *Fogarty catheters* that are inserted in the trachea before the placement of the single-lumen endotracheal tube. A fiberoptic bronchoscope guides the catheter into either the right or left lung; when the balloon of the catheter is inflated, the ipsilateral bronchial lumen is obstructed, and the obstructed lung collapses. The *Univent tube*[*] is a single-lumen endotracheal tube that has a movable and retractable blocker housed in a channel attached to the endotracheal tube wall. A wire-guided low-pressure, high-volume endobronchial blocker is also commercially available.[†]

In general, endobronchial blockers are considered to be *less versatile* and *less easy to manage* than double-lumen tubes (Table 5-11). With bronchial blockers, one cannot easily switch from one lung to the other as it may be required during the pulmonary resection. They have a high failure rate of separation, especially with changes in the patient's position or because of surgical manipulations, and if the blocker slips back into the trachea, it can *obstruct airflow* to the contralateral lung. Bronchial blockers also fail to protect the healthy lung from possible contamination by purulent

---

*Fuji Systems Corporation, Tokyo, Japan.
†Cook Critical Care, Bloomington, Indiana.

bronchial secretions. Finally, they can accidentally be included in the staple line and transected. Advantages of bronchial blockers include more effective exclusion of a lung (or lobe) in case of massive hemoptysis and ease of postoperative ventilation by withdrawal of the blocker. Overall, bronchial blockers are used for patients with "difficult airways" or for *selective lobar blockage* in a patient who cannot tolerate the exclusion of a whole lung.

Most anesthetists use fiberoptic bronchoscopy to confirm that double-lumen tubes or bronchial blockers *are well positioned*. It is first done just after the intubation while the patient is still on the back. The tube is then fixed to the patient's mouth in such a way that it can be accessed and repositioned during the procedure should it be required. Because small movements of the patient's head during the positioning can accidentally provoke significant displacement of the double-lumen tube, fiberoptic bronchoscopy should be repeated after positioning to ensure that the double-lumen tube is still in its original position. During the course of surgery, fiberoptic bronchoscopy is done if there are signs that the position of the catheter needs readjustment.

One-Lung Ventilation

The use of one-lung ventilation implies that there is some degree of arteriovenous shunting because the collapsed lung is nonventilated but still perfused. The importance of this shunt depends on factors such as the hypoxic pulmonary vasoconstriction, a homeostatic mechanism by which pulmonary blood flow is diverted away from hypoxic regions of the lung, and the gravity effect associated with the lateral decubitus position, which helps divert blood away from the nonventilated lung.

Management of the patient under one-lung ventilation includes adequate positioning of the double-lumen tube and regular suctioning of bronchial secretions. Passive oxygenation of the collapsed lung is sometimes helpful, although continuous positive airway pressure (CPAP) with reinflation is the best way to restore adequate oxygenation. Unfortunately, the use of CPAP is not possible during thoracoscopic procedures because distention of the lung being operated on may impair the visibility of the operator.

Positive end-expiratory pressure (PEEP) on the ventilated (down) lung is now an accepted technique for improving oxygenation throughout the operation. When hypoxia is not corrected with the previously described maneuvers, intermittent ventilation of the nonventilated lung or pulmonary arterial clampage (to eliminate the AV shunt) may allow the pursuit of the surgery with better arterial oxygenation.

Fluid Management and Temperature Control

During pulmonary resection and especially during pneumonectomy, it is recommended that *fluid intake be kept at a minimum* to avoid increased pulmonary filtration pressure and fluid extravasation in the alveoli. Central venous pressure measurements and urine output are helpful in monitoring and readjusting fluid balance.

Body temperature must be kept *within normal range* throughout the procedure to facilitate early extubation. This is done by use of a heating mattress over the lower extremities or by heating intravenous fluids administered to the patient. The loss of heat secondary to the breathing of anesthetic gases can also be lowered through the use of a heat and moisture exchanger inserted inside the respiratory circuit.

Emergence from General Anesthesia

At completion of the procedure, the patient is reintubated with a single-lumen tube. The surgeon or anesthetist performs *fiberoptic bronchoscopy* to aspirate blood and mucus as well as to check sites of bronchial closure or bronchial anastomosis. If the body temperature is below 37°C, most anesthetists recommend *gradual warming* with thermal blankets before extubation.

When a pneumonectomy has been carried out, many surgeons use intrathoracic aspiration to balance the mediastinum and prevent excessive mediastinal shift. During this maneuver, the anesthetist must monitor the arterial blood pressure because, on occasion, excessive mediastinal shift will compromise venous return, which can initiate significant hemodynamic perturbations.

IMMEDIATE POSTOPERATIVE CARE

Most patients are extubated either in the operating room or shortly after their arrival in the recovery room. This *early extubation* is recommended to prevent continuous positive pressure from putting undue stress on parenchymal or bronchial suture lines. A portable chest radiograph is always obtained before extubation so that pneumothoraces, atelectasis, hemothoraces, or other problems can be diagnosed and dealt with while the patient is still under general anesthesia. If the mediastinum is not adequately balanced when a pneumonectomy has been done, the situation can also be corrected before extubation.

Postoperative epidural analgesia is adjusted before the patient leaves the recovery room.

POSSIBLE COMPLICATIONS DURING ANESTHESIA FOR PULMONARY RESECTION

On occasion, a *pneumothorax* in the down lung will develop. This may happen quickly, and the signs that suggest this diagnosis include an increase of airway pressure, a deterioration in hemodynamic parameters, and a decrease in the intensity of breath sounds over the involved side. In such cases, the surgeon must *quickly drain the opposite pleural space* either through the mediastinal pleura or through a small intercostal incision over the side of the pneumothorax. Risk factors for intraoperative pneumothoraces include the presence of bullous or diffuse emphysema and high ventilating pressures.

Episodes of hypotension frequently occur during pulmonary resections. These may be due to sudden blood loss or more frequently to traction on mediastinal structures by the surgeon. Unfortunately, such episodes are often severe because the patient has been kept hypovolemic throughout the procedure. When this occurs, the anesthetist will usually ask the surgeon to release traction on the lung and stop all manipulations. Most often, these simple maneuvers quickly correct the situation.

Several problems can be related to double-lumen tube *malposition*. These include accidental direction of a tube down the wrong main stem bronchus, *inadequate separation*, increased airway pressure, and several combinations of malpositions.

Supraventricular arrhythmias are not uncommon during pulmonary resection, but most are easy to control with medication.

Significant hemorrhage due to laceration of blood vessels is rare but can be catastrophic. Major pulmonary vessels, arterial or venous, have thinner walls than systemic arterial blood vessels, but unfortunately, they carry *just as much blood as the aorta* does. When a major pulmonary vessel has been lacerated, the anesthetist must be ready for rapid volume repletion. This includes getting blood units from the blood bank and making sure that the venous lines are available for infusion.

CONCLUSION

Overall, anesthesia for pulmonary resection is safe and free of complications. Good communication between surgeon and anesthetist and team work are prerequisites for successful outcomes.

SUGGESTED READINGS

Review Articles

Slinger PD: Anaesthesia for lung resection. Can J Anaesth 1990; 37:s15-s24.

Slinger P: Choosing the appropriate double-lumen tube: a glimmer of science comes to a dark art [editorial]. J Cardiothorac Vasc Anesth 1995;9:117-118.

Brodsky JB: Thoracic anesthesia. Semin Respir Crit Care Med 1999;20:419-427.

Dunn PF: Physiology of the lateral decubitus position and one-lung ventilation. Int Anesthesiol Clin 2000;38:25-53.

Campos JH: Lung isolation techniques. Anesthesiol Clin North Am 2001;19:455-474.

Double-Lumen Tubes

Benumof JL, Partridge BL, Salvatierra C, Keating J: Margin of safety in positioning modern double-lumen endotracheal tubes. Anesthesiology 1987;67:729-738.

Lewis JW, Serwin JP, Gabriel FS, et al: The utility of a double-lumen tube for one-lung ventilation in a variety of noncardiac thoracic surgical procedures. J Cardiothorac Vasc Anesth 1992;6:705-710.

Desiderio DP, Burt M, Kolker AC, et al: The effects of endobronchial cuff inflation in double-lumen endobronchial tube movement after lateral decubitus positioning. J Cardiothorac Vasc Anesth 1997;11:595-598.

5

Intraoperative Care

Klein U, Karzai W, Bloos F, et al: Role of fiberoptic bronchoscopy in conjunction with the use of double-lumen tubes for thoracic anesthesia. A prospective study. Anesthesiology 1998;88:346-350.

Campos JH, Massa FC, Kernstine KH: The incidence of right upper-lobe collapse when comparing a right-sided double-lumen tube versus a modified left double-lumen tube for left-sided thoracic surgery. Anesth Analg 2000;90:535-540.

Bronchial Blockers

Ginsberg RJ: New technique for one-lung anesthesia using an endo-bronchial blocker. J Thorac Cardiovasc Surg 1981;82:542-546.

Karwande SV: A new tube for single lung ventilation. Chest 1987; 92:761-763.

Ransom ES, Carter SL, Mund GD: Univent tube: a useful device in patients with difficult airways. J Cardiothorac Vasc Anesth 1995;9: 725-727.

Garcia-Aguado R, Mateo EM, Onrubia VJ, Bolinches R: Use of the Univent System tube for difficult intubation and for achieving one-lung anaesthesia. Acta Anaesthesiol Scand 1996;40:765-767.

Complications

Massard G, Rougé C, Dabbagh A, et al: Tracheobronchial lacerations after intubation and tracheostomy. Ann Thorac Surg 1996;61: 1483-1487.

Mussi A, Ambrogi MC, Menconi G, et al: Surgical approaches to membranous tracheal wall lacerations. J Thorac Cardiovasc Surg 2000;120:115-118.

Hofmann HS, Rettig G, Radke J, et al: Iatrogenic ruptures of the tracheobronchial tree. Eur J Cardiothorac Surg 2002;21:649-652.

ANESTHESIA FOR THE PATIENT WITH AN ANTERIOR MEDIASTINAL MASS

The mediastinum is a median partition of the thorax that separates the lungs in their respective pleural cavities. Although its contour and extent vary from upper to lower, it is tightly packed with organs that are important to the anesthetist. These include cardiovascular structures such as the heart and great vessels and major airways such as the trachea and main bronchi. Dynamically, the mediastinum reflects the intrapleural subatmospheric pressure with respiratory variations.

The anesthetic management of patients undergoing surgery for biopsy or excision of mediastinal tumors *must be planned* and all potential problems must have a *ready solution* permitting their safe management. Appropriate prophylactic measures can also usually be taken so that problems that may be encountered during induction, intubation, positioning, or even recovery are avoided.

In general, anesthesia hazards in patients with anterior mediastinal masses are related to airway obstruction or to compression of major vascular structures such as the superior vena cava, the main pulmonary arteries, or the heart itself. The likelihood of the occurrence of problems is related to *the size and location of the tumor*; often, problems arise only when the patient is in the supine position. A thymoma invading the superior vena cava or a germ cell tumor or lymphoma obstructing the trachea, for instance, must alert the anesthesiologist to the risks of potentially life-threatening events. Ultimately, the anesthesiologist will have to decide if surgery can be safely done or if the risks are prohibitive.

ANESTHESIA OF THE PATIENT WITH AIRWAY OBSTRUCTION

In patients with anterior mediastinal masses, the trachea or main bronchi can be obstructed (extrinsic compression or true airway invasion), distorted, or malacic. In each of these situations, general anesthesia *can precipitate complete obstruction*, whether it is at the time of induction or during the procedure. Tumors most likely to create airway obstruction are those in the anterior mediastinum, such as lymphomas, germ cell tumors, or retrosternal goiters, and lung cancer originating in the right upper lobe and extending to the lateral wall of the trachea. Tracheomalacia may be the result of prolonged external compression (retrosternal goiter) or scarring of the trachea.

As a rule, airway obstruction is *more common* and *more dangerous* in infants and small children. In this population, a small decrease in airway diameter can create a significant decrease in luminal area.

Pathophysiology of Airway Obstruction Related to Anesthesia

Large mediastinal masses, even those without obvious airway compression or invasion, can produce significant obstruction when the patient is induced in the *supine position* (Table 5-12). This phenomenon relates to a reduction in the anteroposterior dimension of the thoracic cage when the patient is supine, thus increasing the likelihood that a space-occupying lesion will cause, precipitate, or exacerbate airway obstruction. General anesthesia also decreases functional residual capacity, and because of that, it decreases expanding forces acting on the tracheobronchial tree, which ultimately

TABLE 5-12

PREDISPOSING FACTORS FOR INADEQUATE VENTILATION DURING ANESTHESIA OF THE PATIENT WITH AN ANTERIOR MEDIASTINAL MASS

Prior airway obstruction (intrinsic or extrinsic compression)
Supine position
Reduction in anteroposterior diameter of thoracic cage with patient lying down
Decrease in functional residual capacity
Loss of chest wall tone
Loss of active inspiration (muscle relaxants)
Loss of diaphragm action (supine position, muscle relaxants)
Airway trauma during intubation or during surgical manipulation

tends to decrease airway diameter. In addition, loss of chest wall tone, loss of active inspiration after the administration of muscle relaxants, and loss of diaphragmatic contraction when the patient is lying down and curarized are factors that may precipitate respiratory difficulties.

The patient with prior airway obstruction is obviously *at greater risk* of complete obstruction. This can occur during intubation, during surgical manipulations of the tumor that may produce edema and bleeding, or during postoperative recovery. These considerations are especially important if the site of obstruction is *distal to the tip of the endotracheal tube* (i.e., around the carina).

The use of mechanical ventilation brings additional problems. For instance, the positive pressure delivered by the respirator can be dissipated proximal to the obstruction, or the increased gas velocity and turbulence across the stenosis can also generate inadequate inflating lung pressures. As higher inspiratory pressures are required, the intrapulmonary pressure will also increase, creating ideal conditions for *overdistention of the lungs and pneumothoraces.*

Preanesthetic Evaluation and Preparation of the Patient

In modern medicine, preexisting airway obstruction should always be documented before general anesthesia. This documentation includes information about the *severity of the obstruction*, its *site and length*, and whether it is *intrinsic or extrinsic.* This last consideration is important because intubation through an area stenotic from mucosal invasion may cause edema or hemorrhage, which can worsen the degree of obstruction.

The anesthetist must review the results of imaging techniques because these are good predictors of the anatomy of the obstruction and of whether anesthetic difficulties with the airway are likely to occur. In addition to confirmation of imaging findings, flexible fiberoptic bronchoscopy will also document dynamic airway obstruction (tracheomalacia).

Two other simple investigations that may provide additional information about the severity of obstruction are (1) the recording of a good clinical history (often done by the surgeon) to see if the patient has noted a worsening of symptoms while lying down and (2) the maximum inspiratory and expiratory flow-volume loops, which can be obtained with the patient in the upright and supine positions (see Chapter 3, "Assessment of the Patient with Possible Airway Obstruction"). These flow-volume curves are simple recordings that are *highly reproducible*.

All of these tests must be done fairly close to the operation because malignant mediastinal tumors *may enlarge rapidly.* Anesthetic concerns should always be discussed with the surgeon, and they should also be discussed with the patient, especially if an awake intervention is contemplated. In all cases, the anesthetist *must inform the patient* of the specific and potential risks of general anesthesia, and such a discussion should be documented in the patient's chart.

Conduct of Anesthesia (Table 5-13)

Premedication should not be given to patients with known tracheobronchial compromise because these drugs have the *potential to decrease the respiratory drive*, thus potentially increasing the functional significance of the obstruction. The equipment for difficult intubation, including a set of rigid bronchoscopes, should be available, and in all instances, *the surgeon should also be in the room* while the patient is being induced. It is expected that the surgeon or the anesthetist will be able to carry on a rigid bronchoscopy should it be required.

The method chosen for induction depends on the preoperative evaluation and likelihood of respiratory obstruction. An inhalation induction (volatile anesthetic) with spontaneous respiration is frequently used. The advantage of spontaneous respiration is that the transpulmonary pressure gradient tends to distend the airway *and maintain its patency,* even in the presence of significant airway obstruction. On occasion, a mixture of helium-oxygen may help overcome obstruction-related flow restriction.

Intubation may have to be carried out with the patient in the sitting position or with the use of a bronchoscope, either flexible or rigid. In these instances, maintenance of spontaneous respiration and *avoidance of muscle relaxants* are important until the anesthetist has full control of the airway. If airway obstruction occurs during intubation, management may require advancing the endotracheal tube beyond the lesion (often into a main bronchus) or changing the patient's position from supine to prone or lateral decubitus. A rigid bronchoscope can also be used to guide the endotracheal tube through the obstruction. In such cases, an extralong thin armored endotracheal tube that can be advanced beyond the carina is helpful.

Although some have suggested that all patients with more than 50% airway obstruction as documented preoperatively should undergo cannulation of their femoral vessels before induction of general anesthesia, in readiness of cardiopulmonary bypass, this is *seldom necessary.* Indeed, the anticoagulation that must be used for cardiopulmonary bypass may increase the degree of obstruction because of hemorrhage within the tumor.

5

Intraoperative Care

TABLE 5-13
CONDUCT OF ANESTHESIA IN PATIENTS WITH ANTERIOR MEDIASTINAL MASSES AND POSSIBLE AIRWAY OBSTRUCTION
No premedication
Equipment for rigid bronchoscopy available
Induction with volatile anesthetic (inhalation) and spontaneous respiration
Avoidance of muscle relaxants
Intubation may have to be done in sitting position
Intubation may have to be done with flexible or rigid bronchoscope
Advancement of the endotracheal tube distal to site of obstruction

Recovery from Anesthesia

It is important *to closely monitor* all patients during the immediate postoperative period because problems may still occur at that time. These can be due to edema or hemorrhage caused by surgical manipulations or unsuccessful decompression of the mediastinum. Anxiety, tachypnea, cough, and pain during emergence from anesthesia may also cause turbulence and worsen airway obstruction. Tracheomalacia may be present after long-standing tracheal compression only to become apparent after the tumor has been resected. Recurrent laryngeal nerve damage may have occurred during operation; if both nerves have been damaged, the vocal cords may be immobile in the medial position, causing airway obstruction. Finally, paralysis of both hemidiaphragms due to phrenic nerve injury may be the source of respiratory distress after extubation.

If any of these complications occurs, *the ready availability of bronchoscopy is essential* because often no alternative method can be used to regain control of the airway.

ANESTHESIA OF THE PATIENT WITH COMPRESSION OF MAJOR VASCULAR STRUCTURES

Pathophysiology of Vascular Compression Related to Anesthesia

Several reports have described the potentially serious consequences of general anesthesia in patients with superior vena cava obstruction or in those with mechanical compression of the pulmonary arteries or cardiac invasion (Tables 5-14 and 5-15).

Superior vena cava (SVC) obstruction is almost always due to a malignant tumor, usually thymoma, lymphoma, or lung cancer with mediastinal nodal involvement. These tumors can directly invade the vein, cause extrinsic compression, or cause a narrowing with subsequent obstruction by a mural thrombus.

General anesthesia in the presence of a chronic SVC obstruction is usually not a problem because *extensive collateral circulation is invariably present.*

TABLE 5-14		
ANESTHETIC IMPLICATIONS OF CARDIOVASCULAR COMPRESSION		
Blood Vessel	Anesthetic Implications	Preoperative Assessment
Superior vena cava	Laryngeal and upper airway edema	Physical examination
		Contrast-enhanced CT
	Cerebral edema	Angiography
	Reduction in cardiac output	Transesophageal ultrasonography
Pulmonary artery	Reduction in cardiac output	Contrast-enhanced CT
	Hypoxemia	Magnetic resonance imaging
		Transesophageal ultrasonography
Pericardium and heart	Restriction of diastolic filling	Echocardiography
		Contrast-enhanced CT

TABLE 5-15

GENERAL PRINCIPLES OF ANESTHESIA FOR THE PATIENT WITH SUPERIOR VENA CAVA OBSTRUCTION

Venous access through lower limb

Avoidance of intravenous infusion in upper extremities

Manipulation of airway should be gentle

Intraoperative administration of steroids or diuretics may be helpful

Avoid coughing, straining, bucking

Supine position to be avoided

By contrast, acute SVC obstruction may create laryngeal and upper airway edema as well as intracranial venous hypertension with secondary cerebral edema. The patient will often have subclinical superior vena cava obstruction that becomes significant in the *supine position*. Worsening of the syndrome can also result from *generous fluid administration*.

The pulmonary arteries are less vulnerable than the superior vena cava to compression and obstruction. When this occurs, however, it may cause significant reduction in cardiac output with subsequent hemodynamic compromise. Compression of the pulmonary arteries may also cause significant underperfusion of the lungs with secondary hypoxia. Not unlike in patients with superior vena cava obstruction, these hemodynamic derangements often relate to posture, *being worse with the patient in the supine position.*

Compression of the pericardium and heart (tamponade) may cause a restriction of diastolic filling. If, in addition to compression, there is tumor infiltration of the cardiac muscle, impairment of systolic function may also occur. Germ cell tumors and lymphomas in the anterior mediastinum are the most common tumors that may involve the heart and pericardium. Thymomas often invade the pericardium or superior vena cava but seldom invade the heart itself.

Preanesthetic Evaluation and Preparation of the Patient

As with airway obstruction, one should *always document the presence or absence of vascular compression* by mediastinal masses *preoperatively*. Although the diagnosis of superior vena cava syndrome can usually be made on clinical grounds, useful imaging techniques include contrast-enhanced CT scanning, venous angiography, and transesophageal ultrasonography, which can delineate the mechanism of obstruction (compression, thrombus).

Patients with masses compressing the pulmonary artery are often asymptomatic, yet life-threatening complications may develop under general anesthesia. If this diagnosis is suspected, it can be demonstrated preoperatively by contrast-enhanced CT, magnetic resonance imaging, or transesophageal echocardiography.

Cardiac invasion is best documented by contrast-enhanced CT. Echocardiography may also be useful to determine the precise site of compression as well as to study the diastolic ventricular filling pattern.

5

Intraoperative Care

In all of those cases, *it is important to plan the operation*, and both surgeon and anesthetist must meet to *discuss the indication for surgery, the risk of operation, and its conduct.* If, for instance, the surgeon plans to resect and reconstruct the superior vena cava, it must be known ahead of time so that the anesthetist is ready for venous clamping. Similarly, cardiopulmonary bypass must be available if the surgeon plans to resect the main pulmonary artery or part of the atrium.

Anesthetic Management

If surgery is necessary in the presence of superior vena cava obstruction, a lower limb venous access is preferred. The patient is brought into the operating room in the sitting position; throughout induction, *the supine position is avoided* because it reduces the pressure gradient across the obstruction. The placement of a central venous catheter in the superior vena cava is generally contraindicated because of the dangers of perforation. It can, however, be extremely useful in patients in whom the surgeon expects to resect the superior vena cava.

Because patients with superior vena cava obstruction often have some degree of laryngeal edema, manipulation of the airway should be done gently if one wants to avoid mucosal trauma, increased edema, or hemorrhage. In such cases, preoperative (or intraoperative) administration of steroids and diuretics may decrease the edema and improve symptoms. One should bear in mind, however, that too much diuresis may further decrease cardiac output and lead to hypotension.

Although there is no information to guide the choice between spontaneous and controlled ventilation in the presence of superior vena cava obstruction, *coughing, bucking, and straining are to be avoided* because they may generate a worsening of the obstruction or provoke a significant increase in intracranial pressure. The patient should be positioned with the head up, with avoidance of cervical flexion or rotation, because this may further obstruct the cervical veins. Intravenous fluid infusion in the upper extremities should be avoided because it may aggravate preexistent airway edema or further increase the intracranial pressure.

If resection of the superior vena cava is to be done, the vein may be cross-clamped for periods that vary from 15 to 30 minutes. Before clamping, the patient is fully heparinized, and 1500 to 2000 mL of intravenous fluid is administered to prevent low-output status during cross-clamping. In these situations, it is extremely useful to monitor the venous pressure proximal to the site of clamping. If the venous pressure *does not rise* above 30 to 35 cm H_2O, cross-clamping time can be prolonged without danger. If, on the other hand, the venous pressure *rises to 50 cm H_2O or more,* duration of cross-clamping must be as short as possible because permanent brain damage can occur. Clamp placement that occludes less than 50% of the circumference of the superior vena cava is usually not associated with significant abnormalities.

Recovery from Anesthesia

On occasion, the patient with superior vena cava obstruction will develop *edema of the upper airway*, including the larynx, during the immediate postoperative period. This may happen when the tumor has not been resected or if a graft used for reconstruction of the superior vena cava has become suddenly occluded. Strict and close observation is therefore mandatory because severe obstruction can occur acutely. Under such circumstances, rapid intervention with reintubation or even tracheotomy may be lifesaving.

ALTERNATIVES TO GENERAL ANESTHESIA IN HIGH-RISK PATIENTS

On occasion, the patient with a mediastinal mass is at high or prohibitive risk for severe respiratory or cardiovascular complications during general anesthesia. Because these patients are usually brought to the operating room for tissue diagnosis only, *other strategies* may have to be considered for general anesthesia to be avoided.

In some cases, surgery can be avoided altogether. This applies to non-seminoma germ cell tumors, for which treatment can be started on the basis of elevated tumor markers (human chorionic gonadotropin β, alpha-fetoprotein, carcinoembryonic antigen). It also applies to other anterior mediastinal masses for which a tissue diagnosis can be made by percutaneous fine-needle or core biopsy. This would be the case, for instance, with lymphomas or invasive thymomas.

A large biopsy specimen must often be obtained, however, so that tumors such as lymphomas or thymomas can be positively diagnosed and subclassified. For those patients, the biopsy procedure can be done under local anesthesia.

Mediastinoscopy should *never be done under local anesthesia* if the patient is at prohibitive risk for general anesthesia. In such cases, the additional pressure created by the mediastinoscope, bleeding, or the patient's agitation is likely to lead to catastrophic complications. Anterior mediastinotomy (see "Positioning and Incisions"), on the other hand, can be done more safely, and most if not all anterior mediastinal masses are accessible through this approach. Procedures done under local anesthesia *should be supervised* by an experienced anesthetist in case complications, such as airway obstruction or bleeding, develop during the operation.

Empirical therapy without a diagnosis used to be recommended if the patient had prohibitive risk for general anesthesia. Other than in unusual circumstances, it is no longer the case because *several of these tumors can be cured* if appropriate treatment based on positive tissue diagnosis is provided.

ANESTHESIA OF THE PATIENT WITH MYASTHENIA GRAVIS

Myasthenia gravis, a neurologic disorder, presents with *weakness* or *fatigability* with repetitive exercise that improves with rest. It is an autoimmune disorder; approximately 85% of patients have demonstrable

5

Intraoperative Care

levels of immunoglobulin G antibody to the acetylcholine receptor. The diagnosis can be made on clinical grounds or by decremental response to repetitive stimulation as documented by electromyography.

Thymectomy is indicated if the patient has a thymoma. In patients without thymoma, therapy includes anticholinesterase medication, immunosuppression usually by steroids, plasmapheresis, and thymectomy.

Operative morbidity is decreased if myasthenia gravis is under optimal control at the time of surgery. Symptoms should be controlled with anticholinesterase therapy, and plasmapheresis should be added if necessary. Because thymectomy is an *elective operation,* it should be performed *during a remission of the disease* and *when respiratory infection is not a problem.*

Patients with severe forms of myasthenia gravis usually benefit from plasmapheresis preoperatively. It is a safe procedure that is used to remove immunologically active plasma proteins to transiently improve voluntary muscle strength and decrease the incidence of postoperative complications. Plasmapheresis may also improve dysphagia and aspiration related to bulbar involvement by the disease.

The basic principles of anesthesia are similar to those in patients who are not myasthenic, except that *muscle relaxants are generally avoided,* or, if they are used, their effects are closely monitored. After completion of the operation, weaning ability is assessed by evaluation of respiratory mechanics (vital capacity, tidal volume), the patient's strength, and arterial blood gases. All patients should be carefully monitored for at least 24 to 48 hours to ensure that adequate spontaneous ventilation can be sustained and that the patient has enough muscle strength to raise secretions. Tracheostomy is *not done* on a routine basis.

ANESTHESIA OF THE PATIENT WITH MEDIASTINAL PHEOCHROMOCYTOMA

This tumor, which is extremely uncommon, is usually not documented preoperatively. The risks of anesthesia are related to *excessive release of catecholamines during surgical manipulations* of the tumor, which can produce arrhythmias or, most important, cause severe hypertensive crisis.

If this phenomenon is anticipated, patients should be pretreated with alpha-adrenergic blocking drugs so that restoration of plasma volume is facilitated. Intraoperatively, the anesthesiologist should be ready to treat significant hypertension swiftly; beta blockers are indicated if tachycardia and arrhythmias develop together.

After ligation of the veins draining the pheochromocytoma, a sudden decrease in catecholamine level may result in hypotension requiring volume repletion and use of vasopressors.

Monitoring of blood glucose levels is also important. Hyperglycemia is typically present before operation, followed by *hypoglycemia* after the tumor has been removed. This sequence is the result of insulin inhibition mediated by the stimulation of alpha-adrenergic receptors, which is abolished after the tumor has been removed.

CONCLUSION

General anesthesia for patients undergoing surgery for anterior mediastinal tumors, whether it is biopsy or excision, needs to be well planned. This planning must include a thorough evaluation of the effects of the lesion on the tracheobronchial tree and major vascular structures.

If general anesthesia is deemed mandatory, the patient should be well monitored. The anesthetist must anticipate and be able to manage potentially serious complications. Postoperatively, the patient should be under close surveillance because complications may still arise.

In high-risk patients requiring a tissue diagnosis, local anesthesia should be considered.

SUGGESTED READINGS

Review Articles

Mackie AM, Watson CB: Anesthesia and mediastinal masses. A case report and review of the literature. Anesthesia 1984;39:899-903.

Pullerits J, Holzman R: Anesthesia for patients with mediastinal masses. Can J Anaesth 1989;36:681-688.

Goh MH, Liu XY, Goh YS: Anterior mediastinal masses: an anaesthetic challenge. Anaesthesia 1999;54:670-674.

Narang S, Harte BH, Body SC: Anesthesia for patients with a mediastinal mass. Anesthesiol Clin North Am 2001;19:559-579.

Anesthesia for Children with Mediastinal Masses

Halpera S, Chatten J, Meadows AT, et al: Anterior mediastinal masses: anesthesia hazards and other problems. J Pediatr 1983; 102:407-410.

Shamberger RC, Holzman RS, Griscom NT, et al: CT quantitation of tracheal cross-sectional area as a guide to the surgical and anesthetic management of children with anterior mediastinal masses. J Pediatr Surg 1991;26:138-142.

Shamberger RC, Holzman RS, Griscom NT, et al: Prospective evaluation by computed tomography and pulmonary function tests of children with mediastinal masses. Surgery 1995;118:468-471.

Shamberger RC: Preanesthetic evaluation of children with anterior mediastinal masses [review]. Semin Pediatr Surg 1999;8:61-68.

Clinical Reports

Neuman GG, Weingarten AE, Abramowitz RM, et al: The anesthetic management of the patient with an anterior mediastinal mass. Anesthesiology 1984;60:144-147.

Younker D, Clark R, Coveler L: Fiberoptic endobronchial intubation for resection of an anterior mediastinal mass. Anesthesiology 1989;70:144-146.

Hnatiuk OW, Corcoran PC, Sierra A: Spirometry in surgery for anterior mediastinal masses. Chest 2001;120:1152-1156.

Bechard P, Létourneau L, Lacasse Y, et al: Perioperative cardiorespiratory complications in adults with mediastinal mass. Incidence and risk factors. Anesthesiology 2004;100:826-834.

Anesthesia for Patients with Myasthenia Gravis

Spence PA, Morin JE, Katz M: Role of plasmapheresis in preparing myasthenic patients for thymectomy: initial results. Can J Surg 1984;27:303-305.

d'Empaire G, Hoaglin DC, Perlo VP, Pontoppidan H: Effect of prethymectomy plasma exchange on postoperative respiratory function in myasthenia gravis. J Thorac Cardiovasc Surg 1985;89: 592-596.

Mussi A, Lucchi M, Murri L, et al: Extended thymectomy in myasthenia gravis: a team-work of neurologist, thoracic surgeon and anaesthetist may improve the outcome. Eur J Cardiothorac Surg 2001;19: 570-575.

Anesthesia for Patients with Pheochromocytoma

van Heerden JA, Sheps SG, Hamberger B, et al: Pheochromocytoma: current status and changing trends. Surgery 1982;91:367-373.

Cardiopulmonary Bypass

Tempe DK, Arya R, Dubey S, et al: Mediastinal mass resection: femorofemoral cardiopulmonary bypass before induction of anesthesia in the management of airway obstruction. J Cardiothorac Vasc Anesth 2001;15:233-236.

AIRWAY MANAGEMENT DURING TRACHEAL RESECTION

Diseases of the major airways requiring diagnostic or therapeutic interventions are not uncommon. The management of anesthesia during such interventions can, however, be difficult for both the anesthetist and the surgeon because they must share the airway. Hence, experience and a thorough knowledge of tracheal anatomy and surgical techniques are prerequisites before this type of work is undertaken.

In recent years, anesthesia for airway surgery has been facilitated through the use of new anesthetic agents with rapid onset and short duration of action. Not only do these agents enable the anesthetist to deepen the level of anesthesia rapidly and allow the surgical procedure to be carried out, but the patient can also rapidly regain consciousness and spontaneous breathing at the end of the operation.

PREANESTHETIC EVALUATION

A thorough understanding of the problem is essential to the planning of anesthesia for patients who are to undergo tracheal resection. To achieve this objective, the anesthetist must review all bronchoscopic and radiologic studies that were used to determine the *location, nature, and extent* of the

TABLE 5-16	
ANESTHETIST AND PREANESTHETIC EVALUATION	
Must know location, extent, and nature of lesion	
Must be aware of planned surgical approach	
Must meet and discuss plan with surgeon	
Must explain the procedure to the patient	

tracheal lesion (Table 5-16). The anesthetist must also know about the planned surgical approach (Table 5-17). In general, lesions of the upper third of the trachea are approached through a cervical collar incision with or without full or partial median sternotomy; lesions of the lower third and those of the carina are best approached through a right posterolateral thoracotomy or through a median or transverse (clamshell incision) sternotomy. If a posterolateral thoracotomy is done, epidural analgesia should be used in conjunction with a short-acting general anesthetic to allow early extubation and effective postoperative analgesia.

The anesthetist must be aware of the *presence or absence of significant comorbidities*, such as chronic obstructive pulmonary disease or coronary artery disease, which may have the potential to create life-threatening situations perioperatively. Unless surgery has to be done urgently, these conditions *must be investigated* and their treatment *must be optimized* before operation. Any neurologic deficit that may interfere with the mechanical function of respiratory muscles must also be looked at and investigated carefully.

The anesthetist must meet with the surgeon, and each must be aware of *the other's plan and approach* before induction. Finally, the anesthetist must carefully explain the procedure to the patient, especially if an awake intubation is planned.

IMMEDIATE PREOPERATIVE ANESTHETIC MANAGEMENT

The beneficial effects of premedication, including analgesia and relief of anxiety, must be balanced against the potentially detrimental results of oversedating a patient with significant narrowing of the airway. Preoperative medication should be given to patients who have an adequate airway, but in all other cases, *it should be avoided*. In general, it is safer *not to give* the premedication until the patient is under the direct supervision of the anesthetist in the operating room.

TABLE 5-17	
SURGICAL APPROACHES FOR TRACHEAL RESECTION	
Lesions of upper trachea	Cervical collar incision with or without sternotomy (full or partial)
Lesions of middle trachea	Cervical collar incision with full sternotomy
Lesions of lower trachea	Right thoracotomy
Lesions of carina	Right thoracotomy, median sternotomy, or transverse sternotomy (clamshell incision)

Although some anesthetists advocate the use of steroids to decrease the severity of tracheal edema, most surgeons think that these compounds should be avoided because they can potentially have a detrimental effect on the healing of the tracheal anastomosis.

Because of the risk of aspiration during induction or during the operation itself, gastric acid secretion blockers, antiemetics, and gastric prokinetic agents should be used to lower the incidence and severity of such events.

CONDUCT OF ANESTHESIA

Anesthetic Equipment

A number of specialized pieces of equipment must be available before induction of anesthesia, including a wide variety of polyvinyl chloride tubes, armored tubes, and ventilating catheters. On occasion, small endotracheal tubes such as the microlaryngeal tubes may be useful.

Sterile anesthesia corrugated tubing, connectors, and armored tubes must be *on the operating table* and ready to be used by the surgeon during reconstruction of the airway. At the appropriate time, the tubing will be passed up to the anesthetist so that it can be connected to the anesthesia machine.

An anesthesia machine capable of delivering *high flows of oxygen*, approximately 20 L/min, is desirable, especially during rigid bronchoscopy or when the airways are open. Under such conditions, the air leak with low-flow equipment may be associated with inadequate ventilation. Jet injectors and high-frequency positive-pressure ventilators able to deliver respiratory rates of 60 to 120 breaths/minute must also be available.

New short-acting intravenous agents and the equipment necessary to administer these drugs must finally be available.

Monitoring

Routine monitoring includes electrocardiography and arterial cannulation for blood gas analysis and continuous arterial pressure measurements. Because the innominate artery lies anterior to the trachea and sometimes has to be retracted, the arterial line is *usually inserted on the left side*. For the same reason, venous access is generally obtained through central venous cannulation installed on the left side of the neck, through the left antecubital vein, or less commonly through the femoral vein.

Following intubation, an esophageal stethoscope can be used to monitor breath and heart sounds. These devices are also useful to the surgeon for the identification of the esophagus.

A variety of monitoring devices can be used to record ventilation and gas exchange during tracheal reconstruction. These include the monitoring of oxygen saturation and blood gas analysis as well as the equipment necessary to monitor end-tidal carbon dioxide waveform and pressure-volume curves of the inspiratory lines of the ventilatory system.

Position of the Patient

Patients with respiratory compromise often breathe more effectively in a sitting position. Hence, the operating table should be *adjustable* so that the patient can be induced in the sitting position if required.

Once the airway is under control, the patient is placed in a supine position if a cervical or sternotomy approach is to be used. An inflatable bag is then placed transversely underneath the scapulae so that flexion or extension of the neck is permitted. It is important that the anesthetist has *unrestricted access* to the patient's head and neck areas at all times because in most cases of tracheal resection, the neck will have to be maximally flexed during the reconstruction.

Induction and Maintenance of Anesthesia

When there is a significant degree of airway obstruction, anesthesia can be induced with a *spontaneous inhalation technique*, best accomplished with low blood gas solubility agents such as sevoflurane. Such agents allow for rapid induction and, most important, for rapid emergence should difficulties arise during induction.

If a benign stenosis or a tumor narrows the airway to a diameter of 5 mm or less, dilatation must be performed before an endotracheal tube is advanced beyond the lesion. This is best accomplished with rigid bronchoscopy done immediately prior to induction. For bronchoscopy, the patient is preoxygenated; this preoxygenation is followed by slow inhalation induction, the patient breathing spontaneously. During bronchoscopy, it is important that a sufficient level of anesthesia be maintained *to prevent coughing or bucking*, which could result in endoluminal trauma with secondary edema or hemorrhage. At the termination of bronchoscopy, endotracheal intubation is carried out in standard fashion; the ideal endotracheal tube is a long, flexible, and reinforced tube with a cuff rotated as close as possible to its extremity.

With modern techniques of anesthesia, it is *seldom necessary* to perform an awake intubation under topical anesthesia. If it becomes necessary, however, it can be done with a small orotracheal tube, preferably under the guidance of fiberoptic bronchoscopy. The laryngeal mask airway can also be used for the same purpose; it permits fiberoptic bronchoscopy with little increase in airway resistance.

Once the tracheal obstruction has been bypassed and intubation safely performed, *muscle relaxants may be used.* Anesthesia and ventilation are then maintained in the usual way until surgical transection of the airway. Once the airways are opened, anesthesia is maintained with intravenous anesthetic agents.

Ventilation Techniques during Reconstruction of the Airway

Several anesthetic techniques can be used during the resection and reconstruction of the trachea. Ideally, these techniques must ensure the maintenance of adequate oxygenation, ventilation, and anesthesia while providing optimal and uninterrupted surgical access to the airways.

Orotracheal Intubation

This is a relatively *standard technique* that is recommended when the severity of airway obstruction is minimal. After induction of anesthesia, a long armored endotracheal tube is placed proximal to the stenotic area. Once the surgeon has opened the airway, the tube is advanced under direct vision into the distal trachea. The surgeon then completes the resection and performs the anastomosis around the endotracheal tube. The two main *disadvantages* of this technique are that the *surgical field is intermittently obstructed* and that the tip of the tube may traumatize the lesion, causing bleeding or dislodgment of tissue.

Distal Tracheal Intubation and Intermittent Apnea (Fig. 5-4)

This technique is the most widely used and most reliable method of providing adequate oxygenation during tracheal reconstruction.

After rigid bronchoscopy, the patient is intubated with a small endotracheal tube that is advanced beyond the lesion (Fig. 5-4A). Once the trachea (cervical or thoracic) has been fully mobilized and before surgical resection, anesthesia tubing and connectors are passed from the operating area to the anesthetist so that they can be connected to the anesthesia machine.

The trachea is then transected at a point below the obstruction, and the oral endotracheal tube is pulled back into the proximal trachea (Fig. 5-4B). A stitch is often sewn to the distal tip of the orotracheal tube so that it can be retrieved if necessary. The distal trachea is then intubated (operative tube [OT]) from the surgical field and ventilation resumed (Fig. 5-4B). If tracheal resection is performed near the carina, the OT is advanced into the left main bronchus and one-lung ventilation instituted. Before the anastomosis is performed, an inflatable bag that had been placed beneath the scapula is deflated so that the neck can be maximally flexed to reduce tension at the level of the anastomosis.

Interrupted sutures are then placed through both tracheal ends; short periods of apnea with the OT pulled out of the distal trachea generally facilitate the placement of these sutures (Fig. 5-4C). Once all sutures are in place, the OT is withdrawn from the distal trachea and the original oral endotracheal tube *re-advanced through the anastomosis* under direct vision. Anesthesia is then restarted through the oral tube as the sutures are tied (Fig. 5-4D). While performing the reconstruction, the surgeon must make sure that the orotracheal tube is in the distal trachea (versus being in a main bronchus) and that blood and other debris are regularly aspirated from the distal airway.

Short and intermittent periods of apnea are usually *well tolerated* by the patient. Often, preoxygenation of the patient with 100% oxygen and added positive end-expiratory pressure will allow prolonged periods of apnea (up to 6 to 7 minutes).

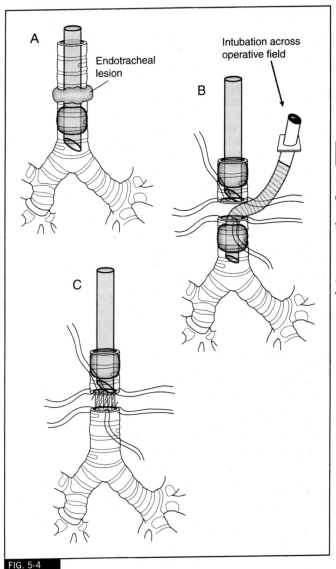

FIG. 5-4

A, Placement of a small oral endotracheal tube beyond the lesion. **B,** The oral endotracheal tube is pulled back, and the distal airway is intubated with a tube from the operative field. **C,** Intermittent periods of apnea facilitate surgical reconstruction and suture placement.   *Continued*

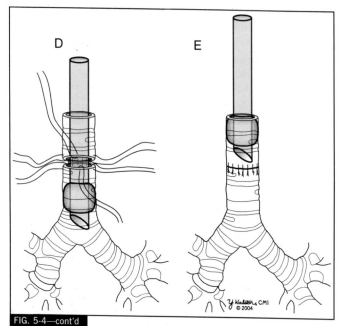

FIG. 5-4—cont'd

D, Anesthesia is restarted through the original oral endotracheal tube as the sutures are tied. **E,** After completion of the anastomosis, the oral endotracheal tube is pulled back well above the anastomosis.

After completion of the tracheal anastomosis, the orotracheal tube is *pulled back* well above the tracheal anastomosis (Fig. 5-4*E*).

Catheter Ventilation

Ventilation through a small catheter can be valuable during airway surgery. The small size of the catheter provides optimal surgical access to the circumferences of transected airways and facilitates the uninterrupted reconstruction. These catheters (one can use a nasogastric tube) are inserted into the distal airway through the endotracheal tube. Two different modes of catheter ventilation can be used during airway reconstruction.

High-Flow Jet Ventilation. Injector jet ventilation delivers a *large tidal volume*—500 to 1500 mL—at a *slow respiratory rate* of 10 to 30 breaths/minute. The technique achieves adequate gas exchange by bulk flow similar to that of conventional positive-pressure ventilation. Jet insufflation also generates a negative pressure around the tip of the catheter, which causes entrainment of air and provides an *enlarged tidal volume* necessary for adequate ventilation (Venturi effect).

Potential disadvantages of the technique include *barotrauma to the lung,* pneumothorax, surgical emphysema, air embolism, and *aspiration* of blood and mucus or other debris in the open airway because of the Venturi effect.

Low-Flow, High-Frequency Ventilation. This technique uses *small tidal volumes* (50 to 250 mL/min) delivered at a *rapid respiratory rate* of 50 to 150 breaths/minute. This method achieves gas exchange by a combination of convective flow and acceleration of gas diffusion. The repeated insufflations of small volumes at high velocity may also generate a continuously positive airway pressure, which increases functional residual capacity, improves gas mixing and distribution, and lowers the chances of alveolar collapse. Other advantages include *minimal lung and mediastinal movements* as well as *less entrainment of* blood or mucus in the open airway.

Cardiopulmonary Bypass

Cardiopulmonary bypass is almost never required during tracheal reconstruction, the main disadvantages of the technique being its complexity and *need for systemic anticoagulation,* which has the *potential for intrapulmonary hemorrhage.*

Emergence after Airway Surgery

At the conclusion of the procedure, resumption of *spontaneous respiration* and *early extubation* are important objectives for the anesthetist. Prompt extubation is particularly important for the surgeon because the endotracheal tube has the potential to cause *direct trauma to the suture line.* An infusion of propofol during the final stages of the procedures often permits rapid emergence to a wakeful state without agitation. At this stage, the surgeon will often perform *flexible bronchoscopy* to inspect the anastomosis and aspirate blood or mucus that might still be in the airway.

The anesthetist must remember that patients will likely have their neck extremely flexed at the end of operation and therefore will be prone to have some postoperative inability to clear secretions. Aspiration can also be a significant early problem after tracheal surgery, especially in those patients who have had a laryngeal release as part of the operation.

If there is some concern about the patency of the reconstructed trachea or about upper airway or glottic edema, most surgeons will have left a tracheostomy tube or a silicone Montgomery T tube. Obviously, these tubes will facilitate safe emergence from anesthesia.

Immediate Postoperative Care and Possible Postoperative Complications

Postoperative monitoring with electrocardiography, arterial blood pressure recording, and serial blood gas determinations is mandatory. A chest radiograph must also be obtained in the immediate postoperative period to rule out the presence of pneumothorax.

Patients will sometimes experience *some degree of respiratory difficulties* after extubation. Because this is most likely due to *local edema,* racemic epinephrine 1:200 (0.5 mL in 2 mL saline) can be nebulized to reduce such edema. Helium mixed with oxygen (He/O_2, 70% to 80%/ 20% to 30%) can also be given through a facemask in the hope of increasing ventilation. Finally, dexamethasone (4 to 10 mg) can also be added to the drug regimen.

If reintubation is required, this is best accomplished under direct vision with a fiberoptic bronchoscope, and the oroendotracheal or nasoendotracheal tube should be positioned well away from the anastomosis. Whenever possible, an attempt should be made to keep the tube proximal to the anastomosis because this location has less potential for suture line damage.

Standard postoperative care includes supplemental oxygen delivered with a high-flow humidified system. Chest physical therapy and routine nursing procedures *may be difficult if not impossible* when the head is maintained in an extreme flexed position.

In some cases, the acute relief of airway obstruction may result in a marked increase in transpulmonary pressure, and this may be the cause of *acute pulmonary edema episodes*. When this complication occurs, treatment is supportive; the majority of patients will require reintubation usually for a short time. If the patient is not intubated, he or she must receive oxygen supplementation and diuretics.

One of the most significant but underestimated problems that often occurs after tracheal surgery relates to *dysphagia and possible microaspiration*. Although there may be many potential causes for the dysphagia (Table 5-18), it is usually secondary to an incoordination between swallowing, initiation of the pharyngeal motor wave, and relaxation of the cricopharynx. Treatment of this condition must be supportive; often, the patient will not be allowed to drink or eat for several days postoperatively. On occasion, bronchoscopy may be required for removal of particulate matters.

ANESTHESIA FOR TRACHEOTOMY

The anesthetic technique used during tracheotomy depends on whether the surgery is done on an *elective or emergency* basis. Fortunately, most tracheotomies are done electively in good operating and anesthetic conditions. If the airway is compromised or not under total control, tracheotomy can be done under local anesthesia supplemented with intravenous sedation and narcotics. Standard monitoring is usually *enough* for stable patients.

Elective Tracheotomy

Elective tracheotomy is done with the neck *hyperextended and the head firmly attached* to a supporting pillow. Before the patient is draped, the in-place endotracheal tube is loosened and made ready to be withdrawn. Both mouth and pharynx are then suctioned so that contaminated secretions are not pushed back in the trachea during tube manipulations.

During the opening of the trachea the cuff of the endotracheal tube is often damaged, thus creating an air leak that can be significant in patients

TABLE 5-18

CAUSES OF DYSPHAGIA AFTER TRACHEAL RESECTION

Motor incoordination at the cricopharyngeal sphincter
Recurrent nerve paralysis
Extreme neck flexion
Presence of a tracheostomy or Montgomery T tube
Laryngeal release

with diseased lungs. This *can be prevented* by deflation of the cuff while the surgeon incises the trachea, or, if it has occurred, ventilation can be improved by increasing the tidal volume or by ventilating the patient manually. The pulling back of the endotracheal tube in the larynx must be coordinated with the surgeon, who should be ready to insert the tracheostomy tube. It is important not to pull the endotracheal tube all the way back into the mouth because, on occasion, this tube *may have to be readvanced distally*.

Once the tracheostomy tube is properly positioned and is functional as demonstrated by *chest wall expansion, end-tidal carbon dioxide waveform,* and *maintenance of adequate oxygen saturation,* the original endotracheal tube can be pulled back in the mouth and removed.

Emergency Tracheotomy

On rare occasions, such as in a patient with acute airway obstruction, an emergency tracheotomy will be necessary. In such cases, the anesthetist will provide some level of sedation while the surgeon quickly performs the tracheotomy under local anesthesia. Once the cannula is in (usually through the cricothyroid membrane), the anesthetist will take over the ventilation.

CONCLUSION

Because surgical resection of the trachea is done infrequently, few centers have expertise and experience in the anesthetic management of such patients. The anesthetist must have a clear understanding of the intended surgery and on the basis of this understanding must be able to determine a specific plan for each individual patient. This planning is essential to ensure adequate oxygenation and safe delivery of anesthetic agents throughout the procedure.

SUGGESTED READINGS

Review Articles

Geffin B, Bland J, Grillo HC: Anesthetic management of tracheal resection and reconstruction. Anesth Analg 1969;48:884-890.
Wilson RS: Anesthetic management for tracheal reconstruction. In Grillo HC, Eschapasse H, eds: International Trends in General Thoracic Surgery, vol 2. Major Challenges. Philadelphia, WB Saunders, 1987:3-12.

Young-Beyer P, Wilson RS: Anesthetic management for tracheal resection and reconstruction. J Cardiothorac Anesth 1988;2:821-835.

Pinsonneault C, Fortier J, Donati F: Tracheal resection and reconstruction. Can J Anaesth 1999;46:439-455.

Sandberg W: Anesthesia and airway management for tracheal resection and reconstruction. Int Anesthesiol Clin 2000;38:55-75.

Jet Ventilation

El-Baz N, El-Ganzouri A, Gottschalk W, Jensik R: One-lung high-frequency positive pressure ventilation for sleeve pneumonectomy: an alternative technique. Anesth Analg 1981;60:683-686.

Biro P, Hegi TR, Weder W, Spahn DR: Laryngeal mask airway and high-frequency jet ventilation for the resection of a high-grade upper tracheal stenosis. J Clin Anesth 2001;13:141-143.

Case Series, Case Reports

Magnusson L, Lang FJW, Monnier P, Ravussin P: Anesthesia for tracheal resection: report of 17 cases. Can J Anaesth 1997;44:1282-1285.

Licker M, Schweizer A, Nicolet G, et al: Anesthesia of a patient with an obstructing tracheal mass: a new way to manage airway. Acta Anaesthesiol Scand 1997;41:84-86.

Mentzelopoulos SD, Romana CN, Hatzimichalis AG, et al: Anesthesia for tracheal resection: a new technique of airway management in a patient with severe stenosis of the midtrachea. Anesth Analg 1999;89:1156-1160.

THORACIC ANATOMY

The importance of detailed knowledge of thoracic anatomy cannot be underestimated in the practice of general thoracic surgery. This knowledge will ensure *complete control in the operating room,* despite the intricacies of the surgery. By contrast, intrathoracic dissection without such knowledge is likely to lead to technical accidents. A *clear understanding* of the lymphatic drainage of the lungs or esophagus is also important for the surgical staging of thoracic malignant neoplasms as well as for their management.

The anatomic information that every thoracic surgeon must know may not appear as such in standard anatomic textbooks, the main reason being that the drawings are those seen through the eyes of an anatomist rather than those of a surgeon. The information attached to the drawings is also often presented from an anatomic rather than from a surgical viewpoint. There finally may be considerable difficulties in correlating what one sees in a cadaver lying on its back to what is seen in the operating room, where most patients are in different positions.

ANATOMY OF THE CHEST WALL

Surface Landmarks and Skin Creases

The size and shape of the thorax are largely determined by the ribs, costal cartilages, sternum, and chest wall muscles. There are 12 pairs of ribs. Each rib forms a *continuous arch* that extends from the spine, turns forward at the angle (point of greatest change in curvature) and extends toward the sternum, where all but the eleventh and twelfth pairs (floating ribs) articulate, directly or indirectly. All ribs have an inferior inclination from the back to the front so that they are two interspaces lower anteriorly than posteriorly. For instance, *the sternal angle,* which is an important landmark because it is where the second costal cartilages articulate with the sternum, is at the level *of T4-5 posteriorly.*

In general, the skin creases of the chest wall follow the inferior inclination of the ribs. This is why the posterolateral thoracotomy incision is not horizontal but gently curves downward from the tip of the scapula to the anterior end of the incision.

Musculature

A number of large muscles have their origins in the chest wall. Knowledge of their anatomy including blood supply *is important* because some of these muscles have to be divided during routine thoracotomy; others may be used to reconstruct soft tissues of the chest wall, to close bronchopleural fistulas, or to obliterate chronic empyema spaces.

The *pectoralis major* (Fig. 5-5) arises from the lower costal cartilages and ribs (two to six), sternum, and clavicle (medial half) to form a unified muscle that inserts in the intertubercular sulcus of the humerus. It is a *thick fan-shaped muscle* whose lower margin forms the anterior fold of the axilla. The primary blood supply is from thoracoacromial vessels (axillary artery); an important secondary blood supply is from multiple perforators from the internal mammary. The pectoralis major is the workhorse for sternal reconstruction (sternal infection after cardiac surgery) and mediastinal coverage.

The *latissimus dorsi* (Fig. 5-6) arises by broad aponeurotic origins from the lower six thoracic vertebrae, lumbodorsal fascia, and iliac crest to form a large muscle that inserts into the intertubercular groove of the humerus. The dominant vascular supply is from the *thoracodorsal artery* (axillary artery); secondary blood supply is from multiple paraspinous perforators. Thoracotomy incisions that divide this muscle (posterolateral thoracotomy) may cause significant alterations in its physiology. The latissimus dorsi is particularly useful for full-thickness reconstruction of chest wall defects anteriorly and laterally. It also functions well for intrathoracic use.

The *serratus anterior* (Fig. 5-7) arises from major muscle slips from the upper eight ribs and attaches on the anterior surface and medial border of the scapula. In thin and muscular individuals, the serratus anterior can be seen along the anterolateral aspect of the chest wall. Its blood supply comes from the lateral thoracic artery (branch of thoracodorsal artery),

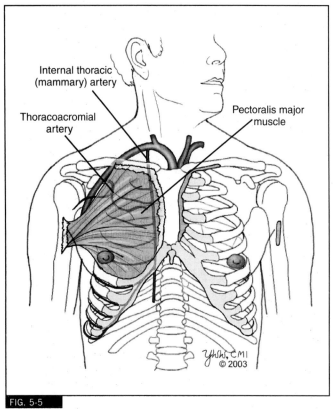

Surgical anatomy of the pectoralis major. *(Modified from a drawing from Dr. Joseph I. Miller, Jr.)*

which travels over the surface of the muscle, parallel to the long thoracic nerve. The serratus anterior is usually preserved during posterolateral thoracotomy; it is most frequently used for intrathoracic problems, such as coverage of bronchopleural stumps. *Scapular winging* can result from its functional loss.

Two additional muscles have their origins on the posterior aspect of the thoracic wall. These muscles are seldom used for reconstruction of thoracic defects, but they may have to be divided during the course of a posterolateral thoracotomy. The *trapezius* is more superficial and more cephalad; it originates from the spinous processes of C7 to C12 and from the occiput and courses laterally to insert on the scapula.

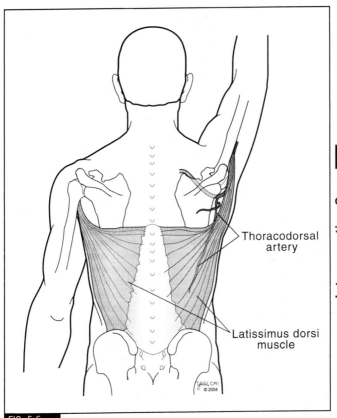

Intraoperative Care

5

FIG. 5-6

Surgical anatomy of the latissimus dorsi. *(Modified from a drawing from Dr. Joseph I. Miller, Jr.)*

The *rhomboid* lies directly beneath the trapezius and courses laterally to insert on the scapula.

Intercostal Space

Every thoracic surgeon must have a clear understanding of the anatomy of the intercostal space because it is the *most common site of surgical entry* into the pleural space. It is also the *most common site of placement of chest tubes*.

Each intercostal space is traversed by three layers of intercostal muscles (external, internal, innermost) that are attached to the periosteum at the upper and lower borders of the rib. Thus, an electrocautery incision over the body of the rib with subsequent elevation of the periosteum *will not*

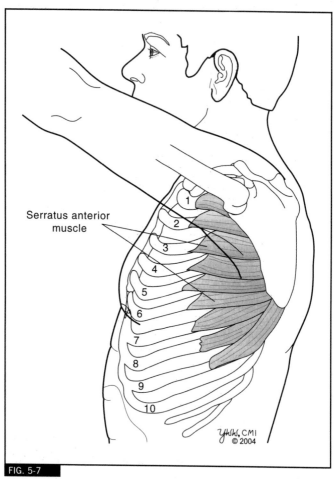

FIG. 5-7

Surgical anatomy of the serratus anterior. *(Modified from a drawing from Dr. Joseph I. Miller, Jr.)*

violate the contents of the intercostal space. The external intercostal muscle fibers run obliquely and inferiorly from the rib above to the rib below. Because of the angle formed by these muscles and the ribs, their detachment must be done from the back to the front on the superior border of the ribs and from the front to the back on the inferior border.

Understanding the anatomy of the intercostal space (Fig. 5-8) is also important if one is to avoid injury to the neurovascular structures located in

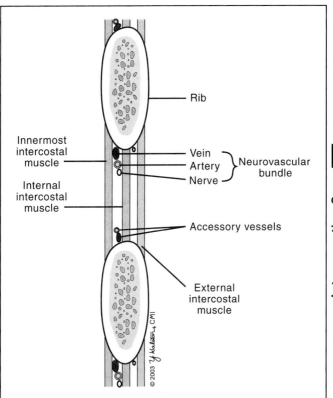

FIG. 5-8

Cross-sectional diagram of the chest wall demonstrating the anatomic relationship of the intercostal space, rib, neurovascular bundle, and accessory vessels. Observe that a chest tube inserted above the superior border of the rib will avoid trauma to the main neurovascular bundle. *(From McFadden PM, Jones JW: Tube thoracostomy: anatomical considerations, overview of complications, and a proposed technique to avoid complications. Milit Med 1985;150:681-685.)*

the costal groove in close relation to the lower border of each rib. Chest tubes should be inserted along the upper margin of the rib because if accessory vessels are injured at that level, *chances of a major hemorrhage are negligible*.

The intercostal nerves provide sensory innervation to the entire chest wall. The first six or seven intercostal nerves supply the sensory innervation from the posterior aspect of the back to the midline of the sternum; the eighth nerve supplies the anterior chest wall around the xiphoid. The ninth intercostal nerve supplies the upper portion of the epigastrium, and the tenth intercostal is responsible for sensation at the level of the umbilicus. Because there is considerable overlap of contiguous dermatomes, results of local anesthesia are poor unless two or more dorsal roots are infiltrated.

ANATOMY OF THE PLEURAL SPACE

The pleura is formed of two membranes, one covering the inner chest wall (parietal pleura) and one covering the lung (visceral pleura). The *transition between parietal pleura and visceral pleura is at the level of the hilum.* At this level, the reflection covers the constituents of the hilum except inferiorly, where the reflection extends down to the diaphragm to form the inferior pulmonary ligament.

The parietal pleura is attached to the inner surface of the thoracic wall by a fibrous layer known as the *endothoracic fascia*. This fascia is a cleavage layer within which the parietal pleura can be separated from the chest wall. The thickness and strength of the endothoracic fascia vary with location. It is strongest over the inner surface of the ribs; in that location, the parietal pleura can easily be stripped from it (pleurectomy, pleural tent, extrapleural pulmonary resection). Posterior to the sternum and over the pericardium, the endothoracic fascia is almost nonexistent, and this makes the detachment of the pleura in these locations impossible. *The visceral pleura* covers the surface of the lung and extends into the fissures. It is thin, transparent, and adherent to the lung.

The *projection* of the pleural sinuses over the chest wall is important because it provides landmarks that must be known before insertion of a chest tube. Anteriorly, the lung extends no lower than the sixth rib in the midclavicular line, whereas the pleural costophrenic sinus extends to the seventh rib. Laterally in the midaxillary line, the lung descends to the eighth rib; the lateral costophrenic sinus descends to the ninth rib. Posteriorly, the lung extends to the eleventh rib and the pleura to the twelfth rib.

The visceral pleura is devoid of somatic innervation; in contrast, the *parietal pleura is innervated through a rich network of somatic, sympathetic, and parasympathetic fibers*. It is therefore very sensitive, and it must be thoroughly infiltrated when one is inserting a chest tube under local anesthesia.

ANATOMY OF THE LUNG

Pulmonary Hilum

The hilum of the lung is where the main bronchi, main pulmonary vessels (arteries and veins), bronchial vessels, and lymph vessels enter and leave the lung. It is surrounded by a reflection of the pleura off the lung (visceral pleura) onto the mediastinum (parietal pleura). At this level, the parietal pleura is called the mediastinal pleura. The hilum *is an important radiologic* landmark.

The position of the hilar structures, mainly the pulmonary arteries, is somewhat different on the two sides (Figs. 5-9 and 5-10). *On the left,* the pulmonary artery, which is a direct continuation of the main pulmonary artery,

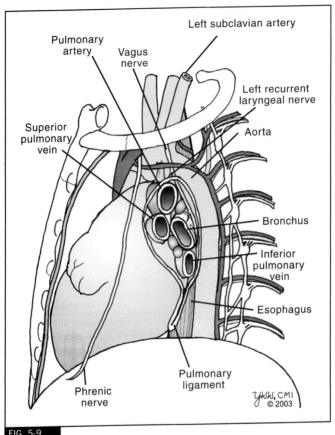

FIG. 5-9

Left pulmonary hilum.

lies anterior and superior to the main bronchus, and it runs in a slightly posterior direction before curving around the upper lobe bronchus. On the right side, it is anterior but inferior to the main bronchus. In both hila, the *superior pulmonary veins are the most anterior structures*; the inferior pulmonary veins are on a more posterior plane.

On both sides, the hilum is bordered by a vascular arch. On the right side, *the azygos vein* arches over the hilum to enter the superior vena cava; on the left, *the arch of the aorta* curves around the hilum superiorly, and the descending thoracic aorta lies behind it. Both are in close contact with the pericardium and phrenic nerves anteriorly (the phrenic nerve

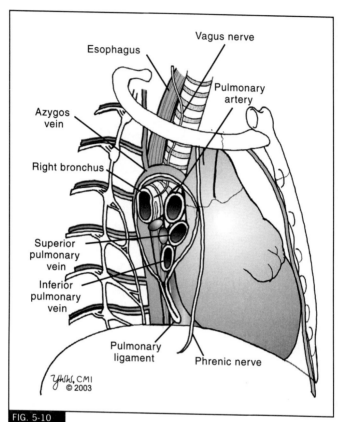

FIG. 5-10

Right pulmonary hilum.

is 1.5 cm anterior to the hilum) and with the vagus nerves and bronchial arteries posteriorly.

Lobes, Segments, and Fissures

The right lung, which is the larger of the two lungs, has three lobes: upper, middle, and lower. The right upper lobe could have easily been named *upper anterior lobe* because it has a large contact anteriorly and a small contact posteriorly. The middle lobe has contact only anteriorly, whereas the lower lobe mostly projects posteriorly. The right *major fissure* runs obliquely (oblique fissure) from the level of T3 posteriorly to the sixth costochondral junction anteriorly. This major fissure separates the lower lobe from the upper and middle lobes. The minor fissure (horizontal) that separates the middle and upper lobes starts from the oblique fissure in the midaxillary

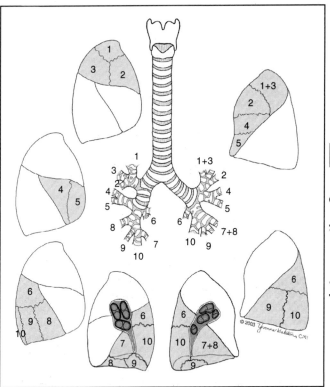

FIG. 5-11

The lobes and segments of the lung. Right upper lobe segments: 1, apical; 2, anterior; 3, posterior. Right middle lobe segments: 4, lateral; 5, medial. Right lower lobe segments: 6, superior; 7, medial basal; 8, anterior basal; 9, lateral basal; 10, posterior basal. Left upper lobe segments: 1 and 3, apical posterior; 2, anterior; 4, superior lingula; 5, inferior lingula. Left lower lobe segments: 6, superior; 7 and 8, anteromedial basal; 9, lateral basal; 10, posterior basal. *(Courtesy of Dr. Thomas W. Rice.)*

line at the level of the sixth rib and runs transversely to the fourth costal cartilage. The right lung is composed of *ten segments* (Fig. 5-11).

The left lung has two lobes, the upper and the lower, which are separated by a major oblique fissure that follows approximately the same course as the one on the right side. The left lung is composed of *eight segments* (Fig. 5-11).

Each segment has its own bronchus and pulmonary artery and vein. The respective bronchi and pulmonary arteries are in close association (Fig. 5-12) and centrally placed in the segment, whereas the pulmonary

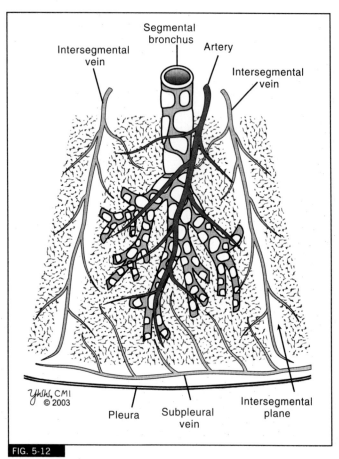

Intersegmental vein

Segmental bronchus

Artery

Intersegmental vein

Pleura

Subpleural vein

Intersegmental plane

YhShj, CMI © 2003

FIG. 5-12

Anatomy of the bronchopulmonary segment. *(Modified from Wareham EE, Huse WM: Surgical anatomy of the lungs. Surg Clin North Am 1964;44:1191-2000, with permission.)*

veins are peripheral and intersegmental. The pulmonary segments are held together by delicate connective tissue, and *no bronchi or major pulmonary artery crosses intersegmental planes.*

Trachea, Main Bronchi, and Lobar Bronchi

The trachea begins as a continuation of the larynx and extends down to its bifurcation (level of T5) into right and left main bronchi. It is approximately 11 cm in length (longer in men). The *right main bronchus is shorter, wider, and more vertical than the left.* The right upper lobe bronchus arises within 2.5 cm of the carina; the bronchus between the origins of right upper lobe and middle lobe is termed the bronchus intermedius. The further continuation of the bronchus intermedius is the lower lobe bronchus. The middle lobe bronchus often arises at the same level as or even below the superior segmental bronchus.

The left main bronchus is *considerably longer* than the right main bronchus. The left upper lobe bronchus arises 5 to 6 cm from the carina. The left lower lobe bronchus is very short, giving off the superior segmental bronchus less than 1 cm from the upper lobe orifice. There is no bronchus intermedius on the left side.

Pulmonary Arteries and Veins

The segmental branches of the pulmonary arteries lie close to the segmental bronchi, usually on the superior and lateral surfaces; in general, they have the same names as the bronchi (Fig. 5-12). The venous tributaries occupy an *intersegmental* rather than a central position.

The right pulmonary artery enters the lung anterior and inferior to the right main bronchus, then enters the horizontal fissure and continues inferolaterally in a fairly straight line. The right superior vein lies anteriorly in the hilum and receives all the tributaries from the *right upper and middle lobes.* The inferior vein lies posterior and inferior to the upper lobe vein and receives the venous drainage from the *lower lobe.*

The left pulmonary artery arches over the upper lobe bronchus, making a sharp turn to enter the floor of the interlobar fissure. The left superior vein is the most anterior structure of the left hilum and drains the left upper lobe. The left inferior pulmonary vein is posterior and inferior to the superior vein and drains the lower lobe.

Pulmonary Lymphatics

The classic drainage pathway of the pulmonary lymphatics is from subpleural lymphatic vessels and then along lymphatic channels that are associated with the pulmonary veins to reach larger channels that run with the arteries and bronchi. These deeper channels drain into segmental, lobar, interlobar, hilar, and mediastinal nodes.

Lymph nodes located in the lymphatic sump of each lung are *constant.* These nodes are important because tumors in any lobe of either lung *must drain through these areas.* On the right side, sump nodes are located in the angle between right upper lobe bronchus and bronchus intermedius; the left lymphatic sump lies between the upper and lower lobes in the major fissure. The obvious *clinical implication* of a sump node is that one may have to consider pneumonectomy (versus lobectomy) if these nodes contain metastatic tumor.

From the hilum, lymphatic channels reach the mediastinum along their respective main bronchus. In the mediastinum, there are two major and one alternate lymphatic pathways. The first pathway follows the superior border of each main bronchus to the tracheobronchial angle. It then travels up to the supraclavicular regions alongside the trachea. This pathway is named *laterotracheal,* and *nodes are those of the superior mediastinum.* The second pathway follows the inferior border of each main bronchus to the subcarinal space. In that space, nodes connect with those of the posterior mediastinum (alongside the esophagus) and with those of the inferior pulmonary ligament. This pathway is named *posteroinferior,* and *nodes are those of the posterior mediastinum.* On the left side, there is an alternate pathway to the subaortic (aortopulmonary), periaortic, and anterior mediastinal nodes. This pathway is named *anterior,* and *nodes are those of the anterior mediastinum.*

The usual drainage of each pulmonary lobe is shown in Figure 5-13 and listed in Table 5-19. In approximately 10% of cases, lymphatic drainage of the left lower lobe and lingula will spread to contralateral nodes.

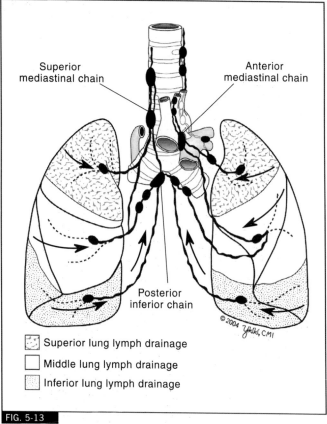

Superior mediastinal chain

Anterior mediastinal chain

Posterior inferior chain

© 2004 *Yghshs,* CMI

⬚ Superior lung lymph drainage

☐ Middle lung lymph drainage

⬚ Inferior lung lymph drainage

FIG. 5-13

Drainage of the parenchymal lymphatic channels to mediastinal lymph nodes. It is generally ipsilateral and directed toward the trachea.

TABLE 5-19

USUAL LYMPHATIC DRAINAGE OF EACH LOBE

Right lung
    Upper lobe: superior mediastinum
    Middle lobe: superior or inferior mediastinum
    Lower lobe: inferior mediastinum
Left lung
    Upper lobe: superior and anterior mediastinum
    Lower lobe: inferior mediastinum

Bronchial Circulation

Most bronchial arteries arise from the anterolateral aspect of the aorta within 2 to 3 cm of the origin of the left subclavian artery. Although they vary in number from one to three to each lung, the *most common distribution* is two arteries on the left and one on the right.

Before reaching the airway, the bronchial arteries give off esophageal branches to supply the midthoracic esophagus. The arteries then pass posteriorly to the airway to lie on the membranous portion of the main stem bronchi.

ANATOMY OF THE MEDIASTINUM

Thoracic Duct (Fig. 5-14)

The thoracic duct is the *left main collecting vessel of the lymphatic system,* and it is far larger than the right terminal lymphatic duct (Table 5-20). It originates from the cisterna chyli in the abdomen (level of L2) and ascends through the chest before it drains in the left subclavian–internal jugular junction.

The thoracic duct enters the thorax through the aortic hiatus (T12) just to the right of the aorta. From there, it ascends on the left posterior aspect of the esophagus between the aorta and azygos vein.

At the level of T4, the thoracic duct *crosses behind the aorta to the left posterior side of the mediastinum,* and from there it ascends on the left side of the esophagus. At the thoracic inlet, the thoracic duct arches behind the innominate vein to enter the venous system.

Esophagus

The esophagus is a muscular tube that extends from the lower end of the pharynx to the cardia (level of T11). It has cervical, thoracic, and abdominal parts (Fig. 5-15). It enters the superior mediastinum between the trachea and spine. Within the mediastinum, it is *posterior to the left main bronchus* and then descends posteriorly and to the right of the aorta and posterior to the pericardium. It then deviates to the left and enters the abdomen through the esophageal hiatus, which is located within the right crus of the diaphragm.

The two vagus nerves are closely attached to the esophagus. *In the upper and mid esophagus,* they are arranged as right and left; *at the lower end,* the left vagus becomes posterior and the right vagus anterior.

5

Intraoperative Care

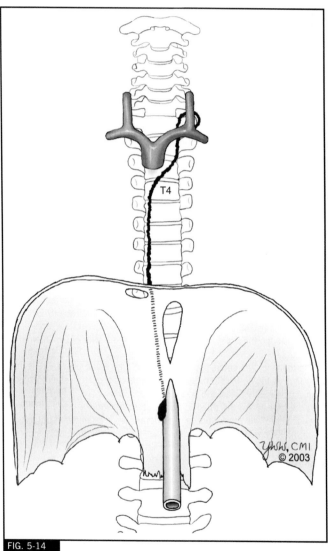

FIG. 5-14

Anatomy of the thoracic duct. *(Reza Mehran.)*

TABLE 5-20

ANATOMY OF THE THORACIC DUCT

Originates from cisterna chyli (L2)

Enters the chest through aortic hiatus (T10)

Ascends extrapleurally to the left of the esophagus between aorta and azygos vein

Crosses to the left at the level of T4

Ascends on the left posterior side of esophagus to thoracic inlet

Arches to the left behind innominate vein

Drains in left subclavian–internal jugular vein junction

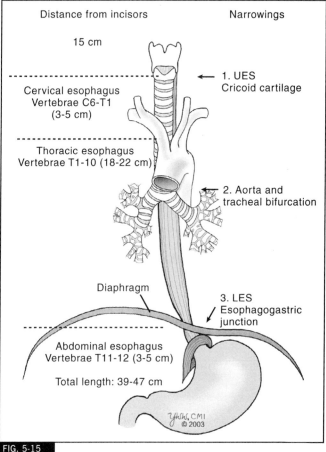

FIG. 5-15

Classical divisions of the esophagus. UES, upper esophageal sphincter; LES, lower esophageal sphincter. (Courtesy of Dr. Dorothea Liebermann-Meffert.)

The thoracic esophagus is supplied by branches from the right and left inferior thyroid arteries and from branches of the bronchial arteries. Lymph node drainage is through posterior mediastinal nodes and celiac nodes.

Nerves and Sympathetic Trunks

The right recurrent laryngeal nerve originates from the right vagus nerve *in front of the right subclavian artery* and then hooks around this vessel to ascend in the neck. This nerve is not at high risk for trauma during thoracic procedures. By contrast, the left recurrent laryngeal nerve arises from the vagus nerve to the left of the aortic arch and hooks *inferior to the arch to the left of the ligamentum arteriosum.* It then ascends to the larynx in the groove between trachea and esophagus. Because of this location, the left recurrent laryngeal nerve is at risk for injury during several thoracic procedures.

The *phrenic nerves* have both motor and sensory functions. They arise from C3-5 and enter the mediastinum between the ipsilateral subclavian artery and innominate vein. The left phrenic nerve descends between the left subclavian and common carotid arteries and then courses along the pericardium superficial to the left atrium and left ventricle. The right phrenic nerve is posterolateral to the superior vena cava and then courses along the pericardium in front of the right hilum. Both phrenic nerves are at risk for injury during any type of pulmonary resection.

The *sympathetic trunks* provide efficient sympathetic fibers to the levator muscles of the eyelids and sweat glands. These trunks are located *over the prevertebral fascia in the paravertebral gutter.* They run in a vertical line that courses the necks of the ribs. The stellate ganglion (inferior cervical ganglion) lies at the level of the superior border of the neck of the first ribs.

ANATOMY OF THE DIAPHRAGM

The mature diaphragm is a flat muscle that is anchored to the bony structures of the floor of the thorax. Posteriorly, its insertion arises from the lumbar vertebrae (L1-3) by two musculotendinous pillars called crura. The two crura are connected in front of the aorta by the fibrous median arcuate ligament. This posterior origin is lower than the anterior attachments to the xiphoid and lower six ribs and costal cartilages. From the costal muscular portions of the diaphragm, fibers are directed upward to join the central tendon. By doing so, each hemidiaphragm takes the shape of a dome that is visible on chest radiographs.

Between the dome and the parietal chest wall, there is a deep sinus called the costodiaphragmatic sinus. Posteriorly, this depression is low and deep; anteriorly, it is more superficial and higher. This is the reason why pleural effusions tend to accumulate posteriorly.

The three major openings in the normal diaphragm are the aortic hiatus (T12, aorta, thoracic duct, azygos vein), the esophageal hiatus (T10, esophagus, vagus nerves), and the inferior vena cava hiatus (T8), which is in the central tendon.

The diaphragm is innervated by the phrenic nerve and is an important inspiratory muscle. The phrenic nerve divides at the level of the diaphragm into four branches. Circumferential incisions in the periphery of the diaphragm or in the central tendon do not interrupt any major branch of the phrenic nerve and result in no loss of diaphragmatic function. By contrast, a radial incision from the costal margin to the esophageal hiatus will almost certainly result in total diaphragmatic paralysis.

CONCLUSION

The clinical practice of thoracic surgery requires the surgeon to have thorough knowledge of chest wall, pleura, pulmonary, mediastinal, and diaphragm anatomy. Attempts to perform thoracic procedures without this knowledge can only result in incomplete operations or technical mishaps. Similarly, knowledge of the lymphatic drainage pathways between lung and mediastinum will ensure that each patient gets the best possible operation for his or her thoracic malignant disease.

SUGGESTED READINGS

Textbook of Anatomy

Moore KL: Clinically Oriented Anatomy, 2nd ed. Baltimore, Williams & Wilkins, 1985.

Intercostal Space

Moore DC: Anatomy of the intercostal nerve: its importance during thoracic surgery. Am J Surg 1982;144:371-373.

McFadden PM, Jones JW: Tube thoracostomy: anatomical considerations, overview of complications, and a proposed technique to avoid complications. Milit Med 1985;150:681-685.

Lungs

Wareham EE, Huse WM: Surgical anatomy of the lungs. Surg Clin North Am 1964;44:1191-1200.

Neef H: Anatomical pathways of lymphatic flow between lung and mediastinum. Ann Ital Chir 1999;70:857-866.

Thoracic Duct

Kausel HW, Reeve TS, Stein AA, et al: Anatomic and pathologic studies of the thoracic duct. J Thorac Surg 1957;34:631-642.

Riquet M, Le Pimpec Barthes F, Souilamas R, Hidden G: Thoracic duct tributaries from intrathoracic organs. Ann Thorac Surg 2002; 73:892-899.

Nerves of Thorax

Aquino SL, Duncan GR, Hayman LA: Nerves of the thorax: atlas of normal and pathologic findings. Radiographics 2001;21:1275-1281.

Diaphragm

Fell SC: Surgical anatomy of the diaphragm and the phrenic nerve. Chest Surg Clin North Am 1998;8:281-294.

Panicek DM, Benson CB, Gottlieb RH, Heltzman ER: The diaphragm: anatomic, pathologic, and radiologic considerations. Radiographics 1988;8:385-425.

Lymphatics

Riquet M, Hidden G, Debesse B: Direct lymphatic drainage of lung segments to the mediastinal nodes. An anatomic study on 260 adults. J Thorac Cardiovasc Surg 1989;97:623-632.

Riquet M, Saab M, Le Pimpec Barthes F, Hidden G: Lymphatic drainage of the esophagus in the adult. Surg Radiol Anat 1993;15:209-211.

POSITIONING AND INCISIONS

The selection of the surgical incision is the *responsibility of the surgeon,* who needs the best possible exposure to complete the proposed operation. In the case of pulmonary resection, for instance, the incision must provide exposure of the hilum so that mobilization of pulmonary vessels can be done safely or a proposed lobectomy can be converted to a pneumonectomy should circumstances dictate. Indeed, a poorly planned incision is likely to lead to a difficult and frustrating operation, increasing the chances of technical misadventures.

The selection of the surgical incision should also be based on *the surgeon's experience and familiarity* with the exposure that a particular incision provides. For example, anatomic pulmonary resections through a midline sternotomy incision can be safely performed, but for the surgeon unfamiliar with the anatomy seen from the front, these can turn out to be nightmares.

Finally but not the least, the incision must be *acceptable* to the patient, who will have postoperative pain or may suffer from long-term muscular, neurologic, or even cosmetic disabilities.

A clear understanding of proper positioning of the patient for the selected incision is also important if one is to achieve maximum use of the incision. A recent radiograph or CT scan must always be available in the operating room to ensure that the patient is positioned on the proper side. Although the surgeon does not necessarily have to be in the operating room while the patient is being positioned, it is important that the personnel who actually position the patient be familiar with the technique.

CERVICAL INCISIONS (TABLE 5-21 and FIG. 5-16)

Cervical incisions are used by thoracic surgeons to access the *cervical trachea, thyroid, cervical esophagus,* and *superior mediastinum* (Table 5-21). Patients are placed in a supine position on the operating table and arms are tucked at the sides. In general, cervical exposure is augmented by neck hyperextension, which is best achieved with a sandbag placed underneath the shoulders.

TABLE 5-21

COMMON PROCEDURES DONE BY THORACIC SURGEONS THROUGH CERVICAL INCISION (see Fig. 5-16)

Type of Incision	Organ Accessed	Operation
Suprasternal	Superior and middle mediastinum	Mediastinoscopy
		Drainage of mediastinal abscesses
	Trachea	Tracheotomy
	Thymus	Thymectomy for myasthenia gravis
Transverse cervical	Trachea	Resection
	Thyroid	Resection of substernal goiters
Supraclavicular	Prescalenic space	Biopsy of nodes
	Thoracic duct	Ligation
Oblique anterior border of sternocleidomastoid	Cervical esophagus	Resection, reconstruction, Zenker diverticulum
Anterior transcervical (hockey stick)	Lung (apex)	Resection of Pancoast tumors

5

Intraoperative Care

Cervical Approach to the Trachea and Thyroid

When tracheal or thyroid operations are planned, the *entire anterior chest wall* should be prepared and draped in case a sternotomy is required. Surgery is done through a standard transverse incision (Fig. 5-16A) usually made midway between thyroid cartilage and suprasternal notch. Once the strap muscles are identified, they are retracted laterally to expose the thyroid gland and cervical trachea. In cases of tracheal surgery (resection or tracheotomy), the thyroid isthmus may have to be divided for better exposure.

Mediastinoscopy, Scalene Node Biopsy

Mediastinoscopy is done through a small incision just *above the suprasternal notch (Fig. 5-16B).* Once the pretracheal fascia is elevated, one has access to the entire superior mediastinum, where nodal biopsy specimens can be taken. For proper mediastinoscopic examination, the surgeon should be positioned (standing, sitting, or on the knees) at the head of the table, which must be elevated.

For scalene node biopsy (Fig. 5-16C), the neck is extended and turned on the contralateral side. A transverse incision is started at the lateral border of the sternocleidomastoid muscle and carried laterally across the supraclavicular fossa.

Oblique Incision for Exposure of the Esophagus

The cervical esophagus is exposed with an oblique incision *along the anterior border* of the sternocleidomastoid muscle (Fig. 5-16D). Once this muscle is retracted laterally, the carotid sheath is mobilized. With both carotid sheath and sternocleidomastoid muscle retracted laterally, the cervical esophagus is approached along the anterior border of the spine.

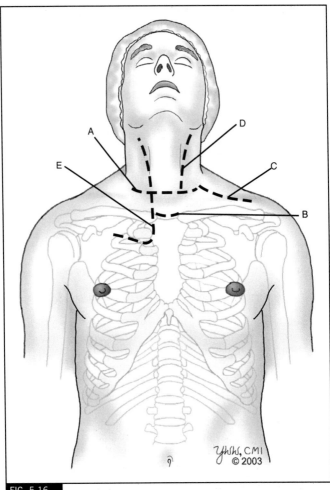

FIG. 5-16

Variety of common cervical incisions. **A,** Transverse cervical. **B,** Suprasternal. **C,** Supraclavicular. **D,** Oblique (anterior border of sternocleidomastoid). **E,** Anterior transcervical.

Anterosuperior Approaches

A variety of anterosuperior approaches (Table 5-22) can provide exposure for safe resection of tumors invading structures of the thoracic inlet, such as Pancoast tumors. In general, an L-type incision (Fig. 5-16*E*) is made

TABLE 5-22

ANTEROSUPERIOR APPROACHES

Approach	Description
Anterior transcervical thoracic (Dartevelle)	Incision made along anterior border of sternomastoid muscle and extended in curved fashion laterally beneath clavicle toward deltopectoral groove; medial half of clavicle resected
Transmanubrial osteomuscular	Leaves clavicle–manubrium joint intact
Sparing approach (Grunenwald)	Leaves clavicle intact

along the anterior border of the sternocleidomastoid and transversely across the inferior border of the clavicle. This approach provides excellent exposure to the subclavian vessels and brachial plexus. The transmanubrial approach has the advantage of leaving the clavicle–manubrial joint intact, thus reducing the chances of postoperative disabilities and deformities.

Again, one of the keys to the successful use of these approaches is the familiarity of the surgeon with the local anatomy and his or her experience with the incision.

ANTERIOR THORACIC INCISIONS

Anterior incisions can be used for a wide variety of thoracic procedures (Table 5-23), whether they are lung resections or cardiac operations.

TABLE 5-23

COMMON PROCEDURES DONE THROUGH ANTERIOR THORACIC INCISIONS (see Fig. 5-17)

Type of Incision	Organ Accessed	Operation
Parasternal mediastinotomy	Anterosuperior mediastinum	Mediastinotomy for biopsy of hilar or anterior mediastinal abnormalities
Anterolateral thoracotomy	Lung	Limited resection of nodules
		Resection of bullae
		Open lung biopsy in critically ill patients
	Pericardium	Pericardial window
Median sternotomy	Anterior mediastinum	Resection of anterior mediastinal tumors
	Trachea and carina	Resection
	Lung	Almost any type of resection
		Bilateral resections
Partial sternotomy	Anterior mediastinum	Resection of anterior mediastinal tumors
	Trachea	Resection and reconstruction
Transverse sternotomy (clamshell)	Anterior mediastinum	Resection of anterior mediastinal tumors
	Lung	Bilateral resections
		Lung transplantation
		Excision of cervicothoracic tumors

Advantages (Table 5-24) of these incisions are that the patient is in a supine or almost supine position, which greatly facilitates surgical positioning; the incisions do not transect any major muscle; and postoperative morbidity and pain are reduced. This last consideration may allow surgical procedures to be done in patients with severe comorbidities, especially respiratory disabilities.

Anterior Mediastinotomy

This is a classic incision that is mostly used for biopsy of hilar or mediastinal nodes or primary anterior mediastinal tumors, such as lymphomas, thymomas, or germ cell tumors.

The skin incision (Fig. 5-17A) is made over the second interspace parasternally, and the fibers of the pectoralis major muscle are separated. The second or third costal cartilage is often removed, preserving the perichondrium. If one elects to remain extrapleural, the anterior mediastinal pleura is dissected from underneath the sternum and deflected laterally. The *internal mammary pedicle is also distracted laterally* and the mediastinum entered bluntly. The pleura may be opened if exposure is inadequate, and in such cases, the pleural cavity is entered lateral to the mammary pedicle.

Anterolateral Thoracotomy

This incision, which can be used for anatomic lung resection, has the advantage of a *pleasing cosmetic appearance.* Its main indications are limited resection of lung nodules, removal of emphysematous bullae, and open lung biopsy in critically ill individuals. Bilateral anterior thoracotomies can be used for volume reduction surgery or double-lung transplantation.

The patient is placed in a supine position, and the operative side is elevated by 20 to 30 degrees with a padded sandbag placed behind the back. The ipsilateral arm is positioned at the side or elevated across the body.

The skin incision extends *from the sternum anteriorly to the midaxillary line* at the level of the fourth intercostal space (Fig. 5-17B). The pectoralis major is divided over the desired intercostal space, and if further exposure is necessary, disarticulation of the chondrosternal joint at the anterior margin of the incision can be done. The internal mammary vessels are 1 cm lateral to the sternum, and they are farther away at the lower end of the sternum (1.5 to 2.0 cm). The pleural cavity is entered through cautery incision of the intercostal muscles.

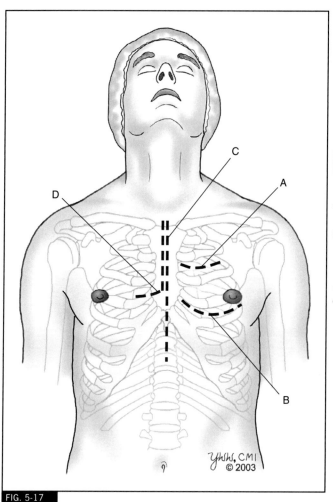

FIG. 5-17

Anterior thoracotomies. **A,** Anterior mediastinotomy (parasternal exploration).
B, Anterolateral thoracotomy. **C,** Median sternotomy. **D,** Partial sternotomy.

Sternotomy

This incision is used for the resection of most tumors in the anterior mediastinum. Through this approach, major pulmonary resections can also be accomplished, and it is the *most direct route* for surgery of the intrathoracic trachea and carina.

Median Sternotomy

Through the median sternotomy approach, upper and middle lobectomies, pneumonectomies, sleeve resections, and carinal resections can be accomplished. This approach is particularly appropriate for bilateral wedge resections of multiple pulmonary metastases or for bilateral excision of emphysematous bullae. The *main advantages* of sternotomy (Table 5-25) over other thoracic incisions are that postoperative pain is reduced and patients have *faster recovery of pulmonary function* after surgery. This is an important consideration because it may allow surgery to be done in patients who would not tolerate posterolateral thoracotomy.

For median sternotomy, the patient lies in a supine position with arms abducted or secured on the sides. The skin incision (Fig. 5-17C) extends in the midline from the suprasternal notch to a point midway between xiphoid and umbilicus. Once the sternum is exposed, the midline is marked with cautery, and a reciprocating saw is used to divide the sternum. A sternal spreader is then used to retract the sternal edges. In uncomplicated cases, six or seven stainless steel wires are used for sternal reapproximation.

Partial Sternotomy

Partial sternotomy can be used for the resection of anterior mediastinal tumors and for some procedures on the trachea.

The incision begins above the suprasternal notch (Fig. 5-17D), or higher over the anterior border of the sternocleidomastoid muscle if needed, and then follows the midline down the sternum before curving laterally over the

TABLE 5-25

ADVANTAGES AND DISADVANTAGES OF STERNOTOMY OVER LATERAL THORACOTOMY FOR PULMONARY RESECTION

ADVANTAGES

Decrease in severity and duration of postoperative pain

Elimination of long-term incisional pain

Decreased hospital stay

Ability to operate on patients with severely compromised pulmonary function or elderly patients who would not tolerate lateral thoracotomy

Easy accessibility to both lungs

Possibility of doing concomitant cardiac procedure

DISADVANTAGES

Less exposure for lower lobectomies

Danger of catastrophic sternal infection

chosen interspace (second to fourth). The sternum is sectioned with the sternal saw vertically in the midline from the suprasternal notch to the level of the intercostal incision. Stainless steel wires are used to reapproximate the sternum.

Transverse Sternotomy (Clamshell Incision)

The clamshell incision and its modification in the form of the hemi-clamshell incision provide excellent exposure to both pleural cavities for the purpose of performing *double-lung transplantation* or *resecting bilateral pulmonary metastases.* It is also an ideal incision for the resection of large and invasive anterior mediastinal or cervicothoracic tumors.

For the clamshell incision (Fig. 5-18A), the patient is placed supine on the operating table. The thoracotomy is performed through a curvilinear *bilateral submammary incision* extending from the midaxillary lines across the anterior aspect of the chest at the level of the fourth interspace. The incision is brought across the sternum at the level of the interspaces entered on either side. At the end of the procedure, the sternum is approximated with two or three sternal wires.

The hemi-clamshell incision is used for the resection of extensive cervicothoracic tumors. For the incision, the patient is positioned supine, usually with the ipsilateral side elevated. A *curvilinear inframammary incision* (Fig. 5-18B) is made and continued superiorly as a partial median sternotomy from the level of the intercostal space entered to the sternal notch. Further exposure can be obtained by continuing the incision over the neck (Fig. 5-18B) or by removing the medial half of the clavicle.

AXILLARY INCISIONS

Axillary incisions represent an efficient approach for a number of procedures (Table 5-26). These include pleurodesis and blebectomy for recurrent pneumothoraces, resection of large bullae, limited resections or even upper lobectomies for lung cancer, excision of some mediastinal tumors, and first rib resection for thoracic outlet syndromes.

Limited Axillary Thoracotomy

The patient is placed in the lateral decubitus position and the arm is anchored to the crossbar of the anesthetic screen. A *transverse incision* is made below the hairline (Fig. 5-19A) from the edge of the latissimus dorsi posteriorly to the pectoralis major anteriorly (submammary fold). The chest wall is quickly reached, and the pleural space is entered through the third intercostal space.

Care must be taken to avoid the long thoracic nerve (innervation of the serratus anterior muscle) and the intercostobrachial nerve, which is in the midportion of the second interspace.

If a *vertical incision* is used (Fig. 5-19B), the patient is usually positioned at a 45-degree angle with a subaxillary roll in place. The incision is made along the *posterior border of the pectoralis major*, and the third interspace is entered.

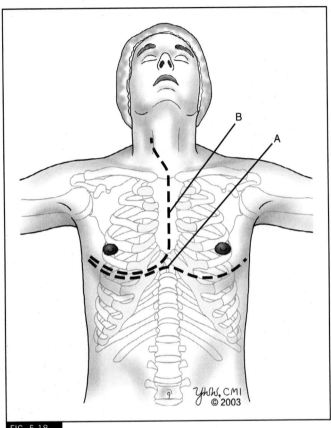

FIG. 5-18
Transverse sternotomy. **A,** Clamshell incision. **B,** Hemi-clamshell incision with possible extension into the neck.

TABLE 5-26

COMMON PROCEDURES DONE THROUGH AXILLARY INCISIONS

Type of Incision	Organ Accessed	Operation
Axillary thoracotomy	Chest wall	First rib and cervical rib resection
	Lung	Limited wedge resection
		Upper lobectomy
		Bleb or bulla resection
	Pleura	Pleurodesis (abrasion, pleurectomy)
	Mediastinum	Resection of tumors
Vertical thoracotomy	Lung	All types of resections

Vertical Axillary Thoracotomy

Vertical axillary thoracotomy is an alternative route of access to entry in the pleural cavity that *minimizes trauma, preserves muscles and shoulder function,* and provides a *satisfactory cosmetic result.* It is useful in patients with impaired pulmonary function.

   The patient is placed in the lateral decubitus position with the arm abducted to 90 degrees and secured to the anesthetic screen. A vertical incision (Fig. 5-19C) is made in the midaxillary line from below the hairline to the ninth intercostal space. The latissimus dorsi muscle is elevated and retracted posteriorly. The serratus anterior muscle is elevated anteriorly

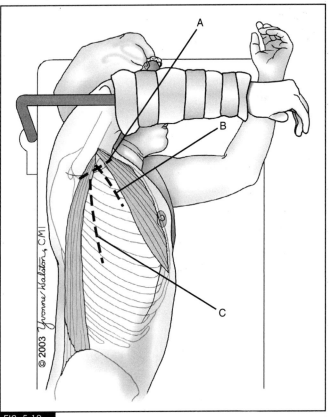

FIG. 5-19

Axillary thoracotomy. **A,** Limited axillary thoracotomy (horizontal). **B,** Limited axillary thoracotomy (vertical incision). **C,** Vertical axillary thoracotomy.

from its rib attachments until the appropriate interspace is exposed. On occasion, the serratus anterior muscle is divided anteriorly, avoiding the long thoracic nerve.

POSTERIOR THORACIC INCISIONS

These are classic incisions for many types of lung procedures (Table 5-27) as well as for operations on the esophagus and diaphragm. They provide extensive exposure and access to virtually any structure in the hemithorax. They have, however, the disadvantage of transecting major muscles.

Posterolateral Thoracotomy

The posterolateral thoracotomy provides excellent access to the lung, hilum, middle and posterior mediastinum, intrathoracic trachea, and esophagus. The *two potential disadvantages* of this incision are that it is painful and that it disturbs respiratory mechanics through division of respiratory muscles. These disturbances can be minimized, however, by meticulous technique and use of modern postoperative analgesia.

The patient is placed in the lateral decubitus position and immobilized with a beanbag to support the back and abdomen (Fig. 5-20A). Strips of adhesive tape or a belt is passed over the hips and secured to the table. The legs are separated with a pillow. The lower leg is flexed at the knee, and the upper leg lies straight over the pillow. To increase the spread of the pleural space, the table is angled or a roll is inserted under the patient's chest.

The incision (Fig. 5-20A) is started at the level of the anterior axillary line over the fifth or sixth interspace. It is gently curved around the tip of the scapula and continued posteriorly along a line between scapula and spine. Anteriorly, the incision follows the rib outline, which has an oblique rather than a horizontal direction. The latissimus dorsi is then opened with the electrocautery (perpendicular to muscle fibers) (Fig. 5-20B); the *serratus anterior muscle is preserved,* being retracted anteriorly.

To identify the fifth intercostal space, which is the space most often used for pulmonary resection, the hand is passed superiorly beneath the scapula (Fig. 5-20C) and the ribs and intercostal spaces are numbered

TABLE 5-27

COMMON PROCEDURES DONE THROUGH POSTERIOR THORACIC INCISIONS

Type of Incision	Organ Accessed	Operation
Posterolateral thoracotomy	Lung	Any type of pulmonary surgery
	Trachea and carina	Resection
	Diaphragm	Hernia repair
	Esophagus	Resection
		Correction of functional disorder
Lateral muscle-sparing thoracotomy	Same as posterolateral thoracotomy	Same as posterolateral thoracotomy
Thoracoabdominal incision	Esophagus	Resection
		Recurrent reflux

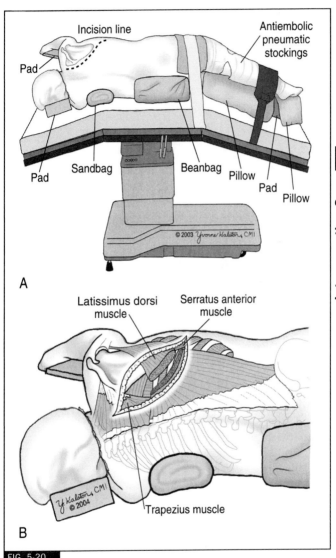

FIG. 5-20

Posterolateral thoracotomy. **A,** Position and skin incision. **B,** Division of latissimus
dorsi muscle. *Continued*

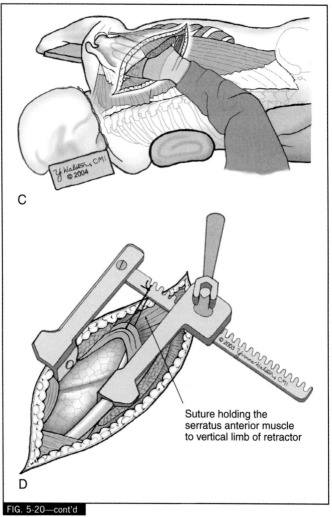

C

D

Suture holding the
serratus anterior muscle
to vertical limb of retractor

FIG. 5-20—cont'd

C, Numbering of ribs and intercostal spaces. **D,** Rib spreader in position.

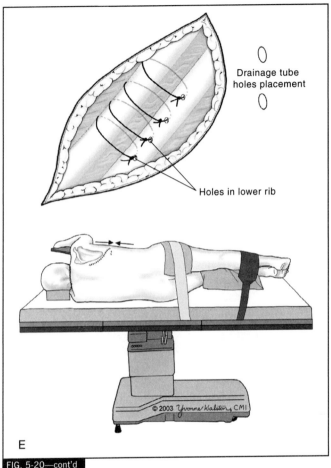

Drainage tube
holes placement

Holes in lower rib

© 2003 Yvonne Walston, CMI

E

5

Intraoperative Care

FIG. 5-20—cont'd

E, Closure of the intercostal space and completion of procedure.

down from the first rib. The pleural cavity is then entered after resection of the full length of a rib (seldom done) or the most posterior 1 cm of the lower rib to allow maximum spread of the interspace without breaking a rib. Many surgeons enter the pleural space by reflecting the periosteum (back to front) from the superior border of the rib with a periosteal elevator.

Once the pleural space is accessed, a chest spreader is placed in such a way as to have its vertical limb anterior to the surgeon. The vertical limb is also used to *hold the serratus anterior muscle* away from the incision (Fig. 5-20D).

ADVANTAGES OF MUSCLE-SPARING THORACOTOMY

Reduced postoperative pain
Decreased long-term neuralgia
Preservation of accessory muscles of respiration
Conservation of muscle strength
Conservation of shoulder girdle movement
Better cosmetic result
Preserved muscles can be used later for transposition flaps if necessary

For closure of the intercostal space, interrupted absorbable sutures are passed through a hole in the lower rib and around the upper rib (Fig. 5-20E).

Muscle-Sparing Thoracotomy

The muscle-sparing lateral thoracotomy spares both the latissimus dorsi and serratus anterior muscles, thus lowering postoperative morbidity with *decreased pain, improved arm motion,* and *earlier ambulation.* Most important, it improves recovery of lung function (Table 5-28). It is generally conceded, however, that muscle-sparing thoracotomies provide inferior access to the chest compared with posterolateral incisions.

The patient is positioned exactly as for a standard thoracotomy. A transverse 10- to 12-cm incision is made from the anterior axillary line to the midportion of the belly of the latissimus dorsi muscle, and generous skin flaps are raised over the surface of the latissimus dorsi (Fig. 5-21). The latissimus dorsi is mobilized and retracted posteriorly; the serratus anterior is exposed and elevated anteriorly from the ribs to gain access to the intercostal space. The serratus anterior must often be divided in line with the direction of its muscle fibers. Access to the pleural space is through the fifth interspace, which is opened by division of intercostal muscles as far anteriorly and posteriorly as possible. Closure is fast because no muscle requires reapproximation.

A muscle-sparing lateral thoracotomy through the auscultatory triangle can also be done by retracting the latissimus dorsi anteriorly and the scapula superiorly. This is the only muscle-sparing incision in which no muscle is actually divided.

Thoracoabdominal Incision

The most recognized uses for thoracoabdominal incisions are *lower esophageal resection* and *reoperation on the esophagus.* The incisions allow simultaneous dissection in pleural and abdominal cavities.

The patient is placed in the lateral position with the hips rotated back 45 degrees to facilitate the abdominal dissection (Table 5-29). The incision is S shaped (Fig. 5-22), opening 4 cm of upper abdomen and 10 cm of anterolateral chest wall (technique of Dr. Robert D. Henderson). In dividing the diaphragm, a 1-cm margin is left attached to the costal margin for use in closure. This circumferential incision avoids injury to the phrenic nerve or its branches.

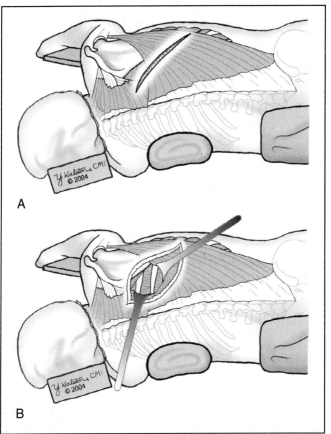

FIG. 5-21

Muscle-sparing lateral thoracotomy. **A,** Transverse 10- to 12-cm skin incision.
B, Latissimus dorsi retracted posteriorly and serratus anterior elevated anteriorly.
(From Mitchell R, Angell W, Wuerflein R, Dor V: Simplified lateral chest incision for most thoracotomies other than sternotomy. Ann Thorac Surg 1976;22:284.)

TABLE 5-29

PRINCIPLES OF THORACOABDOMINAL INCISIONS

Full lateral position with hips rotated back 45 degrees

Seventh or eighth interspace incision

Short abdominal component (rectus muscle not divided)

Circumferential division of diaphragm

No excision of costal cartilage

Pericostal suture only up to costochondral junction; no sutures around or
 through the cartilage

Stabilization of costal cartilage during closure by use of surrounding muscle
 (diaphragm, internal and external oblique, transversus abdominis)

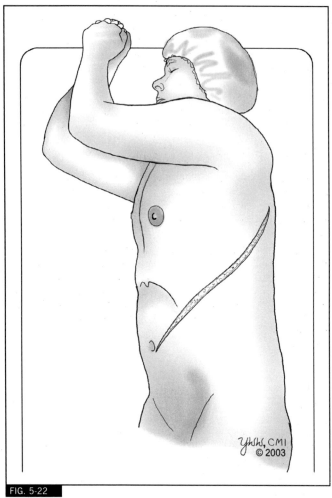

FIG. 5-22

Thoracoabdominal incision. The patient's hips are rotated back 45 degrees to facilitate abdominal dissection.

UPPER MIDLINE ABDOMINAL INCISION

The upper midline abdominal incision has wide application in thoracic surgery. In addition to providing access to abdominal viscera, the pericardium can be drained, and the gastroesophageal junction can easily be exposed.

For the management of pericardial effusions, the patient is placed supine on the operating table with a roll behind the lumbar spine so that a lordotic posture is assumed. A midline incision is made from the xiphoid to 8 or 10 cm below. Once the linea alba is divided, the soft tissue plane behind the xiphoid is developed by blunt dissection until the pericardium is exposed.

COMPLICATIONS OF THORACIC INCISIONS AND THEIR PREVENTION

Fortunately, there are few complications related to thoracic incisions, and most can be prevented. Posterolateral thoracotomy, for example, has a bad reputation because it is painful postoperatively and because it decreases shoulder mobility and respiratory mechanics by the division of large chest wall muscles. Most of these problems *can be avoided,* however, if one is meticulous with the surgical technique.

Wound Complications (Table 5-30)

One of the not so rare complications is that the thoracotomy is done on the wrong side. For prevention of this problem, a chest radiograph must always *be available and looked at* in the operating room before the incision is made.

Wound infection is rare. When it occurs, one should suspect that the problem is related to an undiagnosed empyema draining spontaneously through the wound (empyema necessitatis). Prevention of wound infections includes the use of *prophylactic antibiotics* and, in the case of sternotomy, proper closure and hemostasis. Wound seromas are common with muscle-sparing thoracotomies because of the skin flaps that must be developed. Prevention includes *avoidance of dead spaces* by suturing subcutaneous tissues to muscle and use of soft drains. Wound dehiscence is also uncommon; most cases occur after pneumonectomy. Prevention includes proper closure of the wound and adequate drainage of the pleural cavity *if there are signs of positive pressure within the space.*

Intercostal Complications

Rib fractures should be avoided because they create wound instability, which increases the amount of pain and discomfort and makes effective coughing more difficult. Preventive measures include *a skin incision properly placed* and entrance in the pleural cavity through the *appropriate intercostal space.* For instance, the fourth intercostal space may be better

TABLE 5-30	
WOUND COMPLICATIONS AND THEIR PROPHYLAXIS	
Complication	Prophylaxis
Thoracotomy on the wrong side	Chest radiograph in the operating room
Wound infection	Prophylactic antibiotics
Seromas	Avoidance of dead spaces
Dehiscence	Proper wound closure and adequate pleural space drainage

suited than the fifth space for upper lobectomies. Other prophylaxis includes gradual opening of the chest retracted and, in some cases, resection of a 1-cm segment of the lower rib (posteriorly). On occasion, as in redo surgery, resection of the full length of a rib will provide better access to the lung.

In cases of thoracoabdominal incisions, nonhealing of the costal cartilage can be a source of chronic pain. This can be prevented by resecting a 1-cm segment of costal margin and by avoiding placement of sutures directly through the cartilage.

Persistent or recurrent pain after thoracotomy for a malignant tumor *is often due to recurrent tumor*. This must be ruled out by appropriate imaging techniques.

Neurologic Complications

A variety of neurologic complications can occur after thoracotomy. Among them, the most common are peripheral nerve injuries due to improper positioning or inadequate padding of the extremities during the operation. These include *traction injuries of the brachial plexus* as well as *contact injuries to superficial nerves of the upper or lower extremities*. Lesions of the intercostal brachial nerve or long thoracic nerve are usually associated with axillary thoracotomies. Prevention includes entry in the third interspace rather than in the second to avoid injury to the intercostal brachial nerve characterized by numbness over the inner part of the arm. Denervation of the serratus anterior muscle results in loss of scapula tip stabilization, a syndrome called winged scapula. This syndrome often results in significant and prolonged disability. Trauma to the long thoracic nerve is usually associated with incisions that are cephalad to the scapula tip, especially vertical axillary thoracotomies.

Intercostal nerve injury is a major cause of chronic post-thoracotomy pain. These injuries are mainly related to rib spreading (by retractor) or to techniques of closure in which sutures may erode intercostal nerves. Other contributing factors are rib fracture, trauma to the costovertebral joint posteriorly or to the anterior cartilages, and shoulder dysfunction. Fortunately, chronic pain lasting for more than 1 year is uncommon, being seen in less than 5% of patients.

Paraplegia can occur after posterolateral thoracotomies. It is usually associated with *migration into the spinal canal* of oxidized cellulose that had been used to control venous bleeding at the posterior angle of the thoracotomy incision.

CONCLUSION

The rigidity of the chest wall and lack of mobility of thoracic viscera highlight the importance of selecting the proper incision for a given procedure. This choice must be based on the surgeon's familiarity with the anatomy of the incision as well as his or her experience with it. Above all, the surgeon must understand the advantages and limitations of the incision that has been selected for the operation.

SUGGESTED READINGS

Review Articles

Morrissey NJ, Hollier LH: Anatomic exposures in thoracoabdominal aortic surgery. Semin Vasc Surg 2000;13:283-289.

Dewey TM, Mack MJ: Lung cancer: surgical approaches and incisions. Chest Surg Clin North Am 2000;10:803-821.

Posterolateral Thoracotomy

Mouton W, Fischer G, Striffeler H, et al: Is the function of the serratus anterior muscle disturbed following division during a standard thoracotomy? Thorac Cardiovasc Surg 1999;47:188-189.

Rogers ML, Henderson L, Mahajan RP, Duffy JP: Preliminary findings in the neurophysiological assessment of intercostal nerve injury during thoracotomy. Eur J Cardiothorac Surg 2002;21:298-301.

Deslauriers J, Mehran RJ: Posterolateral thoracotomy. Op Tech Thorac Cardiovasc Surg 2003;8:51-57.

Muscle-Sparing Thoracotomy

Mitchell R, Angell W, Wuerflein R, Dor V: Simplified lateral chest incision for most thoracotomies other than sternotomy. Ann Thorac Surg 1976;22:284-286.

Bethencourt DM, Holmes EC: Muscle-sparing posterolateral thoracotomy. Ann Thorac Surg 1988;45:337-339.

Hazelrigg SR, Landreneau RJ, Boley TM, et al: The effect of muscle-sparing versus standard posterolateral thoracotomy on pulmonary function, muscle strength, and postoperative pain. J Thorac Cardiovasc Surg 1991;101:394-401.

Ponn RB, Ferneini A, D'Agostino RS, et al: Comparison of late pulmonary function after posterolateral and muscle-sparing thoracotomy. Ann Thorac Surg 1992;53:675-679.

Hennington MH, Ulicny KS, Detterbeck FC: Vertical muscle-sparing thoracotomy. Ann Thorac Surg 1994;57:759-761.

Benedetti F, Vighetti S, Ricco C, et al: Neurophysiologic assessment of nerve impairment in posterolateral and muscle-sparing thoracotomy. J Thorac Cardiovasc Surg 1998;115:841-847.

Khan IH, McManus KG, McCraith A, McGuigan JA: Muscle-sparing thoracotomy: a biochemical analysis confirms preservation of muscle strength but no improvement in wound discomfort. Eur J Cardiothorac Surg 2000;18:656-661.

Kutlu CA, Akin H, Olcmen A, et al: Shoulder-girdle strength after standard and lateral muscle-sparing thoracotomy. Thorac Cardiovasc Surg 2001;49:112-114.

Force S, Cooper JD: Horizontal muscle sparing incision. Op Tech Thorac Cardiovasc Surg 2003;8:68-71.

5

Intraoperative Care

Thoracotomy Through the Auscultatory Triangle

Horowitz MD, Ancalmo N, Ochsner JL: Thoracotomy through the auscultatory triangle. Ann Thorac Surg 1989;47:782-783.

Median Sternotomy

Urschel HC, Razzuk MA: Median sternotomy as a standard approach for pulmonary resection. Ann Thorac Surg 1986;41:130-134.

Asaph JW, Handy JR Jr., Grunkemeier GL, et al: Median sternotomy versus thoracotomy to resect primary lung cancer: analysis of 815 cases. Ann Thorac Surg 2000;70:373-379.

Clamshell Incision

Bains MS, Ginsberg RJ, Jones WG II, et al: The clamshell incision: an improved approach to bilateral pulmonary and mediastinal tumor. Ann Thorac Surg 1994;58:30-33.

Hemi-clamshell Incision

Korst RJ, Burt ME: Cervicothoracic tumors: results of resection by the "hemi-clamshell" approach. J Thorac Cardiovasc Surg 1998;115: 286-295.

Axillary Thoracotomy

Becker RM, Munro DD: Transaxillary minithoracotomy: the optimal approach for certain pulmonary and mediastinal lesions. Ann Thorac Surg 1976;22:254-259.

Massimano P, Ponn RB, Toole AL: Transaxillary thoracotomy revisited. Ann Thorac Surg 1988;45:559-560.

Vallières E: Apical axillary thoracotomy. Op Tech Thorac Cardiovasc Surg 2003;8:58-62.

Anterolateral Thoracotomy

Force S, Patterson GA: Anterolateral thoracotomy. Op Tech Thorac Cardiovasc Surg 2003;8:104-109.

Anterosuperior Incision

Vanakesa T, Goldstraw P: Antero-superior approaches in the practice of thoracic surgery. Eur J Cardiothorac Surg 1999;15:774-780.

Dartevelle P, Mussot S: Anterior cervicothoracic approach to the superior sulcus for radical resection of lung tumor invading the thoracic inlet. Op Tech Thorac Cardiovasc Surg 2003;8:86-94.

Thoracoabdominal

Heitmiller RF: The left thoracoabdominal incision. Ann Thorac Surg 1988;46:250-253.

Karakousis CP, Pourshahmir M: Thoracoabdominal incisions and resection of upper retroperitoneal sarcomas. J Surg Oncol 1999;72:150-155.

Sundaresan S: Left thoracoabdominal incision. Op Tech Thorac Cardiovasc Surg 2003;8:71-86.

Morbidity

Landreneau RJ, Pigula F, Luketich JD, et al: Acute and chronic morbidity differences between muscle-sparing and standard lateral thoracotomies. J Thorac Cardiovasc Surg 1996;112:1346-1351.

Cheng KS, Wu RS, Tan PP: Displacement of double-lumen tubes after patient positioning. Anesthesiology 1998;89:1282-1283.

Others

Heitmiller RF: The serratus sling: a simplified serratus-sparing technique. Ann Thorac Surg 1989;48:867-868.

Short HD: Paraplegia associated with the use of oxidized cellulose in postero-lateral thoracotomy incisions. Ann Thorac Surg 1990;50:288-290.

Hayward RH, Knight WL, Baisden CE, Korompai FL: Access to the thorax by incision. J Am Coll Surg 1994;179:202-208.

Salazar JD, Doty JR, Tseng EE, et al: Relationship of the long thoracic nerve to the scapular tip: an aid to prevention of proximal nerve injury. J Thorac Cardiovasc Surg 1998;116:960-964.

5

Intraoperative Care

PRINCIPLES OF VIDEOTHORACOSCOPY

Because of significant technologic developments, widespread availability of video imaging, and better instrumentation, minimally invasive surgical approaches to the chest (video-assisted thoracoscopic surgery [VATS]) became popular in the early 1990s. This popularity *changed the pattern of practice of thoracic surgeons,* and during the subsequent years, VATS found more and more applications.

Well-documented benefits include *reduction in severity and duration of postoperative pain, less respiratory dysfunction, shortened hospital stay,* and *faster recovery* including earlier return to normal activities and work. The role of VATS in the surgical management of thoracic malignant neoplasms remains controversial, however, because many surgeons have expressed concerns about the ability of thoracoscopic procedures to maintain adherence to surgical oncologic principles.

Despite the apparently clear advantages of VATS over open thoracotomy, current limitations include inadequate training and experience of surgeons, lack of instrumentation, and ultimately lack of publications giving results based on a large number of cases.

INDICATIONS FOR VIDEOTHORACOSCOPY APPROACHES

Pleural Diseases (Table 5-31)

Patients with *recurrent pleural effusions* or loculated pleural effusions are best approached by videothoracoscopy when other investigations have been unsuccessful. The entire pleural space can be explored and biopsy of suspicious lesions can be done under direct vision. In cases of malignant effusions, pleurodesis with talc powder or other products can also be done as a complement to the procedure.

ACCEPTED INDICATIONS FOR VIDEOTHORACOSCOPY IN PATIENTS WITH PLEURAL LESIONS

DIAGNOSTIC INDICATIONS

Diagnosis of pleural effusions and undetermined pleural masses

Biopsy for differentiation between mesothelioma and metastatic adenocarcinoma

THERAPEUTIC INDICATIONS

Pleurodesis for recurrent malignant effusions

Deloculation and drainage of stage I and stage II empyemas

Treatment of recurrent spontaneous pneumothorax (pleurodesis, pleurectomy, abrasion, blebectomy)

In patients *with empyemas*, at least those with *stage I (exudative) and stage II (fibrinopurulent) disease,* VATS allows deloculation of the space with removal of pus and fibrin deposits. By doing so, it is helpful in obtaining lung re-expansion. Indeed, VATS débridement of fibrinopurulent empyemas represents *one of the best indications* for therapeutic thoracoscopy. Formal decortication for more mature and organized (stage III) empyemas should probably still be done with an open technique.

Several reports have documented the *safety and efficacy of VATS* in the treatment of recurrent spontaneous primary pneumothoraces. The offending blebs can be resected, and the addition of parietal pleurectomy or parietal pleural abrasion promotes the formation of dense adhesions, which will prevent recurrences. The problems associated with pneumothoraces secondary to chronic obstructive pulmonary disease are different because all of these patients are older, and they often have significant comorbidities. For these individuals, the emergence of thoracoscopy has considerably changed the magnitude of operation, which can now be done with low operative morbidity or mortality, even in high-risk cases.

Thoracoscopic approaches for the management of chylothoraces are used increasingly but require further evaluation.

Lung Diseases (Table 5-32)

There are many indications for VATS in the evaluation and treatment of patients with pulmonary disorders. The VATS approach, for instance, has become the "gold standard" for *elective lung biopsy* in patients with diffuse interstitial diseases. The potential advantages of VATS biopsy over open lung biopsy are its ability to inspect the entire pleural space and the *accessibility of different regions of the lung* for biopsy.

Establishing the diagnosis of *solitary pulmonary nodules* (see Chapter 3) is another indication for thoracoscopy when noninvasive procedures have failed to yield a diagnosis. If the lesion turns out to be malignant, an appropriate surgical resection can then be performed.

In many centers, VATS is used to clinically stage lung cancer, more specifically to recognize *local causes* of unresectability. In such patients,

TABLE 5-32

ACCEPTED INDICATIONS FOR VIDEOTHORACOSCOPY IN PATIENTS WITH PULMONARY DISEASES

DIAGNOSTIC INDICATIONS

Diagnosis of interstitial lung disease and solitary nodules

Staging of lung cancer (tumor and nodes)

THERAPEUTIC INDICATIONS

Surgery for bullous empyema and volume reduction surgery (LVRS)

Limited resection of lung cancer in high-risk patients

?Anatomic resections (lobectomies, pneumonectomies) in low-risk patients

VATS may be useful to demonstrate the cause of an *associated pleural effusion* (malignant effusion or paraneoplastic); for biopsy of *mediastinal nodes;* or to document nonresectability by virtue of mediastinal invasion, esophageal wall invasion, or invasion of the pulmonary artery or heart.

Thoracoscopy is currently the preferred procedure for the resection of giant bullae with evidence of compression of adjacent lung. It is also recommended by some, either unilaterally or bilaterally, for *volume reduction surgery*.

Although several reports advocate the use of VATS for pulmonary metastasectomy, others have shown that thoracoscopy is less likely to yield complete resection of all metastases and thus more likely to compromise long-term survival. By contrast, VATS limited resection (wedge) of small and peripheral lung cancers can be done with good results in *compromised patients*. Although it is also possible to perform anatomic lung resections (lobectomy, pneumonectomy) with VATS technology and even appropriate mediastinal node dissection, there remains major concern that VATS resections may have a detrimental effect on long-term outcome for patients, *especially when the cancer is larger than 4 cm* (Table 5-33).

Mediastinal Diseases (Table 5-34)

Thoracoscopy has an important role in the evaluation of patients with mediastinal masses because it can provide access to *all mediastinal compartments*. Curative resection of mediastinal cysts (foregut cysts, pleuropericardial cysts) or of neurogenic tumors is also possible with a VATS approach. Indeed, neurogenic tumors are ideal lesions for thoracoscopic excision because they are nearly all benign with relatively sparse vasculature. Although thymomas or benign teratomas can be resected by thoracoscopy, the *advisability of such an approach must still be questioned,* and these procedures should be undertaken only by experienced thoracoscopic surgeons. The optimal operative approach for thymectomy in the treatment of myasthenia gravis patients without thymoma (sternotomy, cervical, VATS) still remains a controversial issue.

TABLE 5-33

CONTRAINDICATIONS TO VATS ANATOMIC PULMONARY RESECTION IN CASES OF LUNG CANCER

ABSOLUTE CONTRAINDICATIONS

Inability to tolerate single-lung ventilation
Large tumors (>4 cm diameter)
Dense pleural symphysis
Documented N2 disease
T3 tumors (main bronchus)
Planned sleeve resection

RELATIVE CONTRAINDICATIONS

Hilar lymphadenopathy
Previous surgery
Completely fused fissures
Prior irradiation to hilum
Chest wall involvement

In patients presenting with pericardial tamponade or with a recurrent pericardial effusion, thoracoscopy can be considered a diagnostic and therapeutic option. Recurrent or loculated pericardial effusions can be drained by VATS, and likewise an adequate pericardial window or pericardial sclerodesis can be done.

Esophageal Diseases (Table 5-35)

A variety of esophageal procedures can be done with thoracoscopic exposure. In patients with esophageal carcinomas, a combination of VATS and laparoscopy can be used to determine the N lymph node status. Esophagectomies can also be done by videothoracoscopic approach, but the role of such operations *is still under evaluation.*

Patients with esophageal leiomyomas are well suited for thoracoscopic resection. Thoracoscopic Heller myotomies are rapidly becoming the standard treatment of achalasia.

In experienced hands, *laparoscopic antireflux surgery* provides results superior to those of open techniques and better symptom relief. In patients

TABLE 5-34

ACCEPTED INDICATIONS FOR VIDEOTHORACOSCOPY IN PATIENTS WITH MEDIASTINAL DISEASE

DIAGNOSTIC INDICATIONS

Biopsy of unknown mediastinal tumors
Diagnosis of cause of pericardial effusion

THERAPEUTIC INDICATIONS

Resection of mediastinal cysts and neurogenic tumors
Thymectomy for thymoma or non-thymoma patients with myasthenia gravis
Treatment of recurrent pericardial effusion (pericardial window or sclerodesis)

TABLE 5-35

ACCEPTED INDICATIONS FOR VIDEOTHORACOSCOPY (OR LAPAROSCOPY) IN PATIENTS WITH ESOPHAGEAL DISEASE

DIAGNOSTIC INDICATION

Staging of esophageal cancer

THERAPEUTIC INDICATIONS

Excision of esophageal leiomyomas

Esophageal myotomy for achalasia

Antireflux surgery for uncomplicated gastroesophageal reflux

Repair of giant paraesophageal hernia

Esophagectomy for carcinoma

with complicated reflux, such as those with esophageal shortening, peptic stricture, or a large paraesophageal component, an open approach may be indicated.

Others

Patients with palmar hyperhidrosis, reflex sympathetic dystrophy, and Raynaud phenomenon are good candidates for *thoracoscopic sympathectomy,* and the results are excellent. Similarly, patients undergoing spinal surgery, whether it is for kyphoscoliosis, vertebral abscesses, or neoplasia, can now be approached with thoracoscopy. Another indication for VATS is in the *management of trauma patients,* such as those with clotted hemothoraces or diaphragmatic hernia.

CONTRAINDICATIONS TO THORACOSCOPY

As surgeons are gaining more experience with VATS approaches, there are fewer contraindications specifically applicable to the operation. Even an obliterated pleural space from previous tuberculosis, empyema, or previous surgery is no longer a contraindication to VATS. The inability of the patient to tolerate single-lung ventilation (uncommon) is probably the only true contraindication to VATS techniques.

OPERATIVE TECHNIQUE (TABLE 5-36)

Anesthesia

Thoracoscopic procedures are performed under general endotracheal single-lung anesthesia. This is usually accomplished with use of *a double-lumen left-sided tube,* which is easier to position. For children, a single-lumen tube with bronchial blocker can be used.

Patient Positioning

The patient is turned into a full lateral decubitus position as described in "Positioning and Incisions." Having the patient's back flush with the edge of the operating table makes the manipulation of thoracoscopy instruments much easier. *Maximal flexion of the table* further opens up the intercostal

---

TABLE 5-36

BASIC PROCEDURE OF THORACOSCOPY

Single-lung anesthesia (double-lumen endotracheal tube)
Full lateral decubitus position
Maximal flexion of operating table
Use of two high-resolution video monitors
Placement of access ports at different levels from camera port
   (rectangular or triangular configuration)
Same surgical principles as in open procedure
Use of instruments normally used in open surgery or thoracoscopic instruments
   commercially available
Use of endosurgical staplers

---

spaces and facilitates insertion and manipulation of thoracoscopic instruments, especially in patients with prominent hips. Once the patient is positioned, skin preparation and draping are identical to those of open thoracotomy. Different positioning can, however, be used for surgery of the anterior mediastinum (thymoma) or when bilateral procedures are expected to be carried out.

Ideally, *two high-resolution video monitors* placed on opposite sides of the table should be available so that both the surgeon and his or her assistant can have a direct straight-ahead forward view and therefore be operating in the same direction (avoids mirror imaging). The optimal team for VATS includes the surgeon, a first assistant whose role is to retract the lung and provide better exposure, and a camera operator. Most often, the surgeon stands facing the patient.

Strategies for Port Placement

Although standard positioning of ports may vary from one surgeon to another, we recommend a *rectangular configuration* in which the chest wall is divided into four quadrants by horizontal and vertical lines drawn over the tip of the scapula. In this configuration (Fig. 5-23), the camera port is inserted in the quadrant diagonally opposite the target lesion, usually the sixth or seventh interspace in the midaxillary or posterior axillary line. Because a 10-cm cannula with a 0-degree lens is usually used, a 12-mm skin incision is required for introduction of the access port.

Instrument ports are placed in each other quadrant. The larger one (15 mm), which is used for stapler insertion and tissue extraction, is located anteriorly, where the intercostal space is wider. This port *can easily be enlarged* to ease the removal of larger specimens. The smaller port (5 mm), primarily used for endoscopy forceps, is located posteriorly. These instrument ports should be placed in an arc of 180 degrees with the camera port to afford maximal exposure and maneuverability of the instruments (Table 5-37). Access ports must also be placed at least four fingerbreadths from the camera port to avoid crowding of the instruments within the pleural space. If an operating telescope containing a working channel is available, many procedures can be done with a single 10-mm camera port (Fig. 5-24).

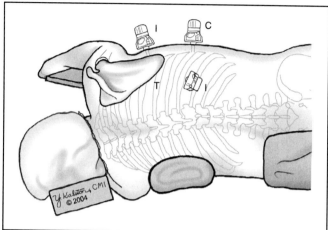

FIG. 5-23

Trocar placement in rectangular configuration for thoracoscopy. The video camera (C) looks directly at the target (T). Instrument access ports (I) are located on each side of the camera.

Another popular configuration is that of an inverted triangle. The camera is placed at the apex of the triangle, and the instrument ports are placed at its base.

Thoracoscopic Instruments

Instruments for videothoracoscopic surgery include those normally used during open surgery. They are inserted directly through the chest wall instead of through an access port, and they have the advantages of being *easy to use and familiar to all surgeons.* Complete sets of disposable or

---

TABLE 5-37

BASIC PRINCIPLES OF THORACOSCOPY

Place trocar sites and thoracoscope at a distance from the lesion to achieve
    a panoramic view and provide room to manipulate the tissue.
Avoid instrument crowding, which may otherwise result in "fencing" during instrument
    manipulation.
Avoid mirror imaging by positioning instruments and thoracoscope within the same
    180-degree arc. (Approach the lesion in the same general direction with
    instruments and camera.)
Move and manipulate instruments (or the camera) serially, rather than randomly or
    synchronously, to avoid operative chaos. Instruments should be manipulated only
    when seen directly through the thoracoscope.

From Landreneau RJ, Mack MJ, Hazelrigg SR, et al: Video-assisted thoracic surgery. Basic technical
concepts and intercostal approach strategies. Ann Thorac Surg 1992;54:800-807.

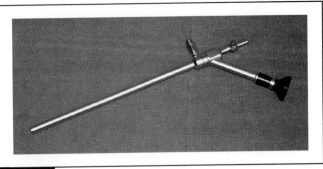

FIG. 5-24

Thoracoscope with a working channel that can be used for the passage of biopsy forceps or for the insufflation of talc powder.

reusable thoracoscopic instruments are also commercially available. Laparoscopic instruments have the advantage of being long and thin and thus can be inserted through smaller trocars.

A variety of percutaneous endosurgical staplers allow the linear stapling of the lung, blood vessels, and bronchi. Their length as well as their size and thickness of rows of staples can be *adapted to the procedure* being performed. In general, thick staples are used for lung parenchyma; thinner staples are used on blood vessels. Vascular staplers usually deliver three rows of staples on both ends of the vessel to be divided. Staplers with a reticulated head are also available.

Tissue Extraction

When a videothoracoscopic approach is used for the resection of malignant neoplasms, tissue extraction is an important part of the procedure if one is to avoid implantation of viable malignant cells into the trocar site.

The safer way to extract such tissue is to use a *commercially available endoscopic plastic bag*. The strength of these endobags allows the tissues to be extracted from the pleural space without tearing them and, most important, without contact with the parietal pleura or soft tissues of the chest wall. Alternatively, the specimen can be retrieved through a utility mini-thoracotomy, usually 5 to 8 cm in length placed over the anterolateral chest wall.

SPECIFICS OF COMMON VIDEOTHORACOSCOPIC PROCEDURES

For pleural procedures, a thoracoscope with a working channel is often used to limit the number of access ports. The thoracoscope is used for inspection of the pleural space, biopsy of suspicious lesions, and sclerotherapy. The port is also used for postoperative tube drainage. If the lesion under investigation is potentially a malignant mesothelioma that may have to be resected, the camera and access ports must be placed in such a way that the *sites can be resected* at the time of thoracotomy. In cases of parapneumonic empyemas, all loculations must be broken down and fibrin deposits must be removed from lung surfaces to improve expansion. Chest tubes must be positioned in the most dependent part of the space. In cases of malignant effusions, talc powder (4 to 5 g) is delivered with a bulb syringe or preferably with an atomizer.

Excisional resection of pulmonary nodules can easily be done if the lesion is on the surface of the lung. If the lesion is deeper, it can be identified through *finger or instrument palpation* and then be wedged out. If difficulties are anticipated before surgery, the lesion can be identified with a hook wire inserted under CT guidance the morning of the operation.

When thoracoscopy is done for recurrent spontaneous pneumothorax, an apical blebectomy is done with an Endo-GIA stapler followed by pleural abrasion or apical parietal pleurectomy. In such cases, the advantages of a VATS approach over an axillary mini-thoracotomy are *questionable*, however.

VATS is an excellent approach for upper thoracic sympathectomy, which is often done in an outpatient setting. Great care must be exercised to avoid use of the cautery near the stellate ganglion because it may result in Horner syndrome.

COMPLICATIONS OF VIDEOTHORACOSCOPY

In general, videothoracoscopic operations are associated with a low complication rate similar to that of open thoracotomy. The rate of conversion to open thoracotomy varies between 4% and 20%, *depending on the procedure and the surgeon's experience.* In general, the reasons for converting are the need for anatomic resection (lobectomy or pneumonectomy), the inability to find a lesion, dense adhesions, and intraoperative hemorrhage.

Common postoperative complications specifically related to VATS include persistent air leak and wound infection. Patients undergoing VATS generally experience less postoperative chest pain and shoulder dysfunction than do those undergoing open operations, although there is no clear evidence that these early benefits translate into improved outcomes. On occasion, patients who have had a VATS procedure will experience *prolonged intercostal neuralgia.*

Port site tumor implantation, implantation into the pleural cavity, and residual neoplastic disease left along staple lines have been reported. These cases are rare and may be related to nonuse of an endoscopic bag during tumor extraction.

CONCLUSION

Thoracoscopy has been used in diagnosis and management of pleural diseases throughout the 20th century, and during those years, it has been performed in different ways. The introduction of video technology and the development of endostaplers in the 1990s have revolutionized the principles of this approach, and in 1991, the councils of the American

Association for Thoracic Surgery and the Society of Thoracic Surgeons appointed a joint committee to develop standards and guidelines pertaining to therapeutic videothoracoscopy. When it is used for appropriate indications and performed with standards applicable to open thoracotomy, thoracoscopy has a *definite role* in general thoracic surgery.

SUGGESTED READINGS

Review Articles

Landreneau RJ, Mack MJ, Hazelrigg SR, et al: Video-assisted thoracic surgery: basic technical concepts and intercostal approach strategies. Ann Thorac Surg 1992;54:800-807.

Landreneau RJ, Mack MJ, Keenan RJ, et al: Strategic planning for video-assisted thoracic surgery. Ann Thorac Surg 1993; 56:615-619.

Allen MS, Trastek VF, Daly RC, et al: Equipment for thoracoscopy. Ann Thorac Surg 1993;56:620-623.

Horswell JL: Anesthetic techniques for thoracoscopy. Ann Thorac Surg 1993;56:624-629.

Little AG: Thoracoscopy: current status. Curr Opin Pulm Med 1996; 2:315-319.

Darling G: Video-assisted thoracoscopic surgery. In Casson AG, Johnston MR, eds: Key Topics in Thoracic Surgery. Oxford, UK, BIOS Scientific Publishers Limited, 1999:275-278.

Dewey TM, Mack MJ: Lung cancer. Surgical approaches and incisions. Chest Surg Clin North Am 2000;10:803-820.

Survey Videothoracoscopy

Mack MJ, Scruggs GR, Kelly KM, et al: Video-assisted thoracic surgery: has technology found its place? Ann Thorac Surg 1997; 64:211-215.

Complications of Videothoracoscopy

Landreneau RJ, Hazelrigg SR, Mack MJ, et al: Postoperative pain-related morbidity: video-assisted thoracic surgery versus thoracotomy. Ann Thorac Surg 1993;56:1285-1289.

Jancovici R, Lang-Lazdunski L, Pons F, et al: Complications of video-assisted thoracic surgery: a five-year experience. Ann Thorac Surg 1996;61:533-537.

Yim APC, Liu HP: Complications and failures of video-assisted thoracic surgery: experience from two centers in Asia. Ann Thorac Surg 1996;61:538-541.

Downey RJ: Complications after video-assisted thoracic surgery. Chest Surg Clin North Am 1998;8:907-917.

Demmy TL, Curtis JJ: Minimally invasive lobectomy directed toward frail and high-risk patients: a case-control study. Ann Thorac Surg 1999;68:194-200.

Endobag

Arzouman DA, Caccavale RJ, Sisler GE, Lewis RJ: Endobag. Ann Thorac Surg 1993;55:1266-1267.

Videothoracoscopy—Pulmonary Resection

McKenna RJ, Wolf RK, Brenner M, et al: Is lobectomy by video-assisted thoracic surgery an adequate cancer operation? Ann Thorac Surg 1998;66:1903-1908.

Yim APC, Landreneau RJ, Izzat MB, et al: Is video-assisted thoracoscopic lobectomy a unified approach? Ann Thorac Surg 1998;66:1155-1158.

Nomori H, Horio H, Naruke T, Suemasu K: What is the advantage of a thoracoscopic lobectomy over a limited thoracotomy procedure for lung cancer surgery? Ann Thorac Surg 2001;72:879-884.

Thomas P, Doddoli C, Yena S, et al: VATS is an adequate oncological operation for stage I non–small cell lung cancer. Eur J Cardiothorac Surg 2002;21:1094-1099.

Yim APC: VATS major pulmonary resection revisited—controversies, techniques, and results. Ann Thorac Surg 2002;74:615-623.

Daniels LJ, Balderson SS, Onaitis MW, D'Amico TA: Thoracoscopic lobectomy: a safe and effective strategy for patients with stage I lung cancer. Ann Thorac Surg 2002;74:860-864.

Rocco G, Martin-Ucar A, Passera E: Uniportal VATS wedge pulmonary resections. Ann Thorac Surg 2004;77:726-728.

Videothoracoscopy—Pulmonary Metastases

McCormack PM, Bains MS, Begg CB, et al: Role of video-assisted thoracic surgery in the treatment of pulmonary metastases: results of a prospective trial. Ann Thorac Surg 1996;62:213-217.

Rusch VW: Surgical techniques for pulmonary metastasectomy. Semin Thorac Cardiovasc Surg 2002;14:4-9.

Videothoracoscopy—Pleurodesis

Cardillo G, Facciolo F, Carbone L, et al: Long-term follow-up of video-assisted talc pleurodesis in malignant recurrent pleural effusions. Eur J Cardiothorac Surg 2002;21:302-306.

Videothoracoscopy—Pneumothorax

Hyland MJ, Ashrafi AS, Crépeau A, Mehran RJ: Is video-assisted thoraco-scopic surgery superior to limited axillary thoracotomy in the manage-ment of spontaneous pneumothorax? Can Respir J 2001;8:339-343.

Videothoracoscopy—Empyema

Waller DA: Thoracoscopy in management of postpneumonic pleural infections. Curr Opin Pulm Med 2002;8:323-326.

Videothoracoscopy—Nodules and Lung Biopsy

Zegdi R, Azorin J, Tremblay B, et al: Videothoracoscopic lung biopsy in diffuse infiltrative lung diseases: a 5-year surgical experience. Ann Thorac Surg 1998;66:1170-1173.

Ciriaco P, Negri G, Puglisi A, et al: Video-assisted thoracoscopic surgery for pulmonary nodules: rationale for preoperative computed tomography–guided hook wire localization. Eur J Cardiothorac Surg 2004;25:429-433.

Videothoracoscopy—Quality of Life

Li WWL, Lee TW, Lam SSY, et al: Quality of life following lung cancer resection. Video-assisted thoracic surgery vs. thoracotomy. Chest 2002;122:584-589.

PREVENTION OF POSTOPERATIVE COMPLICATIONS AFTER PULMONARY SURGERY

Despite advances in the selection of patients for surgery, refinements in surgical techniques, and improvements in postoperative care, the incidence of major complications after pulmonary resection *is still significant*. In large series, the incidence of nonfatal major complications is in the range of 10% to 15%, and that of minor complications is in the range of 20% to 25%. The overall 30-day operative mortality is 2% to 3% after lobectomy and 5% to 6% after pneumonectomy.

Fortunately, a number of measures can be taken to lower this incidence. The use of such prophylactic measures implies, however, a clear understanding of the anatomic and physiologic effects of pulmonary resection as well as thorough knowledge of the added morbidity associated with surgery done in older patients or in those with compromised cardiopulmonary function. The appreciation of such considerations is important not only for the operating surgeon but also for the anesthetist and other specialists involved in the perioperative care of these patients.

Prophylactic measures include appropriate selection for surgery (operability) with special consideration given to *age, weight loss, overall medical status, cardiopulmonary function, extent of resection likely to be required, and appropriate preparation for surgery*. The procedure must be well timed and the type of resection selected. Optimal anesthesia and excellent surgical technique including division of fissures and bronchial stumps and control of the pleural space are also prerequisites for lower operative morbidity. Modern control of postoperative pain, early ambulation and tube removal, and aggressive physiotherapy starting early after surgery are also important issues.

PREVENTION OF RESPIRATORY COMPLICATIONS

Sputum Retention, Atelectasis, Pneumonia

In postoperative patients, atelectasis results from the cumulative effects of decreased tidal volume and functional residual capacity, absence of sigh mechanism, and *ineffective cough* (Table 5-38). The decreased tidal volume is due to the limitation of costal and diaphragmatic excursions secondary to incisional pain and recumbent position for prolonged periods.

TABLE 5-38

MECHANISMS IMPLICATED IN THE DEVELOPMENT OF SPUTUM RETENTION AND ATELECTASIS

PREDISPOSING FACTORS

Smoking

Chronic obstructive pulmonary disease

Older age

Inadequate preoperative preparation

INTRAOPERATIVE FACTORS

Trauma to recurrent or phrenic nerve

POSTOPERATIVE FACTORS

Decreased tidal volume and functional residual capacity

Incisional pain

Prolonged recumbent position

Absence of sigh mechanism

Ineffective cough

The sigh mechanism is an important part of normal respiration and involves the taking of large intermittent breaths, usually three times the normal tidal volume approximately 10 times each hour. Postoperatively, the patient often *loses this sighing mechanism* in favor of shallow breathing that promotes atelectasis.

Ineffective cough with inadequate removal of bronchial secretions is probably the single most important etiologic factor in the development of postoperative atelectasis. It relates not only to *less than optimal pain control* but also to predisposing factors for increased amounts of sputum, such as absence of preparation for surgery, age, presence of chronic obstructive pulmonary disease, and smoking history. Intraoperative trauma to the recurrent laryngeal or phrenic nerve also predisposes to postoperative atelectasis. *Injuries to the recurrent nerve,* for instance, are particularly important because the patient with both a paralyzed vocal cord and a chest tube loses all ability to generate the necessary intrathoracic pressure to bring up and clear secretions. Similarly, the patient with *phrenic nerve paralysis* loses the diaphragmatic contraction that helps move secretions from the distal to the more proximal airway.

Atelectasis can present as "plate" atelectasis in lung bases or as "lobar" atelectasis when secretions are retained and *mucous plugging* occurs. Atelectasis often causes significant arteriovenous shunting with secondary hypoxemia, and it can lead to pneumonia, sepsis, and ultimately postoperative death.

Several methods to assist with removal of secretions are helpful in preventing atelectasis and its consequences (Table 5-39). *Chest physical therapy,* which includes modalities of coughing, deep breathing, chest percussion, and drainage, is probably *the most effective and cost-efficient* technique to prevent atelectasis. It must be delivered by trained and

5

Intraoperative Care

TABLE 5-39

PROPHYLAXIS AGAINST ATELECTASIS AND ITS CONSEQUENCES

Pain control and early ambulation

Physical therapy modalities such as coughing, deep breathing, chest percussion, and drainage

Incentive spirometry

Flexible bronchoscopy, blind nasotracheal suctioning

Mini-tracheostomy

dedicated physical respiratory therapists, and their efficiency is usually proportional to the adequacy of pain control. In general, the therapist coaches the patient to maximally inflate his or her lungs through the taking of deep breaths while applying *pressure over the incision* to reduce the pain associated with vigorous coughing.

Incentive spirometry is a common mode of physical therapy that encourages patients to inflate their lungs and sustain this inflation. It stresses the importance of a *vigorous and sustained inspiratory effort* in reversing alveolar collapse and thereby preventing atelectasis. Various incentive spirometers are commercially available, and they are most effective if the *effort is supervised* by a motivated therapist. Continuous positive airway pressure techniques can also be effective to ensure large inspired volumes, but unfortunately, their use requires trained personnel and cooperative patients.

More invasive methods of prevention include direct aspiration of secretions through flexible bronchoscopy, blind nasotracheal suctioning, and mini-tracheostomy. Fiberoptic bronchoscopy is often used immediately after surgery (in the recovery room) to remove retained secretions and blood and thus prevent later atelectasis. Regular bedside bronchoscopy can also be done in high-risk patients or in patients unable to have an effective cough. Similarly, blind nasotracheal suctioning can be effective, but it requires the skills of an experienced respiratory therapist or nurse and is generally poorly tolerated by patients.

Mini-tracheostomy, a technique of endotracheal suctioning, involves the placement of an indwelling plastic cannula *through the cricothyroid membrane*. The procedure is done at bedside and under local anesthesia. It is particularly useful for patients with copious amounts of secretions, patients unable to cough, and uncooperative patients. Few complications have been reported in centers where this technique is used on a regular basis.

Respiratory Failure

Although transient and mild hypoxemia probably occurs in most patients after any type of lung resection, *severe hypoxemia requiring mechanical ventilation is uncommon* but associated with an increased risk of mortality. In such cases, impaired gas exchange is due to atelectasis, impairment of chest wall mechanics, and diaphragmatic dysfunction, all of

TABLE 5-40
PREDISPOSING FACTORS FOR RESPIRATORY FAILURE
Older age of the patient
Marginal pulmonary reserve
Extended operation
Administration of large amounts of fluids
Silent microaspiration, sputum retention, and atelectasis

which may cause increased work of breathing followed by respiratory failure. Predisposing factors include older age of the patient, magnitude of resection (pneumonectomy), marginal pulmonary reserve as documented by abnormal preoperative $D_{LCO}\%$ and $M\dot{V}o_2$, administration of large amounts of fluids, and possibly *silent microaspiration* in a patient unable to cough (Table 5-40).

Prophylaxis against this complication includes proper selection of patients for surgery; avoidance of extended resections in patients with compromised function; aggressive treatment of sputum retention, atelectasis, and pulmonary infection; and keeping the patient awake so that he or she is able to cough (not "too much" analgesia). One should also *avoid overzealous administration of fluids* because large amounts might be transferred from the pulmonary vascular compartment to the interstitial space.

Postpneumonectomy Edema

Postpneumonectomy edema is a clinical condition in which an early (2 or 3 days) postpneumonectomy patient experiences *rapidly progressing shortness of breath and hypoxemia,* and the contralateral lung develops radiologic infiltration suggesting interstitial pulmonary edema. Once the process has begun, no conventional therapy seems to improve the patient's condition, and the mortality associated with this complication is ultimately in the range of 80% to 100%.

Although the exact pathogenesis of postpneumonectomy edema is not fully understood, several factors are likely to interact to cause this complication (Table 5-41). These factors include a net increase in filtration pressure in the remaining lung that has to accommodate the whole cardiac output, acute hyperinflation of the remaining lung that causes stretching of alveoli (volutrauma) and may promote interstitial accumulation of fluid, and some degree of endothelial damage that contributes to the production of low-pressure pulmonary edema. Other possible factors are transient right ventricular dysfunction, which has been shown to develop on the second postpneumonectomy day, and mediastinal lymphatic interruption with secondary lymph pump capacity reduction. Another possible cause is silent microaspiration related to "too much analgesia." In this situation, *pain control may be at the expense of the patient's awakeness* and ability to prevent the consequences of aspiration by adequate coughing.

Possible prophylaxis measures aimed at preventing this complication are listed in Table 5-41.

TABLE 5-41
POSSIBLE CAUSES AND PROPHYLAXIS OF POSTPNEUMONECTOMY EDEMA

Possible Cause	Possible Prophylaxis
Increased pulmonary capacity and filtration pressure	Fluid restriction and diuretics; if blood pressure and urine output are low, use inotropic agents instead of extra amounts of fluid
Acute hyperinflation of remaining lung	Avoid excessive mediastinal shift by use of balanced drainage systems or no drainage
Microaspiration due to excessive analgesia	Improve the patient's awakeness; keep the patient sitting up in bed and give nothing by mouth for at least 24 hours postoperatively
Endothelial damage and increased vascular permeability	Fluid restriction
Right ventricular dysfunction	None
Mediastinal lymphatic interruption	?Avoid extended operations and mediastinal lymphadenectomy

Deep Vein Thrombosis and Pulmonary Embolism

Although the incidence of deep vein thrombosis in patients undergoing thoracotomy is unknown, several studies have suggested that it is probably underestimated and that it may be in the range of 15%. The incidence of pulmonary embolism is in the range of 4% to 5%. Obviously, pulmonary embolism is a serious complication in patients with chronic obstructive pulmonary disease who just underwent pulmonary resection.

Risk factors for deep vein thrombosis include *age older than 60 years, malignant disease, major surgery, postoperative immobilization,* and *previous history of venous disease* of the lower extremities.

Potential modalities (Table 5-42) to prevent deep vein thrombosis include early ambulation, intermittent pneumatic compression of the lower extremities, and pharmacologic prophylaxis with low-molecular-weight heparin or with aspirin. Most surgeons now use heparin (5000 units given subcutaneously twice a day), which is started at the time of induction of anesthesia and given until the patient is discharged from the hospital.

TABLE 5-42
PROPHYLACTIC MEASURES AGAINST DEEP VEIN THROMBOSIS

Physical methods
  Early ambulation
  Intermittent pneumatic compression of lower extremities
Pharmacologic methods
  Heparin (5000 units subcutaneously twice a day)
  Antiplatelet aggregation treatment with aspirin

PREVENTION OF BRONCHOPLEURAL COMPLICATIONS

Bronchopleural Fistula

It is estimated that bronchopleural fistulas occur in between 3% and 7% of all pulmonary resections. Predisposing systemic factors (Table 5-43) include the patient's underlying nutritional status (hypoalbuminemia); the presence of systemic comorbidities, such as tuberculosis, diabetes, and immunosuppression; and the systemic administration of steroids. Predisposing local factors are listed in Table 5-43.

Several general principles govern a safe and successful bronchial closure. In general, the bronchus should be divided *as close to its origin* as possible, and unnecessary skeletonization of the bronchial stump should be avoided. Unfortunately, this may not be possible after radical mediastinal lymphadenectomy or when the bronchial stump lies in an area that has previously been irradiated. The technique of closure (suture versus staple) is the least important factor in bronchial healing, and there is currently no evidence that one technique is superior to another. The ischemic bronchial stump should be covered by autogenous tissue, such as a pedicled pericardial flap, which can be developed from the pericardium covering the ascending aorta and rotated posteriorly over the right main bronchial stump. Other secure vascularized cover can be provided by *mediastinal fat, intercostal muscle pedicle, omentum, chest wall muscles* (pectoralis major), or *diaphragm*.

Postoperative Spaces and Prolonged Air Leaks

Nearly all patients undergoing lobectomy or a lesser resection are expected to have some degree of postoperative air leakage. Whereas most of these air leaks will stop within 1 week of surgery, some may persist for more

5

Intraoperative Care

TABLE 5-43

PREDISPOSING FACTORS FOR BRONCHOPLEURAL FISTULA

SYSTEMIC FACTORS

Poor underlying nutritional status (hypoalbuminemia)

Systemic comorbidities (tuberculosis, diabetes, immunosuppression)

Steroid administration

LOCAL FACTORS

Poor technique of bronchial closure

Failure to identify a "difficult bronchus"

Presence of a long bronchial stump

Devascularization of the bronchial blood supply

Failure to provide appropriate cover for the bronchus at risk of dehiscence (irradiated or denuded bronchial stump)

Extensive mediastinal node dissection

Residual carcinoma in the bronchial stump

Presence of an empyema

POSTOPERATIVE FACTORS

Mechanical ventilation

Pulmonary infection

TABLE 5-44

RISK FACTORS FOR PROLONGED AIR LEAKS

PREOPERATIVE

Older age (>70 years)

Lower FEV_1 (indicative of chronic obstructive pulmonary disease)

Poor nutritional status (hypoalbuminemia)

Use of steroids

INTRAOPERATIVE

Redo surgery

Segmental resection (versus lobectomy)

Inadequate surgical technique

POSTOPERATIVE

Incomplete lung re-expansion

Mechanical ventilation

---

than 7 days, and these are considered a complication. Air leak persisting for more than 14 days is a major complication. In general, 15% of patients have an air leak for more than 7 days and 2% for more than 14 days. Significant risk factors for prolonged air leaks are listed in Table 5-44.

Persistent air spaces after resection result from the failure of one or more components of normal space obliteration mechanisms (Table 5-45). These include the *shift of adjacent dynamic structures,* such as the heart, mediastinum, and diaphragm; the *hyperinflation* of the residual lung; and the intrapleural accumulation of blood and serum over lung surfaces and in recesses and fissures. This obliteration is facilitated by the negative intrapleural pressure, the lack of air leakage from the lung, and the unimpaired expansibility of the lung.

Known risk factors for post-resectional spaces are listed in Table 5-46. Although the true incidence of post-resectional spaces is not known, it is likely that 100% of patients would have them if a postoperative CT scan were done on everybody. The majority of these spaces are noninfected and asymptomatic, however, and they will become obliterated during a period of weeks. Infected spaces are symptomatic, and their incidence is less than 5%.

The prophylaxis against post-resectional spaces and prolonged air leaks is always more important than any subsequent treatment. Most air leaks can be prevented (Table 5-47) by religious closure of all parenchymal tears. Meticulous attention should be given to the division of intersegmental planes and fissures, and the use of staplers alone or reinforced by bovine

---

TABLE 5-45

MECHANISMS OF SPACE OBLITERATION

Shift of adjacent structures (heart, mediastinum, diaphragm)

Approximation of ribs

Hyperinflation of residual lung

Intrapleural accumulation of blood and serum

TABLE 5-46

RISK FACTORS FOR POST-RESECTIONAL SPACES

Inability of residual lung to fill the hemithorax (previous resection, underlying pulmonary fibrosis)

Extent of resection (bilobectomy versus single lobe)

Presence of a fistula (alveolar or bronchial)

Poor surgical technique

pericardial strips has been advocated. Perhaps *the most important prophylaxis is to make sure that the residual lung re-expands* to fill the space. If, despite these measures, it appears that prolonged air leak might become a problem, a variety of alternative techniques can be used. The creation of a *pleural tent* is useful to prevent apical spaces. The technique involves stripping the parietal pleura from the apex and resuturing it to the lower edge of the wound, thus creating a sterile extrapleural space. An advantage of the pleural tent is that the residual lung can rise to its own level because the parietal pleura is flexible. If a basal space is anticipated, a *pneumoperitoneum* can be initiated intraoperatively. This is done with a catheter placed in the subphrenic space transdiaphragmatically.

Temporary phrenic nerve paralysis can be accomplished by the injection of bupivacaine (Marcaine) in the fatty tissues around the phrenic nerve. This technique will raise the diaphragm, but it has the disadvantage of decreasing pulmonary function. When the potential for post-resectional spaces or prolonged air leak is recognized intraoperatively, *accurate placement of two chest tubes* is of critical importance; immediate *postoperative bronchoscopy* should also be done so that neither mucus nor blood prevents maximal lung re-expansion.

TABLE 5-47

PROPHYLAXIS AGAINST PROLONGED AIR LEAKS

AVOIDANCE OF PARENCHYMAL TEARS

Meticulous division of intersegmental planes and fissures

Use of staplers alone or reinforced

Use of fibrin glue or other sealants applied over surgical surfaces

Use of laser to divide fissures

RE-EXPANSION OF RESIDUAL LUNG

Careful suturing of parenchymal tears

Decortication of residual lung if necessary

Do not resect middle lobe if unnecessary

ALTERNATIVE TECHNIQUES

Creation of a pleural tent (for anticipated apical spaces)

Pneumoperitoneum (for anticipated basal spaces)

Phrenic nerve infiltration

Accurate placement of at least two chest tubes

Bronchoscopy in recovery room

5

Intraoperative Care

TABLE 5-48
PROPHYLAXIS AGAINST POST-RESECTIONAL EMPYEMA
Preoperative antibiotic treatment of pulmonary infection
Sound techniques of bronchial closure and those used to prevent air leaks
Adequate pleural drainage
Postoperative antibiotic prophylaxis

Empyema

Postoperative empyemas are seen almost exclusively after operations in which the *esophageal or bronchial lumens have been entered*. The incidence of this complication is in the range of 2% to 4% after pulmonary resection.

Prophylaxis against postoperative empyema (Table 5-48) includes adequate preoperative antibiotic treatment of pulmonary infection. It also includes careful intraoperative techniques of bronchial handling and closure and techniques to prevent prolonged air leaks. Prophylaxis finally includes adequate pleural drainage and *perioperative antibiotic prophylaxis,* which has been shown to reduce the incidence of wound infection and empyema significantly. A single dose of antibiotic with adequate gram-positive and gram-negative coverage is suggested preoperatively and should be continued for 24 to 48 hours postoperatively.

PREVENTION OF CARDIOVASCULAR COMPLICATIONS

Arrhythmias

The incidence of arrhythmias after resectional lung operation ranges from 10% to 20% after lobectomy and up to 40% after pneumonectomy. Atrial fibrillation, atrial flutter, and paroxistic atrial tachycardia are the most frequently encountered. It is believed that they are the result of a synergistic action between increased vagal tone and hypoxia. In addition to pneumonectomy, *major predisposing factors* for postoperative arrhythmias are older age of the patient and preexisting cardiac disease (Table 5-49).

Several prophylactic antiarrhythmic drug treatments have been studied, but most had no prophylactic efficiency or had a high incidence of severe adverse effects. Digoxin may, in fact, shorten atrial refractoriness, which, in theory at least, could increase the likelihood of atrial fibrillation. Currently, most surgeons *do not advocate* prophylactic digitalization or the use of any other drug such as flecainide or calcium channel blockers. Prophylaxis includes *immediate correction* of risk factors such as hypoxia, hypovolemia, sepsis, electrolyte imbalance, and augmented vagal activity.

TABLE 5-49
PREDISPOSING FACTORS FOR POSTOPERATIVE ATRIAL ARRHYTHMIAS
Older age of the patient (>70 years)
Pneumonectomy (versus lobectomy)
Preexisting cardiac disease including hypertension

Cardiac Herniation (Table 5-50)

Cardiac herniation is an infrequently reported complication of intrapericardial pneumonectomy (right > left). It arises in the immediate postoperative period in patients *with residual and large (>5 cm) pericardial defects* and carries a mortality that approaches 50%.

Prophylactic measures against possible herniation should be taken in all patients in whom a pericardial defect has been created during pneumonectomy. Small defects should be closed by direct suturing; larger defects must be closed by interposition of autogenous tissue, such as pedicled parietal pleura or diaphragm, bovine pericardial patches, or prosthetic meshes.

Myocardial Infarction

Patients with severe coronary artery disease should be identified and treated before thoracotomy, even if such treatment involves coronary artery grafting. Prophylaxis against myocardial infarction also includes proper monitoring and maintenance of adequate arterial blood pressure and oxygen saturation throughout the postoperative period.

PREVENTION OF UNCOMMON COMPLICATIONS

Hemorrhage

Significant intraoperative hemorrhage and postoperative bleeding requiring reoperation are uncommon events, although most surgeons, even the most experienced ones, have had such difficulties at one time or another. Prophylaxis includes meticulous dissection, safe suturing of major blood vessels, and reliable intraoperative hemostasis.

Phrenic and Recurrent Nerve Injuries

Postoperative diaphragmatic dysfunction may occur after division, contusion, or electrocautery trauma of the phrenic nerve. The consequences are respiratory embarrassment and, in some cases, respiratory failure due to fatigue of accessory muscles. Prophylaxis against phrenic nerve palsy includes careful dissection of the nerve, or around it if necessary, and avoidance of use of electrocautery near the phrenic nerve. If the decision is made to infiltrate the nerve, the local anesthetic agent (approximately 10 mL of bupivacaine) should *be infiltrated in the pericardial fat* around the nerve just above the diaphragm.

Because of its anatomic location around the aortic arch, the vagus nerve can be invaded by lung cancer and therefore is at risk of being injured during left hilar or mediastinal node dissection. Lesion of the vagus nerve will result in vocal cord dysfunction (due to recurrent nerve palsy),

5

Intraoperative Care

TABLE 5-50
PREDISPOSING FACTORS FOR CARDIAC HERNIATION
Right pneumonectomy
Median or large pericardial defect
Application of suction to chest tubes
Coughing, tracheal suctioning, mechanical ventilation

which can become a serious problem in compromised patients who have just had a pulmonary resection. Several series have clearly shown a significant increase in operative mortality in patients with vocal cord paralysis as opposed to patients without it.

Unfortunately, there is often no other way to completely remove the tumor than to divide either the vagus nerve or the recurrent nerve. In such cases, some surgeons advocate *immediate vocal cord medialization* by type I thyroplasty.

Lobe Torsion and Lobe Gangrene

Lobe torsion represents a rotation of the bronchovascular pedicle with resultant venous compromise and hemorrhagic necrosis. It usually affects the middle lobe after right upper lobectomy.

Prophylaxis is simple. The remaining lobes (middle and lower lobes) should be attached lightly together after right upper lobectomy.

Chylothorax

The thoracic duct lies posterior to the descending aorta and courses to the right of the spine. At the level of T5 to T7, the duct crosses behind the aorta to the left posterior side of the mediastinum and ascends on the left side of the esophagus posterior to the left subclavian artery. The presence of *multiple collateral channels* and its *highly variable anatomic location* can lead to an injury during lung resection with mediastinal node dissection (incidence of 1% to 2%).

The only prophylaxis measure is to clip lymphatic vessels when they are seen during the course of radical mediastinal node dissection. Most commonly, injuries to the thoracic duct or to collateral vessels occur below the carina or above the aortic arch on the left side.

Thoracic Wound Infection

Although thoracic wound infection is *uncommon*, it has been shown that antibiotic prophylaxis can reduce this complication in patients undergoing pulmonary resection. A wound infection often reflects an empyema that is draining spontaneously through the chest wall.

CONCLUSION

Potential modalities to prevent postoperative complications in thoracic operations are numerous, and each one must be understood and used in conjunction with the others. Most postoperative complications are preventable, and they are directly related to inadequate preparation before surgery and poor surgical technique.

Accurate and complete knowledge of the various techniques for prophylaxis should be part of every general thoracic surgeon's armamentarium.

SUGGESTED READINGS

Review Articles

Kirsh MM, Rotman H, Behrendt DM, et al: Complications of pulmonary resection [collective review]. Ann Thorac Surg 1975;20:215-236.

Pearson FG: Managing the difficult bronchus. Proceedings of the University of Toronto Postgraduate Course in Thoracic Surgery. Toronto, June 1984.

Anderson TM, Miller JI: Use of pleura, azygos vein, pericardium, and muscle flaps in tracheobronchial surgery. Ann Thorac Surg 1995; 60:729-733.

Air Leaks, Spaces, Infection

Olak J, Jeyasingham K, Forrester-Wood C, et al: Randomized trial of one-dose versus six-dose cefazolin prophylaxis in elective general thoracic surgery. Ann Thorac Surg 1991;51:956-958.

Ratto GB, Fantino G, Tassara E, et al: Long-term antimicrobial prophylaxis in lung cancer surgery: correlation between microbiological findings and empyema development. Lung Cancer 1994;11:345-352.

Brunelli A, Al Refai M, Muti M, et al: Pleural tent after upper lobectomy: a prospective randomized study. Ann Thorac Surg 2000;69:1722-1724.

De Giacomo T, Rendina EA, Venuta F, et al: Pneumoperitoneum for the management of pleural air space problems associated with major pulmonary resections. Ann Thorac Surg 2001;72:1716-1719.

Arrhythmias

Cardinale D, Martinoni A, Cipolla CM, et al: Atrial fibrillation after operation for lung cancer: clinical and prognostic significance. Ann Thorac Surg 1999;68:1827-1831.

Recurrent Nerve Injury

Filaire M, Mom T, Laurent S, et al: Vocal cord dysfunction after left lung resection for cancer. Eur J Cardiothorac Surg 2001;20:705-711.

Mom T, Filaire M, Advenier D, et al: Concomitant type I thyroplasty and thoracic operations for lung cancer: preventing respiratory complications associated with vagus or recurrent laryngeal nerve injury. J Thorac Cardiovasc Surg 2001;121:642-648.

Chylothorax

Le Pimpec Barthes F, D'Attellis N, Dujon A, et al: Chylothorax complicating pulmonary resection. Ann Thorac Surg 2002;73;1714-1719.

Pulmonary Complications

Stock MC, Downs JB, Gauer PK, et al: Prevention of postoperative pulmonary complications with CPAP, incentive spirometry, and conservative therapy. Chest 1985;87:151-157.

Wain JC, Wilson DJ, Mathisen DJ: Clinical experience with minitracheostomy. Ann Thorac Surg 1990;49:881-886.

Thromboembolism

Ziomek S, Read RC, Tobler HG, et al: Thromboembolism in patients undergoing thoracotomy. Ann Thorac Surg 1993;56:223-227.

Lobe Torsion

Wong PS, Goldstraw P: Pulmonary torsion: a questionnaire survey and a survey of the literature. Ann Thorac Surg 1992;54:286-288.

PREVENTION OF POSTOPERATIVE COMPLICATIONS AFTER ESOPHAGEAL SURGERY

Operations on the esophagus, especially those involving esophageal resection, require an approach different from operations on other parts of the digestive tract and more meticulous technique. Indeed, there is probably *no greater challenge* in surgery of the gastrointestinal tract than resection and reconstruction of the esophagus. This is, at least in part, because the organ that will be used to replace the esophagus must be able to transport food, must prevent reflux and aspiration, and finally must allow vomiting and belching.

Similarly, operations for functional disorders or even for gastroesophageal reflux must be done with a *clear understanding* of the pathologic process being treated as well as of potential functional disorders that can result from such procedures.

Because esophageal resection is associated with significant operative mortality (5% to 10%) and morbidity (20% to 40%), mostly in older patients or in patients who have had induction therapies, it is important that these individuals be well prepared for the operation and that the surgeon operating be familiar with the selected approach, the method of reconstruction, and the technique of anastomosis.

PREVENTION OF COMPLICATIONS AFTER ESOPHAGEAL RESECTION

Preparation for Surgery

For most patients, preoperative assessment of "medical operability" is similar to that done before pulmonary resection. The general objectives are to assess *comorbidities, especially cardiopulmonary diseases,* and to identify patients at increased or prohibitive risk of complications. These patients should be looked at *very carefully,* and sometimes they are just not candidates for esophagectomy.

"High-risk" patients, such as those with significant weight loss, older patients, or patients who have had induction therapies, may benefit from preoperative correction of nutritional deficiencies. Obvious dehydration and anemia should be treated before surgery. The role of nutritional supplementation is *controversial*, but short-term (<2 weeks) nutritional therapy *does not appear* to be beneficial. Longer nutritional support (>2 weeks) done through a nasogastric tube advanced distal to the tumor or by intravenous hyperalimentation *may help correct deficiencies.*

Because patients with esophageal carcinoma are at risk of aspiration, any pulmonary infection should be identified and treated vigorously before the operation. Similarly, the use of perioperative antibiotic prophylaxis is mandatory not only because all patients can aspirate but also because extensive dissection of the mediastinum and possible opening of the contaminated esophagus can cause severe mediastinitis.

In patients in whom the stomach may not be suitable for reconstruction (i.e., because of previous surgery), the *possible use of the colon* should be investigated preoperatively with barium enema study and possibly angiography. It should then be prepared in the event that colonic interposition is required.

Prevention of Complications during Removal of the Esophagus
(Table 5-51)

The average intraoperative blood loss for esophagectomy is in the range of 700 to 800 mL, and significant bleeding is seldom encountered even during transhiatal resection. This is because esophageal arteries originating from the aorta branch into small capillaries before reaching the esophagus and because most surgeons carry their dissection close to the esophageal wall. If, during transhiatal esophagectomy, the esophagus seems to be fixed to the aorta or other major intrathoracic vascular structure, the best prophylaxis against hemorrhage is *to exercise judgment and convert to open thoracotomy.*

Tracheobronchial tears (incidence < 2%) can occur during open dissection of midesophageal carcinomas or during mediastinal dissection associated with transhiatal esophagectomy. Tracheal invasion will sometimes have been diagnosed by preoperative bronchoscopy, and those patients should not undergo surgery. Tumors at or proximal to the carina may be approached by *open thoracotomy* rather than by transhiatal esophagectomy. As described by Hulscher, the pressure of the dissecting finger should always be on the esophagus rather than on the airway during esophageal mobilization. If true tracheal invasion is identified, resection should be abandoned. Similarly, the surgeon must again be prepared to convert to open thoracotomy if the esophagus is found to be fixed to the trachea during transhiatal esophagectomy.

Both recurrent nerves can be injured during esophagectomy. Such injuries and the resultant nerve palsy are serious complications because they alter cricopharyngeal motor function and predispose to aspiration pneumonia. The left recurrent nerve can be injured in its course around the aortic arch or more likely during the cervical part of the operation. The right recurrent nerve is at risk during the esophageal dissection at the apex of the right side of the chest during an Ivor-Lewis-McKeon three-stage esophagectomy. Most of these injuries are *preventable* by familiarity with local anatomy, careful technique of dissection, and avoidance of the use of metal retractors or other instruments against the tracheoesophageal groove.

5

Intraoperative Care

TABLE 5-51

STRUCTURES AT RISK DURING ESOPHAGECTOMY

Major blood vessels: aorta, azygos vein

Trachea and main bronchi

Right and left recurrent nerves

Thoracic duct

Spleen

The close anatomic relationship of the thoracic duct with the esophagus makes inadvertent injury possible during esophagectomy, and the diagnosis of thoracic duct injury is often difficult to make intraoperatively. If it is diagnosed, however, *the thoracic duct must be ligated* above and below the point of injury. Several authors recommend routine ligation of the thoracic duct to prevent this complication. Whether this strategy improves outcome is unclear.

Prevention of Complications Related to the Organ Used for Reconstruction (Fig. 5-25)

The intact stomach (Table 5-52) is the *most convenient* organ for reconstruction of the esophagus because it can easily be advanced to the neck and because its use requires *only one anastomosis.* Its blood supply is based on the right gastroepiploic artery as well as on numerous submucosal microvascular channels. On occasion, the blood supply can be optimized by dissecting into the splenic hilum to preserve anastomosis between the gastroepiploic and short gastric vessels or by fashioning a narrow gastric tube from the greater curvature. Reversed and nonreversed gastric tubes offer *few advantages* and are *seldom used.*

During positioning of the stomach within the chest, care should be taken to ensure correct orientation for avoidance of volvulus.

According to Bathisen, delayed gastric emptying can be due to a *pyloric obstruction; an obstruction at the level of the hiatus;* or a *redundant intrathoracic stomach* lying in the posterior costophrenic gutter, resulting in a J-shaped configuration of the intrathoracic stomach. These problems are best avoided by an adequate drainage procedure at the time of operation (pyloromyotomy, pyloroplasty), by enlarging the hiatus, and by avoiding excess stomach in the chest.

In some patients, the thoracic inlet is too small to allow advancement of the stomach without excessive compression. If such a problem is

TABLE 5-52

PREVENTION OF COMPLICATIONS WHEN THE STOMACH IS USED FOR RECONSTRUCTION

Complication	Prevention
Vascular insufficiency	Preservation of right gastroepiploic artery and gastroepiploic arcades Dissection into splenic hilum Use of a narrow gastric tube instead of the intact stomach
Volvulus	Ensure correct orientation of the stomach
Delayed gastric emptying	Enlarge hiatus Avoid redundancy of intrathoracic stomach Pyloromyotomy or pyloroplasty
Obstruction at thoracic inlet	Enlarge thoracic inlet
Reflux	Cervical anastomosis (versus intrathoracic) Encircle anastomosis with collar of fundus (fundoplication)

Organ	Technique	No. of Anastomoses	Inherent Morbidity Difficulty	Upper Level of Usefulness	Disadvantages
Stomach	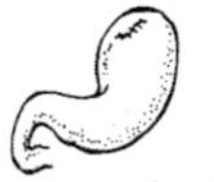	1	+	Cervical esophagus and pharynx	Bulky Reflux risk
Greater curvature tube	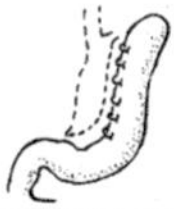	1	+	Cervical esophagus and pharynx	Reflux risk
Reversed gastric tube	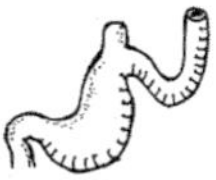	1	+++	Cervical esophagus and pharynx	Long suture line Limited blood supply
Non-reversed gastric tube	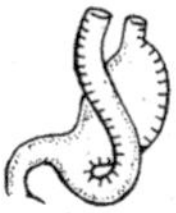	1	++	Lower cervical esophagus	Long suture line
Right colon	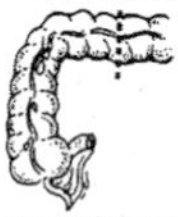	3	+++	Lower cervical esophagus	Thin-walled Bulky Shot pedicle
Left colon	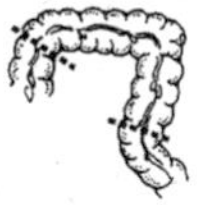	3	++++	Most versatile organ for use at any level Lower third to pharynx	Extensive operation Redundancy over time
Jejunum	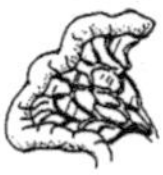	2 (Roux loop) 3 (Interposition)	++	Lower third	Limited graft length without revision of pedicle or bowel
Free graft	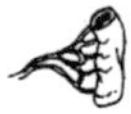	5 (2 micro-vascular)	+++++	Pharynx and cervical esophagus	Microvascular anastomoses required

FIG. 5-25

Comparative usefulness of various esophageal substitutes. *(Courtesy of Dr. Clement A. Hiebert.)*

anticipated, the thoracic inlet can be enlarged by *splitting the upper sternum and dividing clavicles and first and second costal cartilages.*

Another long-term complication of use of the stomach for esophageal replacement is reflux esophagitis with secondary strictures or aspiration. This problem can be prevented by a cervical anastomosis versus an

TABLE 5-53
PREVENTION OF COMPLICATIONS WHEN THE COLON IS USED FOR RECONSTRUCTION
Respect for contraindications to colon use (intrinsic colon disease, compromised vascular supply)
Bowel preparation begun the day before surgery
At operation, reascertain adequacy of communications between left and middle colic vessels
Operation should not be done by inexperienced surgeons

intrathoracic anastomosis (the higher the anastomosis, the less reflux) or by encircling the anastomosis with a collar of fundus (fundoplication).

Despite articulate technique, only a *minority of patients will be symptom free* at long-term follow-up. The most common symptoms are those of reflux, dumping, and swallowing difficulties.

The colon is commonly used as an alternative to the stomach. The most popular technique uses the left and transverse colon (isoperistaltic) based on the ascending branch of the left colic artery. Transposed left colon reaches easily to the neck. Prevention against complications (Table 5-53) includes *avoiding use of the colon when there is intrinsic disease,* such as Crohn disease or diverticulitis, or when compromised vascular supply (severe mesenteric arteriosclerosis, anatomic discontinuity of the marginal artery) is suspected. All of these issues must be evaluated preoperatively by barium enema examination, colonoscopy, and angiography if necessary; at operation, the surgeon must reascertain the adequacy of communications between left and middle colic vessels. A bowel preparation begun the day before surgery will lessen the chances of postoperative infection, whether it is empyema or wound sepsis. Because colon interposition requires extensive mobilization and three anastomoses, it *should not be done* by inexperienced surgeons.

Prevention of Complications Related to the Anastomosis

The reported incidence of anastomotic leaks is 0% to 12%. In general, anastomotic leaks are *more common* with neck anastomosis, but the *mortality is higher* when the leak occurs with an intrathoracic anastomosis.

Prevention against anastomotic dehiscence includes atraumatic handling of the tissues, preservation of blood supply of the esophagus and organ used for replacement, avoidance of crushing clamps, and avoidance of tension at the level of the anastomosis. There is no evidence that performing the anastomosis with staplers or with hand-sewing technique (manual anastomosis) makes much difference as long as the surgeon is *thoroughly familiar with the technique* that she or he is using. If the anastomosis is done between esophagus and stomach, most surgeons advocate the placement of a few sutures between stomach and paravertebral fascia to reduce the downward pull on the anastomosis. In cases in which the stomach has been used, the *omentum* that has been mobilized with it can be placed over the anastomosis anteriorly to provide an additional layer of coverage.

Postoperatively, a nasogastric tube advanced through the anastomosis will lessen the chances of distraction at the suture line by a distended stomach. Late strictures are uncommon, and they can be prevented by early dilatation of high-risk anastomoses, such as those that have leaked early postoperatively.

Prevention of Other Postoperative Complications

Respiratory events such as atelectasis, pneumonia, aspiration, and adult respiratory distress syndrome are the most serious postoperative complications associated with esophagectomy. Risk factors include older age, malnutrition before surgery, induction therapies, and, most important, recurrent laryngeal nerve injuries.

In general, the incidence of respiratory complications can be lowered by optimal pain control, physiotherapy, bedside bronchoscopy, and even mini-tracheostomy when necessary. The role of mini-tracheostomy is controversial, however, because a cannula in the airways *may aggravate difficulties in swallowing.*

Pleural effusions can occur if the pleural spaces have been opened. Prophylaxis against these includes adequate postoperative tube drainage.

PREVENTION OF COMPLICATIONS AFTER SURGERY FOR MOTOR DISORDERS OF THE ESOPHAGUS

Achalasia (Table 5-54)

Pneumatic dilatation of the esophagus achieves mechanical disruption of esophageal smooth muscle fibers through the use of pneumatic balloon dilators. In experienced hands, complications are minimal, and the incidence of perforation is less than 2%. After pneumatic dilatation, however, patients should be observed closely (for at least 24 to 48 hours) for any clinical signs of perforation; if this complication is suspected, a Gastrografin swallow study should be obtained. If an esophageal perforation is documented, *operative repair should be carried out without delay* to minimize the severity of mediastinitis.

Esophagocardiomyotomy is the most definitive means of treatment for achalasia. The goal of the operation is to relieve the functional obstruction of the lower esophageal sphincter without destroying the mechanisms responsible for the prevention of reflux. The operation can be done through

Intraoperative Care

5

TABLE 5-54
PREVENTION OF COMPLICATIONS OF ESOPHAGEAL MYOTOMY FOR ACHALASIA

Clear diagnosis of achalasia made preoperatively
Clear understanding of surgical indications
Consultation with gastroenterologist
Adequate preoperative preparation
Separate muscle layers laterally for distance of 1 cm
Extend proximal myotomy to level of inferior pulmonary vein
Extend distal myotomy into the stomach 1-2 cm below the gastroesophageal junction
Add antireflux procedure of the partial wrap type if myotomy is extended
Avoid total fundoplication

the left side of the chest (open myotomy), through the abdomen, or through thoracoscopic-laparoscopic approaches. *Adequate preoperative preparation is important,* especially if the patient has documented food retention or a history of aspiration pneumonia. This preparation includes liquid diet for 48 hours before surgery and antibiotics and active chest physiotherapy in cases of aspiration pneumonia. If the patient is severely malnourished, enteral hyperalimentation may have to be given for a few weeks preoperatively.

To prevent complications, one must have a clear indication for surgery, and the motor disorder has to have been well documented. It is strongly recommended that the decision be made jointly by the gastroenterologist and the surgeon. At operation, the myotomy must be done through all muscle layers, and to prevent late rehealing at the myotomy site, the surgeon must laterally separate muscle from mucosa for a distance of 1 cm along the whole length of the myotomy.

The myotomy must extend proximally to the level of the inferior pulmonary vein; distally, it usually extends into the stomach 1 to 2 cm below the gastroesophageal junction. If the myotomy does not extend far enough distally, dysphagia may persist. Whether one should *add an antireflux procedure remains controversial,* although most surgeons believe that it is not necessary if the distal extent of the myotomy (onto the stomach) is limited. If the myotomy is more extended, an antireflux operation will prevent reflux and its complications (esophagitis, peptic stricture, Barrett esophagus). A complete fundoplication of the Nissen type should be avoided because it will create too much resistance for the emptying of the myotomized esophagus. Obviously, the abdominal approach requires full mobilization of the hiatus, and an antireflux operation should always be added.

The main complication of laparoscopic or thoracoscopic esophageal myotomy is a mucosal tear, which becomes uncommon with increasing familiarity of the procedure by the surgeon. If there is any doubt about a possible perforation (during open or endoscopic myotomy), 20 to 50 mL of air can be injected through the nasogastric tube while the myotomy site is submerged with water. A perforation should be repaired primarily and reinforced with a fundoplication.

Other Motor Disorders of the Esophagus

Diffuse esophageal spasm is an uncommon motor disorder of the esophagus characterized by simultaneous nonperistaltic contractions in the body of the esophagus. Other findings include high-amplitude, repetitive, and prolonged duration contractions. Patients usually present with chest pain, which must be differentiated from pain related to cardiac causes, and dysphagia. Surgery is *seldom necessary* and is indicated only for symptomatic patients unresponsive to medical treatment. At operation, which is generally done through open thoracotomy, the myotomy must be high enough to encompass the entire length of disordered motility; distally, the same considerations as previously discussed with achalasia also apply to this procedure.

The majority of the other motor disorders of the body of the esophagus do not require surgical intervention.

Surgery of the Cricopharynx

Cricopharyngeal myotomy may be indicated for a variety of cricopharyngeal disorders. As with all other disorders of the esophagus, prevention of complications begins with *systematic investigation of the disorder, proper diagnosis of the cause of dysphagia,* and *careful selection for operation.* One should always be careful before performing a cricopharyngeal myotomy in patients with acid reflux because the operation may remove the only effective barrier against aspiration.

Complications specific to cricopharyngeal myotomy are recurrent laryngeal nerve injury, mucosal tear, and incomplete myotomy. In most cases, the recurrent nerve is easily visualized in the groove between trachea and esophagus and thus can be protected. The myotomy should extend approximately 6 cm across the posterior pharyngoesophageal junction, and this part of the operation is easier to perform over a 36 Fr mercury bougie. To prevent the consequences of a mucosal laceration, the myotomy site should always be checked by asking the anesthetist to inject 20 to 50 mL of air through the nasogastric tube.

If a Zenker diverticulum is present, it is recommended that a *suspension diverticulopexy* be combined with the myotomy. Large diverticula are excised. Large diverticula can also be drained via a peroral stapling procedure.

PREVENTION OF COMPLICATIONS OF SURGERY FOR GASTROESOPHAGEAL REFLUX

Successful outcome after antireflux surgery depends on establishing a correct diagnosis of gastroesophageal reflux disease, ruling out other motor disorders of the esophagus, and carefully selecting patients for operation. In some cases, this selection process may require esophageal manometry and 24-hour pH monitoring.

The most common indications for surgery are listed in Table 5-55. In general, all antireflux operations are characterized by *repositioning of an intra-abdominal segment of esophagus; prevention of recurrent herniation;* and *creation of an antireflux valvular mechanism* that allows normal swallowing, belching, and vomiting but prevents abnormal reflux of gastric contents.

The most common functional complications seen after fundoplication are recurrent acid reflux, dysphagia, and gas bloat syndrome (inability to belch and postprandial fullness). In general, dysphagia and gas bloat syndromes can be prevented by using a loose wrap around the esophagus

---

TABLE 5-55

MOST COMMON INDICATIONS FOR SURGICAL CORRECTION OF GASTROESOPHAGEAL REFLUX

Inadequate medical control of patients with disabling symptoms

Complications of reflux, such as peptic strictures, aspiration,
   or chronic laryngeal irritation

Barrett esophagus

(requires complete mobilization of the upper stomach), by wrapping the stomach around a 50 Fr Maloney bougie, by only performing a 2-cm wrap, and by taking care not to close the diaphragmatic crura behind the esophagus too tightly. A Belsey Mark IV type of wrap (240-degree wrap) is also less likely to create dysphagia and more likely to retain the capacity for belching and vomiting.

If, at operation, the length of esophagus appears insufficient to permit intra-abdominal repositioning of the esophagus (without tension), an esophageal lengthening procedure must be considered, and a 360-degree Nissen fundoplication can be added to the gastroplasty. Protection of the vagus nerves during surgery is important to prevent pyloric spasm and delayed gastric emptying.

CONCLUSION

No area of thoracic surgery is more challenging or more difficult than esophageal resection and reconstruction. The surgeon's experience, team work with the gastroenterologist, and respect of surgical indications are important features of these operations. Operative morbidity, long-term outcomes, and, most important, quality of life depend on adequate preparation for surgery as well as intraoperative prophylaxis against complications.

SUGGESTED READINGS

Review Articles

Hulscher JB, Tijssen JG, Obertop H, van Lanschot JJ: Transthoracic versus transhiatal resection for carcinoma of the esophagus: a meta-analysis. Ann Thorac Surg 2001;72:306-313.

Urschel JD: Does the interponat affect outcome after esophagectomy for cancer? Dis Esophagus 2001;14:124-130.

Bolton JS, Teng S: Transthoracic or transhiatal esophagectomy for cancer of the esophagus—does it matter? Surg Oncol Clin North Am 2002;11:365-375.

General Articles

Duranceau AC, Jamieson GG, Beauchamp G: The technique of cricopharyngeal myotomy. Surg Clin North Am 1983;63:833-839.

McLarty AJ, Deschamps C, Trastek VF, et al: Esophageal resection for cancer of the esophagus: long-term function and quality of life. Ann Thorac Surg 1997;63:1568-1572.

Peters JH, DeMeester TR, Crookes P, et al: The treatment of gastroesophageal reflux disease with laparoscopic Nissen fundoplication. Prospective evaluation of 100 patients with "typical symptoms." Ann Surg 1998;228:40-50.

Orringer MB, Marshall B, Iannettoni MD: Eliminating the cervical esophagogastric anastomotic leak with a side-to-side stapled anastomosis. J Thorac Cardiovasc Surg 2000;119:277-288.

Karl RC, Schreiber R, Boulware D, et al: Factors affecting morbidity, mortality, and survival in patients undergoing Ivor-Lewis esophagogastrectomy. Ann Surg 2000;231:635-643.

Ohwada S, Ogawa T, Kawate S, et al: Omentoplasty versus no omentoplasty for cervical esophagogastrostomy following radical esophagectomy. Hepatogastroenterology 2002;49:181-184.

Surgical Volume and Complications

Birkmeyer JD: Should we regionalize major surgery? Potential benefits and policy considerations. J Am Coll Surg 2000;190:341-349.

van Lanschot JJB, Hulscher JBF, Buskens CJ, et al: Hospital volume and hospital mortality for esophagectomy. Cancer 2001; 91:1574-1578.

Dimick JB, Pronovost PJ, Cowan JA, Lipsett PA: Surgical volume and quality of care for esophageal resection: do high-volume hospitals have fewer complications? Ann Thorac Surg 2003;75:337-341.

Morbidity and Induction Therapy

Doty JR, Salazar JD, Forastiere AA, et al: Postesophagectomy morbidity, mortality, and length of hospital stay after preoperative chemoradiation therapy. Ann Thorac Surg 2002;74:227-231.

Recurrent Nerve

Baba M, Natsugoe S, Shimada M, et al: Does hoarseness of voice from recurrent nerve paralysis after esophagectomy for carcinoma influence patient quality of life? J Am Coll Surg 1999;188:231-236.

Chylothorax

Alexiou C, Watson M, Beggs D, et al: Chylothorax following esophagogastrectomy for malignant disease. Eur J Cardiothorac Surg 1998;14:460-466.

Airway Injuries

Hulscher JBF, ter Hofstede E, Kloek J, et al: Injury to the major airways during subtotal esophagectomy: incidence, management, and sequelae. J Thorac Cardiovasc Surg 2000;120:1093-1096.

PLEURAL DRAINAGE AFTER THORACIC PROCEDURES

One of the important principles of patient management after partial pulmonary resection is that the *residual lung should be totally expanded.* This is considered essential to prevent complications and can be achieved by "religious" intraoperative closure of parenchymal tears and decortication of the residual lung if necessary, prevention of postoperative atelectasis, and approximation of pleural surfaces, best accomplished *by efficient use of chest tubes,* preferably with active suction.

After pneumonectomy, most surgeons *do not* advocate drainage of the space because balancing of the mediastinum can be achieved by needle aspiration or by leaving a small thoracic catheter that is withdrawn once the thoracotomy incision is closed. Potential advantages of draining the space are the recognition of postoperative hemorrhage, should it happen, and the prevention of catastrophic tension pneumothorax should the bronchial suture line acutely break down. In some cases, *balance drainage* helps maintain the mediastinum in an optimal physiologic position during the critical first few hours that follow pneumonectomy.

PLEURAL DRAINAGE AFTER PARTIAL PULMONARY RESECTION

Overall Considerations (Table 5-56)

When chest tubes are inserted in the pleural space after partial pulmonary resection, the most important goal to be achieved is the prompt drainage of air and fluids so that *lung re-expansion and apposition of pleural surfaces* are promoted. Ultimately, complete lung re-expansion will help seal the peripheral sites of air leakage, obliterate the pleural space, and prevent late complications such as chronic bronchopleural fistulas, clotted hemothoraces, and infected spaces. Pleural drainage is also essential to restore cardio-pulmonary function to its maximum state of efficiency. This is achieved by preventing residual pneumothoraces or lung collapse and by balancing the mediastinum in its normal midline position.

Another important objective of pleural drainage is the *monitoring* of air leakage and, in the early postoperative period, of oozing or actual bleeding from raw parietal or pulmonary surfaces. The tamponading effect of the expanded lung against the chest wall may also help stop the oozing.

Finally, optimal drainage is important to gain control of the pleural space in as short a time as possible. This is not an irrelevant consideration because early tube removal will greatly facilitate postoperative recovery by promoting early ambulation and lessening the amount of analgesia required for pain control and efficient chest physiotherapy.

Number and Size of Chest Tubes (Table 5-57)

The most popular tube size in adult thoracic surgery is 28 Fr; in pediatric thoracic surgery, a range of sizes—from 6 to 24 Fr—is used. Most tubes are made of Silastic. In general, *larger tubes are preferred* because they

TABLE 5-56

OBJECTIVES OF PLEURAL DRAINAGE AFTER PARTIAL PULMONARY RESECTION

Achieve complete re-expansion of residual lung.
Empty the pleural space of air and blood.
Monitor air leaks and bleeding.
Seal air leaks.
Obliterate the pleural space and prevent late complications.
Restore normal cardiopulmonary dynamics.
Attain these objectives in the shortest possible time.

TABLE 5-57

NUMBER AND SIZE OF CHEST TUBES AFTER PARTIAL PULMONARY RESECTION

Preferred tube size in adult thoracic surgery is 28 Fr.
Most surgeons use straight tubes.
Tubes must have multiple fenestrations and radiopaque stripes.
One chest tube is sufficient for routine cases.

have less tendency to become plugged with fibrin or clots, and they limit the kinking and twisting usually associated with smaller tubes. Most surgeons use straight tubes, although some prefer right-angled (90-degree) tubes for drainage of the inferior costovertebral gutter. All tubes must have *multiple fenestrations* and a *radiopaque stripe*.

Whether one or two chest tubes should be used is a matter of opinion. In general, *one tube is sufficient for routine cases*; two may be required when a prolonged air leak, oozing, or difficult lung re-expansion is anticipated. If two tubes are used, the first one, whose primary function is to remove air, is positioned anteriorly and superiorly (tip at extreme apex); the second one, whose purpose is to remove fluid, is directed in the most dependent area of the pleural space posteriorly and inferiorly. Both tubes are connected to a single drainage system through a Y connector.

Obviously, two tubes (versus one) are likely to be associated with more postoperative pain, increased delays in the patient's ambulation, and potentially more chances of tube malfunction.

Site and Technique of Insertion

Ideally, the skin incision for tube insertion should be in line with the *anterosuperior iliac spine*. In this location, patients do not tend to be lying on their tubes (limits kinking and maximizes comfort), and the tubes are not in the way of the physical therapist. If two tubes are used, the two skin incisions should be 1 or 2 inches apart; if a Y connection is used, the length of tube outside the thorax should be about the same for each tube. For prevention of air leakage around the tube, especially if prolonged drainage is anticipated, the *skin incisions* should be approximately the *same length* as the tube diameter.

If one wants to position a tube at the apex and keep it there, it must be placed above the superior border of the rib; a tube to be located at the base is placed against the lower border of the rib. An oblique path of entry through the soft tissues of the chest wall will ensure rapid closure at the time of removal. In most cases, it is unnecessary to anchor the tube to the parietal pleura.

After insertion, a heavy suture fixes the tube to the skin around it, thus preventing its accidental dislodgment. After this suture is tied down, a free loop is left before it is tied to the tube so that if the tube has to be repositioned during the postoperative period, refixing can be accomplished without having to go through the skin again. A *U type of stitch* is then placed around the tube for closure of the skin incision when the tube is removed.

Suction or No Suction

There is still a fair amount of controversy as to whether chest tubes should be placed under water seal or suction, and if they are on suction, whether they should be on low suction (-10 to -20 cm H_2O) or high suction (-40 H_2O or higher) (Table 5-58).

Most surgeons prefer the use of *low suction* at least for the first 24 to 48 postoperative hours because this method provides *more accurate monitoring of fluid and blood losses.* More important, it helps evacuate the air completely from the pleural space, thus favoring lung re-expansion. Suction is usually started in the recovery room because if it is started before extubation, it may generate a significant loss of tidal volume in the drainage system. *High suction* is usually reserved for patients with important air leaks (>15 to 20 L/min) or for patients with restrictive diseases such as fibrosis in the residual parenchyma.

After 24 to 48 hours of low-suction drainage, placement of chest tubes on water seal has been shown to be superior to keeping them on suction for stopping air leaks. Another non-negligible advantage of putting the tubes on water seal is that it allows *early ambulation* of the patient. Should significant lung collapse or progressive subcutaneous emphysema develop while the chest tube is on water seal, it should be put back on low suction.

One possible side effect of suction during the postoperative period is that it may keep the air leak alive when one or more of the side holes of the tube are directly at the site of the alveolar leak. In such cases, pulling the tube out 1 or 2 cm may be helpful.

Tube Management and Removal

A chest radiograph should always be obtained in the recovery room so that lung re-expansion and tube position can be assessed. Thereafter, daily chest radiographs are recommended for as long as the chest tubes are in place. In general, tubes should *never be clamped* other than to rule out an air leak or to change a bottle or connecting tube.

When the functional status of the tube is in question, observation of fluid oscillation in the system is important. Oscillations that are synchronous

TABLE 5-58

SUCTION OR NO SUCTION ON CHEST TUBES AFTER PARTIAL PULMONARY RESECTION

Degree of Suction	Advantages
Water seal	?Earlier stoppage of air leaks and earlier tube removal
	Earlier ambulation
Low suction (-10 to -20 cm H_2O)	Better monitoring of possible bleeding
	Prevents clotting in tubing
	May be necessary to re-expand residual lung
	May prevent surgical emphysema
High suction (-40 cm H_2O and higher)	Better if air leaks are large
	May be better with restrictive disease in residual lung

with respiratory movements (tidaling) indicate tube patency. If there are no oscillations, the tube may be obstructed, or this may result from complete lung re-expansion.

Whether a chest tube should be milked to dislodge clots and debris and to maintain patency is a *question of controversy*. When a chest tube is milked or stripped, clots that may have been attached to the sides of the tube are mechanically pressed toward the collecting chamber. It has been shown that negative intrapleural pressures in excess of 400 cm H_2O can be obtained with milking or stripping of the chest tube. Whether these high pressures cause injury in the lung is unknown.

If the system becomes occluded, some authors have suggested use of saline or fibrinolytic agents to irrigate the tubes. Others have suggested the use of a sterile suction catheter introduced into the chest tube through a sterile port. *We do not recommend* these procedures because each manipulation increases the risk of contaminating the pleural space.

The traditional criteria for tube removal are complete re-expansion of residual lung (no residual space), cessation of air leakage, and daily amount of fluid drainage less than 300 mL. These criteria are usually met within 3 to 5 days after operation. Whether tubes can be removed if one or more of these criteria are not present is a matter of debate. Obviously, tubes can be removed if there is no air leak and minimal fluid drainage, even in the presence of a small residual space.

In a small percentage of patients (around 5%), an air leak will persist for more than 2 weeks postoperatively. In those cases, the lung is nearly always fully expanded and there are no signs of sepsis. Under such circumstances, one has to rule out a bronchopleural fistula through bronchoscopy, and a defective drainage system must also be ruled out by sequential clamping. If these conditions have been satisfactorily eliminated, "provocative clamping" with clinical and radiologic observation can be done. If clamping of the tubes is well tolerated (no dyspnea, no surgical emphysema, no increase in size of the space), the tubes can be removed after 24 hours.

In some patients, the only reason not to remove a chest tube is a large amount of daily fluid drainage. The most common cause (Table 5-59) of this condition is a highly negative intrapleural pressure due to atelectasis or simply to a loss of lung volume. In such cases, the increased intrapleural

5

Intraoperative Care

TABLE 5-59

CAUSES OF LARGE AMOUNT OF FLUID DRAINAGE AFTER PARTIAL PULMONARY RESECTION

Loss of volume and atelectasis

Infection in residual lung or pleural space

Lysis of residual blood clots in pleural space

Abnormal fluid such as chyle or cerebrospinal fluid

negative pressure will modify the Starling equation of fluid movement across the pleural space, and more fluid will be secreted that can be reabsorbed. Other possible causes of increased fluid drainage are the lysis of residual clots and a contaminated pleural space with impending empyema.

If the drainage is not that of an abnormal substance such as chyle or cerebrospinal fluid, it is generally desirable to wait *until the amount of drainage is less than 300 mL/day* before withdrawing the tubes so that fluid does not accumulate within the space and potentially cause entrapment of the lung or empyema.

Chest tubes should nearly always be removed in the morning because inadvertent introduction of air or recurrent pneumothorax may stress nighttime "on call" services. Gloves should be worn!

PLEURAL DRAINAGE AFTER PNEUMONECTOMY

Physiologic Adjustments after Pneumonectomy

During the early postoperative period (0 to 24 hours), the extrusion of air from the pleural space may result in displacement of the mediastinum toward the side of the pneumonectomy, whereas the retention of air added to the accumulation of fluid may deviate the mediastinum toward the remaining lung. A number of *physiologic adverse conditions* can occur if these situations are exaggerated or if they happen too rapidly after thoracotomy closure.

Significant deviation toward the side of surgery can lead to arrhythmias, hypotension, cardiac herniation, and postpneumonectomy edema. Exaggerated shift toward the opposite side may compromise lung function and impair venous return.

Within 24 to 48 hours of the pneumonectomy, air is further reabsorbed from the pneumonectomy side or extruded in the soft tissues of the chest wall, generating a more negative pressure within the pleural space. Because of this negative pressure, elevation of the hemidiaphragm, narrowing of the intercostal spaces, and shift of the mediastinum toward the surgical side will occur.

These factors coupled with the accumulation of fluid will gradually obliterate the space within 3 to 4 weeks, although it may take as long as 7 months.

Methods Commonly Used for Early Postpneumonectomy Space Management

Pleural Aspiration with Needle or Small Chest Tube

With this technique, air is evacuated from the pleural space by means of a *sterile needle connected to a 60-mL syringe and three-way stopcock.* Sufficient air is removed to return the mediastinum to the midline; the usual amount is in the range of 1000 to 1200 mL. Once the patient is in the recovery room, the position of the mediastinum is assessed by portable chest radiograph, and if required, additional air can be evacuated by way of thoracentesis. The same objective can be achieved by the use of a 16-gauge soft catheter that is left in the pleural space during closure and immediately withdrawn once the patient is supine. While the catheter is being removed, the anesthetist is asked to perform a Valsalva maneuver, raising the intrapleural pressure above that of the atmosphere.

Tube Drainage and Underwater Seal

Some surgeons advocate routine tube drainage to monitor blood loss and to evacuate pleural collections. In most instances, the tube is connected to an underwater seal system *but is kept clamped* to avoid excessive mediastinal shift. Periodically, the tube is unclamped by the nursing staff so that the accumulated fluid can be drained out.

If the tube is kept permanently unclamped and connected to an underwater seal system, extreme mediastinal shift is likely to occur rapidly. With each cough, air is expelled from the pleural space, lowering the intrapleural pressure and generating further shift of the mediastinum. Ultimately, this will cause acute overdistention of the remaining lung, which is a significant risk factor for pulmonary edema.

Whether clamped or connected to an underwater seal system, chest tubes should be removed *no later* than 24 to 48 hours postoperatively.

Chest Tube Connected to a Balanced Drainage System

Balanced drainage of the pneumonectomy space was described as a method *to maintain optimal physiologic position of the mediastinum* during the critical first few hours after pneumonectomy. The arrangement of the bottles is shown in Figure 5-26. The first bottle serves as a trap, and the other two bottles serve as pressure regulators; the second bottle (positive pressure regulator) is a simple water seal, so arranged that any pressure within the system (pleural space) exceeding 1 cm H_2O will be vented; the

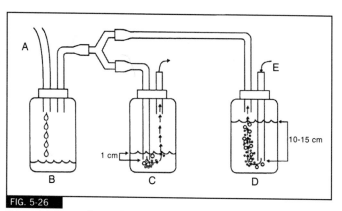

FIG. 5-26

Balanced drainage unit used after pneumonectomy. **A,** Connecting tube from patient. **B,** Collecting bottle. **C,** Positive pressure regulator. **D,** Negative pressure regulator. **E,** Air entering system from outside.

TABLE 5-60

ADVANTAGES OF AND INDICATIONS FOR
POSTPNEUMONECTOMY DRAINAGE

Monitoring of possible postoperative bleeding

Prevention of acute tension pneumothorax should bronchial dehiscence occur

Drainage of excessive fluid formation

Safeguard against wound dehiscence after pneumonectomy and chest wall resection

Drainage of contaminated or infected space

Possible intrapleural infusion of chemotherapy agents

---

third bottle (negative pressure regulator) is a reverse water seal, so
constructed that any pressure more negative than −10 to −15 cm H_2O
(average −13 cm H_2O) that may develop into the system will automatically
be reduced to the desired level by a compensatory ingress of air.
The average of those two levels (1 cm H_2O and −13 cm H_2O) is the
presumed optimal intrapleural pressure (−6 cm H_2O).

Most balanced drainage systems are homemade, although such units
are commercially available.

Advantages of and Indications for Postpneumonectomy
Drainage (Table 5-60)

Although there are virtually no absolute indications for drainage of the
postpneumonectomy space, the presence of a chest tube may be useful
or even lifesaving in several instances. One of these situations is when
postoperative bleeding is anticipated; another is when the bronchus is at
risk of dehiscence, such as after radiotherapy, for instance.

It may also be useful to have a chest tube when there is a possibility
of excessive postoperative fluid accumulation in the space. Not only is this
fluid an excellent culture medium for microorganisms, but it may also help
shift the mediastinum toward the opposite side.

Chest tube drainage may also be a safeguard against wound dehiscence
if a large portion of the chest wall has been resected in conjunction with
the pneumonectomy. Chest tube drainage is also recommended if the
pneumonectomy space has been contaminated intraoperatively or is frankly
infected. In infected spaces, we leave two chest tubes for irrigation, which is
started 48 to 72 hours postoperatively. Chest tube drainage may finally be
indicated for possible intrapleural infusion of chemotherapy agents.

Disadvantages and Complications of Postpneumonectomy
Drainage (Table 5-61)

For most surgeons, the main disadvantage of draining the pneumonectomy
space is that it is not required. Other disadvantages include *limitations to
early ambulation, increased amount of chest pain,* and possible
contamination of the pleural space. The use of water seal drainage can
also impair the cough mechanism because the pressure to bring up the
secretions is often lost in the drainage bottle.

TABLE 5-61

DISADVANTAGES AND COMPLICATIONS OF POSTPNEUMONECTOMY DRAINAGE

It is not required

Limitation to early ambulation

Increased amount of pain

Potential contamination of pleural space

Impaired mechanism of cough

Excessive subcutaneous emphysema with balanced drainage units

Room air has access to pleural space with balanced drainage units

One possible complication of the balanced drainage system is the *extensive subcutaneous emphysema* that may occur when air is pushed into the soft tissues of the chest wall as a result of coughing. This emphysema tends to progress as additional air is made available from the system. Another possible complication of the balanced drainage system is that room air has access to the pleural space, thus increasing the risks of *secondary infection*.

As a rule, chest tubes used in pneumonectomy spaces should never be connected to a suction system. This maneuver may precipitate cardiac herniation if the pericardium has been entered or sudden death if an acute bronchopleural fistula develops.

PLEURAL DRAINAGE AFTER ESOPHAGEAL PROCEDURES

The principles of drainage after esophageal procedures are identical to those recommended after partial pulmonary resections. If the esophagus or site of an anastomosis is at risk for postoperative leakage, it may be wise to anchor the tube in such a way as to have its tip close to the area at risk.

CONCLUSION

Careful attention to details, either intraoperatively or during the postoperative period, is of great importance in thoracic surgery. Although chest tube drainage is one of the most important of those details, there is little consensus among surgeons as to how one should use and manage those tubes.

If confronted with a persistent air leak, each surgeon has his or her method of dealing with the problem, and most are eventually successful with their method. As we have all been taught during our residency training, *patience on the part of the surgeon is a key asset* to successful management of chest tubes after thoracic procedures.

5

Intraoperative Care

SUGGESTED READINGS

Review Articles

Perkins R: Early management of the pleural space following partial pulmonary resection. Am Surg 1957;23:555-567.

Munnell ER, Thomas EK: Current concepts in thoracic drainage systems. Ann Thorac Surg 1975;19:261-268.

Cerfolio RJ: Chest tube management after pulmonary resection. Chest Surg Clin North Am 2002;12:507-527.

Physiology of Postoperative Pleural Drainage

Batchelder TL, Morris KA: Critical factors in determining adequate pleural drainage in both the operated and nonoperated chest. Am Surg 1962;28:296-302.

Storey CF: Intrapleural suction. Is it being used to best advantage? [editorial]. Ann Thorac Surg 1968;6:196-198.

Kirschner PA: "Provocative clamping" and removal of chest tubes despite persistent air leak [letter]. Ann Thorac Surg 1992;53:740-741.

Nonaka M, Kadokura M, Yamamoto S, et al: Analysis of the anatomic changes in the thoracic cage after a lung resection using magnetic resonance imaging. Surg Today 2000;30:879-885.

Cerfolio RJ, Bass C, Katholi CR: Prospective randomized trial compares suction versus water seal for air leaks. Ann Thorac Surg 2001;71:1613-1617.

Drainage after Pneumonectomy

Laforet EG, Boyd TF: Balanced drainage of the pneumonectomy space. Surg Gynecol Obstet 1964;118:1051-1054.

Deslauriers J, Grégoire J: Techniques of pneumonectomy. Drainage after pneumonectomy. Chest Surg Clin North Am 1999;9:437-448.

Wolfe WG, Lewis CW Jr.: Control of the pleural space after pneumonectomy. Chest Surg Clin North Am 2002;12:565-570.

Principles of Postoperative Care

MONITORING OF THE THORACIC SURGICAL PATIENT

The rationale for the monitoring of thoracic surgical patients is the *prevention, early identification,* and *early treatment* of cardiopulmonary complications. Because these events are more likely to occur during the first 3 postoperative days, this time interval should be the period of most intensive monitoring. Whether monitoring is done in an intensive care environment or in an intermediate care facility does not seem to be of great importance as long as the unit allows *close and reliable observation* of clinical and hemodynamic parameters.

A good sense of observation, competency in the interpretation of clinical and biologic signs, and experience in the supervision of postoperative surgical patients are *important attributes* that the staff (nursing and medical) providing postoperative care must possess. Indeed, early postoperative care done by highly trained nurses and through modern devices for monitoring and resuscitation has contributed significantly to the reduction of postoperative morbidity and mortality.

CLINICAL MONITORING (TABLE 6-1)

Several clinical parameters must be closely observed during the first 48 to 72 post-thoracotomy hours. These include the *patient's state of consciousness and alertness;* too much drowsiness can be caused by either inappropriate analgesia or inefficient ventilation with secondary elevation of the arterial Pco_2. As a general rule, effective analgesia must provide adequate pain control without excessive sedation. This is an important consideration because highly sedated patients hypoventilate and are unable to use efficient cough to clear the airway. If a patient is thought to be too sedated, the staff nurse must notify the surgeon or anesthetist, who will reduce the rate of infusion of analgesic drugs.

Nurses must take note of the *color* of lips, nails, or fingers. Cyanosis (blue discoloration) may indicate inefficient oxygenation; white discoloration

TABLE 6-1
CLINICAL MONITORING
State of consciousness
Skin coloration
Respiratory rate, amplitude of respiratory movements
Amount of surgical emphysema
Response to pain therapy (visual analog scale)

may be a sign of significant blood loss. Similarly, the surgeon must be able to determine the respiratory rate and the amplitude of respiratory movements. *Fast and shallow respirations* associated with decreased amplitude of respiratory movements may indicate underlying atelectasis.

Retained secretions can be heard from a distance, or they can be palpated by putting a flat hand over the hemithorax and asking the patient to cough. Palpation of the chest wall can also identify surgical emphysema. If it is present, monitoring should be done by *serial measurements* (every 1 to 3 hours) of the diameter of upper arms or neck. Often, the trachea will deviate toward the side of atelectasis, a phenomenon easily perceived by finger palpation.

The dressing over the thoracotomy wound and the sites of chest tube insertion should be looked at periodically for signs of oozing or wetness.

There should be regular assessment of pain (by patient and nurses) and of the response to pain therapy. The visual analog scale (see Chapter 6) is a useful tool, but it must have been clearly explained to the patient preoperatively. The patient should also be monitored for side effects of pain therapy, such as nausea and itching, and these are treated accordingly.

HEMODYNAMIC AND RESPIRATORY MONITORING (TABLE 6-2)

For a high level of care to be provided, frequent observation of *heart rate, arterial blood pressure, urine output,* and *oxygen saturation* is necessary, at least initially. In most postoperative units, this entails real-time electrocardiographic and arterial line monitoring. Oxygen saturation is readily measured noninvasively.

Arterial blood gas determinations provide information on postoperative ventilatory status. As a rule, oxygen supplementation is guided by saturation recordings and measurements of arterial Po_2.

Continuous cardiac rhythm monitoring should be available because cardiac arrhythmias are common after pulmonary or esophageal operations. If they are diagnosed early, the majority of these arrhythmias can easily be managed. More invasive cardiopulmonary monitoring is reserved for the ventilated patient, in whom a widened alveolar-arterial oxygen gradient ($PAo_2 - Pao_2$), hypotension, or both necessitate regular assessment of cardiac output and oxygen transport.

Because fluid replacement is important after pulmonary surgery, fluid status is monitored through meticulous recording of fluid *intake and losses, urine output,* and *daily weight.*

TABLE 6-2
HEMODYNAMIC AND RESPIRATORY MONITORING
Heart rate, blood pressure, urine output
Continuous cardiac monitoring
Oxygen saturation and arterial blood gases
Fluid status (recording of intake and losses)

CHEST TUBE MONITORING

Precise monitoring of events occurring in the pleural space is important for the thoracic surgeon. This is best accomplished through *the use of properly sized and located chest tubes.*

Chest tubes are initially needed for the mechanical removal of pleural space contents, such as fresh or clotted blood, other fluids, and air. Volume flow of air and actual amount of liquid drainage can be precisely monitored. If the patient is actively hemorrhaging, blood drainage should be monitored every 30 minutes or more often if necessary.

Once active hemorrhaging has stopped, chest tubes are mainly used to evacuate air from the pleural space. Unfortunately, the size of the air leak is difficult to monitor, although commercially available drainage systems have now incorporated air leak meters that can quantify it relatively accurately. *Type of air leaks* (qualitative aspect of the air leak) can also be monitored and recorded (Table 6-3). Both size and type are important determinants for how quickly the air leak will cease.

Two more features of chest tube drainage are useful for monitoring of thoracic surgical patients. *Fluid oscillations* in the water seal or in the tubing are important recordings postoperatively. Oscillations that are synchronous with the respiration indicate tube patency; increased oscillations are a sign of high negative intrapleural pressures, such as with atelectasis, with incomplete lung re-expansion, or after pneumonectomy.

The amount of daily fluid drainage is also important to monitor. Persistently *large amounts of drainage* (>300 mL/24 h) may indicate atelectasis (increased negative intrapleural pressure), infection (empyema), or residual clots that have started to become lytic. In some cases, the appearance of the fluid is indicative of an abnormal fluid. Chyle, for instance, is easy to diagnose once the patient has started oral feedings. It is milky white, and the amount increases in direct proportion to oral intake.

MONITORING BY CHEST RADIOGRAPHS

A postoperative chest radiograph is usually taken routinely in the recovery room. The purpose of this early radiograph is to check tube position and lung re-expansion as well as other potential problems that may be present in either the lungs or pleural space. After that initial radiograph, there is some controversy as to whether daily chest radiographs are necessary (Table 6-4).

Several studies have shown that the policy of obtaining daily chest radiographs as long as chest tubes are in is unnecessary because the

TABLE 6-3	
QUALITATIVE MONITORING OF AIR LEAKS	
Continuous	Present throughout respiratory cycle
Inspiratory	Usually observed in ventilated patients
Expiratory	Present during expiration
Forced expiratory	Present during forced expiration or cough

TABLE 6-4	
VALUE OF DAILY CHEST RADIOGRAPHS	
Should Be Done	Should Not Be Done
Earlier diagnosis of potential complications	Results are unlikely to change treatment
	Lower costs
Avoidance of consequences of missed findings	Lower risk of carcinogenic radiation effect to staff and patients

findings are unlikely to change treatment strategies. This is even more so in the absence of abnormal clinical findings. It has also been shown that daily chest radiographs significantly increase the costs of care as well as expose patients and staff to increased doses of radiation.

The main argument in favor of daily chest radiographs is that *potential complications* such as atelectasis, pneumonia, adult respiratory distress syndrome (ARDS), and abnormal air or fluid collections can be detected and treated at an earlier stage, thus with more chances of being successfully managed. A similar argument says that a large volume of "unnecessary radiographs" is justified to find one life-threatening complication that could be treated early. A typical example is that of a postpneumonectomy bronchopleural fistula diagnosed by a decrease in the amount of pleural fluid accumulation in a patient with relatively few symptoms.

MONITORING BY BIOLOGIC EXAMINATIONS

Although the potential exists for electrolytic imbalance or renal failure, these complications are uncommon in the practice of thoracic surgery and can be evaluated on an individual basis. Our policy is to monitor serum chemistry values and blood count in the recovery room and on the morning after the operation. Thereafter, no further blood testing is done unless there are clinical signs of untoward events (oliguria) or there is use of medications that could generate electrolytic imbalances (diuretics).

CONCLUSION

In many respects, monitoring of patients after thoracic procedures is one of the most important aspects of the operation. If it is done properly and in a systematic fashion, monitoring will *help diagnose early postoperative problems* and complications that can be of special significance to the patient. In many cases, it will provide relevant information not only about changes in the patient's cardiopulmonary status but also for the evaluation and appreciation of the results of the therapeutic interventions.

SUGGESTED READINGS

Review Articles

Henschke CI, Yankelevitz DF, Wand A, et al: Accuracy and efficacy of chest radiography in the intensive care unit. Radiol Clin North Am 1996;34:21-31.

Naunheim KS: Postoperative care and monitoring. Chest Surg Clin North Am 1999;9:501-513.

Cerfolio RJ: Chest tube management after pulmonary resection. Chest Surg Clin North Am 2002;12:507-527.

Vincent JL: Evidence-based medicine in the ICU. Important advances and limitations. Chest 2004;126:592-600.

Chest Radiographs

Silverstein DS, Livingston DH, Elcavage J, et al: The utility of routine daily chest radiography in the surgical intensive care unit. J Trauma 1993;35:643-646.

Fong Y, Whalen GF, Hariri RJ, Barie PS: Utility of routine chest radiographs in the surgical intensive care unit. A prospective study. Arch Surg 1995;130:764-768.

O'Brien W, Karski JM, Cheng D, et al: Routine chest roentgenography on admission to intensive care unit after heart operations: is it of any value? J Thorac Cardiovasc Surg 1997;113:130-133.

Graham RJ, Meziane MA, Rice TW, et al: Postoperative portable chest radiographs: optimum use in thoracic surgery. J Thorac Cardiovasc Surg 1998;115:45-52.

General Reading

Wright CD, Wain JC, Grillo HC, et al: Pulmonary lobectomy patient care pathway: a model to control cost and maintain quality. Ann Thorac Surg 1997;64:299-302.

Zehr KJ, Dawson PB, Yang SC, Heitmiller RF: Standardized clinical care pathways for major thoracic cases reduce hospital costs. Ann Thorac Surg 1998;66:914-919.

Cerfolio RJ, Pickens A, Bass C, Katholi C: Fast-tracking pulmonary resections. J Thorac Cardiovasc Surg 2001;122:318-324.

PAIN CONTROL

Acute post-thoracotomy pain can be severe and cause alterations in the pattern of breathing. Often, the patient will generate low tidal volumes, functional residual capacity will fall, and atelectasis will occur. This is compounded by cough suppression, which in the presence of augmented secretions will further aggravate atelectasis. In addition to lung-related morbidity, poorly controlled pain will lead to prolonged immobilization with increased risks of deep vein thrombosis, to more complicated rehabilitation, and to lower individual satisfaction.

In the past, control of post-thoracotomy pain was achieved by intramuscular narcotic administration. In recent years, however, the advent of *patient-controlled analgesia* and of *spinal narcotics* and the use of *adjuvant pain therapy* with nonsteroidal compounds have provided significant improvements in pain control. Other strategies, such as intercostal nerve block therapy, extrapleural paravertebral analgesia, and

TABLE 6-5	
PATHOPHYSIOLOGY OF POST-THORACOTOMY PAIN	
Structure Involved	Nerve Supply
Skin incision	Intercostal nerves 4-6
Division of muscles of chest wall	
Latissimus dorsi	Thoracodorsal nerve (C6-7-8)
Serratus anterior	Long thoracic nerve (C5-6-7)
Fractured ribs	Intercostal nerves
Damaged costovertebral structures (muscles, ribs, skin)	Dorsal rami of intercostal nerves
Intercostal nerves (stretching, damage by retractors or trocars)	Intercostal nerves
Chest tubes	Intercostal nerves 5-8
Ipsilateral shoulder	Brachial plexus (C5-8, T1)
Parietal pleura (costal pleura)	Intercostal nerves
Mediastinal and diaphragmatic pleura	Phrenic nerve (C3-4-5)

transcutaneous electrical nerve stimulation, are also available. Often, the choice of which modality to use is based on the team's experience and hospital resources.

PATHOPHYSIOLOGY OF POST-THORACOTOMY PAIN

The pain experienced after thoracic surgery is a phenomenon that results *from several causes* (Table 6-5). Because multiple sensory afferents transmitting nociceptive stimuli are involved, *no one analgesia technique* is applicable in all situations.

Most often, stimuli are transmitted *through intercostal nerves* that supply predictable areas of the chest wall (dermatomes). Unfortunately, there is considerable overlap of contiguous dermatomes so that intercostal nerve blocks, for instance, result in complete analgesia only if two or more consecutive intercostal nerves are anesthetized.

Fractured ribs are particularly painful because of their movement with each respiration and during cough. Irritation of the parietal pleura (costal) causes pain that is referred to the corresponding thoracic abdominal wall dermatome (intercostal nerves). Irritation of the mediastinal pleura or of the central part of the diaphragmatic pleura will cause pain that may be referred to the shoulder because of phrenic nerve innervation.

The visceral pleura is insensitive. Its nerve supply is derived from the autonomic nerve system.

MANAGEMENT OF POSTSURGICAL THORACIC PAIN

Preoperative Considerations

Because well-informed patients generally cooperate better than uninformed patients do, taking the time to explain the operation and expected outcome is a major factor in alleviating the patient's distress. Kind reassurance that the pain will be addressed promptly and effectively, for instance, is a major tension-relieving factor. Essentially, the patient is told to expect some pain but that the surgical and anesthetist teams can effectively deal with it through a variety of methods. When patient-controlled analgesia will be used, the patient must clearly understand the technique and its use before the operation.

It is also useful to explain the type of pain intensity scales (Fig. 6-1) that will be used to document the amount of pain the patient is likely to have. The *possible side effects* that may occur, such as nausea, pruritus, and urinary retention, must also be explained to the patient.

Intraoperative Surgical Considerations

Proper techniques of positioning and of opening and closing the chest wall are important factors in minimizing the amount of post-thoracotomy pain. There appears to be *less postoperative pain with muscle-sparing thoracotomies* than with standard thoracotomies, although these incisions are more likely to be associated with rib fractures. *Excessive spreading of the ribs should be avoided* because it often results in rib fractures either at the costovertebral junction or at the site of direct contact between rib spreader and rib. The surgeon must understand that rib fractures not only

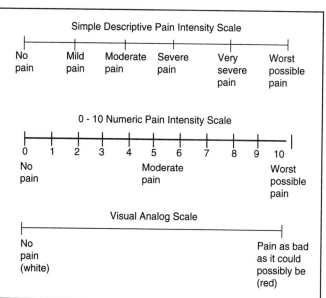

FIG. 6-1

Examples of pain intensity scales to standardize the amount of pain and to follow its intensity over time.

produce significant local pain but also make coughing difficult and ineffective because of the instability of the chest wall.

Care should be exercised while inserting chest tubes to minimize intercostal nerve injury. Properly placed and functioning tubes will also help evacuate local collections, which may themselves be the source of post-thoracotomy pain.

When video-assisted thoracoscopic surgery (VATS) is performed, *careful introduction of trocars and instruments* will minimize trauma to intercostal nerves, thus reducing the risks of significant postoperative discomfort.

Perioperative Anesthetic Considerations: Preemptive Analgesia

Preemptive analgesia refers to analgesic interventions that are started before the surgical incision is made. In such situations, the medication is aimed at *blocking neuronal pathways* between site of incision and central nervous system (medulla) with the hope of altering the propagation of stimuli, thus reducing the intensity of both acute and chronic types of post-thoracotomy pain. The most basic method of preemptive analgesia is to infiltrate local anesthetics into the surgical wound before the incision is made.

Currently, a wide variety of drugs can be used (Table 6-6) for preemptive analgesia, and most are given in conjunction with thoracic epidural analgesia also started before the surgery. Among them, *nonsteroidal anti-inflammatory drugs (NSAIDs)* are the most commonly used. These drugs act by inhibiting the production of byproducts of inflammation, such as prostaglandins and prostacyclins, which are known to stimulate and amplify nociceptive impulses from the incision.

Potentially significant side effects of NSAIDs are *peptic ulceration and renal failure,* both of which are related to the inhibition of prostaglandin-mediated blood flow. All patients receiving NSAIDs should therefore also receive histamine H_2 blockers or proton pump inhibitors, and they should be kept normovolemic. Despite these potentially serious side effects, NSAIDs are beneficial in thoracic surgical patients because they have *no sedative action* as well as *no depressant effects* on respiration or cough.

TABLE 6-6		
MOST COMMONLY USED DRUGS FOR PREEMPTIVE ANALGESIA		
Category	Drug	Usual Dose for Adults
Simple analgesic	Acetaminophen	650-1300 mg q 4 h per os or rectally
Nonsteroidal anti-inflammatory drug	Ibuprofen (Motrin)	400 mg q 4-6 h per os or rectally
	Indomethacin (Indocin)	50-100 mg q 12 h rectally
	Ketorolac	IM: 30-60 mg initially followed by 5-30 mg q 6 h
		IV: 10-30 mg q 6 h
		Orally: 10 mg q 6-8 h

METHODS AVAILABLE FOR POSTOPERATIVE PAIN CONTROL (TABLE 6-7)

A variety of methods are available to control thoracotomy pain during the first few postoperative days. In broad terms, these can be divided into regional techniques, such as spinal administration of narcotics, and systemic techniques, such as opioid administration. A multimodal approach is often preferred. In theory, the advantage of a multinodal approach is that different drugs will act at different levels, thus being overall more effective than each one separately. Another advantage is that the *combined effect of several drugs* given in smaller doses *decreases the potential side effects* of each.

Locoregional Analgesia

Epidural Analgesia

Epidural analgesia is currently the *most commonly employed method* for pain management after thoracic procedures. Epidural catheter infusion of opioids or of local anesthetics allows the establishment of optimal analgesia without resulting in high systemic levels of opioids.

Two types of drugs can be used for epidural analgesia. *Hydrophilic drugs such as morphine* transfer slowly across the dura, leading to a slow onset of analgesia. These drugs, however, remain in the cerebrospinal fluid for long periods, leading to more prolonged duration of analgesia and

TABLE 6-7

METHODS COMMONLY USED FOR POST-THORACOTOMY PAIN MANAGEMENT

Method	Use[1]	Difficulty of Technique[2]	Efficiency for Pain Control[3]	Side Effects[4]	Complications[5]
LOCOREGIONAL TECHNIQUES					
Epidural	+ + + +	+ + + +	+ + + +	+ + +	+ +
Extrapleural, intrapleural	+	+ +	+ + +	+ +	+ +
Paravertebral nerve blocks	+ +	+	+ +	+	+ +
Cryoanalgesia	+	+ + + +	+ +	+ + + +	+ + + + +
TENS	+	+	+	+	+
SYSTEMIC NARCOTIC THERAPY					
Opioid analgesia	+ + +	+	+ +	+ + + +	+ + + +
Patient-controlled analgesia	+ + +	+	+ + +	+ +	+ +

[1]Use: rarely used, +; very often used, + + + + +.

[2]Difficulty of technique including preparation and administration: very easy, +; very difficult, + + + + +.

[3]Efficiency for pain control: little efficiency, +; very efficient, + + + + +.

[4]Side effects: none, +; several, + + + + +.

[5]Complications related to technique: none, +; several, + + + + +.

potentially higher risks of respiratory depression. Because cerebrospinal fluid flows in a cephalad direction, morphine can be administered at the lumbar level to provide analgesia in the thoracic area.

By contrast to morphine, *lipid-soluble lipophilic drugs such as fentanyl* transfer rapidly across the dura to interact with spinal cord receptors, thus providing rapid segmental analgesia at the exact level of administration. This effect is *of short duration,* however, lasting approximately 4 hours. The use of local anesthetics in synergy with fentanyl provides better analgesia; bupivacaine is currently the most commonly used local anesthetic because it has prolonged analgesic effects. These medications are given at the thoracic level and in the form of a constant infusion that can be readjusted according to the patient's needs and tolerance. They can also be administered through patient-triggered dosage (patient-controlled epidural analgesia).

Relative contraindications (Table 6-8) to epidural analgesia include a documented *coagulopathy, systemic infection with sepsis,* and spinal abnormalities that would prevent safe introduction of the catheter. Common side effects are urinary retention, itching, and nausea and vomiting. All of these side effects are easily managed, although most patients require the insertion of a urinary catheter.

The use of local anesthetics can cause hypotensive episodes (due to sympathetic blockade), which may lead to excessive fluid loading. This is best avoided by being aware of this potential and being very careful in treating hypotensive episodes during the first 1 or 2 postoperative days.

Infusion of diluted solutions of local anesthetics in synergy with low-dose fentanyl *minimizes the risk* of respiratory depression and hypotensive episodes. The physicians and nursing staff must understand that these

TABLE 6-8
LIMITATIONS OF EPIDURAL ANALGESIA
CONTRAINDICATIONS
Coagulation abnormalities
Systemic infection (sepsis)
Anatomic abnormalities of the spine
POTENTIAL SIDE EFFECTS
Nausea, vomiting
Itching
Urinary retention (most patients require urinary catheter)
Hypotension
Respiratory depression
Imbalance between sedation and analgesia
POSSIBLE COMPLICATIONS
Epidural hematoma with possible paraplegia
Dislodgment of the catheter
Unsuccessful catheter placement
Dura perforation and headache
Radicular pain

medications are given to control pain (analgesia effect), not to sedate and put the patient to sleep.

Although several puncture- or catheter-related complications are possible (Table 6-8), these are rare (<5% of cases), and most are reversible with early diagnosis and proper treatment. Epidural analgesia is usually continued until the third or even fourth postoperative day.

Extrapleural and Intrapleural Analgesia

Alternative routes for the administration of local anesthetics (0.5% bupivacaine at a rate of 0.1 mL/kg body weight) are through intrapleural or extrapleural catheters. The *intrapleural catheter* lies between visceral pleura and parietal pleura paravertebrally; *the extrapleural catheter* is located between parietal pleura and endothoracic fascia (paravertebral blockade) also in the paravertebral position. Catheters *are positioned by the surgeon* at completion of the procedure. The rationale of these techniques is based on the assumption that local anesthetics given by these routes (continuous infusion) are readily absorbed by the pleura and will affect the underlying sensory structures.

Proponents of these techniques claim that side effects such as respiratory depression and hypotension *are less common* than with epidural analgesia while pain control is comparable. Overall, extrapleural analgesia seems to be more efficient than intrapleural analgesia. In patients receiving intrapleural analgesia, part of the medication is often lost through the chest tube.

Paravertebral Nerve Blocks

Paravertebral nerve blocks are excellent to interrupt pain pathways traveling through intercostal nerves, dorsal rami, and sympathetic chain to the spinal cord. They can be done intraoperatively at a single level or at multiple levels, and they can be repeated as required. Most often, *paravertebral nerve blocks are used in association with systemic agents* such as intravenous patient-controlled analgesia, systemic opioids, NSAIDs, or acetaminophen.

One of the main drawbacks of intercostal nerve blocks is that *they must be repeated every 6 to 12 hours postoperatively*. Because of that problem, many surgeons prefer the use of an extrapleural catheter, which allows continuous infusion of lidocaine or bupivacaine. Another concern with the technique relates to the possibility of toxicity because high concentrations and high volumes of local anesthetic may be required for adequate intercostal nerve blockade. Signs of bupivacaine toxicity include central nervous system irritation and arrhythmias.

Cryoanalgesia

Cryoanalgesia is a specialized block of the intercostal nerves achieved by freezing them with a cryoprobe. The exposure to freezing temperature results in nerve damage that is most of the time reversible. The cryoprobe is *surgically applied to the nerve* of the exposed interspace as well as to the nerves one space above and one space below.

The problems associated with cryoanalgesia relate to the *intensity of the low temperature that must be applied* (–60°C) and to *the duration of application of the cryoprobe.* Because none of these parameters is standardized, cryotherapy, even if it is effective for pain control, is associated with chronic neuralgia, failure of sensation to return, and chronic dermatitis and muscle atrophy. Because there is a significant incidence of these adverse effects (20%), few surgeons currently use the technique.

Transcutaneous Electrical Nerve Stimulation

In general, transcutaneous electrical nerve stimulation (TENS) is effective to control postoperative pain when pain is mild. It is a safe technique with virtually no side effects. TENS is usually associated with other methods of pain control, and sometimes it helps reduce opioid requirements after thoracic operations.

Parenteral Systemic Narcotic Therapy

Opioid Analgesia

Systemic opioids given intramuscularly, intravenously, or subcutaneously are generally efficient to control post-thoracotomy pain. The problem is the *extreme variability* from patient to patient in *rate of absorption, serum level, intensity,* and *duration of effect of the drugs.* Because of such variability, systemic opioids have a narrow therapeutic range. Significant side effects, such as respiratory depression, excessive sedation, and nausea, are common. Drowsiness and respiratory depression are of particular concern after thoracic surgical procedures because patients often have borderline respiratory function.

Systemic opioids must be given with a loading dose to quickly reach the minimum effective analgesia concentration. Thereafter, the optimal method to avoid fluctuations in the minimum effective analgesia concentration is continuous intravenous delivery of the drug. The most commonly used drug is morphine.

In most centers, systemic opioids are given only as a replacement for epidural analgesia by postoperative day 3 or 4.

Patient-Controlled Analgesia

Patient-controlled analgesia is effective to maintain a serum concentration of opioids as close to the effective analgesia requirement as possible. It is administered intravenously by use of an infusion pump programmed to deliver a set dose of drug when the patient activates a control button. One major advantage of the technique is that there is *no delay between perception of pain and administration of drug*. Although the usual prescription of morphine is 1 to 3 mg every 5 to 10 minutes after a loading dose of 3 to 5 mg, parameters may vary according to the patient's age, gender, and weight and the magnitude of the operation. In general, patient-controlled analgesia may have the same adverse effects as opioid analgesia, but these effects are more predictable and can be reversed quickly. Disadvantages of

TABLE 6-9

MULTIMODAL BALANCED ANALGESIA AFTER THORACIC OPERATIONS

Action	Method
Preemptive analgesia (before surgical incision is made)	Acetaminophen
	Epidural analgesia (narcotic and local anesthetic administered at thoracic level)
Day 1-3 postoperatively	Epidural analgesia (continuous infusion or patient controlled)
Day 4-10	Opioids initially subcutaneously and then orally when intensity of pain subsides

patient-controlled analgesia are that it requires the patient's understanding and cooperation and that patients cannot administer the drug while they are sleeping.

BALANCED ANALGESIA REGIMEN

For most patients, a multimodal balanced analgesia is recommended (Table 6-9). This approach includes preemptive analgesia through an epidural catheter with the addition of an adjunctive NSAID. Postoperatively, analgesia is controlled with *continuous infusion of fentanyl combined with a local anesthetic* administered by thoracic epidural technique. Once pain subsides, usually by day 3 or 4, systemic opioids are administered initially subcutaneously or intramuscularly and later orally.

CONCLUSION

Modern techniques of postoperative analgesia are numerous, but ultimately their goals are to ensure the patient's comfort and lower the incidence of respiratory complications. It is important that pain control be initiated preoperatively by winning the patient's confidence and reducing his or her feeling of anxiety toward postoperative pain. Intraoperatively and postoperatively, a multimodal and balanced analgesia has the best chance of providing optimal pain control.

SUGGESTED READINGS

Review Articles

Moore KL: Clinically Oriented Anatomy, 2nd ed. Baltimore, Williams & Wilkins, 1985.

Coleman DL: Control of postoperative pain. Nonnarcotic and narcotic alternatives and their effect on pulmonary function. Chest 1987;92: 520-528.

Sabanathan S, Richardson J, Mearns AJ: Management of pain in thoracic surgery. Br J Hosp Med 1993;50:114-120.

Kavanagh BP, Katz J, Sandler AN: Pain control after thoracic surgery. A review of current techniques. Anesthesiology 1994;81:737-759.

Jain S, Datta S: Postoperative pain management. Chest Surg Clin North Am 1997;7:773-799.

Ballantyne JC, Carr DB, deFerranti S, et al: The comparative effects of postoperative analgesic therapies on pulmonary outcome: cumulative meta-analyses of randomized, controlled trials. Anesth Analg 1998;86: 598-612.

Peeters-Asdourian C, Gupta S: Choices in pain management following thoracotomy. Chest 1999;115:122s-124s.

Richardson J, Sabanathan S, Shah R: Post-thoracotomy spirometric lung function: the effect of analgesia. A review. J Cardiovasc Surg 1999;40:445-456.

Kruger M, McRae K: Pain management in cardiothoracic practice. Surg Clin North Am 1999;79:387-399.

Hazelrigg SR, Cetindag IB, Fullerton J: Acute and chronic pain syndromes after thoracic surgery. Surg Clin North Am 2002;82:849-865.

Soto RG, Fu ES: Acute pain management for patients undergoing thoracotomy. Ann Thorac Surg 2003;75:1349-1357.

Physiology of Pain

Benedetti F, Amanzio M, Casadio C, et al: Postoperative pain and superficial abdominal reflexes after posterolateral thoracotomy. Ann Thorac Surg 1997;64:207-210.

Case Series

Miguel R, Hubbell D: Pain management and spirometry following thoracotomy: a prospective, randomized study of four techniques. J Cardiothorac Vasc Anesth 1993;7:529-534.

Salzer GM, Klinger P, Klinger A, Unger A: Pain treatment after thoracotomy: is it a special problem? Ann Thorac Surg 1997;63:1411-1414.

Epidural Analgesia

Lubenow TR, Faber LP, McCarthy RJ, et al: Postthoracotomy pain management using continuous epidural analgesia in 1,324 patients. Ann Thorac Surg 1994;58:924-930.

Burgess FW, Anderson DM, Colonna D, Cavanaugh DG: Thoracic epidural analgesia with bupivacaine and fentanyl for postoperative thoracotomy pain. J Cardiothorac Vasc Anesth 1994;8:420-424.

Singh H, Bossard RF, White PF, et al: Effects of ketorolac versus bupivacaine coadmiustration during patient-controlled hydromorphone epidural analgesia after thoracotomy procedures. Anesth Analg 1997;84:564-569.

Slinger PD: Pro: every postthoracotomy patient deserves thoracic epidural analgesia. J Cardiothorac Vasc Anesth 1999;13:350-354.

Mahon SV, Berry PD, Jackson M, et al: Thoracic epidural infusions for post-thoracotomy pain: a comparison of fentanyl-bupivacaine mixtures vs. fentanyl alone. Anaesthesia 1999;54:641-646.

Schumann R, Shikora S, Weiss JM, et al: A comparison of multimodal perioperative analgesia to epidural pain management after gastric bypass surgery. Anesth Analg 2003;96:469-474.

Intercostal and Paravertebral Blocks

Deneuville M, Bisserier A, Regnard JF, et al: Continuous intercostal analgesia with 0.5% bupivacaine after thoracotomy: a randomized study. Ann Thorac Surg 1993;55:381-385.

Karmakar MK: Thoracic paravertebral block [review article]. Anesthesiology 2001;95:771-777.

Takamori S, Yoshida S, Hayashi A, et al: Intraoperative intercostal nerve blockade for postthoracotomy pain. Ann Thorac Surg 2002;74:338-341.

Wurnig PN, Lackner H, Teiner C, et al: Is intercostal block for pain management in thoracic surgery more successful than epidural anaesthesia? Eur J Cardiothorac Surg 2002;21:1115-1119.

TENS

Benedetti F, Amanzio M, Casadio C, et al: Control of postoperative pain by transcutaneous electrical nerve stimulation after thoracic operations. Ann Thorac Surg 1997;63:773-776.

Extrapleural Analgesia

Kaiser AM, Zollinger A, De Lorenzi D, et al: Prospective randomized comparison of extrapleural versus epidural analgesia for postthoracotomy pain. Ann Thorac Surg 1998;66:367-372.

Bimston DN, McGee JP, Liptay MJ, Fry WA: Continuous paravertebral extrapleural infusion for post-thoracotomy pain management. Surgery 1999;126:650-657.

Preemptive Analgesia

McQuay HJ: Pre-emptive analgesia. Br J Anaesth 1992;69:1-3.

Møiniche S, Kehlet H, Dahl JB: A qualitative and quantitative systematic review of preemptive analgesia for postoperative pain relief. The role of timing of analgesia [review article]. Anesthesiology 2002;96:725-741.

Intra(inter)pleural Analgesia

Silomon M, Claus T, Huwer H, et al: Interpleural analgesia does not influence postthoracotomy pain. Anesth Analg 2000;91:44-50.

FLUID MANAGEMENT

Intraoperative and postoperative fluid replacement in patients undergoing pulmonary resection is a difficult task because ideal strategies have yet to be determined. On the one hand, patients *should not receive excessive fluids* because it may overload the circulation of those with significantly reduced pulmonary arterial capillary beds, such as those undergoing pneumonectomy. On the other hand, *minimizing fluid administration* in patients who are hemodynamically stable can limit the accumulation of lung water and potentially create difficulties in oxygenation.

By contrast to patients who undergo pulmonary resection, all esophagectomy patients have had considerable dissection and mobilization of tissue planes. Owing to the significant third-space accumulations that result from such dissections, these patients are more likely *to require large amounts of perioperative fluid.*

Although it is sometimes necessary to give blood products, a *restrictive strategy* is generally recommended.

OVERALL PATHOPHYSIOLOGY OF SURGICAL FLUID BALANCE

The general objective of fluid therapy during or after any major thoracic surgical procedure is *to maintain or restore* intravascular volume and to ensure *adequate organ perfusion*. Thus, ideal fluid management must be individualized and based on giving required standard maintenance fluids in addition to replacing any losses. Patients with chylothoraces, for instance, may lose large amounts of extracellular fluids, and these must be replaced almost on an hourly basis.

Fluid management must also take into account the precept that many drugs given intraoperatively or postoperatively may lead to *abnormal shifts in fluid balance* or may simply blunt normal physiologic responses to hypovolemia. This is the case, for example, of epidural analgesic techniques, which are often associated with vasodilatation and hypotension related to the blockade of sympathetic outflows from the spinal cord. These physiologic responses often contribute to excessive fluid loading.

Another important consideration in managing fluid balance is that *significant third-space* (fluid still in the body but not contributing to intravascular volume) *losses* may occur, and the *magnitude* of these losses may be difficult to appreciate. Although third-space losses are uncommon after pulmonary resection, they are routine after esophageal resectional procedures. In such patients, simple restoration of blood volume may thus be inadequate.

Other clinical considerations that may influence fluid therapy are the *age* of the patient and the status of *renal and cardiac functions*. Adults with poor underlying cardiac function, for instance, are highly susceptible to fluid challenges and should be kept relatively hypovolemic. Elderly patients, such as those operated on for lung cancer, may have age-related abnormalities of renal function, and, because of these abnormalities, they are more susceptible to volume depletion and drug-induced nephrotoxicity. Some of the preventive measures useful to avoid renal failure in aging patients are listed in Table 6-10.

Measurements routinely used as markers of intravascular volume status (Table 6-11) include arterial blood pressure and pulse rate,

TABLE 6-10
PREVENTIVE MEASURES TO AVOID RENAL FAILURE IN AGING PATIENTS
Appropriate dosing of all medications
Avoidance of imaging techniques with contrast material
Maintenance of euvolemia
Avoidance of rapid shifts in volume status
Avoidance of medication known to be nephrotoxic

From Kellerman PS: Perioperative care of the renal patient. Arch Intern Med 1994;154:1674-1688.

TABLE 6-11

MARKERS USED FOR THE MONITORING OF INTRAVASCULAR VOLUME STATUS

Routinely used
    Arterial blood pressure and pulse rate
    Central venous pressure
    Urine output
Occasionally used
    Body weight
Seldom used
    Pulmonary capillary wedge pressure (Swan-Ganz)
    Cardiac output

6

central venous pressure, and urine output. It is generally agreed that urine outputs of 0.5 to 1.0 mL/kg/h (30 to 60 mL/h) in normal adults are consistent with adequate intravascular fluid volume. From time to time, measurements such as pulmonary capillary wedge pressure and cardiac output will also be used with the understanding that pulmonary artery capillary wedge pressure may be falsely low after pneumonectomy and that these low abnormal readings can lead to erroneous clinical decisions.

Daily measurements of *body weight* may be helpful, particularly in patients who require parenteral nutrition for prolonged periods. Under normal postoperative conditions, a daily weight loss of 0.2 to 0.4 kg is anticipated in adult patients receiving conventional fluid therapy. A stable or an increasing body weight may thus imply excessive fluid administration.

FLUID REPLACEMENT SOLUTIONS

Intravenous fluids commonly used during or after surgical procedures are generally classified according to their ability to penetrate barriers separating body fluid compartments. Crystalloid solutions are predominantly located in the extravascular space (interstitial and intracellular spaces). Colloid fluids are retained within the intravascular space, where they act to expand blood volume.

Crystalloid Solutions

Crystalloids (Table 6-12) are solutions that contain water and electrolytes, but their principal component is *sodium chloride*. Based on the concentration of sodium chloride, they are classified as balanced, hypertonic, or hypotonic salt solutions. Balanced salt solutions (lactated Ringer solution, Normosol) have an electrolytic composition similar to that of extracellular fluid, but with respect to sodium, they are hypotonic.

Normal saline (0.9% sodium chloride) is isotonic but contains more chloride than extracellular fluid. Hypertonic salt solutions (7.5% sodium chloride) are occasionally used to correct hyponatremia.

TABLE 6-12

CLASSIFICATION OF CRYSTALLOID SOLUTIONS

Type of Solution	Commonly Used Product
Balanced salt solutions	Lactated Ringer solution
	Normosol solution
Normal saline	0.9% sodium chloride
Hypertonic salt solutions	7.5% sodium chloride
Isosmotic solutions	5% dextrose in water

Colloid Solutions (Table 6-13)

Because they increase the oncotic pressure of the intravascular space, colloid solutions act as *blood volume expanders* (water migrates from extracellular fluid space into the blood). They are generally administered in a volume equivalent to that of blood loss. Human albumin solutions are available in 5% and 25% solutions. The 5% solution causes an increase in intravascular volume equal to the volume infused; the 25% solution can expand the plasma volume up to five times the volume infused. Potential transmission of infection is negligible because these solutions have been heat treated.

Pentastarch (Pentaspan) is a lower molecular weight hetastarch (synthetic colloid solution) that gives an effective plasma volume increase of *twice the volume infused*. Potential adverse effects are extremely rare but may include allergic reactions and coagulation disorders.

Dextran solutions are water-soluble glucose polymers synthesized by bacteria grown on sucrose media. The numbers 40 and 70 refer to their average molecular weight. Plasma volume is usually increased by up to twice the volume infused. The main clinical use of dextran solutions is in the prevention of deep vein thrombosis and low blood viscosity status.

Blood Products (Table 6-14)

Blood products should be given with caution. In the absence of ischemic heart disease or significant blood loss, *they are seldom required* after pulmonary resections. Blood products are beneficial (Table 6-15) in correcting intravascular volume and improving tissue oxygenation, but they can be associated with the transmission of infection (AIDS, hepatitis) and with hemolytic transfusion reactions. In addition, the nonspecific immunosuppression induced by blood transfusions might favor tumor growth and predispose to higher rates of cancer recurrence.

Blood is usually given as packed red cells (volume of 250 mL), which is blood that has been centrifuged and plasma drawn off. It can also be

TABLE 6-13

CLASSIFICATION OF COMMONLY USED COLLOID SOLUTIONS

Albumin 5%, 25%

Hetastarch (Pentaspan)

Dextran 40, 70

TABLE 6-14

COMMONLY USED BLOOD PRODUCTS

Product	Characteristic
Whole blood	Seldom used
Packed red cells	Plasma drawn off blood
Leukocyte-depleted blood	Decreases immunosuppressive effect of whole blood
Fresh frozen plasma	Provides coagulation factors

given as leukocyte-depleted blood (leukocyte-depleting blood filters can remove 99.9% of white blood cells from whole blood), which may be beneficial in decreasing the immunosuppressive effect of whole blood.

FLUID MANAGEMENT AFTER SPECIFIC THORACIC PROCEDURES

Lobectomy and Lesser Resections

In uncomplicated cases of lobectomy or of more limited pulmonary resections, there is no significant third-space loss so that postoperative fluid requirements are at a minimum. Simple restoration of blood volume is achieved with crystalloid solutions such as normal saline (0.9% sodium chloride) or lactated Ringer solution given at 1.5 mL/kg/h (90 mL/h in a 60-kg patient). Other electrolytes such as potassium can be added if necessary.

Most lobectomy patients will resume a normal diet *the day after surgery* and will no longer require meticulous fluid management.

Pneumonectomy

Pneumonectomy patients have always been known to be *more susceptible* than lobectomy patients to complications arising from fluid overload. Indeed, fluid overload and increased pulmonary capillary hydrostatic pressure are thought to be the driving forces involved in the pathogenesis of *postpneumonectomy edema.* On the basis of some experimental results, it is thought that after pneumonectomy, the remaining lung has to accommodate the whole cardiac output, which is always elevated because of catecholamine release, operative stress, and fluid overload. This elevated cardiac output increases the capillary pressure (Fig. 6-2) and results in a net increase in fluid filtration pressures with subsequent pulmonary edema

TABLE 6-15

POTENTIAL BENEFITS AND DISADVANTAGES OF BLOOD TRANSFUSION

BENEFITS

Correction of intravascular volume

Improvement in tissue oxygenation

DISADVANTAGES

May be associated with transmission of AIDS or hepatitis

May generate hemolytic transfusion reaction

May predispose to higher rates of cancer recurrence

May predispose to higher rates of postoperative infections

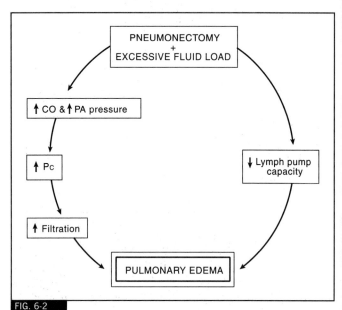

FIG. 6-2

The interaction of increase in cardiac output (CO) and pulmonary artery (PA) pressure results in increase in pulmonary capillary pressure (Pc). The increased Pc increases filtration. Removal of one lung decreases lymph pump capacity for fluid resorption. The combination of increased filtration and decreased pump capacity results in pulmonary edema. *(Courtesy of Dr. Richard M. Peters.)*

and ARDS. On the basis of these concepts, most surgeons advise that *moderation in fluid therapy or even fluid restriction* should be the mean in patients undergoing pneumonectomy.

Current information, however, shows that although postpneumonectomy edema may indeed be associated with fluid overload, there is *no clear cause-effect relationship*. For instance, significant positive fluid balance (e.g., >2500 mL in 24 hours) may contribute to the development of postpneumonectomy edema, but severely restricting fluid intake (e.g., <1000 mL in 24 hours) does not completely eliminate it. Some authors even believe that minimizing fluid intake in hemodynamically stable patients can limit the accumulation of lung water in the capillary bed and potentially compromise oxygenation, especially if the remaining lung is acutely hyperinflated (see Chapter 7).

In the end, fluid management of uncomplicated pneumonectomy patients is similar to that of lobectomy patients with maintenance fluids of 1.5 mL/kg/h in fasting individuals. If the blood pressure is low or if the urine output has decreased, however, it may be advisable to use inotropic agents rather than to give extra amounts of blood, plasma, or other colloids. Intermittent bolus infusion of 250 mL of normal saline or colloid solutions can also be used when urine output falls below the 20 to 30 mL/h mark.

Just like lobectomy patients, pneumonectomy patients are usually started on a *progressive diet the day after surgery.* At that stage, they no longer require careful fluid management.

Esophagectomy

Esophagectomy patients typically require *large volumes of fluid replacement* as water escapes from the intravascular space into the third space (small and large bowel, peritoneal cavity) during and after the operation. Because this fluid will move back into the intravascular space at 3 to 5 days postoperatively (resolution of ileus), it can potentially create problems with fluid overload.

Intraoperatively and during the immediate postoperative period, sufficient fluids (crystalloids, balanced salt solutions) must therefore be administered to maintain a relatively normal blood pressure and a urine output of 0.5 to 1.0 mL/kg/h (30 to 60 mL/h in a 60-kg patient). Starting the day after surgery, the same amount of fluids is still required, but half of it can be given intravenously and the other half through jejunostomy enteral feedings. During the following few days, jejunostomy feedings will gradually be increased until the minimum calorie requirements of the patient are met (1 kcal/kg/h). Intravenous infusions are then proportionally decreased.

When the patient enters the fluid mobilization phase of recovery, fluid intake is decreased and gentle diuresis may be initiated with the help of diuretics. Uncomplicated esophagectomy patients will usually start oral intake (fluids initially) by day 5 to 7.

CONCLUSION

During and after pulmonary operations, fluid management is straightforward because patients can regulate themselves when they resume oral alimentation, usually the day after surgery. One word of caution, however, concerns pneumonectomy patients, in whom the administration of large fluid loads must be avoided if one wants to prevent pulmonary congestion and edema. After esophageal resection, early enteral jejunostomy nutrition is well tolerated and should be used to regulate fluid balance.

SUGGESTED READINGS

Review Articles

Twigley AJ, Hillman KM: The end of the crystalloid era? A new approach to peri-operative fluid administration. Anesthesia 1985;40:860-871.
Kellerman PS: Perioperative care of the renal patient. Arch Intern Med 1994;154:1674-1688.

Vermeulen LC, Ratko TA, Erstad BL, et al: A paradigm for consensus. The University Hospital consortium guidelines for the use of albumin, nonprotein colloid, and crystalloid solutions. Arch Intern Med 1995;155:373-379.

Slinger PD: Perioperative fluid management for thoracic surgery: the puzzle of postpneumonectomy pulmonary edema. J Cardiothorac Vasc Anesth 1995;9:442-451.

Schierhout G, Roberts I: Fluid resuscitation with colloid or crystalloid solutions in critically ill patients: a systematic review of randomized trials. Br Med J 1998;316:961-964.

Choi PTL, Yip G, Quinonez LG, Cook DJ: Crystalloids vs. colloids in fluid resuscitation: a systematic review [special article]. Crit Care Med 1999;27:200-210.

Naunheim KS: Postoperative care and monitoring. Chest Surg Clin North Am 1999;9:501-513.

Fluid Management in the Acutely Ill. An Evidence-Based Educational Program (Bayer Health Care Division). Concord, Ontario, Canada, Core Health Services, 2001.

Holmes CL, Walley KR: Bad medicine: low-dose dopamine in the ICU. Chest 2003;123:1266-1275.

Monitoring

Shippy CR, Appel PL, Shoemaker WC: Reliability of clinical monitoring to assess blood volume in critically ill patients. Crit Care Med 1984; 12:107-112.

Wittnich C, Trudel J, Zidulka A, Chiu RCJ: Misleading "pulmonary wedge pressure" after pneumonectomy: its importance in postoperative fluid therapy. Ann Thorac Surg 1986;42:192-196.

Fluid and ARDS

Hutchin P, Terzi RG, Hollandsworth LA, et al: Pulmonary congestion following infusion of large fluid loads in thoracic surgical patients. Ann Thorac Surg 1969;8:339-347.

Zeldin RA, Normandin D, Landtwing D, Peters RM: Postpneumonectomy pulmonary edema. J Thorac Cardiovasc Surg 1984;87:359-365.

Bishop MH, Jorgens J, Shoemaker WC, et al: The relationship between ARDS, pulmonary infiltration, fluid balance, and hemodynamics in critically ill surgical patients. Am Surg 1991;57:785-792.

Schuster DP: The case for and against fluid restriction and occlusion pressure reduction in adult respiratory distress syndrome. New Horizons 1993;1:478-488.

Arieff AI: Fatal postoperative pulmonary edema. Pathogenesis and literature review. Chest 1999;115:1371-1377.

Blood Transfusions

Moores DWO, Piantadosi S, McKneally MF, for the Lung Cancer Study Group: Effect of perioperative blood transfusion on outcome in patients with surgically resected lung cancer. Ann Thorac Surg 1989;47:346-351.

Enteral Nutrition

Aiko S, Yoshizumi Y, Sugiura Y, et al: Beneficial effects of immediate
    enteral nutrition after esophageal cancer surgery. Surg Today
    2001;31:971-978.

PHARMACOLOGIC INTERVENTIONS IN THE THORACIC SURGICAL PATIENT

Pharmacologic interventions have always been an important component
of the perioperative care of thoracic surgical patients. During the past
30 years, however, these interventions have become even more important
not only because thoracic surgical procedures are more complex but also
because patients submitted to those operations are *older* and often have
significant associated cardiorespiratory morbidities.

Better postoperative monitoring has also increased the demands for
new pharmacologic interventions. This is the case, for instance, of the
demands for oxygen supplementation, which have increased notably since
noninvasive saturometry has become widely available. It is also the case
for supraventricular arrhythmias, which are now readily diagnosed through
the electrocardiographic monitoring that has become standard in most
thoracic surgical postoperative units.

Although hundreds of drugs are available and indeed are recommended
by drug company representatives, experience and wisdom suggest that
patients are better served if the surgeon uses only drugs for which she or
he has *complete knowledge of pharmacology, indications for use and
limitations,* and, most important, *potential adverse effects.*

RESPIRATORY PHARMACOLOGY

Oxygen

Oxygen is one of the most commonly used drugs in thoracic surgical
patients because some degree of hypoxemia is almost universal during
the early postoperative period.

Mechanisms (Table 6-16) and Consequences of Hypoxemia

Hypoxemia, defined as low oxygen saturation of arterial blood (Sao_2),
is almost always associated with low arterial partial pressure of oxygen
(Pao_2). Hypoxia occurs when *tissue delivery of oxygen is insufficient* to
meet its demand.

In the postoperative thoracic surgical patient, the two most important
mechanisms of hypoxemia are those related to *disturbances of ventilation-
perfusion ratio (V/Q)* and those related to *diffusion abnormalities.*
Ventilation/perfusion mismatches are due to atelectasis, in which alveoli
are underventilated in relation to their perfusion; ARDS and pulmonary
edema are characterized by impaired oxygen diffusion across the
alveolocapillary membrane. Preexisting chronic obstructive pulmonary
disease (COPD) or excessive narcotic use can also result in alveolar

TABLE 6-16	
COMMON CAUSES OF ARTERIAL HYPOXEMIA IN THE THORACIC SURGICAL PATIENT	
Mechanism	Common Cause
Ventilation/perfusion mismatch	Atelectasis, pneumonia
Diffusion defect	ARDS, pulmonary edema
Alveolar hypoventilation	Preexisting chronic obstructive pulmonary disease, excessive sedation
Increased metabolic demand	Increased work of breathing, fever

hypoventilation and hypoxemia in association with hypercapnia (elevated $Paco_2$). Other less common mechanisms of hypoxemia are those of increased metabolic demands and decreased oxygen delivery due to heart failure.

For most patients, temporary or mild hypoxemia has no clinical repercussions. For hypoxemia-sensitive patients and for those with moderate to severe hypoxemia, however, possible clinical responses (Table 6-17) include confusion and somnolence, tachycardia, hypotension due to peripheral vasodilatation, dyspnea, and tachypnea. These symptoms may be discreet, but often they precede radiographic changes.

From a physiologic standpoint, severe arterial hypoxemia may lead to decreased Pao_2 (see oxygen-hemoglobin dissociation curve, Fig. 6-3) with secondary tissue hypoxia. This tissue hypoxia may in turn be detrimental to cardiac or renal function, especially if those organs are the sites of *preexisting disease*. In the pulmonary arterial circulation, hypoxia may cause vasoconstriction and pulmonary hypertension.

Indications for Supplemental Oxygen

After pulmonary resection, supplemental oxygen may be given *to correct the hypoxemia* that is often present when physiologic readjustments are taking place in the residual lung. Oxygen therapy is also indicated to relieve hypoxemia secondary to atelectasis or diffusion defects. It has finally been shown that supplemental oxygen may be useful to reduce the incidence of wound infections in high-risk patients.

Methods of Oxygen Delivery (Table 6-18)

Because oxygen is considered pharmacotherapy, the *concentration* to be given and the *method of delivery* should be clearly defined by the surgeon.

TABLE 6-17	
POSSIBLE CLINICAL RESPONSES TO ARTERIAL HYPOXEMIA	
System	Response
Respiratory system	Dyspnea, tachypnea
Central nervous system	Somnolence, confusion
Cardiovascular system	Tachycardia, hypotension

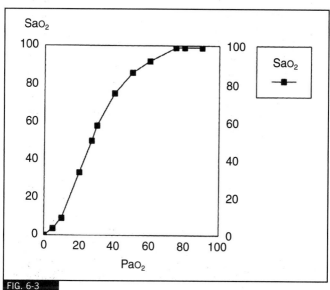

FIG. 6-3

Oxygen-hemoglobin dissociation curve. Given the shape of the curve, the higher the Sao_2, the greater is the Pao_2.

In most hospitals, oxygen is available from central sources in gaseous or liquid forms or from portable cylinders (compressed gas).

Oxygen can be administered by means of *nasal cannulas* (nasal prongs), *facemasks* designed to fit over mouth and nose, and *masks with a reservoir*. Oxygen concentrations (Fio_2) delivered to the patient

TABLE 6-18

DELIVERY OF OXYGEN IN POSTOPERATIVE THORACIC PATIENTS

NASAL PRONGS

Advantages
   Cheap, well tolerated
   Patient can eat, talk, expectorate

Disadvantages
   Fio_2 unreliable
   High Fio_2 not possible
   Can become displaced during sleep

FACEMASKS

Advantages
   Humidified gas
   Allows increase in Fio_2 up to 70%

Disadvantages
   Difficult to wear for long periods
   Can lead to hypercapnia

are generally less than 40%, except with reservoir high-concentration masks, where the F_{IO_2} can be as high as 70%. Nasal prongs are well tolerated, but the amount and concentration of oxygen received by the patient are lower than with facemasks. High oxygen flow through nasal prongs can also be a *source of irritation of nasal and upper airway mucosa*.

Oxygen delivery should be monitored by clinical responses and oxygen saturation of arterial blood (Sao_2) as documented by oxymetry. In patients with COPD and in hypercapnic patients, monitoring should also include *measurements of $Paco_2$* in arterial blood samples.

Toxicity and Adverse Effects (Table 6-19)

The most important toxicity related to oxygen supplementation is the *depression of the ventilatory drive,* which in turn may initiate significant carbon dioxide retention. Although normal individuals can tolerate this effect quite well, the loss of respiratory drive in patients with recent lung resection, especially those with prior COPD, can lead to respiratory depression, secondary hypoventilation, and severe respiratory acidosis.

Adverse effects that may be significant in postoperative patients are listed in Table 6-19. They include drying of nasal passages and upper airways; drying of bronchial secretions, which makes them more difficult to expectorate; nausea and vomiting; and gastric dilatation secondary to oxygen swallowing. Some patients also think that because they receive supplemental oxygen, they *no longer need* to make the extra effort to cough vigorously.

Airway Pharmacology

In postoperative patients, airway pharmacology is mainly concerned with managing small airway obstruction secondary to preexisting COPD. This problem may indeed have been magnified by surgical manipulations of the lung, especially if the patient has hyperreactive airways.

Pharmacologic efforts are thus aimed at achieving optimal airflow through the use of *bronchodilators,* which cause relaxation of airway smooth muscles, and *anti-inflammatory drugs* such as corticosteroids, which are suppressive of the inflammatory response.

TABLE 6-19
OXYGEN TOXICITY AND ADVERSE EFFECTS IN POSTOPERATIVE THORACIC SURGICAL PATIENTS
TOXIC EFFECT
Depression of ventilatory drive and retention of carbon dioxide
ADVERSE EFFECTS
Immobilization of the patient
Drying and irritation of nasal and upper airway mucosa
Discomfort
Drying of secretions
Nausea, vomiting, gastric dilatation due to air hunger and oxygen swallowing
Patients think that they no longer need to cough (psychological effect)

TABLE 6-20		
INHALED BRONCHODILATORS IN POSTOPERATIVE PATIENTS		
Category of Medication	Proprietary Name	Duration of Action
Beta$_2$ agonists	Ventolin (albuterol and salbutamol are two generic names applicable to Ventolin)	4-6 hours (peak of action at 30 minutes)
Anticholinergics (ipratropium bromide)	Atrovent	6-8 hours (peak of action at 1 hour)

Bronchodilators

In pulmonary resection patients, pharmacologic agents causing rapid reversal of airway obstruction are the mainstay of treatment.

Inhaled short-acting beta$_2$ agonists such as salbutamol (Table 6-20) are the agents of choice because they provide a *rapid response with few side effects.* In the immediate postoperative setting, they are often given with intermittent positive pressure ventilation every 4 to 6 hours (Ventolin, 0.5 mL, mixed with normal saline, 2 mL). The *main advantage* of this method of administration is that the *inhalation therapist giving the treatment will make sure* that the patient expectorates once the treatment is over.

Anticholinergic drugs inhibit vagally mediated airway tone. Ipratropium bromide (Atrovent) is the most widely used of these products. Inhaled anticholinergic drugs have few side effects, but they have a *slower onset* of bronchodilatation than Ventolin.

The response to a combination of Ventolin and Atrovent given together with intermittent positive pressure ventilation at submaximal doses appears *to be better* than with either agent alone.

Corticosteroids

Because some patients may have preoperatively shown a marked improvement in FEV$_1$ with corticosteroids given orally (30 to 40 mg/day for 2 weeks), the drug (10 mg/day) is often added to the postoperative therapeutic regimen of patients with COPD.

Important toxicities of systemic steroids include the *suppression of normal healing processes* with higher incidences of prolonged air leaks and bronchopleural fistulas and the *increased susceptibility to opportunistic infections.* Other potentially significant adverse effects are listed in Table 6-21.

Antidotes Against Respiratory Depression

Excessive postoperative sedation or analgesia can sometimes result in profound neurologic depression, which may jeopardize airway protection and lead to reintubation or aspiration pneumonia. The thoracic surgeon faced with such adverse effects must promptly consider use of the appropriate antidote.

TABLE 6-21
TOXICITY AND ADVERSE EFFECTS OF SYSTEMIC CORTICOSTEROIDS
TOXIC EFFECTS
Suppression of normal healing process
Increased susceptibility to opportunistic infections
ADVERSE EFFECTS
Fluid retention
Peptic ulceration
Psychiatric disorders (delirium and others)
Hyperglycemia

Naloxone (Narcan) is an *opiate antagonist* that will reverse the respiratory depression, hemodynamic effects, sedation, and analgesia associated with opiate derivatives. It has a rapid onset of action (less than 2 minutes) and can be administered intravenously, intramuscularly, or subcutaneously. In adults, doses of 0.1 to 0.4 mg every 2 to 3 minutes should be used. Considering the potential cardiotoxicity of the drug and the abrupt reversal of postoperative sedation, *one should always use the minimal effective dose.* In addition, one should stop giving the drug if it does not reverse the condition for which it is administered (i.e., respiratory depression).

If postoperative sedation includes the use of *benzodiazepines,* these drugs can also be the source of both altered mentation and depression of the respiratory drive. In such cases, flumazenil (Anexate), 0.2 mg given intravenously followed by 0.1 mg intravenously given every minute if necessary (up to a total dose of 1 mg), can be used to reverse these adverse effects. One should be cautious when using flumazenil in patients with epileptic disorders or pharmacodependence to benzodiazepine because the drug can induce seizures in such patients.

ANTIMICROBIAL PHARMACOLOGY

Wound infections and empyemas are *uncommon after elective thoracic surgical procedures* except for operations in which the esophageal lumen has been entered. Indeed, a wound infection occurring after pulmonary resection is more often related to an empyema draining through it than to a primary infection (see Chapter 7). One reason for this low incidence is that bronchial mucus is sterile except in patients with bacterial pneumonia at the time of operation. Another reason is that the dynamic re-expansion of the residual lung tends to prevent the occurrence of intrapleural spaces or fluid collections that may become infected. Despite this low incidence, however, infections can still occur, and it has been shown that *perioperative antibiotic prophylaxis* can further reduce their occurrence. Whether the use of prophylactic antibiotics also lowers the incidence of postoperative pneumonia remains a controversial issue.

Best Prophylactic Regimen

For most patients, a *single agent with adequate gram-positive and gram-negative sensitivity* given at the onset of the operation and continued for 24 hours postoperatively is adequate prophylaxis. In the event that the surgical procedure lasts for more than 3 to 4 hours, antibiotics can be readministered.

Because of its wide antibacterial spectrum and low incidence of side effects, *cefazolin (1 g every 6 hours) is the antibiotic of choice* for most pulmonary operations. In patients with preexistent pneumonia, obstructive pneumonitis, or bronchiectasis, specific antibiotics should be started a few days before surgery and continued for at least 1 week to 10 days postoperatively.

Surgery for Tuberculosis

With the advent of effective antituberculous medication, the role of surgery in the management of active tuberculosis has greatly diminished. Operations are now mostly indicated for the *management of complications or late sequelae* of the disease.

In active cases of tuberculosis, no patient should be operated on without proper antituberculous drug coverage for at least 3 months preoperatively. Operations should also be followed by complete courses of antituberculous drugs. In patients with normal immune systems, such postoperative courses should include at least two drugs (isoniazid and rifampin) (Table 6-22) given for 6 months. In immunocompromised hosts, such as patients with human immunodeficiency virus infection, postoperative treatments should be *prolonged* for periods of 9 to 12 months.

ANTICOAGULATION

Preoperative Management of the Anticoagulated Patient

All patients receiving systemic warfarin anticoagulation are at risk of significant bleeding should they undergo diagnostic procedures, invasive staging techniques, or thoracotomy. It is thus recommended that these patients be admitted to the hospital, where intravenous heparin can be started and warfarin stopped. In general, *heparin is stopped 4 to 6 hours* before the planned procedure. An alternative method is to keep the patient anticoagulated with *low-molecular-weight heparin* given subcutaneously once or twice a day on an outpatient basis. The low-molecular-weight heparin injections are stopped the day before the scheduled intervention.

TABLE 6-22	
DOSAGE OF COMMONLY USED ANTITUBERCULOUS DRUGS	
Drug	**Daily Dosage (adults)**
Ethambutol	15-25 mg/kg (by mouth)
Isoniazid	5-10 mg/kg (by mouth)
Pyrazinamide	20-40 mg/kg (by mouth)
Rifampin	10 mg/kg (by mouth)
Streptomycin	15 mg/kg (intramuscularly)

6

Principles of Postoperative Care

If the patient is taking aspirin (usually 80- to 160-mg tablet daily) because of coronary artery or cerebrovascular disease, it does not need to be stopped before thoracic operations. If the patient is taking inhibitors of platelet function, such as clopidogrel bisulfate (Plavix), *the drug should be stopped 7 to 10 days preoperatively.*

Prophylaxis Against Deep Vein Thrombosis

Prophylactic anticoagulation as a means of preventing deep vein thrombosis is an important part of the postoperative care for most types of surgery. Such prophylaxis consists of administering 5000 international units of unfractionated heparin subcutaneously two or three times a day during and after the operation, *the first dose being given by the anesthetist.* Such low doses of heparin are not associated with increased risks of bleeding, but they can substantially reduce the risks of deep vein thrombosis.

Alternatively, low-molecular-weight heparins can be used with possible better prophylaxis and lower incidence of heparin-induced thrombocytopenia. Their routine use in thoracic surgery is still controversial, however, because *they may increase the risks of epidural hematomas* in patients with epidural catheters.

Other helpful measures that can reduce the risks of deep vein thrombosis include *early ambulation* of the patient and *intermittent pneumatic compression* of the lower extremities for 2 or 3 days postoperatively.

Indications for and Technique of Systemic Anticoagulation in the Postoperative Thoracic Patient

In the postoperative thoracic patient, systemic anticoagulation can be indicated either for acute thromboembolic events or for atrial fibrillation or flutter. If the initial operation has been uncomplicated, systemic anticoagulation can be safely started within 3 to 4 days of the surgery. If, by contrast, the initial operation has been difficult or bloody, it may be wise to wait longer. Systemic heparin anticoagulation is usually begun with a bolus of 3000 to 5000 IU given intravenously, which is followed by the continuous intravenous infusion of 800 to 1000 units per hour. The dosage is then *readjusted according to the results* of the activated partial thromboplastin time. If the patient is at risk of bleeding, no bolus should be given. When the patient resumes oral alimentation, warfarin therapy is started in parallel to the heparin, which can be discontinued once the prothrombin time has reached stable values of about 2.0 to 3.0. It usually takes 4 or 5 days to complete the conversion, and the long-term duration of anticoagulation varies with its indication (Table 6-23).

Complications of Anticoagulants

The most significant complications of systemic heparin are an increased risk of hemorrhage, especially during the early postoperative period, and heparin-induced thrombocytopenia.

TABLE 6-23

DURATION OF ORAL ANTICOAGULATION IN THE THORACIC
SURGICAL PATIENT

Indication for Anticoagulants	INR	Duration of Anticoagulation
Deep vein thrombosis	2.0-3.0	4-6 months
Atrial arrhythmias	2.0-3.0	Variable and dependent on the clinical setting

INR, international normalized ratio.

Heparin-induced thrombocytopenia, which occurs in 2% to 5% of patients, can be divided into a nonimmune and an immune variety. *Nonimmune thrombocytopenia* is the most common variety, and it generally occurs within the first 4 to 5 days of heparin therapy. It is usually mild and not associated with bleeding or thrombotic events. It is spontaneously reversible and does not warrant any therapy besides monitoring of the platelet count. Heparin can be safely continued if it is still indicated.

Immune thrombocytopenia usually occurs after 5 to 7 days of treatment. It *may be severe and is often associated with thrombotic events, both arterial and venous.* On recognition, all heparin infusions must be stopped and confirmation of the diagnosis should be obtained. If anticoagulation is still warranted, it should be done by nonheparin agents. Patients with immune thrombocytopenia should never be re-exposed to any form of unfractionated heparin or low-molecular-weight heparin.

MANAGEMENT OF FLUID AND ELECTROLYTE DISTURBANCES

Patients undergoing pulmonary resection, especially those requiring pneumonectomy, should not receive excessive fluids because this strategy may result in water accumulation in the residual lung (see Chapter 6). When patients have signs of fluid overload, such as crepitations and decreased Sao_2, or if they have radiographic images suggestive of lung edema, they *should be given diuretics,* usually furosemide (Lasix) orally or intravenously (Table 6-24).

Electrolyte imbalances are uncommon after thoracic procedures because most patients are able to resume a normal diet the day after the operation. Hyponatremia usually reflects *excess water in the intravascular space* (dilution factor), and it is of no clinical importance unless the level falls below 120 mEq/L. In such cases, the hyponatremia should be slowly

TABLE 6-24

PHARMACOLOGY OF FUROSEMIDE (LASIX)

Method of Administration	Usual Dose	Onset of Action	Peak of Action	Duration of Action
Orally	40 mg daily	30-60 minutes	1-2 hours	Up to 6 hours
Intravenously	20-40 mg as indicated	5-15 minutes	30-60 minutes	Up to 2 hours

corrected with small amounts of hypertonic solutions (lactated Ringer or normal saline). Indeed, *correcting the hyponatremia too rapidly can lead to permanent neurologic sequelae.* Hypernatremia reflects a relative deficiency of water in the intravascular space (concentration factor); under normal circumstances, this problem will quickly resolve once the patient resumes oral alimentation.

Hypokalemia can be due to several causes, but in the postoperative setting, it is usually secondary to excessive administration of diuretics. A serum potassium concentration lower than 3.0 mEq/L should be considered significant and must be corrected by giving the patient two or three infusions of potassium chloride (10 mEq potassium chloride diluted in 100 mL of normal saline infused in 1 hour). These can be repeated until the serum potassium value is normalized. Potassium supplements can also be added (20 to 40 mEq/L) to intravenous solutions, or they can be given orally in the form of suspension three times a day. Hypomagnesemia should be considered when one is faced with refractory hypokalemia.

PERIOPERATIVE MANAGEMENT OF THE DIABETIC PATIENT

In diabetic patients, blood glucose levels must be followed carefully to prevent such complications as hypoglycemia or hyperglycemia with possible ketoacidosis. In patients with type II diabetes (adult diabetes) previously treated by diet and oral hypoglycemic agents, the medication should be stopped the day of surgery and insulin given according to an insulin sliding scale (Table 6-25) protocol.

Insulin-dependent patients should receive an intravenous dextrose infusion in addition to 50% of their regular insulin dose the morning of surgery.

MANAGEMENT OF NAUSEA AND VOMITING

Postoperative nausea and vomiting are common complications of thoracic surgery, especially in patients who are receiving epidural analgesia (see "Pain Control"). Once mechanical factors such as gastric dilatation or bowel obstruction have been ruled out, *management is mainly symptomatic.* The two most commonly used medications are ondansetron (Zofran), 1 mg

TABLE 6-25

EXAMPLE OF AN INSULIN SLIDING SCALE*

Blood Glucose (mmol/L)	Insulin (Humulin R)†
≤8	No insulin
8.1-10.0	4 units
10.1-12.0	6 units
12.1-14.0	8 units
14.1-16.0	10 units
16.1-18.0	12 units
>18.0	Call physician

*Blood glucose concentration measured every 6 hours and followed by therapy.
†Given subcutaneously.

TABLE 6-26			
DRUGS COMMONLY USED TO TREAT NAUSEA AND VOMITING			
Type of Drug	Generic Name	Commercial Name	Usual Dose
Serotonin receptor antagonists	Ondansetron	Zofran	2-4 mg IV q 8 h
Antihistamine	Dimenhydrinate	Gravol (Canada)	50-100 mg IV or intrarectally q 4-6 h

given intravenously supplemented with dimenhydrinate if necessary, and dimenhydrinate, 50 to 100 mg given intravenously or intrarectally every 4 to 6 hours (Table 6-26).

CONCLUSION

Because the practice of general thoracic surgery encompasses a wide breadth of varied operations, it is important for the surgeon to have a firm understanding of the pharmacotherapy that can be associated with such procedures. Most important, *the surgeon must be mindful that drug administration can have deleterious effects.*

SUGGESTED READINGS

Review Article

Nelson HS: Drug therapy—β-adrenergic bronchodilators. N Engl J Med 1995;333:499-506.

Antibiotics

Classen DC, Evans RS, Pestotnik SL, et al: The timing of prophylactic administration of antibiotics and the risk of surgical-wound infection. N Engl J Med 1992;326:281-286.

Page CP, Bohnen JMA, Fletcher JR, et al: Antimicrobial prophylaxis for surgical wounds. Guidelines for clinical care. Arch Surg 1993;128:79-88.

Bernard A, Pillet M, Goudet P, Viard H: Antibiotic prophylaxis in pulmonary surgery. A prospective randomized double-blind trial of flash cefuroxime versus forty-eight-hour cefuroxime. J Thorac Cardiovasc Surg 1994; 107:896-900.

Evans JT, Green JD, Carlin PE, Barrett LO: Meta-analysis of antibiotics in tube thoracostomy. Am Surg 1995;61:215-219.

Boldt J, Piper S, Uphus D, et al: Preoperative microbiologic screening and antibiotic prophylaxis in pulmonary resection operations. Ann Thorac Surg 1999;68:208-211.

Kernodle DS, Kaiser AB: Postoperative infections and antimicrobial prophylaxis. In Mandell GL, Bennett JE, Dolin R, eds: Principles and Practice of Infectious Diseases, 5th ed. New York, Churchill Livingstone, 2000:3177-3191.

Chronic Obstructive Pulmonary Disease

Greening A: Pharmacotherapy in COPD. Eur Respir Rev 1997;7:45, 243-248.

Canadian Thoracic Society recommendations for management of chronic obstructive pulmonary disease—2003 [executive summary]. Can Respir J 2003;10(suppl A):11A-31A.

Oxygen

Fisher AB: Oxygen therapy. Side effects and toxicity. Am Rev Respir Dis 1980;122:61-69.

Fairley HB: Oxygen therapy for surgical patients. Am Rev Respir Dis 1980;122:37-44.

Greif R, Akça O, Horn EP, et al: Supplemental perioperative oxygen to reduce the incidence of surgical-wound infection. N Engl J Med 2000;342:161-167.

Pépin JL, Levy P: Principles of oxygen therapy. In Gibson GJ, Geddes DM, Costabel U, et al, eds: Respiratory Medicine, 3rd ed, vol 1. Philadelphia, WB Saunders, 2003:502-521.

Nausea and Vomiting

Gan TJ, Meyer T, Apfel CC, et al: Consensus guidelines for managing postoperative nausea and vomiting. Anesth Analg 2003;97:62-71.

Other

Dhand R, Tobin MJ: Inhaled bronchodilator therapy in mechanically ventilated patients. Am J Respir Crit Care Med 1997;156:3-10.

Management of Postoperative Complications after Pulmonary Surgery

ATELECTASIS AND PNEUMONIA

Atelectasis is a disorder characterized by the collapse of a segment or lobe of the lung or of the entire lung. Its incidence after pulmonary resection is approximately 40%. It is the result of decreased tidal volume, absence of sigh mechanism, and ineffective cough. Although most cases of postoperative atelectasis are not clinically significant, perfusion of underventilated areas of the lung *may result in shunting,* with resultant hypoxemia. Once symptomatic atelectasis has developed, active respiratory therapy, including bedside bronchoscopy, is the mainstay of treatment; optimal pain control will facilitate vigorous coughing and deep breathing.

Atelectasis can predispose the lung to pneumonia not only because retained mucus is an ideal medium for bacterial growth but also because decreased blood flow affects local defense mechanisms. In most patients with documented pneumonia, antibiotics must be added, and they should be directed specifically against causative organisms. When no pathogens are identified, large-spectrum antibiotics should be given.

ATELECTASIS

Atelectasis is one of the most common respiratory complications seen after pulmonary resection. Although the majority of patients have only "plate-like atelectasis" in lung bases, approximately *5% to 10% of resected patients* will develop clinically significant lobar collapse related to retained secretions. The risk of atelectasis is highest 24 to 48 hours after the operation, and in the majority of cases, it is ipsilateral.

Pathogenesis

Factors thought to play a role in the pathogenesis of postoperative atelectasis are numerous and summarized in Table 7-1. The most common direct cause of atelectasis, however, relates to the *patient's inability to cough efficiently.* Because of that, secretions are retained; mucous plugging occurs, and it is soon followed by lobar collapse. This cascade also relates to postoperative *limitations of costal and diaphragmatic excursions* (splinting) as well as to the *absence of sigh mechanisms* (deep breathing), both related to inadequate pain control.

It has also been shown that deficient transport of secretions because of abnormal ciliary function as well as kinking of residual bronchi due to anatomic rearrangements also contributes to mucous plugging. *Intraoperative injuries* to either the recurrent laryngeal or phrenic nerves may finally interfere with the patient's ability to clear secretions.

TABLE 7-1

FACTORS INVOLVED IN THE PATHOGENESIS OF SPUTUM RETENTION AND ATELECTASIS

Factor	Pathogenesis
Increased production of mucus	Preoperative smoking history and COPD (chronic bronchitis)
	Intraoperative airway manipulations
Decreased clearance of mucus	Ineffective cough
	Limitation of costal and diaphragmatic movements
	Inadequate pain control
	Possible paralysis (or paresis) of phrenic or recurrent laryngeal nerves
	Absence of sigh mechanism
	Abnormal ciliary transport
	Anatomic rearrangement after lobectomy (kinking of residual bronchi)
	?Bronchial denervation

Diagnosis (Table 7-2)

Clinical findings suggestive of postoperative atelectasis include tachypnea, decreased breath sounds over the involved hemithorax, and bronchial breathing. On radiologic examination, there may be direct evidence of loss of volume or only indirect signs, such as elevation of the hemidiaphragm and mediastinal shift toward the atelectatic side. Perhaps the most important observation is an *increased fluid oscillation* in the water seal bottle. Another easily observed sign is an *abrupt cessation of air leakage* through the chest tube when there had been one before.

Consequences of Atelectasis

Most patients, especially those with limited basilar atelectasis, will not suffer clinically significant consequences. Spontaneous improvement will occur through deep breathing and active chest physiotherapy.

In some patients, however, acute atelectasis may be the cause of severe hypoxemia not only because of further decrease in vital capacity and

TABLE 7-2

DIAGNOSIS OF ATELECTASIS

CLINICAL SIGNS

Tachypnea, tachycardia

Hemithorax retracted and immobile

Decreased breath sounds, bronchial breathing

RADIOLOGIC SIGNS

Direct: loss of volume, crowding of lung vessels

Indirect: elevation of hemidiaphragm, mediastinal shift

THORACOSTOMY TUBE SIGNS

Increased fluid oscillations

Abrupt cessation of air leakage

functional residual capacity but also because of the resulting ventilation/perfusion ($\dot{V}/\dot{Q}$) mismatching with intrapulmonary right-to-left shunt (perfusion of nonventilated lung). In patients with *an already impaired function,* these physiologic derangements can lead to frank respiratory failure with its own set of complications.

Failure to control atelectasis will finally predispose the lung to pneumonia with or without systemic sepsis. In such cases, infection results from the cumulative effects of ineffective mucociliary clearance of bacteria, decreased local pulmonary arterial blood flow, and decreased antibacterial function of alveolar macrophages.

Management

Most patients who have undergone pulmonary resection will have transient radiographic abnormalities suggestive of atelectasis during the first 2 or 3 postoperative days. Although these abnormalities do not usually translate into clinically significant problems, they *must be recognized and treated vigorously* if one hopes to prevent their progression into significant atelectasis.

Prophylaxis

Chest physiotherapy is the mainstay of all regimens intended to prevent atelectasis (Table 7-3) and physically aid in the expulsion of retained endobronchial secretions. Breathing exercises, such as inhaling deeply before coughing, are meant to increase total lung capacity and therefore cough force. Patients should be encouraged to be sitting rather than supine because they are more likely to develop vigorous coughing in the supine position. They should also be encouraged to use maneuvers and devices (incentive spirometry) that will intermittently maximize lung inflation (sighing). At the outset, postural drainage and vibration are important further adjuncts. Because patients are often unable to raise sputum by themselves, they should receive *assistance from physiotherapists.*

TABLE 7-3
COMPONENTS OF PREOPERATIVE AND POSTOPERATIVE PHYSIOTHERAPY
Breathing exercises
Maximum inhalation
Intermittent deep breathing (sighing)
Sitting position (rather than supine)
Coughing exercises
Active coughing
Assisted coughing with wound support
Arm and leg exercises
Mobilization of secretions
Postural drainage
Vibrations to all areas of the chest
Humidification of inspired air or oxygen
Inhalations
Albuterol (Ventolin)

Management of Postoperative Complications

If the patient receives oxygen, it should be warmed and moistened so that thick and tenacious secretions can be broken down, thus making physiotherapy more productive. Albuterol *(Ventolin) given every 4 to 6 hours* (0.5 mL of Ventolin delivered in 2 mL of normal saline) may help alleviate bronchospasm and potentiate more effective coughing and clearing of secretions.

Management of Significant Atelectasis

Significant atelectasis is defined as one that requires at least one bronchoscopy to re-expand the lung and improve oxygenation. Because all of these patients are unable or unwilling to raise sputum, treatment must be more aggressive, and often it entails blind nasotracheal suctioning or bedside flexible bronchoscopy. Flexible bronchoscopy is currently the preferred method because mucous plugs can be aspirated under direct vision from main, lobar, or segmental bronchi. Individual segments or lobes can also be lavaged with sterile saline solutions. Because hypoxemia may worsen during the procedure, constant monitoring of oxygen saturation by pulse oximetry is a valuable adjunct during bronchoaspiration.

Cricothyroidotomy and mini-tracheostomy can also be used to treat sputum retention and atelectasis (see Chapter 5). The advantages of these techniques are that aspiration through the cannula can be performed as often as necessary. There are few complications related to these techniques, which can be done prophylactically in patients at high or very high risk of sputum retention.

PNEUMONIA

Pathogenesis

Nosocomial pneumonias are infections that are acquired in the hospital (versus community-acquired pneumonia). They are usually caused by gram-negative bacteria, and in most cases, they are the *immediate and direct consequence of sputum retention* with secondary atelectasis that either has been left untreated or is recurrent. The same pathogenesis as described for atelectasis thus applies to pneumonia. In general, infection will occur when the host defense mechanisms are locally depressed; when the global immunologic response is inadequate, such as after major surgery or in cancer patients; and when the virulence of the organisms simply overwhelms these defenses.

The sources of pathogenic organisms are usually the oral cavity, pharynx, and hypopharynx. Bacteria reach the distal airways and lung through *microaspiration.*

Diagnosis

Diagnostic criteria for pneumonia involve various combinations of clinical, radiographic, and laboratory evidence of infection. Often, the diagnosis of pneumonia will be based on the presence of worsening pulmonary infiltrates during several days, high temperature, high white blood cell count, and purulent secretions (Tables 7-4 and 7-5).

Although the pathogenic organisms can be isolated from the sputum, bronchial aspirates, or blood, this is not always possible because the

TABLE 7-4

CRITERIA FOR PNEUMONIA

Chest radiographic examination shows new or progressive infiltrate, consolidation, cavitation, or pleural effusion and any of the following:

New onset of purulent sputum or change in character of sputum

Organism isolated from blood culture

Isolation of pathogen from specimen obtained by transtracheal aspiration, bronchial brushing, or biopsy

Modified from CDC definitions for nosocomial infections, 1988. Am Rev Respir Dis 1989;139:1058-1059.

patient has already been given antibiotics for several days. Protected specimen brush sampling is precise with reliable results, but *the technique is impractical* in postoperative patients. The same applies to bronchoalveolar lavages, which are sensitive but can be dangerous if done postoperatively.

Consequences of Pneumonia

The two immediate consequences that are associated with postoperative pneumonia are *sepsis* and *hypoxemia.* In both cases, the patient may require intubation and mechanical ventilation.

Management

Antibiotics

If clinical or radiologic findings suggest that a pneumonia is developing, a sputum sample should be obtained and the patient started *on empirical antibiotherapy.* Whether monomicrobial therapy or multidrug therapy is necessary remains controversial. In most centers, however, combination therapy with a second- or third-generation cephalosporin and clindamycin is entertained as initial treatment. This combination is effective not only against gram-negative bacteria but also against aerobic and anaerobic gram-positive cocci.

Once the causative agent has been identified, the initial empirical therapy can be narrowed and directed at the specific pathogens. The optimum duration of intravenous antibiotherapy, the timing of conversion to

7

Management of Postoperative Complications

TABLE 7-5

PRACTICAL DIAGNOSTIC CRITERIA FOR POSTOPERATIVE NOSOCOMIAL PNEUMONIA

CLINICAL

Fever, tachypnea

Purulent sputum

RADIOLOGIC

Progressive pulmonary infiltrate

LABORATORY

Leukocytosis

Positive result of Gram stain and bacterial culture of sputum oral therapy, and the duration of treatment are variables for which there is no consensus. In general, however, postoperative pneumonia should be treated for a minimum of 10 to 14 days.

Supportive Measures

Supportive measures include hydration, nutrition, and the entire spectrum of physical therapy maneuvers described for the management of atelectasis. *Incentive spirometry, intensive chest physiotherapy,* and *regular bedside flexible bronchoscopic aspirations* are particularly important in these patients. Continuous positive airway pressure (CPAP) techniques may be useful in some individuals, but in general, they are poorly tolerated by postoperative patients. The best method is still to encourage the patient to cough deeply and expectorate and to provide adequate pain control.

If hypoxemia persists, patients should be given supplemental oxygen to maintain oxygen saturations between 90% and 100%. If hypoxemia persists despite a high fraction of inspired oxygen, or if the patient becomes exhausted or hemodynamically unstable, intubation and mechanical ventilation will be needed.

Most patients do not require mechanical ventilation because of early diagnosis, adequate response to antibiotic therapy, and good supportive measures. Complications of pneumonia, such as lung abscess and empyema, are uncommon in postoperative patients.

CONCLUSION

Although many factors predispose patients to postoperative atelectasis, these factors can, in most instances, be *identified and corrected,* thus preventing the complication from occurring or minimizing its impact. Neglected atelectasis is likely to deteriorate into pneumonia. This deterioration relates to microaspiration and greatly diminished host defense mechanisms. Once pneumonia has developed, treatment must be supplemented by antibiotics, more aggressive techniques of sputum aspiration, and maintenance of oxygenation.

SUGGESTED READINGS

Review Articles

O'Donohue WJ: Prevention and treatment of postoperative atelectasis. Can it and will it be adequately studied? [editorial]. Chest 1985;87:1-2.

Centers for Disease Control and Prevention. CDC definitions for nosocomial infections, 1988. Am Rev Respir Dis 1989;139:1058-1059.

Scheld WM, Mandell GL: Nosocomial pneumonia: pathogenesis and recent advances in diagnosis and therapy. Rev Infect Dis 1991; 13(suppl 9):s743-s751.

Polk HC Jr., Heinzelmann M, Malangoni MA, et al: Pneumonia in the surgical patient. Curr Probl Surg 1997;34:119-201.

Massard G, Wihlm JM: Postoperative atelectasis. Chest Surg Clin North Am 1998;8:503-529.

Ferdinand B, Shennib H: Postoperative pneumonia. Chest Surg Clin North Am 1998;8:529-539.

Kreider ME, Lipson DA: Bronchoscopy for atelectasis in the ICU. A case report and review of the literature. Chest 2003;124: 344-350.

Kollef MH: Appropriate empirical antibacterial therapy for nosocomial infections. Getting it right the first time. Drugs 2003;63: 2157-2168.

Risk Factors

Fujita T, Sakurai K: Multivariate analysis of risk factors for postoperative pneumonia. Am J Surg 1995;169:304-307.

Bonde P, McManus K, McAnespie M, McGuigan J: Lung surgery: identifying the subgroup at risk for sputum retention. Eur J Cardiothorac Surg 2002;22:18-22.

Prophylactic Mini-tracheostomy

Merkle NM, Schlüter M, Foitzik T: Minitracheotomy: a new interventional technique for treatment of sputum retention. Surg Endosc 1992;6:199-204.

Bonde P, Papachristos I, McCraith A, et al: Sputum retention after lung operation: prospective, randomized trial shows superiority of prophylactic minitracheostomy in high-risk patients. Ann Thorac Surg 2002;74:196-203.

Case Series

Korst RJ, Humphrey CB: Complete lobar collapse following pulmonary lobectomy. Its incidence, predisposing factors, and clinical ramifications. Chest 1997;111:1285-1289.

Sok M, Dragaš AZ, Eržen J, Jerman J: Sources of pathogens causing pleuropulmonary infections after lung cancer resection. Eur J Cardiothorac Surg 2002;22:23-29.

Air Insufflation

Haenel JB, Moore FA, Moore EE, Read RA: Efficacy of selective intrabronchial air insufflation in acute lobar collapse. Am J Surg 1992;164:501-505.

7

Management of Postoperative Complications

RESPIRATORY FAILURE

In patients undergoing pulmonary resection, the incidence of early postoperative respiratory failure is low, but when it occurs, it is always associated with significant mortality. Management includes mechanical ventilation, advanced critical care, and nutritional support.

Late respiratory failure usually relates to progression of chronic obstructive pulmonary disease (COPD), development of pulmonary hypertension, occurrence of mechanical complications exclusively observed after pneumonectomy, or locoregional recurrences of previously resected lung cancer. For most of these patients, treatment options are limited and prognosis is poor.

EARLY RESPIRATORY FAILURE

Terminology and Classification (Table 7-6)

Early respiratory failure usually occurs *during the first 2 to 3 days after pulmonary resection.* For most patients, it is characterized by transient and mild hypoxemia (decreased PaO_2) and hypercapnia (elevated $PaCO_2$). These are self-limited conditions that do not require mechanical ventilation. In some instances, however, the clinical picture will be characterized by worsening of gas exchange and development of pulmonary infiltrates.

Pure ventilatory failure is characterized by an *elevated $PaCO_2$* and is a sign of *alveolar hypoventilation.* When it occurs rapidly, it may produce significant respiratory acidosis, which in turn may necessitate ventilatory assistance. In the setting of recent pulmonary surgery, carbon dioxide retention is usually transient and secondary to unrecognized central nervous system depression due to inadequate reversal of anesthesia or excessive analgesia. Later in the postoperative period, ventilatory failure is often associated with hypoxemia (mixed failure); the most common causes are respiratory muscle fatigue, bronchospasm, and exacerbation of already present COPD.

Hypoxemic failure is characterized by a *decreased PaO_2* and is secondary to right-to-left shunting of blood flow and severe ventilation/perfusion ($\dot{V}/\dot{Q}$) mismatching. It is the hallmark of adult respiratory distress syndrome (ARDS), and in general, the *severity of hypoxemia is a reasonable index of the severity of the patient's illness.* Hypoxemic failure may also be caused by atelectasis with or without pneumonia, excessive fluid administration with or without heart failure, and pulmonary embolism. Inadequate lung expansion, such as may occur with bronchopleural

TABLE 7-6

COMMON CAUSES OF EARLY RESPIRATORY FAILURE

Type	Measurement	Etiology
Ventilatory failure	Elevated $PaCO_2$ (hypercapnia)	Narcotic overdosage
		Inadequate reversal of anesthesia
		Fatigue
		Bronchospasm and exacerbation of already present COPD
Hypoxic failure	Decreased PaO_2 (hypoxemia)	Atelectasis, pneumonia
		Pulmonary embolism
		Pulmonary edema due to fluid overload
		Heart failure
		Acute lung injury, ARDS
Mixed failure	Elevated $PaCO_2$ and decreased PaO_2	Respiratory fatigue
		Large pulmonary embolus
		Acute or chronic respiratory failure

fistulas, and large air leaks are additional factors that may contribute to the hypoxemia.

Pathophysiology, Risk Factors, and Diagnosis of Common Causes

In the setting of lung surgery, most causes of early respiratory failure can be diagnosed by careful observation of the patient and judicious use of diagnostic modalities.

Ventilatory Failure

Bronchospasm and Exacerbation of Already Present COPD. In a patient with *limited pulmonary reserve,* respiratory fatigue and ventilatory failure can occur at any time after lung resection. Preoperative documentation of the degree of pulmonary impairment (see Chapter 2, "Assessment of Pulmonary Reserve") (Table 7-7) and its reversibility is thus important not only to determine if the patient can tolerate resection but also to guide the surgeon as to what extent of resection can be done. Forced expiratory volume in 1 second (FEV_1) is a practical criterion for prediction of early respiratory failure and so are the results of arterial blood gas analysis, split perfusion lung scanning, and exercise testing (MVo_2). Arterial blood gas analysis is particularly useful because it identifies patients with resting hypercapnia ($Paco_2 > 45$ mm Hg) who essentially have *no pulmonary reserve.*

Early ventilatory failure may develop in patients with COPD because they do not have enough functional reserves to adjust to the amount of parenchyma that has been resected or because of alterations in chest wall mechanics and respiratory muscle fatigue due to the operation. It will often be precipitated by phrenic or recurrent nerve palsy, diminished hypoxic ventilatory drive due to oxygen supplementation, or excessive analgesia.

The usual clinical manifestations of impending ventilatory failure are rapid shallow pattern of breathing (tachypnea), tachycardia, anxiety, and somnolence. Arterial blood gas measurement may show a normal Pao_2, especially if the patient is receiving oxygen, but characteristically, the $Paco_2$ will be elevated and rising. At this early stage, *the chest radiograph is often normal.*

Because of the high incidence of coexisting reactive airway disease in this population, patients may also experience severe bronchospasm during the early postoperative period. Indeed, the bronchospasm may have been aggravated by airway manipulations during the operation, airway edema, and retained secretions.

TABLE 7-7
RISK FACTORS FOR EARLY RESPIRATORY FAILURE IN PATIENTS WITH COPD
$FEV_1 < 1.2$ L
Arterial $Paco_2 > 45$ mm Hg
$D_{LCO} < 50\%$ predicted
$MVo_2 < 10$ mL/kg/min
Older age
Need for pneumonectomy

Hypoxic Failure

Atelectasis and Pneumonia. In postoperative patients, atelectasis predisposes to early respiratory failure because perfusion of underventilated areas of the lung results in *shunting of blood, with resultant hypoxemia.* The significance of the physiologic consequences related to hypoxemia depends on the *amount of lung involved, the clinical response to treatment,* and the presence or absence of systemic sepsis. Often, ARDS will have its onset after an episode of respiratory failure that has occurred because of sputum retention and pneumonia.

Clinical signs of pneumonia (see earlier, "Atelectasis and Pneumonia") include fever, tachypnea, tachycardia, and crackles or bronchial breathing on auscultation. The majority of such patients also have leukocytosis (15 to 30×10^8/L) and a lobar pulmonary infiltrate on the chest radiograph.

Pulmonary Embolism. Pulmonary embolism occurs in 1% to 2% of patients undergoing pulmonary resection, and most of the time, it arises from thrombosis in the deep veins of the leg. Lung cancer patients are at particularly high risk because they may have several risk factors for deep vein thrombosis (Table 7-8), including advanced age, malignant disease, prolonged duration of anesthesia, and prolonged preoperative and postoperative immobilization.

Although small pulmonary emboli may only lead to mild hypercapnia, recurrent or large emboli often *produce significant hypoxemia* because partially oxygenated blood mixes with fully oxygenated blood originating from normally perfused parenchyma.

The symptoms of pulmonary embolism can be variable, but most patients will complain of sudden-onset dyspnea, tachypnea, tachycardia, increased cough, and apprehension. More subtle manifestations of possible postoperative pulmonary embolism are listed in Table 7-9. Unlike respiratory failure due to other causes, which usually occurs by postoperative days 2 to 4, most pulmonary emboli are seen by postoperative days 5 to 10.

Suspected pulmonary embolism mandates urgent investigation and treatment. Patients should have ventilation/perfusion scans or spiral computed tomographic (CT) scanning enhanced by contrast media for diagnosis. Angiographic CT scanning is particularly useful not only for the

---

TABLE 7-8

RISK FACTORS FOR POSTOPERATIVE DEEP VEIN THROMBOSIS IN LUNG CANCER PATIENTS

Older age
Known history of heart disease
Known history of previous deep vein thrombosis
Prolonged hospitalization before surgery
Immobilization (preoperative and postoperative)
Surgery for malignant disease
Prolonged duration of anesthesia

TABLE 7-9

SUBTLE MANIFESTATIONS OF PULMONARY EMBOLISM

Worsening arterial hypoxemia and respiratory alkalosis in a spontaneously
   ventilating patient

Persistent dyspnea and hypoxemia unresponsive to bronchodilators

Unexplained fever, atelectasis, or pleura-based infiltrates

Sudden development of pulmonary hypertension

Unexplained elevation of central venous pressure

Unexplained tachycardia or tachypnea

Worsening hypoxemia, hypercapnia, and respiratory acidosis in a sedated
   patient on mechanical ventilation

From Zwischenberger JB, Alpard SK, Bidani A: Early complications. Respiratory failure.
   Chest Surg Clin North Am 1999;9:543-564.

fast diagnosis of pulmonary emboli but also to detect other pathologic processes, such as pneumonia or ARDS.

Pulmonary Edema Due to Fluid Overload and Heart Failure. Intraoperative or postoperative excessive fluid administration (Table 7-10) may result in pulmonary edema with secondary hypoxemia. *Intraoperatively,* large volumes of fluid may have been given to counteract hypotension (i.e., during induction of anesthesia) or to replace overestimated insensible and third-space fluid losses. Postoperatively, the vasodilatation associated with epidural analgesia may be treated with more fluids. Often, there is also a standing order for patients to receive boluses of colloid solutions if their urine output falls below the 15 to 20 mL/h mark.

Although fluid overload may be of little consequence in a patient without preexistent cardiovascular disorders, it can lead to pulmonary edema in elderly patients with known congestive heart failure or poorly controlled hypertension (Table 7-11). Pneumonectomy patients are particularly vulnerable to pulmonary edema not only because the residual lung has to accommodate the whole cardiac output, but also because the associated (temporary) right ventricular dysfunction may lead to an increase in central venous pressure and inhibit fluid clearance from the lung.

TABLE 7-10

**REASONS WHY PULMONARY RESECTION PATIENTS MAY
HAVE RECEIVED TOO MUCH FLUID**

Counteraction of hypotension after induction of anesthesia

Overestimation of insensible or third-space fluid losses during surgery

Overzealous replacement of calculated intraoperative losses

Counteraction of hypotension that may follow rewarming after long operations

Correction of hypotension due to epidural analgesia

Correction of low urine output during postoperative period

TABLE 7-11

RISK FACTORS FOR PULMONARY EDEMA

Advanced age
Known coronary artery disease with or without congestive heart failure
Poorly controlled systemic hypertension
Diabetes mellitus
Fluid overload
Pneumonectomy

Patients with pulmonary edema usually present with *acute respiratory distress,* tachycardia, and diaphoresis and are unable to lie down. Often, they are also unable to speak more than one sentence at a time because of their shortness of breath. Arterial blood gas analysis, a portable chest radiograph, and a bedside echocardiogram will confirm this diagnosis. When *furosemide (Lasix) is given intravenously,* the symptoms will usually subside rapidly.

Acute Lung Injury and Adult Respiratory Distress Syndrome. Postoperative acute lung injury (ALI) and adult respiratory distress syndrome (ARDS) are clinical conditions in which an early postoperative patient experiences rapidly progressive shortness of breath and hypoxemia; the lung develops radiologic infiltrates suggestive of interstitial pulmonary edema. Although this usually occurs after pneumonectomy, where it is termed postpneumonectomy edema, it can also be encountered after lesser resections such as lobectomies.

In 1994, the American-European Consensus Committee on ARDS recommended that ALI be defined *as a syndrome of inflammation and increased permeability* that cannot be explained but may coexist with left atrial or pulmonary hypertension and that the term ARDS be reserved for the *most severe end of the spectrum* (Table 7-12). Both conditions are characterized by arterial hypoxemia resistant to conventional therapy, such as oxygen supplementation and diuretics, and both are associated with significant mortality, which is in the range of 75% after pulmonary resection.

TABLE 7-12

RECOMMENDED CRITERIA FOR THE DIAGNOSIS OF ACUTE LUNG INJURY AND ADULT RESPIRATORY DISTRESS SYNDROME

	Timing	Oxygenation (Pao_2/Fio_2)*	Chest Radiograph	Pulmonary Artery Wedge Pressure
Acute lung injury	Acute	≤300	Diffuse infiltrates†	<18 mm Hg‡
ARDS	Acute	≤200	Diffuse infiltrates	<18 mm Hg

*Regardless of positive end-expiratory pressure level.
†Infiltrates are diffuse but unilateral in cases of pneumonectomy.
‡Or no evidence of left atrial hypertension.
Reprinted from Bernard GR, Artigas A, Brigham KL, et al: The American-European Consensus Conference on ARDS. Definition mechanisms, relevant outcomes, and clinical trial coordination. Am J Respir Crit Care Med 1994;149:818-824.

TABLE 7-13

FACTORS INVOLVED IN THE PATHOGENESIS OF ACUTE LUNG INJURY AND ADULT RESPIRATORY DISTRESS SYNDROME

PROBABLE FACTORS

Elevated pulmonary capillary pressure and fluid filtration pressure

Reduced lymphatic capacity for interstitial fluid resorption

Endothelial damage with increased vascular permeability

POSSIBLE FACTORS

Acute hyperinflation of residual parenchyma

Microaspiration and silent aspiration (?due to excessive analgesia)

One-lung ventilation during surgery

PRECIPITATING FACTOR

?Perioperative fluid overload

The incidence is approximately 5% after pneumonectomy and 2% after lobectomy.

Although the pathogenesis of ALI and ARDS is not fully understood, *several factors are likely to interact to cause these complications* (Table 7-13). Among them, elevated capillary pulmonary pressure, endothelial damage with increased permeability, inability of the lymphatics to transport the fluid out of the lung, hyperinflation of the residual lung parenchyma, and microaspiration have been implicated. Other possible factors include the use of one-lung anesthesia, when the ventilated lung may be subjected to volutrauma and hyperinflation, and the temporary right ventricular dysfunction observed after pneumonectomy.

For a long time, fluid overload and increased capillary hydrostatic pressure were thought to be the main forces behind the pathogenesis of ALI and ARDS, especially when it occurred after pneumonectomy. Indeed, it had been shown that after pneumonectomy, the elevated capillary pressure observed in the residual lung resulted in a net increase in fluid filtration pressures that precipitated fluid transudation. Currently, however, the theory that ALI and ARDS are always associated with fluid overload is *challenged,* and several reports have shown *no correlation* between fluid balance and ALI or ARDS.

Classically, ALI and ARDS develop 2 to 3 days after an otherwise uncomplicated postoperative period (honeymoon period) (Table 7-14). At that time, patients become short of breath and hypoxemic and experience great difficulties in bringing up sputum. Despite what appears to be adequate treatment, the dyspnea quickly worsens, and within 12 hours, *virtually all patients require positive-pressure mechanical ventilation.* On radiologic examination, the first signs of impending ALI and ARDS can be subtle and are often missed. Rapidly, however, the initial discrete infiltration progresses to diffuse interstitial edema and frank ARDS. Hemodynamically, the main pulmonary artery pressure can be moderately elevated, but the wedge pressure remains normal, ruling out left ventricular failure.

TABLE 7-14

KNOWN FACTS ABOUT POSTOPERATIVE ACUTE LUNG INJURY AND ADULT RESPIRATORY DISTRESS SYNDROME

More common after pneumonectomy than after lesser resection

Appears 2 to 3 days after otherwise uncomplicated postoperative period

Radiologic onset may precede symptoms by 12 to 24 hours

Radiologic image of interstitial pulmonary edema

Unresponsive to conventional therapies

Mortality of 50% to 75% after lobectomy and 80% to 100% after pneumonectomy

Histology compatible with ARDS

Assessment of the Patient with Early Respiratory Distress

When respiratory distress occurs after pulmonary resection, most possible causes can be assessed by *careful observation of the patient, physical examination, blood gas analysis,* and *use of imaging modalities.* All patients must be transferred to an intensive care unit (ICU) environment where investigation and monitoring can be done by experienced staff.

The clinical signs (Table 7-15) that may indicate impending respiratory failure are often subtle. They include tachypnea, tachycardia, high supplemental oxygen to maintain a saturation above 90%, and discrete pulmonary infiltrates. The development of hypercapnia (elevated $Paco_2$) is an ominous sign that signifies respiratory fatigue. *The rapidity of changes in Pao_2 and $Paco_2$ usually reflects the severity of the problem.*

Pulmonary edema occurs in patients fluid overloaded and usually in those with risk factors, and it has a good response to diuretics and oxygen. By contrast, diuretics and fluid restriction often aggravate ALI or ARDS rather than improve it. When the diagnosis of heart failure is doubtful, two-dimensional bedside echocardiography may be of value.

Pulmonary embolism can be difficult to diagnose by clinical history alone; but if it is a possibility, the patient should be anticoagulated until it is well documented that he or she does not have the complication. If a bronchopleural fistula is suspected by radiographic changes or increased air leakage through the chest tube, *bedside bronchoscopy* should also be done.

Management

General Measures

During the period of assessment, general measures that may help the patient and ultimately avoid the need for mechanical ventilation include

TABLE 7-15

CLINICAL SIGNS OF IMPENDING EARLY RESPIRATORY FAILURE

Tachypnea, tachycardia, somnolence

High supplemental oxygen to maintain saturation ≥90%

Discrete pulmonary infiltrates

Hypercapnia

Rapidity of changes reflects severity of problems

supplemental oxygen administration with an oxygen rebreathing mask or with CPAP. Unfortunately, most patients have difficulty tolerating the CPAP mask, although this modality may *temporarily* improve their oxygenation.

Diuretics are also given, especially if the chest radiograph shows generalized alveolar infiltrates suggestive of pulmonary edema. *Broad-spectrum antibiotics* are added to treat possible bronchopneumonia, and if pulmonary embolism is suspected, *anticoagulants* are also added to the regimen.

Because most patients experiencing early respiratory failure have associated small airway disease, they should receive *albuterol (Ventolin)* therapy through an ultrasonic nebulizer with the hope of relieving the associated bronchospasm.

Mechanical Ventilation

The majority of patients with established early respiratory failure will require endotracheal intubation *and mechanical ventilation.* Often, mechanical ventilation will increase volutrauma to the residual parenchyma, thus exacerbating the lesions of ARDS, so that it is not unusual for patients with ALI or ARDS to require Fio_2 of 80% to 100% to maintain an arterial Pao_2 of 60 to 70 mm Hg. Early institution of *nitric oxide* (10 to 20 parts per million) to reduce pulmonary hypertension and to improve ventilation and perfusion matching should be considered as well as use of *positive end-expiratory pressure (PEEP)* to decrease shunting and to maintain Fio_2 at the lowest possible level. Although the use of steroids remains unproven during the early phases of ARDS, consideration should be given to the addition of a short course of intravenous steroid therapy.

Finally, maintenance of *adequate nutrition* and of sedation to decrease oxygen demand and to permit more effective mechanical ventilation is also important.

LATE RESPIRATORY FAILURE

The occurrence of late respiratory failure is seen almost exclusively after pneumonectomy. These complications are difficult to predict and also difficult to manage once they are manifest. Ultimately, late respiratory failure is an important cause of death.

Classification and Pathogenesis (Table 7-16)

Progressive Lung Disease: COPD and Pulmonary Hypertension

Progressive lung disease is the *most common cause* of late respiratory failure both in the lobectomy and in the pneumonectomy patient. It relates to the *normal physiologic decline* of respiratory function due to aging, to the *accelerated decline* in individuals with ongoing smoking habits, and to the *destructive changes* in the alveoli by overdistention (compensatory emphysema) that follows pulmonary resection. Clinically, patients present with dyspnea, decreased exercise tolerance, and often symptoms of chronic bronchitis even if they no longer smoke. Their pulmonary function studies show both restrictive and obstructive lung disease, and although they may

7

Management of Postoperative Complications

TABLE 7-16	

CLASSIFICATION OF COMMON CAUSES OF LATE RESPIRATORY FAILURE AFTER PULMONARY RESECTION

PROGRESSIVE LUNG DISEASE

Chronic obstructive pulmonary disease

Pulmonary hypertension

MECHANICAL SYNDROMES

Postpneumonectomy syndrome

Platypnea-orthodeoxia syndrome

RECURRENT CANCER

Pleural effusion

Lymphangitic carcinomatosis

Airway obstruction

have normal blood gas values at rest, *hypoxemia and hypercapnia will occur during minimal exercise.* Most patients with progressive COPD are managed in the same fashion as they would be if they had not had pulmonary resection. This includes pharmacologic interventions with bronchodilators and steroids, rehabilitation, and ultimately home oxygen therapy. Smoking cessation is obviously important.

A number of alterations concerning the pulmonary circulation have been proposed to explain the pulmonary hypertension that sometimes occurs late after pneumonectomy. In a patient who has undergone pneumonectomy, for instance, the blood flow through the residual lung is substantially increased, but the total capillary bed is unchanged. When the oxygen requirements and pulmonary blood flow further increase during exertion, the capillary bed may not be able to accommodate the demand, and this may result in pulmonary hypertension. Another hypothesis is that exercise may have an active motor effect on the lung, thus creating dynamic pulmonary hypertension. Another *more likely* explanation is that pulmonary hypertension is simply the consequence of *hypoxemic respiratory failure with secondary pulmonary capillary vasoconstriction.*

Clinically, patients present with dyspnea often at rest, cyanosis, and signs of right-sided heart failure. They are severely hypoxic, and an echocardiogram will confirm the elevated pulmonary artery pressure. The natural history of pulmonary hypertension secondary to pulmonary resection may vary according to its pathogenesis, but in general, this condition carries a poor prognosis. Pulmonary hypertension is best managed by supplemental oxygen, anticoagulation, and maximum treatment of the right-sided heart failure.

Mechanical Syndromes

Postpneumonectomy Syndrome. The postpneumonectomy syndrome is caused by airway obstruction, which is itself secondary to the extreme mediastinal shift and rotation after pneumonectomy. In this situation, the main stem bronchus becomes compressed between the spine and aorta posteriorly and the pulmonary artery anteriorly. This syndrome mainly occurs in *younger patients* in whom the bronchus is softer and thus more compressible; it has been described almost exclusively after right pneumonectomy. The low incidence of 0.1% reflects the older age of patients undergoing pneumonectomy for lung cancer.

The interval between pneumonectomy and onset of symptoms is variable and ranges from 6 months to as long as 15 years. Patients can present with acute onset of dyspnea and airway obstruction, or they can present with a more insidious onset of symptoms, such as repeated bouts of pulmonary infection, persistent cough, and stridor. The diagnosis of postpneumonectomy syndrome is *made by CT scanning and bronchoscopy.*

Therapy for the postpneumonectomy syndrome is directed toward correcting the tracheobronchial compression and diminishing the extreme mediastinal shift and rotation by repositioning the mediastinum. This is best accomplished by the use of a Silastic prosthesis that is inserted in the pleural space and filled with the necessary amount of fluid *to reposition the mediastinum* in a more central position. The operation is fairly simple, and the improvement is often dramatic and immediate.

Platypnea-Orthodeoxia Syndrome. This syndrome, which also occurs almost exclusively after pneumonectomy, is due to a right-to-left shunt through an existing atrial septal defect or through *reopening of a foramen ovale.* Although there are many hypotheses to explain the platypnea-orthodeoxia syndrome, it appears to be related to the mediastinal shift and distortion that follow pneumonectomy. In this situation, the right atrium and inferior vena cava remain fixed in their original anatomic position, and this may favor reopening of a previously closed foramen ovale.

Platypnea-orthodeoxia syndrome mostly occurs after right pneumonectomy and most often within a year of the operation. It is characterized by dyspnea and desaturation related to the position of the patient, being worse in the sitting or standing position than when the patient is lying down. The diagnosis can be made by measuring oxygen saturation and Pao_2 while the patient is in different positions or by cardiac catheterization, which will dynamically demonstrate the shunt at the atrial level.

All patients with platypnea-orthodeoxia syndrome require closure of the foramen ovale either by open surgery or through heart cathetherization techniques.

Recurrent Cancer

Probably the most common cause of late respiratory failure in a patient who previously had pulmonary resection for lung cancer is a locoregional recurrence of the tumor. Causes of respiratory difficulties include *lymphangitic carcinomatosis* in the remaining lung, occurrence of a *malignant pleural effusion* with lung compression, and *airway obstruction* due to endobronchial recurrence or extrinsic compression related to nodal disease.

All of these entities can lead to rapid deterioration of the respiratory status. Their diagnosis is usually straightforward with CT scanning, bronchoscopy, and thoracentesis. Treatment is primarily palliative.

CONCLUSION

Management of patients with early postoperative respiratory failure requires a clear understanding of the pathogenesis involved in the complication as well as of its natural history. The mortality associated with such events is high because most patients have an already compromised pulmonary function that has been further impaired by the surgery itself. When the patient requires mechanical ventilation, recovery is always expected to be prolonged.

SUGGESTED READINGS

Review Articles

Bernard GR, Artigas A, Brigham KL, et al: The American-European Consensus Conference on ARDS. Definitions, mechanisms, relevant outcomes, and clinical trial coordination. Am J Respir Crit Care Med 1994;149:818-824.

Zwischenberger JB, Alpard SK, Bidani A: Early complications. Respiratory failure. Chest Surg Clin North Am 1999;9:543-564.

Jordan S, Mitchell JA, Quinlan GJ, et al: The pathogenesis of lung injury following pulmonary resection. Eur Respir J 2000;15:790-799.

Alpard SK, Duarte AG, Bidani A, Zwischenberger JB: Pathogenesis and management of respiratory insufficiency following pulmonary resection. Semin Surg Oncol 2000;18:183-196.

Editorial

Bauer P: Postpneumonectomy pulmonary oedema revisited. Eur Respir J 2000;15:629-630.

Pulmonary Complications (General)

Dales RE, Dionne G, Leech JA, et al: Preoperative prediction of pulmonary complications following thoracic surgery. Chest 1993;104:155-159.

Busch E, Verazin G, Antkowiak JG: Pulmonary complications in patients undergoing thoracotomy for lung carcinoma. Chest 1994;105:760-766.

Wang J, Olak J, Ultmann RE, Ferguson MK: Assessment of pulmonary complications after lung resection. Ann Thorac Surg 1999; 67:1444-1447.

Filaire M, Bedu M, Naamee A, et al: Prediction of hypoxemia and mechanical ventilation after lung resection for cancer. Ann Thorac Surg 1999;67:1460-1465.

Arieff AI: Fatal postoperative pulmonary edema. Pathogenesis and literature review. Chest 1999;115:1371-1377.

Stéphan F, Boucheseiche S, Hollande J, et al: Pulmonary complications following lung resection. A comprehensive analysis of incidence and possible risk factors. Chest 2000;118:1263-1270.

Kutlu CA, Williams EA, Evans TW, et al: Acute lung injury and acute respiratory distress syndrome after pulmonary resection. Ann Thorac Surg 2000;69:376-380.

Ruffini E, Parola A, Papalia E, et al: Frequency and mortality of acute lung injury and acute respiratory distress syndrome after pulmonary resection for bronchogenic carcinoma. Eur J Cardiothorac Surg 2001;20:30-37.

Pilling JE, Martin-Ucar AE, Waller DA: Salvage intensive care following initial recovery from pulmonary resection: is it justified? Ann Thorac Surg 2004;77:1039-1044.

Pulmonary Complications after Pneumonectomy

Zeldin RA, Normandin D, Landtwing D, Peters RM: Postpneumonectomy pulmonary edema. J Thorac Cardiovasc Surg 1984;87:359-365.

Williams EA, Evans TW, Goldstraw P: Acute lung injury following lung resection: is one lung anaesthesia to blame? Thorax 1996; 51:114-116.

Vaporciyan AA, Merriman KW, Ece F, et al: Incidence of major pulmonary morbidity after pneumonectomy: association with timing of smoking cessation. Ann Thorac Surg 2002;73:420-426.

Algar FJ, Alvarez A, Salvatierra A, et al: Predicting pulmonary complications after pneumonectomy for lung cancer. Eur J Cardiothorac Surg 2003;23:201-208.

Alvarez JM, Panda RK, Newman MAJ, et al: Postpneumonectomy pulmonary edema [case conference]. J Cardiothorac Vasc Anesth 2003;17:388-395.

Pulmonary Embolus

Kalweit G, Huwer H, Volkmer I, et al: Pulmonary embolism: a frequent cause of acute fatality after lung resection. Eur J Cardiothorac Surg 1996;10:242-247.

Kameyama K, Cheng-long H, Liu D, et al: Pulmonary embolism after lung resection: diagnosis and treatment. Ann Thorac Surg 2003; 76:599-601.

Sakuragi T, Sakao Y, Furukawa K, et al: Successful management of acute pulmonary embolism after surgery for lung cancer. Eur J Cardiothorac Surg 2003;24:580-587.

Nitric Oxide

Mathisen DJ, Kuo EY, Hahn C, et al: Inhaled nitric oxide for adult respiratory distress syndrome after pulmonary resection. Ann Thorac Surg 1998; 65:1894-1902.

Case Series

Lowell JA, Schifferdecker C, Driscoll DF, et al: Postoperative fluid overload: not a benign problem. Crit Care Med 1990;18:728-733.

Late Complications

Grillo HC, Shepard JAO, Mathisen DJ, Kanarek DJ: Postpneumonectomy syndrome: diagnosis, management, and results. Ann Thorac Surg 1992;54:638-651.

Wihlm JM, Massard G: Late complications. Late respiratory failure. Chest Surg Clin North Am 1999;9:633-654.

7

Management of Postoperative Complications

MECHANICAL VENTILATION FOR THE SURGEON

The management of patients on the ventilator is often a *shared responsibility* between intensivist and surgeon. On several occasions, however, *the lines of responsibility are blurred,* and, as stated by Dr. F. G. Pearson, the attending surgeon must have a clear understanding of the most common modes of mechanical ventilation that can be used. The surgeon must also have good knowledge of the *vocabulary* used by intensivists so that he or she is able to clearly communicate with them.

Most important, the surgeon must be able to act as an intermediate between the intensivist, who may strive for normality of gas exchange *at whatever cost,* and the patient, who requires *pressure-limited ventilation* to avoid complications of mechanical ventilation or oxygen therapy. The surgeon must finally be able to understand and discuss intelligently the many crisis situations that are likely to arise during the course of mechanical ventilation.

Although it is admittedly difficult for surgeons to remain abreast of all management techniques in this field, they must at least understand the objectives of mechanical ventilation, the available options and modes of ventilatory assistance, and the approaches to weaning the patient from the ventilator.

OBJECTIVES OF AND INDICATIONS FOR VENTILATORY ASSISTANCE (TABLES 7-17 and 7-18)

The primary objective of mechanical ventilation is to *support inefficient gas exchange.* Indications may thus be manifested by ventilatory failure (carbon dioxide retention), hypoxemia (oxygenation failure), or a combination of both (see earlier, "Respiratory Failure").

Other perhaps secondary objectives of ventilatory assistance include substitution for respiratory muscles (intercostals, diaphragms) when those muscles are tired and reversal of atelectasis, which may have increased both shunt fraction and hypoxemia.

Clinical judgment rather than laboratory numbers often determines the need for mechanical ventilation. The increased work of breathing, for instance,

---

TABLE 7-17

GENERAL OBJECTIVES OF MECHANICAL VENTILATORY ASSISTANCE

Improvement in pulmonary gas exchange
    Reverse hypoxemia (optimize $\dot{V}/\dot{Q}$)
    Reverse acute respiratory acidosis
Relieve respiratory distress
    Decrease work of breathing
    Reverse respiratory muscle fatigue
Alter pressure-volume relationship
    Prevent and reverse alveolar atelectasis
    Improve pulmonary and thoracic compliance

Modified from Tobin MJ: Mechanical ventilation. N Engl J Med 1994;330:1056-1061.

TABLE 7-18

COMMON INDICATIONS FOR VENTILATORY ASSISTANCE

Alveolar hypoventilation (elevated $Paco_2$; >50 mm Hg)
Severe hypoxemia (reduced Pao_2; <55 mm Hg with Fio_2 > 0.6)
Diminished respiratory drive
Excessive work of breathing (respiratory rate > 35 breaths/minute)

may be signaled by *recruitment of accessory muscles* and *discoordinated breathing patterns.* In other patients, the onset of tachypnea, confusion, agitation, or somnolence may indicate that intubation is imminent. In general, the combination of hypoxemia and hypercapnia as documented by analysis of arterial blood gases and of increased respiratory rate (Table 7-18) should signal the need for immediate intubation. Indeed, positive-pressure ventilation can be *lifesaving* when the $Paco_2$ rises rapidly or when severe hypoxemia is associated with hemodynamic instability.

INTUBATION (TABLE 7-19)

During intubation, the operator must have *easy access* to all the equipment (usually in an intubating tray) that may be required for the procedure. In most cases, intubation is done in an awake but sedated patient (intravenous midazolam, 2 to 5 mg), and for this reason, the procedure must be explained in a reassuring and clear manner. A short-acting intravenous analgesic such as fentanyl (50 to 100 μg) is often added to further reduce the patient's awareness.

The mouth is first suctioned and the back of the throat sprayed with a 1% lidocaine aerosol. The laryngoscope blade is then inserted, and the vocal cords are also sprayed with the lidocaine aerosol. During this part of the procedure, the patient's respiration is *supported with an Ambu bag.*

During intubation, the patient is generally positioned in a high Fowler position. This position facilitates assisting the patient's respiratory efforts in addition to making intubation easier (the oropharynx and glottis are in alignment).

TABLE 7-19

PREREQUISITES FOR SUCCESSFUL INTUBATION

Operator must have easy access to all equipment that may be required.
Operator must be experienced or under direct supervision of somebody
  who is experienced.
Procedure should be explained to the patient in a reassuring manner.
Patient must be adequately monitored.
Patient must be sedated (midazolam, 2-5 mg; fentanyl, 50-100 μg).
Patient is best positioned in a high Fowler position (pillow behind head).
Suction mouth and spray back of throat and vocal cords with 1% lidocaine aerosol.
Assist patient with Ambu bag during procedure.
Size of endotracheal tube is individualized.
Unless it is a life-threatening situation, take your time.

7

Management of Postoperative Complications

TABLE 7-20

POSSIBLE COMPLICATIONS OF INTUBATION

Ventricular arrhythmias
Exacerbation of hypoxemia
Hemodynamic instability and hypotension
Aspiration
Laryngeal or tracheal trauma
Barotrauma to the lungs
Increased intracranial pressure

Two of the most important aspects of intubation are that the patient must be adequately monitored during the procedure and that, unless it is a life-threatening situation, *the operator must take the necessary time* to carry out the technique safely. Possible complications (Table 7-20) that may occur during intubation include ventricular arrhythmias, exacerbation of hypoxemia, hemodynamic instability (hypotension), and aspiration.

If the intubation is difficult, *flexible bronchoscopy* through either the oral or the nasal route can facilitate the procedure. The bronchoscope is first passed through the endotracheal tube and then advanced through the vocal cords into either main stem bronchus. In this position, the bronchoscope acts as a stylet over which the endotracheal tube can easily be advanced.

VENTILATORY MODES AND SETTINGS

Once the patient has been intubated, the first decision concerns the *selection of an appropriate ventilatory mode.* The clinician must then determine the specifics of ventilation management, such as respiratory rate (breaths/minute [f]), tidal volume (VT), inflation pressure, level of PEEP, and FIO_2.

Common Modes of Mechanical Ventilation (Tables 7-21 and 7-22)

In general, assisted modes that are triggered by the patient's inspiratory efforts are preferred. These include assist-control ventilation, intermittent mandatory ventilation, and pressure support ventilation.

Pressure-targeted modes guarantee pressure, but they allow variable tidal volume. The major advantage of these respirators is that peak inspiratory pressures are maintained at a constant level, thus decreasing the likelihood of localized overdistention, associated volutrauma, and lung injury (Tables 7-21 and 7-22). In addition, pressure ventilation is able to respond on a breath-to-breath basis to changes in ventilatory demand, thus increasing patient-ventilator synchronicity and potentially reducing the patient's effort.

Volume-targeted modes guarantee flow and volume, but they allow peak airway pressure to vary. Major advantages of this mode are the capacity to deliver a fixed tidal volume, ensuring a constant level of alveolar ventilation ($PaCO_2$ constant), and the flexibility of possible flow and volume adjustments. However, volume ventilation is unable to respond to changes in the patient's demand, thus possibly creating *patient-ventilator dyssynchrony* and increased effort by the patient.

TABLE 7-21

MOST COMMON MODES OF MECHANICAL VENTILATION

Ventilatory Mode	Type of Ventilatory Support	Benefits	Risks
VOLUME-TARGETED MODES			
Assist-control ventilation (ACV)	Assisted*	Minimal ventilatory work load	Hyperventilation Auto-PEEP
Synchronized intermittent mandatory ventilation (SIMV)	Assisted	Well tolerated Can be used for weaning	Increased work of breathing
PRESSURE-TARGETED MODES			
Pressure control ventilation (PCV)	Control/assisted†	Possibly better oxygenation in ARDS patients	Difficult to tolerate Auto-PEEP is used with inverse ratio ventilation
Pressure support ventilation (PSV)	Supported‡	Reduction in time necessary for weaning Can be used noninvasively	Limited support Increased work of breathing

*Assisted ventilation: Ventilator is used to amplify patient's own ventilatory efforts to achieve prescribed target.
†Controlled ventilation: Ventilator dictates both the rhythmicity and work of breathing without input from patient.
‡Supported ventilation: Ventilator provides a fixed pressure to help patient with his or her own spontaneous ventilatory targets.

TABLE 7-22

ADVANTAGES AND DISADVANTAGES OF PRESSURE- AND VOLUME-TARGETED VENTILATION

PRESSURE-TARGETED VENTILATION

Advantages
    Peak alveolar pressure is limited
    Flow responds to patient's demand
    Increased patient-ventilator synchrony
Disadvantages
    Tidal volume variable
    $Paco_2$ variable

VOLUME-TARGETED VENTILATION

Advantages
    Tidal volume constant
    $Paco_2$ constant
    Easily identifiable changes in peak inspiratory pressure as impedance changes
Disadvantages
    Peak alveolar pressure variable
    Inability to respond to changes in patient's ventilatory demand

From Kacmarek RM: Current status of new modes of mechanical ventilation. Can Respir J 1996;3:357-360.

A number of ventilators combining the beneficial effects of both pressure and volume ventilation are now commercially available.

Controlled Mechanical Ventilation (CMV)

Controlled mechanical ventilation involves *complete control of the patient's respiration* by delivery of fixed ventilation at defined time intervals. With this mode, there is no provision for spontaneous ventilatory efforts, which are inhibited by either sedation or paralysis. Controlled mechanical ventilation is generally limited to intraoperative and immediate postintubation ventilation.

Assist-Control Ventilation (ACV)

Assist-control ventilation is the *most commonly used mode of ventilation in critically ill patients.* The ventilator guarantees minute ventilation by delivering a set tidal volume at a fixed respiratory rate. Patient-triggered breaths are sensed and assisted by the respirator and may thus contribute to the minute ventilation.

Assist-control ventilation can be used to minimize the work of breathing, and it is generally *well tolerated* by sedated patients. In awake patients who breathe over the set respiratory rate, however, there is a potential risk for hyperventilation and secondary respiratory alkalosis.

Intermittent Mandatory Ventilation (IMV) and Synchronized Intermittent Mandatory Ventilation (SIMV)

In this mode, a mandatory minute ventilation (V_T and f) is preset, but patients are *free to breathe spontaneously* (by means of a demand valve) between set ventilator breaths. Mandatory breaths may be synchronized with the patient's spontaneous efforts (synchronized intermittent mandatory ventilation).

The main advantage of this mode is that it is well tolerated by the awake patient (less sedation required) so that it can be used as a weaning mode. In this setting, the set mandatory rate is gradually reduced as spontaneous rate increases. One potential disadvantage of intermittent mandatory ventilation and synchronized intermittent mandatory ventilation is that spontaneous breathing can result in a *significant increase in the overall work of breathing,* which may override potential benefits related to the patient's comfort.

Pressure Support Ventilation (PSV)

In this mode, a preset inspiratory pressure (rather than volume) is applied to the ventilator circuit during inspiration in spontaneously breathing patients. Tidal volume is determined by this preset inspiratory pressure and the patient's effort. Pressure support ventilation provides the greatest patient-ventilator interaction of the conventionally used ventilatory modes and thus is *useful to wean* the patient off the respirator.

Ventilator Settings

Once the ventilatory mode has been determined, the clinician must next determine the specifics of ventilator management. As described by Dr. Thomas R. J. Todd, it is useful to remember the rule of the "lowest therapeutic intervention" involving the *lowest F_{IO_2}* to achieve satisfactory

TABLE 7-23

INITIAL SETTING UP OF MECHANICAL VENTILATION

Parameter	Setting
FIO_2	0.8-1.0
Tidal volume (V_T)	10 mL/kg
Respiratory rate (f)	10-15 breaths/minute
Inspiratory/expiratory ratio	1:3
Peak airway pressure	<35 cm H_2O
PEEP	5-7 cm H_2O

arterial oxygenation, the *lowest inflation pressure* to achieve the lowest peak airway pressure, and the *lowest level of PEEP*.

Initial settings are estimated on the basis of the patient's size and clinical condition (Table 7-23). These settings are then assessed repeatedly and readjusted to achieve optimal gas exchange (Table 7-24). Inverse ratio ventilation may be used to improve gas exchange without inflicting damage to the lung. *Prolonged expiration* (normal setting of respirator) can be useful in patients with COPD. By contrast, *prolonged inspiration* (inverse ratio ventilation) may be preferred in patients with ARDS because it increases the mean airway pressure without increasing the peak alveolar pressure, allowing more time for gas exchanges.

Fractional Inspired Oxygen Concentration (FIO_2)

Immediately after intubation, it is best to provide the patient with an FIO_2 of 80% to 100%; but once the patient has stabilized, the FIO_2 should be lowered to meet a target of a PaO_2 approximating 60 to 70 mm Hg or an arterial oxygen saturation (SaO_2) of 90%. Because prolonged (>24 hours) exposure to FIO_2 greater than 50% *exposes the lungs to oxygen toxicity,* every effort should be made to decrease the FIO_2 to 50% or lower as soon as possible.

A list of the possible options that can be used to lower the FIO_2 is given in Table 7-25. *Diuretics* may help improve lung compliance and $\dot{V}/\dot{Q}$ matching if excessive lung water has accumulated. Changes from *supine to prone position* may bring well-ventilated areas in a more dependent position in which perfusion will be improved. *Nitric oxide,* administered by inhalation through a circuit coupled with the respirator, is an endothelium-derived relaxing factor that decreases the pulmonary vascular resistance and results in a better flow distribution (improves matching of ventilation and perfusion),

TABLE 7-24

RESULTS OF CHANGES IN VENTILATORY SETTING

Change in Ventilator Setting	Expected Result
FIO_2, PEEP	Alteration in PaO_2
V_T, respiratory rate	Alteration in $PaCO_2$
Prolonged expiration (insp/exp: 1:3)	Useful in COPD patients
Prolonged inspiration* (insp/exp: 1:1, 2:1)	Possibly useful in ARDS patients

*Inverse ratio ventilation.

7

Management of Postoperative Complications

POSSIBLE OPTIONS TO LOWER F_{IO_2} IN MECHANICALLY VENTILATED PATIENTS

Use of PEEP

Use of diuretics if excessive lung water has accumulated

Use of prone position (versus supine)

Use of nitric oxide

Modify inspiration-to-expiration ratio (I:E ratio)

Look at alternative means of ventilation

especially in patients with ARDS. Although there is no evidence that the use of nitric oxide improves outcome in the general population of mechanically ventilated patients, it may be useful in the patient who had recent pulmonary resection and who is expected eventually to adjust to modified conditions of ventilation and redistribution of pulmonary blood flow.

Permissive Hypercapnia

The problem of alveolar overdistention and barotrauma has led many clinicians to speculate that prevention could be accomplished by reducing alveolar pressure and tidal volume, thus *accepting lower ventilation and elevated $Paco_2$*. This ventilation strategy is called permissive hypercapnia, and it is recommended for patients with ARDS. When there is no concomitant arterial oxygen desaturation, $Paco_2$ in the range of 75 to 90 mm Hg is well tolerated, and indeed, clinically significant adverse effects are unusual at these $Paco_2$ levels.

Positive End-Expiratory Pressure

Although there is no consensus on the use of PEEP and at what level it should be set, this modality is helpful in *improving Pao_2 and hence allowing a decrease in F_{IO_2}* in patients with alveolar processes such as ARDS, pneumonia, and pulmonary edema. This effect appears to be related to alveolar recruitment of atelectatic regions with reduction in intrapulmonary shunting as well as to a redistribution of lung water from the alveoli to the interstitial space.

TABLE 7-26

POSSIBLE ADVERSE EFFECTS OF PEEP

Effect	Consequence
Barotrauma	Pneumothorax, mediastinal or subcutaneous emphysema, parenchymal damage
Barotrauma in postoperative patients	Bronchopleural fistulas
	Prolonged air leaks
Decreased cardiac output	Hypotension
	Decreased renal and portal blood flow
Increased hyperinflation	May be detrimental in asthma patients
Decreased cerebral venous blood flow	May be detrimental in patients with intracranial injuries
Increased intracranial pressure	May be detrimental in patients with intracranial injuries

Adverse effects of PEEP are listed in Table 7-26. They include barotrauma in the form of pneumothorax, mediastinal or subcutaneous emphysema, and volutrauma manifested by parenchymal damage. High levels of PEEP can also reduce venous return to the heart (preload), thus reducing cardiac output with secondary systemic hypotension.

Institution of PEEP should be done *in a systematic manner,* with small stepwise increments of 3 to 5 cm H_2O. There is no consensus on the ideal level of PEEP, but in general, one must aim at a PEEP level that will optimize the Pao_2 without creating hemodynamic instability (usually between 5 and 12 cm H_2O).

COMPLICATIONS OF MECHANICAL VENTILATION (TABLE 7-27)

Several adverse events can occur while patients are receiving mechanical ventilation, but often these events are *as much due to the underlying illness as to the mechanical ventilation itself.*

Positive-pressure ventilation can lower the cardiac output because of reduced venous return and increased pulmonary vascular resistance. This effect can be minimized by reducing airway pressures, avoiding high PEEP, avoiding prolonged inspiratory times, maintaining intravascular volume, and sedating the patient. Indeed, patients who actively fight the respirator raise their intrathoracic pressures, and this may significantly decrease the venous return to the heart.

Endotracheal tube malfunction is rare, but it can arise when the tube becomes obstructed by secretions or if it becomes dislodged. Prophylaxis against those problems includes use *of humidified gases, frequent suctioning, and adequately securing the tube.*

Positive-pressure ventilation may result in *worsening of V̇/Q̇ mismatching* because gravitational forces favor perfusion in the dependent lung zones, but gas delivered by positive-pressure ventilation is greatest in the nondependent zones. Barotrauma in the form of life-threatening *pneumothoraces* or *pneumomediastinum* may result from alveolar rupture.

Dynamic hyperinflation occurs when the expiration phase of the inspiration-expiration (I:E) ratio is too short to allow the lung to deflate itself properly. With every subsequent breath, the alveolar pressure at end-expiration increases further until injury occurs. Volutrauma is related to alveolar overdistention, and it may further exacerbate lung damage.

Prolonged muscle weakness and atrophy of respiratory muscles and others are related to prolonged mechanical ventilation, use of steroids, and muscle relaxants (neuromuscular blockers). Prophylaxis includes avoidance of steroids, curare, and aminoglycosides and maintenance of good glycemic control. Long-term use of muscle relaxants *is particularly harmful* because it has a deconditioning effect on the striated muscles, including the diaphragm.

Ventilation-associated pneumonia complicates the course of mechanical ventilation *in approximately 10% to 20% of patients.* The predominant organisms responsible for these infections are *Staphylococcus aureus, Pseudomonas aeruginosa,* and *Enterobacter* species. The proper use of hand washing, sterile techniques, bronchial toilet, maintenance of oral and

7

Management of Postoperative Complications

TABLE 7-27

POSSIBLE COMPLICATIONS OF MECHANICAL VENTILATION

System	Complication	Possible Result	Prophylaxis
Cardiovascular	Reduction in venous return‡	Reduced cardiac output	Reduce inflation pressures
	Increased pulmonary vascular resistance‡	Hypotension	Avoid high PEEP
			Avoid prolonged inspiratory times
			Keep patient sedated
	Hemorrhage due to erosion of innominate artery by endotracheal tube*	Usually fatal	Use of soft and low-pressure cuff tubes
			Use minimum cuff pressure to achieve a seal (<25 mm Hg)
Respiratory (airway and lung)	Laryngeal injury,* deep tracheal ulcerations*	Subglottic stricture, tracheal stricture, tracheomalacia	Proper technique of intubation, low-pressure cuff tubes
	Endobronchial tube malfunction* (blockage by secretions, dislodgment)		Use humidified air
			Adequate suctioning and securing of tube
	Ventilator circuit malfunction*	Hypoxemia	
	Worsening of $\dot{V}/\dot{Q}$ mismatch†	Hypoxemia	
	Barotrauma*	Pneumothorax, pneumo-mediastinum	Avoid high VT
			Avoid high PEEP
	Volutrauma†	Exacerbation of lung injury	Avoid high inflation pressure
	Disuse atrophy of respiratory muscles*	Muscle atrophy	Avoid steroids and curare
	Oxygen toxicity*	Pulmonary fibrosis	Decrease FIO$_2$
	Ventilator-associated pneumonia	Sepsis	Antibiotics
			Use of sterile techniques
			Bronchial, oral, and nasal hygiene
Renal	Release of antidiuretic hormone, renin, vasopressin*	Reduced urine output	
		Water retention	
Neuromuscular	Peripheral neuropathies and myopathies‡	Prolonged disability	Avoid steroids and curare
			Nutritional support
			Active and passive physiotherapy (muscle reconditioning)

*Rare.
†Common.
‡Very common.

nasal hygiene, prevention of aspiration, maintenance of proper nutrition, and prompt treatment of extrapulmonary septic foci are helpful measures to reduce the amount of contamination and its effect on the airway.

GENERAL CARE OF THE PATIENT DURING MECHANICAL VENTILATION

General aspects of patient care include *oral hygiene, nutritional supplementation,* and *measures to prevent decubitus ulcers.* Maintaining the patient's comfort is helpful to decrease the work of breathing and to allow better oxygenation. For most patients, this objective can be achieved by combining short-acting drugs (fentanyl) given intravenously and optimal adjustment of respirator settings, such as respiratory rate and tidal volume. In patients who require controlled mechanical ventilation, the regimen can be switched to propofol given in a continuous drip.

Reassurance from the staff will contribute to the patient's well-being. In some ICUs, psychologists or psychiatrists are routine members of the team managing patients on the respirator.

DISCONTINUATION OF MECHANICAL VENTILATION

Once the criteria for discontinuation of mechanical ventilation are met and the cause of respiratory failure has been corrected, weaning will be successful in approximately 95% of patients.

Criteria for Weaning (Table 7-28)

The most important issue is to determine that indeed weaning has become possible. In general terms, this assessment requires the clinician to judge the *patient's ability to maintain spontaneous respiration* and her or his *recovery* from the primary illness.

This is usually signaled by a Pao_2 greater than 60 mm Hg on Fio_2 smaller than 0.4, PEEP that is 7 cm H_2O or less, and clearing of infiltrates on the chest radiograph. Measurements of vital capacity and peak inspiratory pressures will assess the patient's ability to generate enough muscle force. Adequacy of ventilation is determined through minute ventilation, respiratory rate, and $Paco_2$. Commonly used objective weaning criteria are listed in Table 7-28.

TABLE 7-28
OBJECTIVE END-OF-WEAN CRITERIA
Recovery from primary illness
Optimization of general medical condition and nutritional status
Adequate oxygenation
$Pao_2 > 60$ mm Hg on $Fio_2 < 0.4$
Adequate ventilation
$Paco_2 < 45$ mm Hg (in non-COPD patients)
Respiratory rate (f) <25-30 breaths/minute
Tidal volume (V_T) >5 mL/kg
Minute ventilation ($V_T \times f$) <10 L/min
Vital capacity >10 mL/kg

7

Management of Postoperative Complications

Methods of Weaning

Patients who require brief periods of ventilatory assistance can resume spontaneous breathing with little difficulty. This is the case, for instance, of surgery patients who are extubated within 24 hours of the operation.

If the patient has been on the respirator for some time or has a tracheotomy, he or she can also *be disconnected from the ventilator* and *receive supplemental oxygen through a T-tube system.* If the patient does not have signs of intolerance, extubation can then be performed safely.

Weaning the patient through intermittent mandatory ventilation involves a gradual reduction in the amount of support being provided by the respirator and a progressive increase in the amount of respiratory work being performed by the patient, who remains connected to the ventilation until weaning is complete.

An alternative method is to use *pressure support ventilation.* The patient is switched to spontaneous breathing with positive-pressure inspiratory assist, and the inspiratory pressure level is progressively decreased as tolerated.

Although all of these methods are likely to be successful if the patient is ready to be weaned, it is good practice to follow a set protocol before extubation (see Appendix, "Weaning Protocol").

Tracheostomy

The most common indication for tracheostomy is the facilitation of prolonged mechanical ventilation. Although there is no consensus as to the appropriate time to perform tracheostomy, the recommendation of most intensivists is to *carry out the procedure after 7 to 10 days* if the patient's clinical picture suggests that the duration of mechanical ventilation will be prolonged.

Open Tracheostomy

Most tracheostomies are performed under general anesthesia by *an open technique in the operating room.* The tracheal incision is made over the second and third tracheal cartilages, and a No. 8 tube is generally used in the adult population. The advantage of open tracheostomy is that the operation is done in optimal conditions of exposure with readily available equipment if it is required. Another advantage is that a feeding jejunostomy can be done during the same setting. The main disadvantage is the risk of transporting a critically ill patient to the operating room. Elective open cricothyroidostomy is a valuable alternative to tracheostomy, especially after median sternotomy, because the incision is higher with theoretically *less risk* of sternal contamination.

Open bedside tracheostomy in the setting of the ICU *should almost never be done.*

Percutaneous Tracheostomy

The most widely accepted alternative to open tracheostomy is the technique of *progressive dilation over a percutaneously inserted guide wire (Ciaghia technique).* Potential advantages of this procedure over open surgical tracheostomy are listed in Table 7-29. The need for conversion to open tracheostomy is rare when the operator is familiar with the technique, and

---

TABLE 7-29

POSSIBLE ADVANTAGES OF PERCUTANEOUS TRACHEOSTOMY VERSUS OPEN TRACHEOSTOMY

Self-sufficiency of ICU medical staff (reduced delay for intervention)
Less disruption of patient's care
Does not require transfer of critically ill patients out of the ICU
Easier technically
Can be performed expeditiously
Lower cost (no operating room cost)
?Lower short-term and long-term complication rate

---

the rate of complications, such as airway bleeding or perforation of the posterior tracheal wall, is lower. In terms of morbidity, *the influence of the learning curve* should be recognized, particularly as those who usually perform percutaneous tracheostomy are not surgeons. Contraindications include conditions in which the neck cannot be manipulated, significantly enlarged thyroid gland, and coagulation disorders.

Complications of Tracheostomy

The most common complications of tracheostomy are listed in Table 7-30. Early bleeding occurs in approximately 5% of patients and is due to lacerations of the anterior jugular vein or thyroid veins. Tracheostomy tube displacement is caused by *inadequately securing the tube* around the neck. When it happens, it is best to reintubate the patient orally rather than try to force the cannula into an unsecure neck wound.

Tracheal-innominate fistulas generally occur 2 to 3 weeks after tracheostomy. This complication is due to low tracheostomy (below fourth tracheal ring), high position of the innominate artery (usually seen in women), or excessive movement of the tracheostomy tube, or it is the result of a high-pressure cuff causing erosion of the anterior tracheal wall.

Tracheal stenosis is a long-term complication of tracheostomy; strictures develop in the subglottic region, at the stoma, or at the level of the cuff. These lesions, which are the result of ischemic damage to the tracheal mucosa, *have become uncommon* since the advent of low-pressure cuffs.

Tracheoesophageal fistula can follow open or percutaneous tracheostomy. When it is associated with open tracheostomy, the tracheoesophageal

---

TABLE 7-30

MOST COMMON COMPLICATIONS OF TRACHEOSTOMY

EARLY

Bleeding (anterior jugular vein, thyroid veins)
Inadvertent tube displacement

DELAYED

Fistula with innominate artery
Subglottic and tracheal strictures
Tracheoesophageal fistulas

fistula develops late and is related to erosion of the posterior trachea by the cannula. After percutaneous operation, most fistulas occur early and are due to penetration of the posterior tracheal wall during insertion of the dilator or tube.

ALTERNATIVE MODES OF VENTILATION

Because of the potential disadvantages associated with mechanical ventilation, several alternative modes of ventilation have been introduced during the past 25 years.

Noninvasive Ventilation

Noninvasive ventilation is the delivery of positive-pressure ventilation with facemasks or nasal masks. These techniques are most useful for patients in acute respiratory failure, such as those with *pulmonary edema.* In those situations, as well as in postoperative patients, noninvasive ventilation can improve pulmonary gas exchange rapidly and sometimes avoid the need for intubation (Table 7-31).

Continuous Positive Airway Pressure

CPAP is the addition of positive pressure (2.5 to 10.0 cm H_2O) during expiration in a spontaneously breathing patient. This is done through a tight-fitting mask, a nasal mask, or the expiratory limb of a T breathing circuit. CPAP may be indicated in hypoxemic patients because *it increases functional residual capacity and reduces $\dot{V}/\dot{Q}$ mismatch.* It is most useful in patients with pulmonary edema due to left ventricular failure.

Bi-level Ventilation

Bi-level ventilation applies *two different levels of airway pressurization* during the respiratory cycle. Inspiratory positive airway pressure (IPAP) is used during the inspiratory phase, assisting respiratory muscles and increasing minute ventilation. A lower level of pressurization is used during expiration (EPAP), acting much like PEEP to recruit alveolar spaces and to reduce the shunt effect. Ventilatory assistance is proportional to the IPAP-EPAP gradient, whereas oxygenation is mainly a factor of the EPAP level.

TABLE 7-31
CHARACTERISTICS OF PATIENTS SUCCESSFULLY TREATED WITH NONINVASIVE POSITIVE-PRESSURE VENTILATION
Cooperative patient
Intact neurologic function
Able to coordinate breathing with respirator
Moderate to moderately high (but not very high) severity of illness
Intact dentition
Able to control oral and pulmonary secretions
Moderate hypercapnia
Moderate respiratory acidosis (pH > 7.20)

Modified from Hill NS: Noninvasive ventilation. In Albert RK, Spiro SG, Jett JR, eds: Comprehensive Respiratory Medicine. London, Mosby, 1999:12.1-12.10.

High-Frequency Ventilation

High-frequency positive-pressure ventilation essentially delivers *small tidal volumes (1 to 3 mL/kg) at a high frequency of 60 to 120 breaths/minute.* Expiration remains passive, and PEEP may be added to the circuit.

High-frequency ventilation differs from conventional ventilation in that benefits are thought to be related to enhanced diffusivity of gas through increased turbulent flow and convective mixing in upper airways and at bronchial bifurcations and increased lung volume. These effects are achieved without generating the large peak airway pressures that would occur with conventional mechanical ventilation.

This mode of ventilation is particularly useful in patients with large bronchopleural fistulas because with conventional ventilation, the inspired air tends to take the path of low resistance and exit through the fistula. Other than to manage such patients, the role of high-frequency ventilation is unclear at present.

Extracorporeal Membrane Oxygenation

On occasion, maximum ventilatory support is insufficient to reverse hypoxemia, hypercapnia, or both. Although extracorporeal membrane oxygenation may salvage a few of these patients, multicentric National Institutes of Health trials have shown *no survival advantage* with extracorporeal membrane oxygenation over continued conventional ventilatory support.

CONCLUSION

Ventilatory support is primarily a therapeutic measure to supplement deficient gas exchange. Despite the availability of numerous commercial ventilators all performing satisfactorily, most clinical situations can be successfully managed by use of a limited number of ventilatory modes. The surgeon clinician must thus concentrate her or his expertise on these modes so that she or he is able to complement the expertise of the intensivist.

7

Management of Postoperative Complications

SUGGESTED READINGS

Review Articles

Cunningham DG: Mechanical ventilation—practice and pitfalls. Med North Am 1986;3:504-508.

Plummer AL, Gracey DR: Consensus conference on artificial airways in patients receiving mechanical ventilation. Chest 1989;96:178-180.

Hubmayr RD, Abel MD, Rehder K: Physiologic approach to mechanical ventilation. Crit Care Med 1990;18:103-113.

Tobin MJ: Mechanical ventilation. N Engl J Med 1994;330: 1056-1061.

Slutsky AS: Consensus conference on mechanical ventilation. Intensive Care Med 1994;20:64-79 (part I), 150-162 (part II).

Kacmarek RM: Current status of new modes of mechanical ventilation. Can Respir J 1996;3:357-360.

Stewart TE: Establishing an approach to mechanical ventilation. Can Respir J 1996;3:403-408.

Kalia P, Webster NR: Conventional ventilation and weaning. New modes of respiratory support. In Goldhill DR, Withington PS, eds: Textbook of Intensive Care. London, Chapman Hall Medical, 1997:401.

Gao F: Mechanical ventilation. In Casson AG, Johnston MR, eds: Key Topics in Thoracic Surgery. Oxford, UK, BIOS Scientific Publishers Limited, 1999:166-169.

Conrad SA, Bidani A: Management of the acute respiratory distress syndrome. Chest Surg Clin North Am 2002;12:325-354.

Cordingley JJ, Keogh BF: The pulmonary physician in critical care. 8: Ventilatory management of ALI/ARDS. Thorax 2002; 57:729-734.

Ventilation Modes

Feihl F, Perret C: Permissive hypercapnia. How permissive should we be? Am J Respir Crit Care Med 1994;150:1722-1737.

Marini JJ: Inverse ratio ventilation—simply an alternative, or something more? Crit Care Med 1995;23:224-228.

Villar J, Slutsky AS: PEEP or no PEEP: that is not the question. Can Respir J 1996;3:361-366.

Lee DL, Chiang HT, Lin SL, et al: Prone-position ventilation induces sustained improvement in oxygenation in patients with acute respiratory distress syndrome who have a large shunt. Crit Care Med 2002;30:1446-1452.

Monitoring

Hess D: Monitoring during mechanical ventilation. Can Respir J 1996;3:386-394.

Nitric Oxide

Fullerton DA, McIntyre RC: Inhaled nitric oxide: therapeutic applications in cardiothoracic surgery. Ann Thorac Surg 1996;61:1856-1864.

Kacmarek RM: Update on the use of inhaled nitric oxide. Can Respir J 1996;3:373-376.

Extracorporeal Membrane Oxygenation

Morris AH, Wallace CJ, Menlove RL, et al: Randomized clinical trial of pressure-controlled inverse ratio ventilation and extracorporeal CO_2 removal for adult respiratory distress syndrome. Am J Respir Crit Care Med 1994;149:295-305.

Demajo W: Update on extracorporeal oxygenation in adults. Can Respir J 1996;3:377-379.

Noninvasive Ventilation

Auriant I, Jallot A, Hervé P, et al: Noninvasive ventilation reduces mortality in acute respiratory failure following lung resection. Am J Respir Crit Care Med 2001;164:1231-1235.

Esteban A, Frutos-Vivar F, Ferguson ND, et al: Noninvasive positive-pressure ventilation for respiratory failure after extubation. N Engl J Med 2004;350:2452-2459.

Complications

Haake R, Schlichtig R, Ulstad DR, Henschen RR: Barotrauma. Pathophysiology, risk factors, and prevention. Chest 1987;91:608-613.

Chastre J, Fagon JY: Ventilator-associated pneumonia. Am J Respir Crit Care Med 2002;165:867-903.

Tracheotomy

Heffner JE, Miller KS, Sahn SA: Tracheostomy in the intensive care unit. Part 2: complications. Chest 1986;90:430-436.

Heffner JE: Medical indications for tracheotomy. Chest 1989; 96:186-190.

Ciaglia P, Graniero KD: Percutaneous dilatational tracheostomy. Results and long-term follow-up. Chest 1992;101:464-467.

Toursarkissian B, Zweng TN, Kearney PA, et al: Percutaneous dilational tracheostomy: report of 141 cases. Ann Thorac Surg 1994;57:862-867.

Powell DM, Price PD, Forrest LA: Review of percutaneous tracheostomy. Laryngoscope 1998;108:170-177.

Gysin C, Dulguerov P, Guyot JP, et al: Percutaneous versus surgical tracheostomy. A double-blind randomized trial. Ann Surg 1999;230:708-714.

Khalili TM, Koss W, Margulies DR, et al: Percutaneous dilatational tracheostomy is as safe as open tracheostomy. Am Surg 2002;68:92-94.

Engoren M, Arslanian-Engoren C, Fenn-Guderer N: Hospital and long-term outcome after tracheostomy for respiratory failure. Chest 2004;125:220-227.

ARRHYTHMIAS

Supraventricular tachyarrhythmias, especially atrial fibrillations, are common after all types of thoracic surgical procedures including pulmonary and esophageal operations. Their etiology is unclear, but several risk factors, such as older age, preexisting cardiac disease, and pneumonectomy, have been identified.

Most arrhythmias occur *within the first 3 postoperative days* with a peak incidence at 48 hours. These arrhythmias are generally a transient phenomenon that seldom leads to hemodynamic instability. It has been suggested, however, that atrial fibrillation may be associated with increased mortality and longer postoperative hospital stay.

General principles of management include the *identification and correction of causative factors, the control of heart rate, the restoration and maintenance of sinus rhythm,* and *the prevention of complications* such as cardiac failure and thromboembolism.

ATRIAL ARRHYTHMIAS

Etiology

Much speculation still exists with regard to the underlying mechanisms involved in the production of postoperative atrial arrhythmias. It is likely, however, that they result from the *synergistic action of several factors* (Table 7-32).

Autonomic imbalance with increased vagal tone, excessive production of catecholamines, and possibly direct damage to sympathetic and parasympathetic nerves innervating the heart are probably important mechanisms. Similarly, interstitial mobilization of fluids and generous intraoperative fluid administration may result in *atrial dilatation,* which may affect its electrical properties.

Other mechanisms likely to be involved include pulmonary hypertension and dilatation of the right side of the heart more commonly seen after pneumonectomy, hypoxemia, and local inflammation of the pericardium.

Risk Factors

The identification of risk factors (Table 7-33) for postoperative atrial arrhythmias has been attempted in several studies, but unfortunately, authors often have different or even contradictory data about the clinical significance of each factor.

Patients with a *previous history of atrial arrhythmia* are at definite increased risk for postoperative atrial arrhythmias. Similarly, *older patients* (>70 years) and patients with a *history of high blood pressure* have an increased risk of postoperative arrhythmias. It is likely that such individuals already have cardiac structural changes, such as atrial dilatation, muscle atrophy, or decreased conduction, that may predispose to atrial arrhythmias. It also seems clear that patients who have had a *pneumonectomy,* especially those with added radical lymphadenectomy, are more at risk than are patients who have had a lobectomy. This is probably related to the extent of cardiopulmonary denervation as well as to the transient pulmonary vasoconstriction and right-sided heart dilatation associated with pneumonectomy.

Concomitant coronary artery disease as evidenced by a clinical history of angina, an abnormal electrocardiogram, or an abnormal exercise test is likely to be a predictor of postoperative dysrhythmias. Another factor probably involved is whether the pulmonary resection was done with

---

TABLE 7-32
UNDERLYING MECHANISMS OF POSTOPERATIVE ATRIAL ARRHYTHMIAS
Autonomic imbalance with increase in vagal tone and excessive production of catecholamines
Mobilization of fluid with resultant atrial dilatation
Hypoxemia
Pulmonary hypertension and dilatation of right side of the heart
Local inflammation of the pericardium

TABLE 7-33		
RISK FACTORS FOR POSTOPERATIVE ATRIAL ARRHYTHMIAS		
FACTORS LIKELY TO BE RELATED		
Preoperative		
Older age		
Previous history of atrial arrhythmias		
High blood pressure		
Intraoperative		
Pneumonectomy (versus lobectomy)		
Radical nodal dissection		
FACTORS POSSIBLY RELATED		
Preoperative		
Concomitant arteriosclerotic heart disease		
Intraoperative		
Intrapericardial pulmonary resection		
FACTORS NOT LIKELY TO BE RELATED		
Preoperative		
Gender		
Pulmonary function		
Intraoperative		
Abnormal hemodynamics (prolonged hypotension)		

intrapericardial ligation of blood vessels. Under such circumstances, it is reasonable to hypothesize that *operative manipulations* of the pericardium or of the atria may play a role in the initiation of postoperative episodes of atrial fibrillation.

Factors *not likely* to be related include gender of the patient, preoperative pulmonary function, and abnormal hemodynamics such as hypotensive episodes that may have occurred during the surgery.

Clinical Manifestations and Consequences

Atrial arrhythmias including paroxistic atrial tachycardia, atrial fibrillation, and atrial flutter usually occur within 3 days of surgery (80% of cases). Their overall incidence is *in the range of 12% to 15%*.

Clinically, a number of patients remain asymptomatic even if they have an irregular and elevated heart rate. In other patients, the loss of atrial contraction and atrioventricular synchronization can present with hypotension, chest pain and discomfort, and palpitations if the heart rate is fast. Signs and symptoms of heart failure can also develop.

The risk of atrial fibrillation–related stroke is 5% per year versus approximately 1% for the general population. This potential develops early after the onset of the arrhythmia, and it is higher in patients who are *on and off* these arrhythmias.

Diagnosis

The diagnosis of atrial arrhythmias is often suspected by an irregular pulse and confirmed by an electrocardiogram. Obviously, if the patient is still being

7

Management of Postoperative Complications

directly monitored, whether in the ICU or by Holter recording, the diagnosis is straightforward.

Once the diagnosis is substantiated, patients should have blood work for hemoglobin and electrolyte values to make sure that there are no important derangements that could have precipitated the arrhythmia. They should also have analysis of arterial blood gases to ensure that there is *no important hypoxemia.* Although cardiac echography may be useful to demonstrate the presence of a preexisting cardiopathy, of atrial dilatation, or of an atrial thrombus, this examination *does not need* to be done before treatment is initiated.

All patients with acute-onset atrial arrhythmias *should be monitored* with the Holter technique. If they are hemodynamically unstable, they should be transferred to an ICU or coronary care unit.

Treatment

Prophylaxis

Prophylactic digitalization has been suggested for older patients (>50 years) undergoing pulmonary resection. Unfortunately, this strategy has a variable effect on the incidence of atrial arrhythmias, and in one study, it was actually found to increase the frequency and severity of arrhythmias.

Other studies using flecainide (class IC antiarrhythmic drug), amiodarone (class III antiarrhythmic drug), and diltiazem (calcium channel blocker) as prophylaxis for postoperative arrhythmias have shown a reduction in the incidence of clinically significant atrial arrhythmias, but *no difference in overall morbidity and length of stay* could be identified in any of these trials.

As a result, most thoracic surgeons *do not* routinely use prophylaxis for atrial fibrillation after pulmonary resection except perhaps in high-risk patients. Individuals receiving antiarrhythmic agents preoperatively should, however, take their regular medication throughout the perioperative period.

Treatment

General Treatment Principles. In the postoperative setting, the triggering factor for the arrhythmia must always be *sought and corrected* if possible. This would apply, for instance, to patients with severe hypoxemia, electrolyte imbalance (hypokalemia), or low hemoglobin. Similarly, if the chest radiograph shows evidence of atelectasis or pneumonia, this should be actively treated.

The urgency of and mode of therapy for the arrhythmia itself are dictated by the *degree of hemodynamic impairment* imposed by the arrhythmia. In actual practice, the ventricular rate has to be controlled (goal of heart rate of around 80 to 100 beats/minute), and sinus rhythm must be restored and maintained by either pharmacologic therapy or electrical cardioversion.

Pharmacologic Therapy (Table 7-34). An attempt should be made to control ventricular response in all patients presenting with postoperative atrial arrhythmias. Patients who are asymptomatic with a normal blood

TABLE 7-34
DRUGS COMMONLY USED TO TREAT POSTOPERATIVE ATRIAL ARRHYTHMIAS

Drugs to Control Heart Rate	IV Bolus	IV Infusion	Oral Dose	Comments
Digoxin	0.5 mg (with subsequent doses of 0.25 mg IV q 6 h)		0.25 mg daily	Less effective when sympathetic nervous system is active
Calcium channel blockers				May cause bradycardia and hypotension
Diltiazem (Cardizem)	0.25 mg/kg*	5-15 mg/h[†]	180-360 mg/day	
Verapamil (Isoptin)	0.15 mg/kg[‡]	0.05 mg/kg/h[§]	120-480 mg/day	
Beta-adrenergic blockers				
Propranolol	1 mg every 5 min (maximum of 5 mg)	2-3 mg/h	10-80 mg q 6-8 h	May cause bradycardia, hypotension, bronchospasm
Antiarrhythmic drugs				
Class IA				
Procainamide	10-15 mg/kg	1-6 mg/min	500-2000 mg twice/day	May cause hypotension
Class III				
Amiodarone (Cordarone)	150 mg[‖]	1000 mg/day	200-400 mg/day	May cause lung toxicity (interstitial fibrosis)

*Initial bolus of 0.25 mg/kg given IV in 2 minutes; if the response is not satisfactory, give a second bolus 15 minutes later.
[†]Initial recommended perfusion of 10 mg/h; to be readjusted according to response.
[‡]Initial bolus of 2.5 to 5.0 mg given IV in 2 minutes; additional boluses of 5 to 10 mg IV can be given every 15 to 30 minutes up to a total of 20 mg. For older patients (>60 years old), give bolus in 5 minutes.
[§]Perfusion at 2.5 to 10 mg/h.
[‖]Initial bolus of 150 mg diluted in 50 mL of 5% dextrose or 0.9% NaCl given IV in 10 minutes.
Modified from Ommen SR, Odell JA, Stanton MS: Atrial arrhythmias after cardiothoracic surgery. N Engl J Med 1997;336:1429-1434.

7

Management of Postoperative Complications

pressure *are easily treated with digoxin,* which decreases ventricular rate by slowing conduction in the atrioventricular node without impairing myocardial contractility (has a positive inotropic effect). The average-size adult should receive 0.5 mg intravenously followed by two or three subsequent doses of 0.25 mg given every 6 hours or more rapidly if indicated. Subsequently, a maintenance dose of 0.25 mg is given daily.

Patients demonstrating evidence of circulatory compromise (hypotension, dizziness, angina) or patients with heart rates above 160 beats/minute require more urgent drug therapy. In such cases, *calcium channel blockers* like verapamil and diltiazem are effective in providing rapid slowing of ventricular response when they are administered intravenously. Calcium channel blockers have a more direct effect on the atrioventricular node than does digoxin, and they are easier to administer because their infusion through the intravenous route *allows better control.* Verapamil may be given at an initial dose of 2.5 mg intravenously, and the dose can be repeated every 10 to 15 minutes to a maximum of 15 mg. Beta-adrenergic blockers (propranolol) can also be given, but these drugs may initiate severe bronchospasm.

In some cases, chemical cardioversion can be attempted, and as a rule, it is more effective in recent-onset atrial fibrillation and flutter (>48 hours). For this purpose, the best-known conventional treatment is intravenous *procainamide,* a class IA antiarrhythmic (see Table 7-34). More recently, *intravenous amiodarone* (class III antiarrhythmic) has also been used. Antiarrhythmia agents may have potentially severe side effects, including pulmonary toxicity from amiodarone.

Pharmacologic therapy of atrial arrhythmias should always be done in a monitored environment, and it is our policy to administer these medications under the advice and supervision of a cardiologist.

Electrical Cardioversion. Patients may occasionally experience severe circulation compromise with new-onset atrial arrhythmias, which may need urgent treatment. In such cases, electrical cardioversion has a success rate of approximately 90%, but it requires a short period of general anesthesia. After cardioversion, digoxin or diltiazem should be given to reduce the risks of recurrence.

Long-term Management

Most patients revert to sinus rhythm once their heart rate has been slowed by digoxin or calcium channel blockers. Even if they have converted to sinus rhythm, they should be discharged home with either *digoxin or diltiazem* for a period of 8 to 12 weeks.

Because of the significant risk of thromboembolic accidents, all patients *should be anticoagulated,* even those who have converted to sinus rhythm. Most physicians initiate anticoagulation with heparin as soon as the risk of bleeding is minimal (usually 48 to 72 hours after routine cases). Warfarin therapy should then be continued for 3 to 6 months, with an international normalized ratio of 2.0 to 3.0 being recommended. This strategy is strongly recommended even if no studies have specifically addressed the issue of risk-benefit ratio of anticoagulant therapy in atrial arrhythmias occurring after general thoracic surgical procedures.

OTHER ARRHYTHMIAS

Ventricular arrhythmias are uncommon after thoracic operations, and they usually consist of isolated ventricular premature beats. These *are not treated,* and they will resolve spontaneously.

Heart block should be managed as it would be in a nonsurgical patient.

CONCLUSION

Although the cause of postoperative atrial arrhythmias is still speculative, this complication is *common* after pulmonary resections. Whether its occurrence can be prevented by prophylactic therapy remains unclear at present. It is likely, however, that improved knowledge of risk factors and advances in antiarrhythmic therapy will allow the surgeon to identify the high-risk patient who could benefit from such prophylaxis.

Because embolic stroke could be a devastating complication of atrial fibrillation, even in the postoperative setting, it seems prudent to add anticoagulation with warfarin to the usual treatment.

SUGGESTED READINGS

Review Articles

Ommen SR, Odell JA, Stanton MS: Atrial arrhythmias after cardiothoracic surgery. N Engl J Med 1997;336:1429-1434.

Amar D: Cardiac arrhythmias. Chest Surg Clin North Am 1998; 8:479-493.

Samson M: Atrial fibrillation: a practical approach to treatment. Can J CME 1999;August:119-127.

De Decker K, Jorens PG, Van Schil P: Cardiac complications after noncardiac thoracic surgery: an evidence-based current review. Ann Thorac Surg 2003;75:1340-1348.

Prophylaxis

Ritchie AJ, Bowe P, Gibbons JRP: Prophylactic digitalization for thoracotomy: a reassessment. Ann Thorac Surg 1990;50:86-88.

Van Mieghem W, Tits G, Demuynck K, et al: Verapamil as prophylactic treatment for atrial fibrillation after lung operations. Ann Thorac Surg 1996;61:1083-1086.

Terzi A, Furlan G, Chiavacci P, et al: Prevention of atrial tachyarrhythmias after non-cardiac thoracic surgery by infusion of magnesium sulfate. Thorac Cardiovasc Surg 1996;44:300-303.

Amar D, Roistacher N, Burt ME, et al: Effects of diltiazem versus digoxin on dysrhythmias and cardiac function after pneumonectomy. Ann Thorac Surg 1997;63:1374-1382.

7

Management of Postoperative Complications

Bayliff CD, Massel DR, Inculet RI, et al: Propranolol for the prevention of postoperative arrhythmias in general thoracic surgery. Ann Thorac Surg 1999;67:182-186.

Amar D, Roistacher N, Rusch VW, et al: Effects of diltiazem prophylaxis on the incidence and clinical outcome of atrial arrhythmias after thoracic surgery. J Thorac Cardiovasc Surg 2000;120:790-798.

Lanza LA, Visbal AI, DeValeria PA, et al: Low-dose oral amiodarone prophylaxis reduces atrial fibrillation after pulmonary resection. Ann Thorac Surg 2003;75:223-230.

Treatment

Ciriaco P, Mazzone P, Canneto B, Zannini P: Supraventricular arrhythmia following lung resection for non–small cell lung cancer and its treatment with amiodarone. Eur J Cardiothorac Surg 2000;18:12-16.

Case Series

Asamura H, Naruke T, Tsuchiya R, et al: What are the risk factors for arrhythmias after thoracic operations? A retrospective multivariate analysis of 267 consecutive thoracic operations. J Thorac Cardiovasc Surg 1993;106:1104-1110.

Amar D, Roistacher N, Burt M, et al: Clinical and echocardiographic correlates of symptomatic tachydysrhythmias after noncardiac thoracic surgery. Chest 1995;108:349-354.

Curtis JJ, Parker BM, McKenney CA, et al: Incidence and predictors of supraventricular dysrhythmias after pulmonary resection. Ann Thorac Surg 1998;66:1766-1771.

Cardinale D, Martinoni A, Cipolla CM, et al: Atrial fibrillation after operation for lung cancer: clinical and prognostic significance. Ann Thorac Surg 1999;68:1827-1831.

Rena O, Papalia E, Oliaro A, et al: Supraventricular arrhythmias after resection surgery of the lung. Eur J Cardiothorac Surg 2001; 20:688-693.

Ventricular Arrhythmias

Amar D, Zhang H, Roistacher N: The incidence and outcome of ventricular arrhythmias after noncardiac thoracic surgery. Anesth Analg 2002;95:537-543.

PROLONGED AIR LEAKS AND SPACE PROBLEMS

Nearly all patients undergoing lobectomies or lesser resections can be expected to have *some degree* of postoperative air leakage. Whereas most of these air leaks will stop within a few days of surgery, those persisting for more than 1 week should be considered a complication because they are associated with increased morbidity and prolonged hospitalization.

Post-resectional spaces are the result of failure of one or more components of normal space obliteration mechanisms, and their occurrence is greatly facilitated by the presence of persistent and significant air leaks. In the majority of cases, however, such spaces are relatively innocuous and will resolve without specific treatment.

PROLONGED AIR LEAKS

Terminology and Incidence

Although prolonged air leaks can be defined as those persisting beyond a normal hospital stay, most surgeons consider that air leaks *lasting more than 7 days* after surgery are significant complications because they delay hospital discharge, increase the possibility of other morbidities, increase costs, and expose the patient to complicating empyemas. After lobectomy, approximately 10% to 15% of patients will have an air leak for more than 7 days, and 5% will have it for more than 14 days.

Pathogenesis and Predictors (Table 7-35)

Postoperative air leaks are related to *surgical disruption of peripheral lung surfaces*, mostly intersegmental planes and fissures, or to damage to residual parenchyma during mobilization, retraction, and manipulation. In general, the duration of an air leak is *directly proportional* to the healing potential of the residual lung as well as its ability to re-expand and come into contact with the parietal pleura. Most surgeons believe that close apposition between lung and parietal pleura promotes healing of the source of the air leak by *initiating an inflammatory reaction* that will subsequently lead to fibrin deposition and granulation formation.

TABLE 7-35
PREDICTORS OF PROLONGED AIR LEAKS
FACTORS AFFECTING HEALING PROCESS OF THE LUNG (PREOPERATIVE FACTORS)
Older age
Chronic obstructive pulmonary disease
Chronic steroid therapy
Malnutrition
SEVERITY OF INTRAOPERATIVE TRAUMA
Reoperations
Incomplete fissures
Aggressive manipulations of the lung
Inadequate suturing of parenchymal tears
Type of operation: upper lobectomies, decortication, lung volume reduction surgery
FACTORS AFFECTING LUNG RE-EXPANSION
Impaired expansibility of residual lung due to interstitial fibrosis or thickening of visceral pleura
Incomplete mobilization of residual lung
Not enough lung to fill up the space
Inadequate control of the pleural space

7

Management of Postoperative Complications

Prolonged air leaks can be related to *factors that affect the normal healing process of the lung.* Indeed, air leaks have been shown to be more prevalent in older patients and among emphysema patients who already have abnormal parenchyma. It is a source of considerable morbidity, for instance, in patients undergoing lung volume reduction procedures. Chronic steroid therapy and malnutrition are also significant predictors because they impair the inflammatory reaction and fibroblast proliferation necessary for the rapid sealing of air leaks.

Reoperations are nearly always associated with significant air leakage because they involve retraction of the lung and lysis of adhesions between lung surface and parietal pleura. Fortunately, this extensive mobilization can also lead to an *increased inflammatory* reaction, which may in turn decrease the duration of the air leak. Incomplete fissures and technical considerations, such as inadequate closure of the pulmonary parenchyma or failure to use reinforced staple lines in severely emphysematous patients, are also predictors of prolonged air leaks. *Upper lobectomies* (versus lower lobectomies) are thought to be associated with an increased incidence of prolonged air leaks because a large apical space often remains. Patients who undergo bullectomy, *lung volume reduction surgery,* and decortication are also at high risk for significant and prolonged air leaks.

Perhaps the most important factors in the pathogenesis of prolonged air leaks are those related to the *re-expansion of the lung.* These include low compliance of the residual lung because of interstitial fibrosis or thickening of visceral pleura; residual lobes that have been incompletely mobilized; and simply insufficient amount of residual lung to fill up the space, a situation that is possible after bilobectomies or overzealous volume reduction procedures.

Prolonged air leaks can finally be facilitated by poor control of the postoperative pleural space. Factors such as inadequate number and location of chest tubes, faulty suction systems, and failure to establish negative pleural pressures, at least initially, are potential predictors of prolonged air leaks because they may prevent lung expansion and pleural apposition.

Management

Intraoperative Techniques to Prevent Air Leaks (Table 7-36)

Prolonged air leaks can be avoided by securing an airtight closure of the pulmonary parenchyma, particularly during dissection of the interlobar fissures or intersegmental planes. Currently, the best means of fulfilling this objective is to staple the fissures and in high-risk cases *to use buttressed staples with bovine pericardium* or other material. Pulmonary sealants such as fibrin glues or polyethylene glycol–based gels that are polymerized on the lung surface can also be used, although their efficacy is as yet unproven. Simple maneuvers such as making sure that the remaining lobe is completely mobilized and that no visceral peel prevents its re-expansion are also useful to stimulate complete re-expansion of pulmonary remnants.

TABLE 7-36
INTRAOPERATIVE TECHNIQUES TO PREVENT AIR LEAKS
Standard closure of parenchymal tears
Buttressed staple closure of fissures in high-risk cases (emphysema patients)
Use of pulmonary sealants
Decortication (when necessary) and complete mobilization of residual lung
Bronchoscopy at conclusion of procedure
Prophylactic space reduction
Infiltration of phrenic nerve
Pleural tent
Intraoperative pneumoperitoneum

7

Bronchoscopy performed at the conclusion of the procedure will help clear the airway and re-expand the residual lung.

Prophylactic space reduction may be helpful in selected high-risk cases. Infiltration of bupivacaine (Marcaine) around the phrenic nerve (usually in the fatty tissues just above the diaphragm) will result in a temporary diaphragmatic paralysis that will last a few hours to several days. After lower lobectomy or bilobectomy, the creation of a pneumoperitoneum by transdiaphragmatic injection of 1000 mL of room air can raise further the hemidiaphragm.

Parietal pleural plasty (pleural tent) is a simple and effective technique most useful in the prevention of apical spaces after upper lobectomy (Fig. 7-1). The parietal pleura is stripped over the apex, and its free edge is resutured over the upper edge of the thoracotomy, *thus leaving an extrapleural space.* The advantage of this procedure is that the remaining lung may rise to its own level as the pleural tent is flexible and may be pushed right back into the apex if the remaining lung expands well.

Older techniques, such as adjunctive tailoring thoracoplasty and diaphragmatic advancement, are *no longer used.* They offer no advantage over the less morbid techniques of apical tenting and pneumoperitoneum.

When the potential for prolonged air leak is recognized intraoperatively, accurate placement of at least two chest tubes is of critical importance.

Immediate Postoperative Techniques to Seal Air Leaks

Obliteration of the pleural space is the most important single factor in the immediate management of air leaks. The chest tube should be connected to an active suction system with an initial negative pressure of 20 cm H_2O, and the surgeon must make sure that the chest tubes are functioning properly and that all connectors and sites of tube insertion are airtight. On occasion, the *negative pressure in the suction system can be increased* to 40 or 50 cm H_2O so that space obliteration is helped by increasing mediastinal shift, evacuating residual air, and counteracting the high intrapleural negative pressure secondary to pulmonary resection.

Management of Postoperative Complications

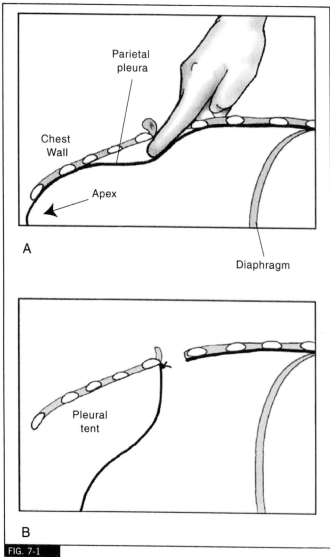

FIG. 7-1

Creation of a pleural tent at thoracotomy. **(A)** The parietal pleura is stripped from the endothoracic fascia beginning at the incision level and going up to the apex. **(B)** Its free edge is resutured over the upper edge of the thoracotomy.

Pain control, active physiotherapy, and even bronchoscopy are exceedingly important to ensure that no mucus or blood prevents maximal re-expansion of the lung.

It has been shown by Dr. Robert J. Cerfolio that terminating suction early (by day 2 or 3) and placing chest tubes to an underwater seal may be helpful not only to decrease the size of the air leak but also to seal it more quickly. If a pneumothorax occurs or subcutaneous emphysema develops, chest tubes can simply be reconnected to an active suction system at lower negative pressure (-10 cm H_2O). The *slight withdrawal* of chest tubes (1 or 2 cm) may often stop the air leak by removing the tube from the actual site of the leak.

If the air leak is small and the lung is fully re-expanded, *provocative clamping* can be tried. This technique involves clamping the tube for 12 to 24 hours and removing it if no pneumothorax or subcutaneous emphysema has developed during the interval. In some cases, the tube can even be removed in the presence of a small and well-tolerated pneumothorax.

Options in the Management of Prolonged Air Leaks

Although several options (Table 7-37) are available to manage prolonged air leaks, the treatment often has to be individualized to a given patient. Overall, however, *patience is the golden rule* not only for the patient and the patient's relatives but also for the surgeon.

All patients with an air leak lasting more than 7 to 10 days *should have bronchoscopy* to rule out stump dehiscence as the source of the leak. If the bronchus is normal, the first possible option is continuous in-hospital observation on an active drainage system with *minimal amount* of suction. This strategy mainly applies to patients with large air leaks or to patients whose lung collapses when suction is discontinued. It is often useful to initiate a pneumoperitoneum with the objective of raising the diaphragm and reducing the size of the space. Initially, 1000 mL of air is insufflated in the peritoneal cavity, and this is followed by the injection of 500 mL of air daily thereafter (Fig. 7-2). Although seldom done, an alternative technique is to inject bupivacaine around the phrenic nerve in the neck to temporarily paralyze the hemidiaphragm.

TABLE 7-37
MANAGEMENT OPTIONS FOR PATIENTS WITH PROLONGED AIR LEAKS DUE TO PERIPHERAL ALVEOLAR FISTULA
Bronchoscopy should always be done to rule out stump dehiscence
Continuous observation on a drainage system
Pneumoperitoneum (mostly effective after lower lobectomy)
Cervical phrenic nerve infiltration with protected needle
Pleurodesis with talc, autologous blood, or doxycycline
Embolization of bronchial tree with Gelfoam or coils
Reoperation
Sending the patient home with a chest tube connected to a Heimlich valve

7

Management of Postoperative Complications

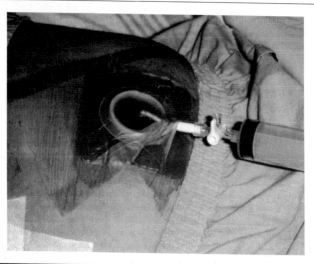

Peritoneal catheter in place. The catheter is used to create a pneumoperitoneum and to maintain the pressure by daily air insufflations.

Another possibility is to attempt *bedside pleurodesis* with asbestos-free talc (2.5 to 5 g diluted in 60 mL of normal saline), autologous blood (150 mL), or other sclerotic agents such as doxycycline. These products are injected in the chest tube, which is then irrigated with 100 mL of normal saline to prevent clogging. All of these techniques are *best used when the lung is fully expanded* because their primary objective is to promote pleural apposition and sealing of air leaks by stimulating a greater inflammatory reaction. Possible side effects include chest pain, fever, and occlusion of the chest tubes.

Embolizing the feeding subsegmental bronchus with Gelfoam or coils can sometimes be useful. This bronchoscopic technique involves localizing the subsegmental bronchus feeding the air leak with a Fogarty catheter and then embolizing it. Unfortunately, these techniques are often unsuccessful, either because air leakage originates from several sites over the residual lung, or because the emboli will become dislocated during vigorous coughing.

Reoperation for persistent air leaks is seldom indicated (0.05% of all cases), especially if the patient is beyond 2 to 3 weeks postoperatively. If an operation is warranted, however, it can be done with the use of video-assisted thoracoscopic surgery (VATS) techniques.

If patients still have an air leak by the time they are ready to be discharged from the hospital, their chest tube can be connected to a Heimlich valve and the valve attached to commercially available drainage bags or alternatively to a Foley leg bag with several holes cut in the top of the bag so that the air can escape. It has been shown that this technique is safe (few complications) and effective (high incidence of resolution of air leaks). In most patients, the chest tube can be removed 2 to 3 weeks later even if there is a small residual pneumothorax.

SPACE PROBLEMS

Terminology and Incidence

Although there is no precise definition of a post-resectional space, it is generally agreed that when *full expansion of the lung is not achieved* after lobectomy or lesser resections, a persistent pleural space exists. The incidence is thought to be approximately 20% to 25%, although if one were to do a CT scan in every lobectomy patient, the incidence would more likely be in the neighborhood of 75% to 90%.

Persistent spaces (Table 7-38) can be apical or basilar and can be further classified as being infected or not. *Noninfected spaces* are characterized by being small and getting smaller on serial radiographs and by their thin walls. Most of these spaces have no or minimal and decreasing amounts of fluid, and they are asymptomatic. Patients with *infected spaces* have fever and leukocytosis, and they are generally ill. These spaces are large and getting larger, have a thick wall, and contain fluid in increasing amounts. Spaces can finally be classified as *having or not having a fistula,* at either the alveolar (persistent air leak) or bronchial (bronchopleural fistula) level.

Pathogenesis and Predictors

Persistent spaces generally result from the *failure of one or more components of the normal space obliteration mechanisms* (Table 7-39). These include the shift of adjacent dynamic structures, such as the heart, mediastinum, and diaphragm; the approximation of ribs with internal bulging of the intercostal muscles; the hyperinflation of the remaining lung and its anatomic rearrangements; and the intrapleural accumulation of blood and serum over the surface of the lung and in recesses and fissures. This obliteration is facilitated by the negative intrapleural pressure generated by active tube

TABLE 7-38
CLASSIFICATION OF PERSISTENT SPACES
Based on anatomy of the space: apical, basilar
Based on status of the space
Infected
Fever, leukocytosis
Space is large and getting larger
Thick walls
Noninfected
Asymptomatic
Space is small and getting smaller
Thin walls
Based on presence or absence of an associated fistula (peripheral, central)

7

Management of Postoperative Complications

TABLE 7-39
NORMAL SPACE OBLITERATION MECHANISMS
Shift of adjacent dynamic structures, such as the heart or diaphragm
Approximation of ribs and narrowing of intercostal spaces
Hyperinflation of residual lung
Intrapleural accumulation of blood and serum

suction, lack of air leakage from the lung, and unimpaired expansibility of the residual parenchyma.

Factors that predispose to space problems (Table 7-40) thus include inability of the residual lung to fill the space due to previous resection, interstitial fibrosis or presence of constricting visceral peel over the lung surface, extent of resection (bilobectomy), and presence of a fixed mediastinum. In the end, the *most important factor* that predisposes to space problems, especially to infected and complicated spaces, *is a persistent and large air leak* and inefficiency of the drainage system to evacuate it.

Management

Intraoperative Techniques to Prevent Spaces

Certain intraoperative maneuvers can be used to prevent postoperative spaces (Table 7-41). First and foremost, the surgeon must *eliminate air leakage* from the residual lung by using all techniques previously described. Second, the surgeon must make sure that the residual lung is given a chance to re-expand. In cases of right lung partial resections (upper or lower lobectomy), this means leaving the middle lobe whenever possible because this lobe, even if it looks small, *helps fill the space.*

It also means decortication of a restrictive visceral pleura peel if it is present and complete freeing of parietal pleura adhesions so that the pulmonary remnants have a chance to be spatially reoriented. If the lower lobe is the residual lobe, the inferior pulmonary ligament must be divided.

If the remaining lung appears too small to fill the space, one can reduce the confines of the pleural space by pleural tenting (after upper lobectomy), pneumoperitoneum (after lower lobectomy), or phrenic nerve infiltration.

When the potential for post-resectional space is recognized intraoperatively, the surgeon must finally ensure that at least *two chest tubes* are accurately positioned and connected to an active drainage system.

TABLE 7-40
RISK FACTORS FOR PERSISTENT SPACES
Inability of residual lung to fill the space
Previous resection
Underlying fibrosis
Visceral peel on lung surface
Extent of resection: bilobectomy
Persistent large air leak
Fixed mediastinum

TABLE 7-41

INTRAOPERATIVE TECHNIQUES TO PREVENT SPACES

Minimize air leaks.
Ensure that residual lung can re-expand.
   Leave middle lobe if possible.
   Decorticate remaining lobe when needed.
   Lyse all parietal adhesions.
   Divide inferior pulmonary ligament.
Reduce confines of pleural space.
Position accurately at least two chest tubes.

Immediate Postoperative Techniques to Obliterate the Space

Given enough time, most residual spaces will be obliterated without complications, and indeed the old belief that all such spaces represent a major problem is unfounded. If a potentially complicated space is noted early, the two most important aspects of management are *to ensure that it is well drained and to achieve maximal lung expansion.* Pain control and effective chest physiotherapy are also important, and any evidence of atelectasis should be managed by bedside flexible bronchoscopy. Once the air leak has stopped and the space is stable, the tubes can be pulled out. If a space is noted after the tubes have been pulled out, nothing further should be done unless there are signs of infection within the space. Thoracentesis or further drainage is not indicated because there are *significant risks* of infecting a previously sterile space.

Options in the Management of Complicated Spaces

Persistent spaces can become a problem if they are *associated with a prolonged air leak* or *if they subsequently become infected.* These problems often occur together because the residual space will prevent sealing of the air leak, and eventually infection will enter the space either from the chest tube or from the upper airway. In such cases, prolonged drainage will be necessary either in a closed fashion (tube drainage) or by open drainage once sufficient adhesions have formed to prevent lung collapse. Conversion to open drainage allows the surgeon to gain time, and given enough time, several of the infected spaces will be obliterated through contraction of the chest wall and lung re-expansion.

Options for further management of infected spaces with or without peripheral fistulas are given in Table 7-42.

Limited five-rib thoracoplasty is ideally suited for apical spaces that can also be filled with either a turnover pectoralis major flap or the latissimus dorsi. Basilar spaces are best obliterated by filling them with a muscle flap or with the greater omentum.

CONCLUSION

For most patients, prolonged air leaks and complicated space problems can be prevented through systematic use of prophylactic measures applied during the operation. If they should nevertheless occur, the surgeon must

TABLE 7-42

OPTIONS FOR FURTHER MANAGEMENT OF CHRONICALLY INFECTED SPACES

Anatomy of the Space	Management
Apical space	Thoracoplasty
	Muscle flap
	Pectoralis major
	Latissimus dorsi
Basilar space	Muscle flap
	Latissimus dorsi
	Serratus anterior
	Rectus abdominis
	Omentoplasty

be not only patient in his or her approach to the complication but also rational and sequential. Most important, the patient and the patient's relatives must be told that resolution of the complication may take a substantial amount of time.

SUGGESTED READINGS

Review Articles

Rice TW, Kirby TJ: Prolonged air leak. Chest Surg Clin North Am 1992;2:803-811.

Barker WL: Natural history of residual air spaces after pulmonary resection. Chest Surg Clin North Am 1996;6:585-613.

Miller JI Jr.: Acute and delayed space problems following pulmonary resection. Chest Surg Clin North Am 1996;6:615-621.

Rice TW, Okereke IC, Blackstone EH: Persistent air-leak following pulmonary resection. Chest Surg Clin North Am 2002;12:529-539.

Loran DB, Woodside KJ, Cerfolio RJ, Zwischenberger JB: Predictors of alveolar air leaks. Chest Surg Clin North Am 2002;12:477-488.

Cerfolio RJ: Treatment of persistent air leaks. Proceedings of the AATS Symposium on General Thoracic Surgery, 2002:132-134.

Air Leaks

Yokomise H, Satoh K, Ohno N, Tamura K: Autoblood plus OK 432 pleurodesis with open drainage for persistent air leak after lobectomy. Ann Thorac Surg 1998;65:563-565.

Cerfolio RJ, Tummala RP, Holman WL, et al: A prospective algorithm for the management of air leaks after pulmonary resection. Ann Thorac Surg 1998;66:1726-1731.

Abolhoda A, Liu D, Brooks A, Burt M: Prolonged air leak following radical upper lobectomy. An analysis of incidence and possible risk factors. Chest 1998;113:1507-1510.

Cerfolio RJ, Bass C, Katholi CR: Prospective randomized trial compares suction versus water seal for air leaks. Ann Thorac Surg 2001;71:1613-1617.

Cerfolio RJ, Bass CS, Pask AH, Katholi CR: Predictors and treatment of persistent air leaks. Ann Thorac Surg 2002;73:1727-1731.

Brunelli A, Monteverde M, Borri A, et al: Predictors of prolonged air leak after pulmonary lobectomy. Ann Thorac Surg 2004;77:1205-1210.

Prophylaxis, Air Leaks

Wong K, Goldstraw P: Effect of fibrin glue in the reduction of postthoracotomy alveolar air leak. Ann Thorac Surg 1997;64:979-981.

Brunelli A, Fianchini A: Prolonged air leak following upper lobectomy. In search of the key. Chest 1999;116:848.

Macchiarini P, Wain J, Almy S, Dartevelle P: Experimental and clinical evaluation of a new synthetic, absorbable sealant to reduce air leaks in thoracic operations. J Thorac Cardiovasc Surg 1999;117:751-758.

Stammberger U, Klepetko W, Stamatis G, et al: Buttressing the staple line in lung volume reduction surgery: a randomized three-center study. Ann Thorac Surg 2000;70:1820-1825.

Porte HL, Jany T, Akkad R, et al: Randomized controlled trial of a synthetic sealant for preventing alveolar air leaks after lobectomy. Ann Thorac Surg 2001;71:1618-1622.

Wain JC, Kaiser LR, Johnstone DW, et al: Trial of a novel synthetic sealant in preventing air leaks after lung resection. Ann Thorac Surg 2001;71:1623-1629.

Toloza EM, Harpole DH Jr.: Intraoperative techniques to prevent air leaks. Chest Surg Clin North Am 2002;12:489-405.

Fabian T, Federico JA, Ponn RB: Fibrin glue in pulmonary resection: a prospective, randomized, blinded study. Ann Thorac Surg 2003;75:1587-1592.

Treatment

Cooper JD: Technique to reduce air leaks after resection of emphysematous lung. Ann Thorac Surg 1994;57:1038-1039.

McKenna RJ, Fischel RJ, Brenner M, Gelb AF: Use of the Heimlich valve to shorten hospital stay after lung reduction surgery for emphysema. Ann Thorac Surg 1996;61:1115-1117.

Rivas de Andrés JJ, Blanco S, de la Torre M: Postsurgical pleurodesis with autologous blood in patients with persistent air leak. Ann Thorac Surg 2000;70:270-272.

Pneumoperitoneum

Yusen RD, Littenberg B: Technology assessment and pneumoperitoneum therapy for air leaks and pleural spaces. Ann Thorac Surg 1997;64:1583-1584.

Cerfolio RJ, Holman WL, Katholi CR: Pneumoperitoneum after concomitant resection of the right middle and lower lobes (bilobectomy). Ann Thorac Surg 2000;70:942-947.

Puc MM, Podbielski FJ, Conlan AA: A novel technique for creation of adjustable pneumoperitoneum. Ann Thorac Surg 2004;77:1469-1471.

Pleural Tent

Robinson LA, Preksto D: Pleural tenting during upper lobectomy decreases chest tube time and total hospitalization days. J Thorac Cardiovasc Surg 1998;115:319-327.

Brunelli A, Al Refai M, Monteverde M, et al: Pleural tent after upper lobectomy: a randomized study of efficacy and duration of effect. Ann Thorac Surg 2002;74:1958-1962.

Post-resectional Spaces

Silver AW, Espinas EE, Byron FX: The fate of postresection space. Ann Thorac Surg 1966;2:311-326.

EMPYEMA AND BRONCHOPLEURAL FISTULA

Early bronchopleural fistula (BPF) is a major source of morbidity and mortality in patients undergoing pulmonary resection. Risk factors such as low FEV_1, steroid therapy, and preoperative irradiation are well documented. Because of bronchial devascularization, radical and extensive mediastinal lymphadenectomy also increases the risk of fistula.

Because BPFs are associated with significant mortality, surgeons must concentrate on prevention, and they must be able to identify bronchi at risk of dehiscence so that these can be protected.

Late BPFs are uncommon; in general, they are secondary to an empyema draining through the bronchial stump. In contrast to early BPF, the mortality associated with late BPF is low, and some of these fistulas will even close spontaneously once the empyema has been evacuated.

Most empyemas without fistulas are due to bacterial contamination of the pleural space at the time of operation. Related mortality is low, but management can be prolonged.

EARLY BRONCHOPLEURAL FISTULAS

Incidence, Pathogenesis, and Risk Factors

With current-day methods of managing bronchial stumps, the incidence of early BPF is in the range of 1% to 2% after lobectomy and 6% to 10% after pneumonectomy. When pulmonary resection is done for benign disease such as bronchiectasis, *the frequency of BPF is even lower* because the bronchial artery hyperplasia associated with the disease process brings additional blood supply to the bronchus. If, on the other hand, pulmonary resection is done in patients with positive sputum for tuberculosis or in patients with active endobronchial tuberculosis, the incidence of BPF can be as high as 20% to 25%.

Two pathogenetic concepts must be appreciated if one hopes to prevent the occurrence of BPF. The first one concerns differential blood supply to main bronchi. The right main bronchus normally *receives less blood* (bronchial and pulmonary) than does its left counterpart, thus exposing it

TABLE 7-43

DOCUMENTED RISK FACTORS FOR POST-RESECTIONAL BRONCHOPLEURAL FISTULA

Low predicted FEV_1 (chronic obstructive pulmonary disease)

Associated comorbidities: diabetes, steroid therapy, poor nutritional status

Preoperative irradiation (>45 cGy)

Endobronchial disease (tuberculosis)

Right main bronchus and bronchus intermedius (versus left main and all other lobar bronchi)

Need for postoperative mechanical ventilation

7

to increased risk of dehiscence. Knowledge of such variations must lead the surgeon to be more careful in dissecting out right main bronchi during pneumonectomy. Preventive coverage should be considered *routine* for these stumps.

The second concept that must be appreciated is that the bronchus has a natural tendency to spring open because of its semicircular cartilaginous rings. This is more so in *older patients* in whom cartilage may have become ossified, in patients with *emphysema* (defective membrane), and in patients with *scarred bronchi* due to previous surgery or irradiation.

Both systemic and local factors have been associated with increased incidence of post-resectional BPF (Tables 7-43 to 7-45). In most series, the coexistence of *low predicted FEV_1* is an independent risk factor, presumably because in those patients, the bronchial mucosa is the site of chronic inflammation. In addition, emphysematous patients have structural abnormalities (elastic component) of the membranous part of the bronchial wall. Other systemic factors thought to increase risks of BPF include the patient's underlying nutritional status, the use of steroids, and comorbidities such as diabetes. The *influence of neoadjuvant therapy is still unclear,* although it is well documented that there is a higher incidence of BPF in patients who have received preoperative irradiation in excess of 45 cGy.

Management of Postoperative Complications

TABLE 7-44

PROBABLE RISK FACTORS FOR POST-RESECTIONAL BRONCHOPLEURAL FISTULA

Older age (>70 years)

Extended operations and reoperations

Long residual stumps in cases of pneumonectomy

Incomplete resection (cancer in bronchial margin)

Extensive mediastinal lymphadenectomy

Inexperienced surgeon

TABLE 7-45

POSSIBLE BUT NOT LIKELY RISK FACTORS FOR POST-RESECTIONAL BRONCHOPLEURAL FISTULA

Induction chemotherapy

Method of bronchial closure (stapled or hand-sewn)

It is generally agreed that there is a higher incidence of BPF after right pneumonectomy than after any other resectional procedure of the lung, including left pneumonectomy. This is not only because the right main bronchus is vascularized by only one bronchial artery (versus two on the left side) but also because once the lung has been removed, *the right main bronchus is left unprotected by mediastinal tissues.* On the left side, the main bronchus retracts underneath the aortic arch and is thus protected by surrounding mediastinal structures. Another contributing factor to an increased risk of bronchial dehiscence is the presence of residual cancer in the bronchial margin. *Long residual stumps* are also considered at risk because local accumulation of mucus may lead to secondary infection and impaired healing.

The actual technique of bronchial closure, whether stapled or hand-sewn, does not have an effect on the incidence of BPF, although *the stapler technique is simpler and much more standardized* and thus easier to use by less experienced surgeons. Overall, the highest risk factor for postoperative BPF is the inability of the operating surgeon to recognize high-risk bronchi (Table 7-46) as well as the surgeon's poor understanding of the benefits of stump coverage in such cases.

Postoperatively, the need for mechanical ventilation is highly predictive of the occurrence of BPF.

Diagnosis (Table 7-47)

Early BPF usually presents during the first 2 postoperative weeks. Clinically, patients often have a *fever* and a *cough productive of serosanguineous fluid.* Because the actual size of the fistula *does not* necessarily correlate with the amount of sputum, some patients with a large fistula may present with only a dry cough. Other physical findings that must alert the surgeon to the possibility of an early BPF are an increase in the amount of subcutaneous emphysema and a bulging of the thoracotomy incision during coughing efforts. If the patient still has a chest tube, *increased bubbling* will be noted.

TABLE 7-46

WHICH BRONCHUS IS AT RISK OF BRONCHOPLEURAL FISTULA?

All right main bronchi

All irradiated bronchi

All bronchi with residual endobronchial disease (tuberculosis, cancer)

All structurally abnormal bronchi (ossified, older age)

All devascularized bronchi (extended resections, extensive lymphadenectomy)

All long residual bronchial stumps

7

TABLE 7-47
DIAGNOSIS OF EARLY POSTOPERATIVE BRONCHOPLEURAL FISTULAS
CLINICAL
Fever, cough productive of sanguineous sputum
Increase in amount of subcutaneous emphysema
Bulging of thoracotomy incision during cough
Increased bubbling through the chest tube
RADIOLOGIC
Postlobectomy bronchopleural fistula
Development of a new air space
Already present air space increases in size
Collapse of residual lung
Postpneumonectomy bronchopleural fistula
Falling air-fluid level
Shift of mediastinum to contralateral side
Increase in amount of subcutaneous emphysema
ENDOSCOPIC
Direct sign
Dehiscence visualized
Indirect signs
Bubbling in bronchial stump
Sighting of staples
Ulcerations of bronchial mucosa

Chest radiographs often demonstrate a new or an increasing air space after lobectomy or a *falling air-fluid level* in a pneumonectomy space. Other findings suggestive of BPF are an increase in the amount of surgical emphysema, a previously expanded residual lobe that is now collapsed, and mediastinal shift toward the contralateral side.

Bronchoscopy is of value in demonstrating the fistula as well as in documenting its exact site and size. Often, however, the presence of a fistula is difficult to ascertain; the *sighting of staples, bubbling in the bronchial stump,* and *ulcerations of the mucosa* are all indirect signs that suggest the diagnosis. On occasion, endobronchial instillation of contrast material will provide positive documentation of a BPF (contrast material in pleural space).

Management

Prevention

The most important factor in the management of postoperative BPF is to prevent it, and this essentially *relates to the technical conduct of the operation.* Appropriate prophylaxis is achieved through *gentle handling of bronchial mucosa,* minimal dissection of peribronchial tissues, avoidance of excessively long stumps, and bronchial closure without tension. *Stump coverage* with vascularized autogenous tissue provides further reassurance, particularly in those patients with risk factors for fistula. In most cases, pericardial fat, parietal pleura, and pericardium provide excellent coverage. In very high risk cases, flaps of intercostal muscles, diaphragm, transposed chest wall muscles, or omentum are also available for coverage of the bronchial stump.

TABLE 7-48
INITIAL MANAGEMENT OF THE PATIENT WITH A BRONCHOPLEURAL FISTULA
Establish immediate and adequate chest tube drainage.
Confirm diagnosis with bronchoscopy.
Stabilize clinical condition.
Attempt bronchial reclosure.

Initial Management (Table 7-48)

Acute BPF, especially that occurring after pneumonectomy, *is a true emergency* because patients can potentially drown from contralateral aspiration. Initial management must therefore include immediate dependent chest tube drainage. Once the patient is clinically stable, bronchoscopy should be performed. When the diagnosis is well documented and the patient medically stabilized, nearly all fistulas are *best managed* by reoperation and reinforced bronchial reclosure.

Further Management

Further management thus follows three basic tenets: reclosure of the BPF, débridement and drainage of the space, and obliteration or sterilization of the space.

A vast array of methods have been employed to close BPF either indirectly or directly (Table 7-49). As a whole, *indirect methods apply only to patients with very small BPF.* On occasion, small fistulas may close spontaneously once chest tube drainage has been initiated. This is not likely to happen, however, because the natural history of early BPF is that it will get larger even if the pleural space is adequately drained. Endoscopic cauterization with 0.5% silver nitrate is no longer done, but *endoscopic closure with fibrin glue or Gelfoam* can be successful from time to time, especially if the fistula is very small.

Most patients, especially those in stable condition, are best managed by direct surgical reclosure of the bronchial stump, a procedure usually done through the reopening of the ipsilateral hemithorax. An alternative method is to approach the stump transsternally, thus avoiding re-entering a potentially contaminated space.

Surgical principles (Table 7-50) involved in the repair include identification of the fistula site (often facilitated by ventilating proximal to the fistula); unroofing of the fistula until normal bronchus is encountered;

TABLE 7-49
METHODS USED FOR BRONCHIAL STUMP RECLOSURE
INDIRECT
Spontaneous closure with tube drainage
Repeated cauterization
Endoscopic application of glues
DIRECT
Ipsilateral thoracotomy
Transpericardial approach

TABLE 7-50
SURGICAL PRINCIPLES INVOLVED IN RECLOSURE OF BRONCHOPLEURAL FISTULAS
Identification of fistula site (often facilitated by ventilating more proximally)
Unroofing of fistula until normal bronchus
Re-resection of long bronchial stumps
Direct reclosure of bronchial stump if possible
Buttressing site of repair with intercostal or chest wall muscles or omentum
Débridement of pleural space of fibrin or necrotic tissue
Drainage with chest tubes and underwater seal system

re-resection of long bronchial stumps; direct reclosure of the bronchus; and buttressing the site of repair with *vascularized tissues,* such as intercostal or chest wall muscles or omentum. For many surgeons, the omentum is superior to other flaps because of its unique ability to induce angiogenesis and neovascularity. We prefer the intercostal muscle not only because of ease of harvesting but also because *it is covered by the parietal pleura,* which provides a nice epithelial surface to cover the bronchus.

The advantage of using chest wall muscles such as the latissimus dorsi or the pectoralis major is that those muscles are bulky and thus contribute to obliteration of the space. In patients in whom the stump is too short to be reclosed, the selected flap is carefully sewn to the edges of the fistula as to achieve an airtight seal. The pleural space is then débrided of all fibrin and necrotic tissues, and *it is drained with an underwater seal system* until the mediastinum becomes stable and the space is sterile (three consecutive negative cultures of pleural fluid).

Management of Residual Cavities (Table 7-51)

The management of residual infected spaces after reclosure of BPF can be accomplished in a number of ways. Simple drainage with closed tubes, irrigation, and systemic antibiotherapy can be successful in up to 70% of cases. In chronic cases, open drainage can be employed until the space is no longer infected and has a smooth and glistening surface. At that time, the space is filled with antibiotics and the chest wall is closed (Clagett procedure). Often, however, properly drained small spaces, such as postlobectomy spaces, will close spontaneously through lung re-expansion, tissue contraction, and skin ingrowth. The advantage of an open thoracic window is that it allows *direct irrigation of the space* and *frequent visual inspections* (see Chapter 10).

TABLE 7-51
OPTIONS IN THE MANAGEMENT OF RESIDUAL CAVITIES
Sterilization
Closed drainage, tube irrigation, systemic antibiotics
Open drainage until space is cleaned of gross infection
Obliteration
Muscle flap or omental transposition
Collapse
Partial or extensive thoracoplasty

7

Management of Postoperative Complications

TABLE 7-52

VENTILATION IN PATIENTS WITH BRONCHOPLEURAL FISTULAS

Conventional ventilation
    Lowest effective tidal volume
    Least number of mechanical breaths
    Lowest PEEP
    Shorten inspiratory time
Endobronchial ventilation
    Use of bronchial blocker
    Use of extralong endotracheal tube in opposite bronchus
High-frequency ventilation

Modified from Baumann MH, Sahn SA: Medical management and therapy of bronchopleural fistulas in the mechanically ventilated patient. Chest 1990;97:721-728, with permission.

The overall success rate for the Clagett procedure is 50% to 60% in postpneumonectomy infected spaces.

Muscle flaps or omental transposition can be used to fill the space, thus allowing it to be obliterated. In some patients with large spaces such as postpneumonectomy spaces, however, multiple flaps and multiple operations may be necessary to accomplish this goal.

Thoracoplasty can finally be used to collapse the chest wall and obliterate residual spaces. Although this operation has received "bad press" because it is considered a mutilating procedure and a procedure associated with late scoliosis, most of these problems can be avoided by not resecting the first rib. Thoracoplasty *remains a valid option* for the management of residual apical spaces and of postpneumonectomy spaces.

Management of Systemic Factors

Systemic factors *such as nutrition* must be corrected, and *specific antibiotic treatment* of infections must be started as soon as BPF has been diagnosed.

If the BPF caused considerable soilage into the contralateral lung, mechanical ventilation may be required. This is a difficult situation because the constant positive pressure associated with mechanical ventilation might reopen the site of bronchial reclosure. If there is a partial dehiscence, the site of dehiscence becomes an area of low resistance to airflow so that a percentage of the delivered tidal volume will escape during conventional positive-pressure ventilation.

Table 7-52 lists some maneuvers that can be tried in patients being mechanically ventilated to maintain their oxygenation while reducing fistula airflow. These options include the use of high-frequency (low-flow) ventilation. If this system is unavailable, the fistula can be controlled with either a bronchial blocker or a balloon catheter or by insertion of an extralong endotracheal tube in the contralateral main stem bronchus.

LATE BRONCHOPLEURAL FISTULAS (TABLE 7-53)

Pathogenesis

Although late BPF and empyemas may occur separately, they generally occur together. In most cases, the BPF is a *direct consequence of the*

TABLE 7-53

CHARACTERISTICS OF EARLY AND LATE BRONCHOPLEURAL FISTULAS

	Early BPF	Late BPF
Time elapsed after pneumonectomy	<2 weeks	>2 months
Clinical features	Acute	Insidious
Empyema at diagnosis of BPF	Rare	Frequent
Full dehiscence of bronchial stump	Possible	Rare
Risk of aspiration pneumonia	High	Low
Mortality	High	Low
Direct surgical closure of BPF	Yes	No
Spontaneous closure of BPF	Rare	Possible

Modified from de Perrot M, Licker M, Robert J, Spiliopoulos A: Incidence, risk factors, and management of bronchopleural fistulae after pneumonectomy. Scand Cardiovasc J 1999;33:171-174.

7

Management of Postoperative Complications

empyema, impairing healing and leading to stump breakdown. This is the reason why such bronchial dehiscences are usually small and why spontaneous closure may occur once the empyema is evacuated.

Clinical Features and Diagnosis

Late BPFs occur after the second postoperative month. Their clinical presentation is usually insidious with low-grade fever and dry cough lasting weeks to months before the correct diagnosis is made. Patients are often debilitated, and in general, factors such as the size of empyema and bacteria involved rather than size of the BPF determine the extent of symptoms.

The diagnosis of late BPF can be made by standard chest radiographs, which in pneumonectomy patients will show a *fall in the fluid level,* presence of new loculated intrapleural gas, and mediastinal shift to the nonsurgical side. After lobectomy, a *new fluid level* may be noted. Bronchoscopy is *helpful* to document the BPF as well as to rule out residual or recurrent cancer in the bronchial stump.

Management

Management of late BPF is considerably different from that of early BPF. Conservative therapy can often be attempted because the risk of aspiration is low, and *spontaneous closure of the BPF might occur.* Management is also different because at this stage (>2 months postoperatively), mediastinal fixation has occurred, and there is a considerable amount of pleural thickening and pleural space contraction.

Initial measures include tube thoracostomy, appropriate systemic antibiotherapy, and nutritional support, which is most important in debilitated patients. Long-term management is then individualized and is based on the success of initial measures, the patient's medical condition, and whether the BPF has closed with tube thoracostomy. Overall, the objectives of treatment are the sterilization of the space, the closure of the BPF, and the obliteration of the remaining space.

If the fistula has closed, the residual cavity can often be sterilized with continuous tube irrigation and systemic antibiotherapy.

MORTALITY ASSOCIATED WITH BRONCHOPLEURAL FISTULAS

Although mortality rates after early postpneumonectomy BPF have been reported to be as high as 70%, 10% to 15% is more realistic, and patients die of aspiration pneumonia with subsequent ARDS. The mortality related to late BPF is low (see Table 7-53) and in the range of 4% to 5%.

The mortality associated with *postlobectomy BPF is low* unless it occurs while the patient is being mechanically ventilated.

EMPYEMA WITHOUT BRONCHOPLEURAL FISTULA

Empyemas without BPF are uncommon, and most of them relate to intraoperative contamination from pulmonary infection or to postoperative contamination from long-standing chest tubes or infection in the lung parenchyma. Empyemas are *more likely* to occur after pneumonectomy or if the pleural space is not completely obliterated after lobectomy. They may occur early during the postoperative period or more than 6 months after the procedure (*late empyema*). In those latter cases, the pleural cavity may have been contaminated during the initial surgery (microorganisms are lodged in small loculations of fluid and lay dormant), or seeding of the space may have occurred through the hematogenous route. *Staphylococcus* is the most frequently observed pathogen.

The diagnosis of postoperative empyema is often difficult because the onset is insidious and most patients will have only nonspecific symptoms. The presence of an empyema is usually confirmed by thoracentesis, which should be considered whenever post-resectional patients are febrile, lethargic, or anorexic.

Once the diagnosis is established, *adequate tube thoracostomy* must be obtained and *appropriate parenteral antibiotics* must be administered. A more planned surgical approach can then be put into effect for long-term management. If no residual space is present (i.e., lung completely re-expands after drainage of a postlobectomy empyema), no further treatment may be necessary. If the lung does not re-expand or if the empyema has occurred after pneumonectomy, the residual space can be sterilized (closed tube drainage, irrigation, open drainage) or the space can be obliterated with muscle flaps. In our experience, *closed tube irrigation and systemic specific antibiotics will sterilize most residual spaces* if no BPF is present. We recommend continuous tube irrigation (50 mL/h) with an antiseptic solution (Dakin $\frac{1}{32}$). Tubes are removed when three consecutive samplings from pleural fluid are bacteriologically negative after 2 to 3 weeks of irrigation. Chest tubes are best inserted under VATS guidance so that they can be properly placed and all necrotic material can be removed from the pleural space. Once the space is sterile, it is filled with normal saline and the tubes are removed.

CONCLUSION

In summary, post-resectional BPF is an extremely serious complication with related mortality as high as 20% when it occurs after pneumonectomy. In this context, emphasis should be given to prevention, including bronchial reinforcement for high-risk bronchi and immediate bronchial reclosure for most cases of early fistulas. Patients who survive this complication are likely to suffer significant morbidity with a prolonged course of management.

SUGGESTED READINGS

Review Articles

Baumann MH, Sahn SA: Medical management and therapy of bronchopleural fistulas in the mechanically ventilated patient. Chest 1990;97:721-728.

Allen MS, Deschamps C, Trastek VF, Pairolero PC: Bronchopleural fistula. Chest Surg Clin North Am 1992;2:823-837.

Pairolero PC, Deschamps C, Allen MS, Trastek VF: Postoperative empyema. Chest Surg Clin North Am 1992;2:813-822.

Wain JC: Management of late post pneumonectomy empyema and bronchopleural fistula. Chest Surg Clin North Am 1996;6:529-541.

Miller JI Jr.: Overview: postresectional bronchopleural fistula. Semin Thorac Cardiovasc Surg 2001;13:27-28.

Cooper WA, Miller JI Jr.: Management of bronchopleural fistula after lobectomy. Semin Thorac Cardiovasc Surg 2001;13:8-12.

Bronchopleural Fistula (General)

Vester SR, Faber LP, Kittle CF, et al: Bronchopleural fistula after stapled closure of bronchus. Ann Thorac Surg 1991;52:1253-1258.

Asamura H, Naruke T, Tsuchiya R, et al: Bronchopleural fistulas associated with lung cancer operations. Univariate and multivariate analysis of risk factors, management, and outcome. J Thorac Cardiovasc Surg 1992;104:1456-1464.

Puskas JD, Mathisen DJ, Grillo HC, et al: Treatment strategies for bronchopleural fistula. J Thorac Cardiovasc Surg 1995;109:989-996.

Hollaus PH, Lax F, Janakiev D, et al: Endoscopic treatment of postoperative bronchopleural fistula: experience with 45 cases. Ann Thorac Surg 1998;66:923-927.

Sonobe M, Nakagawa M, Ichinose M, et al: Analysis of risk factors in bronchopleural fistula after pulmonary resection for primary lung cancer. Eur J Cardiothorac Surg 2000;18:519-523.

Postpneumonectomy Bronchopleural Fistula

Sabanathan S, Richardson J: Management of postpneumonectomy bronchopleural fistulae: a review. J Cardiovasc Surg 1994;35:449-451.

Wright CD, Wain JC, Mathisen DJ, Grillo HC: Postpneumonectomy bronchopleural fistula after sutured bronchial closure: incidence, risk factors, and management. J Thorac Cardiovasc Surg 1996;112:1367-1371.

Hollaus PH, Lax F, El-Nashef BB, et al: Natural history of bronchopleural fistula after pneumonectomy: a review of 96 cases. Ann Thorac Surg 1997;63:1391-1397.

Hollaus PH, Huber M, Lax F, et al: Closure of bronchopleural fistula after pneumonectomy with a pedicled intercostal muscle flap. Eur J Cardiothorac Surg 1999;16:181-186.

de Perrot M, Licker M, Robert J, Spiliopoulos A: Incidence, risk factors and management of bronchopleural fistulae after pneumonectomy. Scand Cardiovasc J 1999;33:171-174.

Algar FJ, Alvarez A, Aranda JL, et al: Prediction of early bronchopleural fistula after pneumonectomy: a multivariate analysis. Ann Thorac Surg 2001;72:1662-1667.

Deschamps C, Bernard A, Nichols FC III, et al: Empyema and bronchopleural fistula after pneumonectomy: factors affecting incidence. Ann Thorac Surg 2001;72:243-248.

Postpneumonectomy Empyema

Pairolero PC, Arnold PG, Trastek VF, et al: Postpneumonectomy empyema. The role of intrathoracic muscle transposition. J Thorac Cardiovasc Surg 1990;99:958-968.

Weber J, Grabner D, al-Zand K, Beyer D: Empyema after pneumonectomy—empyema window or thoracoplasty? Thorac Cardiovasc Surg 1990;38:355-358.

Gossot D, Stern JB, Galetta D, et al: Thoracoscopic management of postpneumonectomy empyema. Ann Thorac Surg 2004;78:273-276.

DELIRIUM

Delirium is an active disorder of attention and cognition that occurs in approximately 10% to 15% of patients aged 70 years or older who undergo major surgery. Since lung cancer patients scheduled for pulmonary resection are getting older, it is likely that delirium will become one of the most common complications of general thoracic surgical procedures.

Because delirium is often overlooked as a complication, risk and precipitating factors are *largely unknown.* Despite this lack of information, it seems clear that delirium is associated with increased rates of other postoperative morbidities, operative mortality, and *longer and costlier hospitalizations.*

Age (>70 years), alcohol abuse and withdrawal, preexisting cognitive impairment, severe illness, and metabolic imbalance have been associated with increased incidence of delirium. Indeed, the risk of delirium arises when one or more of these factors is present in a patient undergoing major surgery. Whether delirium can be totally prevented *is unlikely,* although risk factors such as hypoxemia and fluid and electrolyte imbalances can be monitored and corrected when required.

IDENTIFICATION OF DELIRIUM (TABLES 7-54 and 7-55)

Delirium is a *transient* disorder of cognition and attention that is usually accompanied by disturbances of psychomotor behavior. Symptoms may

TABLE 7-54

CLINICAL FEATURES OF DELIRIUM

Acute onset and fluctuating course (more pronounced at night)

Inattention (distractible and unable to focus)

Disorganized thinking

Altered level of consciousness

Disorientation to time, place, and persons

Memory impairment (short and long term)

Perceptual disturbance (illusions, hallucinations)

Abnormal psychomotor activity

Altered sleep-awake cycle

From Inouye SK, van Dyck CH, Alessi CA, et al: Clarifying confusion: the confusion assessment method. A new method for detection of delirium. Ann Intern Med 1990;113:941-948, with permission.

develop suddenly, although most of the time, *the nursing staff will have noticed behavioral manifestations,* such as reduced level of attention or consciousness, disorientation, and restlessness, for some time before the acute episode. Attention disorders such as inability to concentrate and incoherent speech are often present; these symptoms tend to fluctuate in severity throughout the day, often being *more pronounced during the evening and at night.* On occasion, patients will become so agitated and confused that they have to be restrained to avoid self-injuries or prevented from pulling out chest tubes or intravenous lines. They may have visual or auditory hallucinations interpreted as confusion. Thinking is *disorganized and incoherent,* and as a result, the patient's behavior tends to be erratic and lacking judgment. In most cases, orientation is also defective for time, place, and even persons.

According to the *Diagnostic and Statistical Manual of Mental Disorders,* the diagnosis of delirium has four key features: acute change in mental status with a fluctuating course, inattention, disorganized thinking, and altered level of consciousness (Table 7-55).

Delirium usually starts by day 3 to 5 after operation. Because it is transient, it ends after 5 to 7 days in most cases.

TABLE 7-55

DSM-IV-TR DIAGNOSTIC CRITERIA FOR DELIRIUM

Disturbance of consciousness (i.e., reduced clarity of awareness of environment) with reduced ability to focus, sustain, or shift attention.

A change in cognition (such as memory deficit, disorientation, language disturbance) or the development of a perceptual disturbance that is not better accounted for by a preexisting, established, or evolving dementia.

The disturbance develops over a short period of time (usually hours to days) and tends to fluctuate during the course of the day.

There is evidence from the history, physical examination, or laboratory findings that the disturbance is caused by the direct physiological consequences of a general medical condition.

From American Psychiatric Association: Diagnostic and Statistical Manual of Mental Disorders, 4th ed, text revision. Washington, DC, American Psychiatric Association, 2000:143.

Management of Postoperative Complications

PREDISPOSING AND PRECIPITATING FACTORS

In general, delirium occurs when a *vulnerable and predisposed patient undergoes a significant stress,* such as a major thoracic surgical procedure.

Predisposing Risk Factors

Several risk factors have been identified (Table 7-56), and *age is probably the most significant.* It has been well documented that elderly patients are more likely to have delirium because of "an aging brain," impaired vision and hearing, and higher prevalence and duration of chronic or severe comorbidities. Dementia, preexisting cognitive impairment, and use of antipsychotic medications have also been identified as predictors of delirium. Other factors that are important are *alcohol abuse and sudden withdrawal,* history of delirium after a prior operation, postoperative sleep deprivation, and forced immobilization. The *ICU environment*—with extraneous noises, light, continuous monitoring, movement, unfamiliarity of the patient with this environment, frequent waking of the patient, and sleep deprivation— is also of critical importance in predisposing to delirium.

In one study (Table 7-57), risk groups for delirium were identified. A point system was developed with the hope that high-risk patients could become candidates for preventive interventions.

It is generally acknowledged that if a patient has several predisposing risk factors, delirium can be precipitated by a minor insult; whereas in a normal individual (i.e., no predisposing factors), it may take a more severe stress to initiate delirium. In general, the *risk of delirium increases in proportion to the number of risk factors* present.

Precipitating Factors (Table 7-58)

Precipitating factors are factors that will directly initiate the delirium. Among them, the most important are the *type of surgery in terms of site, magnitude, and duration and the anesthesia.* Invasive and long procedures are more likely than less invasive and short operations to be associated with delirium. Other factors, such as infection (pneumonia, urinary tract infection), dehydration, and metabolic derangements (such as uremia, hypokalemia, or sodium depletion) may also trigger the development of delirium, especially in elderly patients. Similarly, *poor pain control,* whether it is undertreated or overtreated, and *discomfort* due to a nonfunctioning urinary catheter, for instance, can trigger delirium.

TABLE 7-56

PREDISPOSING RISK FACTORS FOR DELIRIUM

Age (>70 years)
Preexisting visual or auditory impairment
Chronic or severe comorbidities
Preexisting cognitive impairment
Alcohol abuse (and withdrawal)
Previous history of delirium after surgery
Postoperative sleep deprivation and forced immobilization
ICU environment

TABLE 7-57

CLINICAL PREDICTORS FOR POSTOPERATIVE DELIRIUM

Risk Factors	Points
Age ≥ 70 years	1
Alcohol abuse	1
Telephone interview score <30*	1
Specific activity scale class IV†	1
Markedly abnormal preoperative sodium, potassium, and glucose levels‡	1
Aortic aneurysm surgery	2
Noncardiac thoracic surgery	1

Total Points	Risk of Delirium (%)
0	2
1 or 2	11
≥3	50

*A score below 30 suggests cognitive impairment.

†Represents severe physical impairment.

‡Defined as follows: sodium <130 or >150 mmol/L; potassium <3.0 or >6.0 mmol/L; glucose <60 or >300 mg/dL.

From Marcantonio ER, Goldman L, Mangione CM, et al: A clinical prediction rule for delirium after elective noncardiac surgery. JAMA 1994;271:134-139, reprinted with permission.

Use of common drugs, such as cardiac medications, antipsychotics, antidepressants, and sedative-hypnotic agents, is often implicated as a precipitating factor, even if these drugs are at therapeutic doses. Again, these events are much more likely to occur in *elderly patients with more than one predisposing factor.*

PATHOGENESIS AND PATHOPHYSIOLOGY

Although delirium is common, scientific information about its pathogenesis is scanty. In general, however, delirium is thought to be related to reduced cerebral oxidative metabolism, with consequent reduction in synthesis of certain neurotransmitters, notably acetylcholine. The other commonly accepted hypothesis is that delirium is a reaction mediated by *elevated levels of plasma cortisol,* secondary to the acute stress of major surgery.

MANAGEMENT

Prophylactic Measures (Table 7-59)

Prophylactic measures include close monitoring of the high-risk patient and correction of documented causes, such as hypoxemia, hypotension, and

TABLE 7-58

PRECIPITATING FACTORS

Magnitude and duration of surgical procedure and anesthesia

Dehydration

Metabolic and electrolytic imbalances

Infection

Drug toxicity

Urinary retention

Significant blood loss

Inadequate pain control (undertreated or overtreated)

TABLE 7-59
MEASURES TO PREVENT DELIRIUM

Preoperative psychiatric consultation in high-risk patients
Close monitoring of patient and of biochemistry
Anticipate the problem and treat before it becomes severe
Avoid restraints
High-risk patient in quiet, well-lit room where family and friends have access

---

fluid and electrolyte imbalances. Indeed, this is most important for the vulnerable patient with several predisposing factors.

Physical restraints should be avoided. Nursing care should be provided, if possible, in a quiet, well-lit room where family and friends have easy access. Often, it is worthwhile to have a *psychiatric consultation* before surgery so that the psychiatrist not only knows about the patient but possibly can readjust the patient's medication or prescribe more appropriate drugs. In many cases, the problem can be easily and quickly solved if it has been anticipated.

Management (Tables 7-60 and 7-61)

When a patient goes into a delirium, careful medical evaluation is necessary and *organic causes should be looked for and treated*. This includes fluid and electrolyte disturbances, infections, drug toxicities, and metabolic derangements (i.e., renal, hepatic failure, or other). On occasion, brain CT scan will be required to rule out a cerebrovascular accident or a metastatic lesion. The patient should be provided with symptomatic and supportive therapy, and a psychiatric consultation should be asked. If the patient is agitated and difficult to control, haloperidol (Haldol) should be given at doses of 2 to 10 mg by mouth or parenterally. This drug is a potent antipsychotic medication with minimal respiratory or cardiac toxicities. The initial dose of haloperidol for an adult is 2 to 5 mg for moderate agitation and 5 to 10 mg for severe agitation. The drug can be repeated at regular intervals (but not before 30 minutes) until the patient is quieter. After the confusion has cleared, the drug is tapered during several days.

Good nursing care is important, and if possible, the patient should be transferred out of the ICU environment. For security reasons, however, the patient may require a sitter to provide supervision. Other features of medical management are listed in Table 7-61.

TABLE 7-60
MANAGEMENT OF DELIRIUM

Organic cause must be sought and treated
Psychiatric consultation useful
Sedation to release severe agitation (haloperidol)
Supportive therapy during episode
Close surveillance
If possible, transfer to a well-lit room with familiar objects

---

TABLE 7-61

MEDICAL MANAGEMENT OF DELIRIUM

MEDICAL CARE

Monitor vital signs, fluid input and output, and oxygenation.

Discontinue nonessential medications.

Avoid addition of multiple medications at one time.

Identify sources of pain.

Avoid interruption of sleep whenever possible.

PREVENT AND MANAGE DISRUPTIVE BEHAVIOR

Place patient in a room near nursing station.

Consider a sitter.

Keep bed in low position and use side rails only if patient insists on getting out of bed.

Use restraints only if necessary.

Avoid placement in a room cluttered with equipment or furniture.

USE OF MEDICATIONS

Use haloperidol for agitation (IV whenever possible).

Avoid use of benzodiazepines as sole agents.

Avoid use of narcotics unless there is significant pain.

Avoid use of anticholinergic agents.

FACILITATE REALITY

Encourage presence of family members.

Provide familiar clues (e.g., clock, calendar).

Provide adequate day and night lighting.

Minimize transfer.

Maximize staff continuity.

Encourage use of personal belongings.

Reassure patient.

From Wise MG, Rundell JR, eds: Textbook of Consultation-Liaison Psychiatry, 2nd ed. Washington, DC, APA Press, 2002, with permission.

Most episodes of postoperative delirium will recover within 3 to 5 days of their beginning, without sequelae.

CONCLUSION

Postoperative delirium is a common complication in thoracic surgical patients not only because most of these individuals are older than 60 years but also because they have to undergo major surgery. Although delirium is considered a minor problem, attending surgeons should learn to identify risk factors as well as to anticipate the problem, recognize its clinical features early, and treat it vigorously. By doing so, they may prevent the development of a full-blown syndrome, thus reducing length of stay and ultimately overall morbidity and mortality.

SUGGESTED READINGS

Review Articles

Lipowski ZJ: Delirium (acute confusional states). JAMA 1987; 258:1789-1792.

7

Management of Postoperative Complications

Inouye SK: The dilemma of delirium: clinical and research controversies regarding diagnosis and evaluation of delirium in hospitalized elderly medical patients. Am J Med 1994;97:278-287.

American Psychiatric Association: Diagnostic and Statistical Manual of Mental Disorders, 4th ed, text revision. Washington, DC, American Psychiatric Association, 2000.

Wise MG, Hilty DM, Cerda GM, Trzepacz PT: Delirium (confusional states). In Wise MG, Rundell JR, eds: Textbook of Consultation-Liaison Psychiatry. Washington, DC, APA Press, 2002:257-272.

Detection

Inouye SK, van Dyck CH, Alessi CA, et al: Clarifying confusion: the confusion assessment method. A new method for detection of delirium. Ann Intern Med 1990;113:941-948.

Case Series

Morse RM, Litin EM: Postoperative delirium: a study of etiologic factors. Am J Psychiatry 1969;126:388-395.

Rogers MP, Liang MH, Daltroy LH, et al: Delirium after elective orthopedic surgery: risk factors and natural history. Int J Psychiatry Med 1989;19:109-121.

Francis J, Martin D, Kapoor WN: A prospective study of delirium in hospitalized elderly. JAMA 1990;263:1097-1110.

Williams-Russo P, Urquhart BL, Sharrock NE, Charlson ME: Post-operative delirium: predictors and prognosis in elderly orthopedic patients. J Am Geriatr Soc 1992;40:759-767.

Inouye SK, Viscoli CM, Horwitz RI, et al: A predictive model for delirium in hospitalized elderly medical patients based on admission characteristics. Ann Intern Med 1993;119:474-481.

Marcantonio ER, Goldman L, Mangione CM, et al: A clinical prediction rule for delirium after elective noncardiac surgery. JAMA 1994;271:134-139.

Inouye SK, Bogardus ST, Charpentier PA, et al: A multicomponent intervention to prevent delirium in hospitalized older patients. N Engl J Med 1999;340:669-676.

Franco K, Litaker D, Locala J, Bronson D: The cost of delirium in the surgical patient. Psychosomatics 2001;42:68-73.

RECURRENT LARYNGEAL NERVE PALSY

Because of their anatomic locations, the left vagus and left recurrent laryngeal nerves are *vulnerable to injury during surgical procedures involving the left lung.* Unfortunately, many of these injuries are unavoidable when one is removing locally invasive lung carcinomas, where wide resection margins are required. In several cases, however, injury is due to the surgeon's inexperience and unfamiliarity with the local anatomy of the nerves or to technical errors during dissection of the aortopulmonary and subaortic regions.

Because of inability to cough and raise secretions, recurrent laryngeal nerve palsy can be devastating during the immediate postoperative period. Some patients, especially older individuals, will also aspirate, making cough failure even more significant. In the long term, the ability of patients to tolerate vocal cord paralysis and its attending hoarseness, shortness of breath, swallowing difficulties, and chronic aspiration is variable and depends on the final position of the paralyzed vocal cord as well as on the degree of compensation by the contralateral hemilarynx. In general, *older patients and patients with COPD* are significantly less tolerant of vocal cord paralysis.

ANATOMY OF RECURRENT LARYNGEAL NERVES (FIG. 7-3) AND MECHANISM OF INJURY

Each recurrent laryngeal nerve arises from the ipsilateral vagus nerve.

Left Recurrent Laryngeal Nerve

The left recurrent laryngeal nerve takes off *close to the ligamentum arteriosum,* where it courses around the aorta from front to back before ascending in the neck in the tracheoesophageal groove. During pulmonary resection, it is vulnerable in opening of the mediastinal pleura, dissection of the aortopulmonary and subaortic regions, or division of the ligamentum arteriosum, which is sometimes necessary to gain control of the left proximal pulmonary artery. The left recurrent nerve is also vulnerable during *mobilization of the carina and lower trachea* in patients undergoing right sleeve pneumonectomies.

Mechanisms of injury (Table 7-62) include *deliberate section* because the nerve cannot be dissected free of the tumor, *stretching* due to excessive traction, accidental section, and *thermal injury* due to electrocoagulation. Some authors are also suggesting that at least in some cases, vocal cord paralysis may be due to perineural vascular injury with secondary recurrent nerve ischemia.

Right Recurrent Laryngeal Nerve

On the right side, the recurrent laryngeal nerve arises at the level of the first portion of the right subclavian artery, around which it loops to ascend in the tracheoesophageal groove to the larynx. It is *almost never* injured during lung surgery except in cases of extensive cervicomediastinal dissection for tumors in or near the thoracic inlet.

LARYNGEAL NERVE FUNCTION (FIG. 7-4) AND CONSEQUENCES OF VOCAL CORD PARALYSIS (TABLE 7-63)

In patients with unilateral recurrent laryngeal nerve palsy, the paralyzed cord is usually *abducted in a paramedian position, thus preventing effective sealing of the airway.* During the immediate postoperative period, this ineffective sealing of the airway makes patients unable to hold their breath as well as unable to generate sufficient subglottic pressure to produce an effective cough and raise secretions. These difficulties are often compounded by the fact that they also lose intrathoracic pressure through the chest tube. The ultimate consequences of these phenomena include *retention of secretions, bronchopneumonia,* and *respiratory failure.*

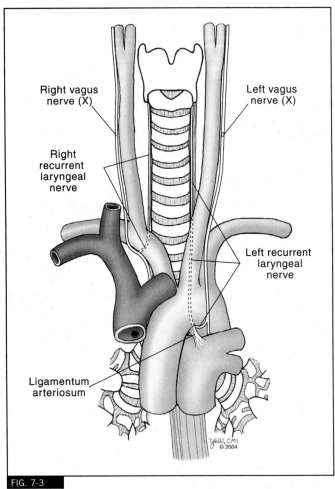

Anatomy of the left and right recurrent laryngeal nerves. *(Courtesy of Dr. Clement A. Hiebert.)*

POSSIBLE MECHANISMS OF INJURY OF RECURRENT LARYNGEAL NERVE

Deliberate section due to tumor proximity

Stretching due to excessive retraction

Accidental section during mobilization of aortopulmonary window or division of ligamentum arteriosum

Thermal injury due to electrocoagulation

Perineural vascular injury with secondary ischemia

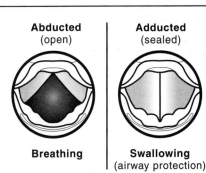

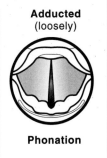

Abducted (open)	Adducted (sealed)	Adducted (loosely)
Breathing	**Swallowing** (airway protection)	**Phonation**

FIG. 7-4

Overview of laryngeal functions. *(Courtesy of Dr. Clement A. Hiebert.)*

Without effective sealing of the airway, patients may also have *swallowing impairment and may be susceptible to aspiration.* Indeed, the cumulative effects of even minimal aspiration and ineffective cough can lead to clinically significant pneumonia, which is always a serious complication.

Patients with unilateral vocal cord paralysis almost invariably have a weak voice or true hoarseness. Although these symptoms are not a worry during the immediate postoperative period, they can become a major disability in the longer term. Patients may also be unable to modulate the expiration phase of their breathing, resulting in significant shortness of breath.

Some patients may finally experience cricopharyngeal dysphagia secondary to impaired swallowing coordination between the pharyngeal propulsion peristaltic wave and the relaxation of the upper esophageal sphincter. This uncoordinated swallowing mechanism can lead to *sudden food choking with or without aspiration.*

TABLE 7-63

POSSIBLE CONSEQUENCES OF VOCAL CORD PARALYSIS

Abnormal Function	Immediate Consequence	Possible End Result
Inadequate sealing of airway	Ineffective cough	Retention of secretions Bronchopneumonia Respiratory failure
	Swallowing impairment	Aspiration pneumonia
Inadequate approximation of cords	Hoarseness	Hoarseness
Inadequate opening of cords	Inability to modulate expiratory phase of breathing	Shortness of breath
Cricopharyngeal motor dysfunction	Food choking	Dysphagia Food choking

7

DIAGNOSIS OF RECURRENT NERVE PALSY AND EVALUATION OF THE PATIENT

More than 90% of patients with vocal cord paralysis related to surgical interruption of the recurrent laryngeal or vagus nerve will have *a flaccid paralysis of the hemilarynx* with abduction of the involved cord (Fig. 7-5). During the early postoperative period, this problem is easy to recognize (Table 7-64) because patients cannot hold air and have difficulties in raising secretions, and when they try to cough, there is almost always a whistling sound (high-pitched noise) coming off the glottis. Interestingly, some patients may have an almost normal voice for 2 or 3 days before they develop hoarseness or aphonia. This is because early on, the paralyzed cord can be in an *intermediate position* allowing partial closure of the glottis. When the diagnosis of vocal cord paralysis is doubtful on clinical grounds, it can be confirmed by laryngeal examination through laryngoscopy or bronchoscopy.

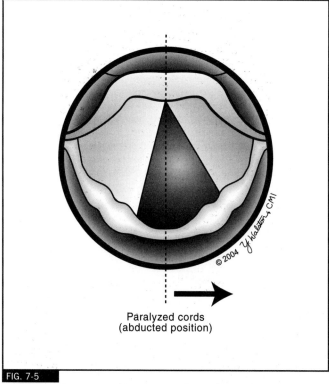

Paralyzed cords
(abducted position)

FIG. 7-5

Paralyzed vocal cord in abducted position. *(Courtesy of Dr. Clement A. Hiebert.)*

TABLE 7-64

CLINICAL FEATURES OF VOCAL CORD PARALYSIS DURING EARLY POSTOPERATIVE PERIOD

Known dissection in aortopulmonary or subaortic region
Patient cannot hold air
Patient cannot raise secretions
Whistling sound during cough efforts
Voice may be normal for first 2-3 days
Diagnosis easy to confirm by laryngeal examination (indirect laryngoscopy
    or flexible bronchoscopy)
Aspiration difficult to demonstrate

Swallowing difficulties (dysphagia or aspiration) are much *more difficult to document,* and their true incidence is unknown. Patients are often completely asymptomatic but they still aspirate (silent aspiration), whereas at other times, they will complain of choking on swallowing (rare in early postoperative period) or have repeated bouts of aspiration pneumonia. These problems are best documented by barium swallow examination, which may clearly demonstrate aspiration or show abnormal residue in the posterior glottis or in the piriform fossae.

The consequences of vocal cord paralysis often *depend on the severity of underlying COPD.* Difficulties in coughing or mild aspiration may, for instance, be of no significance in healthy individuals who only had a lobectomy, but the same symptoms can become catastrophic in pneumonectomy patients with prior evidence of COPD.

NATURAL HISTORY OF RECURRENT LARYNGEAL NERVE PALSY

The natural history of postoperative vocal cord paralysis depends on the site of injury, the type and severity of injury, and whether reinnervation and compensation from the contralateral normal cord will occur.

One of the first questions to be asked is whether the vocal cord palsy is due to an injury of the recurrent laryngeal nerve (distal injury) or to an injury to the vagus nerve more proximally. If the injury occurred on the vagus nerve, *spontaneous recovery is less likely* to happen, and these patients will usually have persistent and at times crippling swallowing difficulties.

For the majority of patients with vocal cord paralysis due to traction or even ischemic injury to the recurrent nerve, spontaneous recovery of voice and of other symptoms is expected to occur because the laryngeal muscles will become reinnervated over time. Although it is less predictable, the same phenomenon is possible when the nerve has been completely divided. This reinnervation process, however, can take *up to 9 to 12 months.* At the time of recovery, laryngeal motor function will return to normal, and the quality and tone of the voice will improve.

MANAGEMENT

Prevention of Injury

It is always better to prevent injuries to the recurrent laryngeal nerves than to treat their consequences. All surgeons performing lung resection must therefore be familiar with the intrathoracic anatomy of recurrent nerves and of the most common site of injury, usually the *subaortic region near the ligamentum arteriosum.* Surgeons must not only avoid extensive dissection in that area but also understand that it is always safer to identify and properly expose the nerve than to perform blind dissections.

Any patient undergoing an operation in the left hemithorax *must be warned beforehand* of the possibility of postoperative recurrent nerve palsy. The patient should be told that her or his voice may change and that these changes may or may not revert over time. Having had a clear discussion about the possibility of such a complication always makes it easier to deal with it postoperatively.

Palliation of Symptoms

For many patients, whether cord function is anticipated to recover or not, palliative measures may be useful. In general, the two symptoms that need to be palliated are the *difficulty to cough and raise secretions* and the *inability to swallow without aspiration.*

Methods to Palliate Ineffective Coughing (Table 7-65)

The choice of techniques that may be used to palliate ineffective coughing depends on the magnitude of the problem. For patients with mild difficulties or with difficulties expected to be temporary, active physiotherapy and frequent bronchoaspirations may be all that is required. For other patients, a mini-tracheostomy (see Chapter 5, "Prevention of Postoperative Complications after Pulmonary Surgery") may be useful because it allows the nursing personnel to aspirate secretions as often as required.

Early medialization of the paralyzed cord by injection of Teflon (nonresorbable) or autologous fat (resorbable) in the vocal fold can also be attempted. By adding bulky material to the abducted cord, these substances create a rigid structure against which the normal cord apposes during cough, thus effectively sealing the airway. Medialization can be performed under topical anesthesia and intravenous sedation or under general anesthesia.

The benefits and disadvantages of commonly used products are listed in Table 7-66. At present, *autologous fat is the preferred material,* although the resorption rate of fat is unpredictable and the volume of the implant may decrease over time. Other less commonly used materials include

---

TABLE 7-65

METHODS USED TO PALLIATE INEFFECTIVE COUGH DUE TO VOCAL CORD PARALYSIS

GENERAL MEASURES

Active physiotherapy

Frequent bronchoaspiration

SPECIFIC MEASURES

Mini-tracheostomy

Early surgical medialization of involved cord

TABLE 7-66

PRODUCTS COMMONLY USED FOR MEDIALIZATION OF
PARALYZED VOCAL CORD

	Benefits	Disadvantages
Nonresorbable (Teflon)	May be more stable over time	May be too heavy for vocal cord
		May create inflammatory reaction with granulomas and poor quality of voice
		Possible migration
		Higher cost
Resorbable (autologous fat)	No inflammatory reaction and better quality of voice	Unpredictable degree of resorption over time
	Easy to harvest	
	No side effects (local or systemic)	
	No cost	
	Readily available	

Gelfoam powder and collagen. Gelfoam lasts up to 3 months; collagen may last as long as 3 years after cord injection.

Methods to Palliate Aspiration

Because the consequences of aspiration can be disastrous, especially after pneumonectomy, all patients with suspected or documented recurrent laryngeal nerve palsy should be monitored closely when they resume eating. As a rule, patients with swallowing difficulties, those with symptoms of aspiration (coughing while eating), and those with radiographic abnormalities suggestive of aspiration pneumonia should stop all oral intake, especially clear liquids. Treatment options (Table 7-67) include trying *thickened liquid or soft diets,* which facilitate upper esophageal sphincter relaxation; performing *early medialization* of the paralyzed cord; and alimenting the patient through a feeding jejunostomy until glottic competence has returned. In all of those patients, it is best to avoid a tracheotomy because the tracheal cannula may increase the swallowing difficulties.

Treatment of Permanent Dysfunction

Hoarseness with impaired ability to communicate is the most common symptom that will bring the patient to seek medical attention. Initially,

TABLE 7-67

TREATMENT OPTIONS IN PATIENTS WITH ASPIRATION AND RECURRENT
NERVE PARALYSIS

Reintroduce oral intake with thickened liquids and soft diet
Early medialization of vocal cord
Jejunostomy feedings preferably without tracheostomy

7

Management of Postoperative Complications

those patients should be told that the quality of their voice may improve over time, as it often does through compensation by the contralateral hemilarynx or because of spontaneous reinnervation. Speech therapists are useful during that waiting period, and indeed they may help avoid further surgical therapy.

For patients whose cord function fails to recover and who are still disabled after 1 year, a number of options are available for permanent treatment. Currently, the most popular surgical technique consists of positioning a *hand-grafted Silastic implant* in a pocket on the deep surface of the thyroid cartilage (type I thyroplasty) to displace the vocal cord toward the midline. The advantages of thyroplasty over injection of material directly into the vocal cord are that the size of the implant is easier to adjust and that the vocal cord can better vibrate because the implant is outside its main body. A possible disadvantage of Silastic medialization is that it may not totally prevent aspiration.

CONCLUSION

Because the most important function of the patient who had a pulmonary resection is his or her ability to have an effective cough, all surgeons must understand the *importance of preserving the recurrent laryngeal nerve,* especially in older patients and in patients with impaired pulmonary function. Not only are patients with vocal cord paralysis exposed to increased retention of secretions and resulting pneumonia, but this complication exposes them to an increased overall perioperative mortality.

SUGGESTED READINGS

Review Articles

Benninger MS, Crumley RL, Ford CN, et al: Evaluation and treatment of the unilateral paralyzed vocal cord. Otolaryngol Head Neck Surg 1994;111:497-508.

Harries ML: Unilateral vocal cord paralysis: a review of the current methods of surgical rehabilitation. J Laryngol Otol 1996;110:111-116.

Liebermann-Meffert DMI, Walbrun B, Hiebert CA, Siewert JR: Recurrent and superior laryngeal nerves: a new look with implications for the esophageal surgeon. Ann Thorac Surg 1999;67:217-223.

Carew JF, Kraus DH, Ginsberg RJ: Early complications. Recurrent nerve palsy. Chest Surg Clin North Am 1999;9:597-608.

Anatomy

Henderson RD, Boszko A, van Nostrand AWP: Pharyngoesophageal dysphagia and recurrent laryngeal nerve palsy. J Thorac Cardiovasc Surg 1974;68:507-512.

Moreau S, Goullet M, Babin E, et al: The recurrent laryngeal nerve: related vascular anatomy. Laryngoscope 1998;108:1351-1353.

Liebermann-Meffert DMI, Walbrun B, Hiebert CA, Siewert JR: Recurrent and superior laryngeal nerves: a new look with implications for the esophageal surgeon. Ann Thorac Surg 1999;67:217-223.

Consequences of Vocal Cord Paralysis

Périé S, Laccourreye O, Bou-Malhab F, Brasnu D: Aspiration in unilateral recurrent laryngeal nerve paralysis after surgery. Am J Otol 1998; 19:18-23.

Treatment

Netterville JL, Stone RE, Luken ES, et al: Silastic medialization and arytenoid adduction: the Vanderbilt experience. A review of 116 phonosurgical procedures. Ann Otol Rhinol Laryngol 1993; 102:413-424.

Kraus DH, Ali MK, Ginsberg RJ, et al: Vocal cord medialization for unilateral paralysis associated with intrathoracic malignancies. J Thorac Cardiovasc Surg 1996;111:334-341.

Laccourreye O, Le Pimpec-Barthès F, Hans S, et al: Traitement de la paralysie récurrentielle unilatérale après chirurgie pulmonaire carcinologique par injection intracordale de graisse autologue. J Chir Thorac Cardiovasc 1999;3:181-184.

Mom T, Filaire M, Advenier D, et al: Concomitant type I thyroplasty and thoracic operations for lung cancer: preventing respiratory complications associated with vagus or recurrent laryngeal nerve injury. J Thorac Cardiovasc Surg 2001;121:642-648.

Abraham MT, Bains MS, Downey RJ, et al: Type 1 thyroplasty for acute unilateral vocal cord paralysis following intrathoracic surgery. Ann Otol Rhinol Laryngol 2002;111:667-671.

Case Series

Filaire M, Mom T, Laurent S, et al: Vocal cord dysfunction after left lung resection for cancer. Eur J Cardiothorac Surg 2001; 20:705-711.

OTHER COMMON AND LESS COMMON COMPLICATIONS OF PULMONARY SURGERY

Despite advances in the perioperative care of pulmonary resection patients, complications still occur. Some of these complications, such as fever and subcutaneous emphysema, are common and indeed are *expected* and *almost unavoidable*. If neglected, however, fever may persist or subcutaneous emphysema may progress, thus becoming serious issues that need to be addressed if one wants to avoid significant morbidity or even mortality.

Other complications, such as cardiac herniation and lobe torsion, are uncommon and often difficult to diagnose, even by experienced surgeons. Unfortunately, missing the diagnosis of such problems is likely to lead to catastrophic and life-threatening situations.

7

Management of Postoperative Complications

COMMON COMPLICATIONS

Fever

Transient fever (38°C to 38.5°C) for 2 or 3 days is a *normal response to surgical trauma.* It is indeed expected in patients undergoing pulmonary resection because of *prior pneumonia, long operative procedures* (>2 hours), and variable degree of postoperative atelectasis. If the fever persists beyond 2 or 3 days, especially if it is higher than 39°C, it is likely to be related to atelectasis or pulmonary infection. If it starts by postoperative days 5 to 7 or after the thoracostomy tubes have been removed, empyemas must be included in the differential diagnosis. Obviously, the possibility of deep wound infections, urinary tract infections, or infections at other sites must be looked into, although these are uncommon causes of fever in the lung resection patient.

Management is based on documenting the source of fever and applying a specific treatment to it. During the first 24 to 72 postoperative hours, however, *only symptomatic treatment* should be applied, especially if the chest radiograph shows adequate lung re-expansion and no residual spaces. If lung consolidation is present, bedside fiberoptic bronchoscopy may be required to relieve bronchial obstruction and to sample bronchial secretions for culture. The spectrum of antibiotherapy may also have to be widened.

If the initial fever persists beyond 3 to 5 days or starts by day 4 or 5, one should investigate its source (Table 7-68) and *strongly resist the urge to systematically order antibiotics* that may mask the source of infection.

Directed patient questionnaire may reveal purulent sputum or increased amounts of secretions indicating lung infection. The patient should be examined for abnormalities of lung auscultation such as crepitations or rhonchi, redness at the sites of thoracotomy or chest tube incisions, and signs of deep vein thrombosis of the lower extremities. The chest radiograph should be looked at because it may show pulmonary consolidation,

TABLE 7-68

BASIC INVESTIGATION OF PERSISTENT FEVER IN POST-THORACOTOMY PATIENTS

Test	Finding	Likely Source of Fever
Clinical history	Purulent sputum	Lung
	Dysuria, burning on urination	Urinary
Physical examination	Bronchial breathing, rhonchi	Lung
	Wound abnormalities	Wound collection or true infection
	Signs of deep vein thrombosis	Acute thrombophlebitis
Chest radiograph	Lung consolidation	Lung
	Persistent space	Pleural (empyema)
White blood cell count	Normal or elevated	Nonspecific
Sputum culture	Positive	Lung
Urine culture	Positive	Urinary

incomplete lung re-expansion, persistent air spaces, or fluid accumulation, all potential sources of fever. An elevated or rising white blood cell count will provide *further evidence* of an active infection. If the white blood cell count is *normal,* it will set a baseline should the fever persist. A positive blood culture always indicates a serious infection, and in such cases, *a consultant in infectious diseases* should be asked to see the patient.

The most important initial therapeutic decision concerning postoperative fever is whether to treat it. If the cause is unknown, the patient should be given antipyretic therapy (acetaminophen, 325 to 650 mg every 4 hours for adults) and further observed, especially if she or he is clinically well. A specific cause will often never be found, and *the fever will subside on its own* during a period of a few days.

If a source of infection is documented or at least likely, specific treatment including both pharmacologic (antibiotics) and nonpharmacologic measures such as pleural space tube drainage, bronchoscopy, or evacuation of wound collections should be initiated immediately. In *rare instances* of persistent high postoperative fever of unknown origin, wide-spectrum antibiotics can be given on an empirical basis.

Surgical Emphysema

Surgical emphysema can occur immediately after surgery or develop during the days after the operation. It is *always secondary to inadequate drainage* of the pleural space as air reaches the subcutaneous tissues through the perforated pleura at the sites of thoracotomy or chest tube insertion. Whereas a minimal and nonprogressive amount of surgical emphysema around the wound is almost normal, a significant amount extending into the arms, neck, and eyelids or down to the abdominal wall and scrotum is of importance, *especially if it is progressive over time.* Fortunately, surgical emphysema, even in large amounts, is seldom life-threatening. It can be the source of significant discomfort for the patient, however, especially if the eyelids are inflated and the eyes are closed or if it is associated with changes in the patient's voice (high pitch or nasal voice).

Etiology (Table 7-69) and Investigation

Surgical emphysema may be due to improper positioning of the chest tubes, to *kinking or occlusion* of those tubes, to obstruction within the

7

Management of Postoperative Complications

TABLE 7-69

COMMON CAUSES OF POSTOPERATIVE SURGICAL EMPHYSEMA

Inadequacy of drainage system
    Tubes are malpositioned in the pleural space.
    Tubes are kinked.
    Patient is lying over the tubes.
    Tubing or connecting system is occluded.
    Tubes have pulled back outside the pleural space.
    One chest tube hole is outside the skin incision.
Large air leak inadequately absorbed by the drainage unit

connecting tubing or drainage system, or to tube pullback in the soft tissues of the chest wall. Progressive surgical emphysema can also be related to a large air leak that *cannot* be completely absorbed by the drainage unit or an air leak that *fuses directly* from the lung into the thoracotomy incision.

When progressive surgical emphysema does occur, the entire drainage system and all thoracostomy sites *should be thoroughly inspected* to make sure that the tubes are not kinked or occluded and that they have not been accidentally pulled out of the pleural space. Sometimes, the incisions around the thoracostomy tubes are not airtight so that atmospheric air can reach the subcutaneous tissues and be the source of the surgical emphysema.

If the system is airtight and functioning properly, a chest radiograph should be obtained to determine if there is a pneumothorax and if the tubes are properly positioned within the pleural space. Ultimately, CT scanning may be required to provide better definitions of undrained spaces.

Treatment

If the thoracostomy tubes are patent and the system is airtight, the amount of active suction can first be increased from 20 cm H_2O to 30 or even 40 cm H_2O. If increasing the suction does not stop the progression of surgical emphysema, as is often the case, or if the thoracostomy tubes are blocked or there is a pneumothorax on the chest radiograph, *another tube should be inserted.* Sometimes pulling out a tube already in place by 1 or 2 cm will restore its patency and solve the problem. Connecting each tube to separate drainage units may also help improve drainage.

If the progression of surgical emphysema still cannot be controlled, dehiscence of the bronchial stump must be suspected and ruled out by bronchoscopy. In rare cases, thoracic re-exploration either by VATS or by reopening the thoracotomy incision may eventually be necessary to locate and suture the site of air leak and to reposition the chest tubes.

Because surgical emphysema is often of some concern to the patient and the patient's relatives, it is important to take some time to explain to them that it is not dangerous and that during a period of days or weeks, it will completely disappear without any sequelae.

Attempts to aspirate air from subcutaneous tissues either with needles or through small incisions may relieve the tension, *but it is generally not indicated and is of little or no use.*

Surgical Emphysema after Pneumonectomy

Surgical emphysema almost always occurs after pneumonectomy because residual air in the pneumonectomy space escapes directly into the wound when the patient coughs. The amount of surgical emphysema is limited, however, and its progression will stop once the pleural space pressure becomes negative, usually by 8 to 12 hours postoperatively. If surgical emphysema progresses beyond that time, a *bronchopleural fistula is likely* and should be ruled out by bronchoscopic examination.

Gastrointestinal Complications

Minor gastrointestinal complications are fairly common after any thoracic operation, especially if the patient has COPD and is anxious about his or her ability to breathe. By contrast, major gastrointestinal complications are unusual.

Upper Gastrointestinal Complications

Most upper gastrointestinal complications, such as gastric dilatation and stress ulcers, can be prevented by an *early return to normal oral alimentation, avoidance of prolonged use of nonsteroidal anti-inflammatory drugs,* and *use of prophylactic medication* against stress or peptic ulcers (Table 7-70). It is also good practice to discuss the issue of air swallowing with every COPD patient undergoing pulmonary resection or lung volume reduction surgery. Teaching the patient how to breathe quietly and how to avoid air swallowing can prevent acute gastric dilatation with its inherent dangers of acid aspiration and secondary chemical pneumonitis.

Lower Gastrointestinal Complications

Intestinal ileus is not uncommon in patients undergoing lung volume reduction surgery. In such cases, it is related to a combination *of excessive air swallowing* and *decreased bowel motility* due to epidural analgesia. This complication is generally self-limited and will resolve without specific treatment within 3 to 4 days. Temporarily, however, intestinal ileus can be a significant problem because it restricts diaphragmatic contraction and lung expansion, delays return to normal alimentation, and prevents early mobilization of the patient. Ogilvie syndrome, characterized by massive colonic distention, *is rare* in the absence of other major postoperative complications.

In recent years, *Clostridium difficile* colitis has become a fairly common complication of surgery, probably because of *increased use of wide-spectrum antibiotics* and *higher number of immunosuppressed patients* undergoing operations. Such colitis, which can become fulminant, is characterized by diarrhea and foul-smelling stool; the diagnosis is easily made by recovering *C. difficile* toxins in the stools. Because this analysis may take up to several days, however, it is recommended to begin treatment with *metronidazole* given orally as soon as the diagnosis is suspected. If metronidazole does

7

Management of Postoperative Complications

TABLE 7-70

PROPHYLAXIS AGAINST UPPER GASTROINTESTINAL COMPLICATIONS

Resume oral alimentation as soon as possible.

Avoid prolonged use of nonsteroidal anti-inflammatory drugs.

Use prophylactic pharmacologic agents.

    Antacids

    Histamine antagonists (H_2 blockers)

    Proton pump inhibitors (omeprazole)

Teach the emphysema patient how to avoid air swallowing.

not control the diarrhea, vancomycin can be added to the regimen. All other antibiotics should be stopped unless absolutely necessary.

Residual Pleural Effusions

Pleural effusions can develop after chest tube removal in relation to either the lysis of undrained blood clots or inflammation of pleural surfaces; more commonly, pleural effusions develop because of *significant negative pleural pressure secondary to atelectasis* or loss of volume of the residual lung. They are usually self-limited, and over time, the accumulated pleural fluid will be completely reabsorbed without any long-term sequelae. Such effusions may be temporarily symptomatic, however, causing fever, chest pain, and dyspnea.

Unless the effusion is or subsequently becomes infected, management should be directed at controlling the symptoms with antipyretic medications and analgesics.

UNCOMMON COMPLICATIONS

Hemorrhage

Hemorrhagic complications can occur during the operation or postoperatively.

Hemorrhage during Pulmonary Resection

Despite significant advances in the techniques of lung resection, intraoperative bleeding can occur. The most commonly injured blood vessels are the *pulmonary artery* or one of its branches, *the pulmonary veins,* and the *superior vena cava.* Risk factors, listed in Table 7-71, include reoperations; surgery for chronic inflammatory conditions; and diseased nodes, such as those affected by histoplasmosis, tuberculosis, or silicosis around the pulmonary blood vessels.

The most important prophylaxis measures against intraoperative hemorrhage are the preoperative identification of patients at risk and the use of meticulous surgical technique. If hemorrhage still occurs, vascular clamps should be applied and the site of laceration repaired with 4-0 or 5-0 Prolene suture material. However, when bleeding is profuse, *blind application of vascular clamps may be dangerous* because such application may increase the size of the laceration with further aggravation of the problem.

Postoperative Hemorrhage

Significant postoperative hemorrhage requiring reoperation occurs in about 5% of all lung resection patients. The most common sources of bleeding are *the bronchial arteries, the systemic vessels within divided adhesions,*

TABLE 7-71
RISK FACTORS FOR INTRAOPERATIVE HEMORRHAGE
Redo surgery (completion pneumonectomy)
Surgery for chronic inflammatory conditions (late sequelae of tuberculosis, bronchiectasis)
Surgery in the presence of dense and diffuse adhesions
Nodal disease such as histoplasmosis, broncholithiasis, silicosis
Coagulation abnormality

TABLE 7-72

RISK FACTORS FOR POSTOPERATIVE HEMORRHAGE

Redo surgery

Surgery for bronchiectasis or other chronic benign lung disorders

Significant pleural adhesions

Extrapleural pulmonary resection

Associated parietal pleurectomy

Complex procedures

Incomplete fissures

Inadequate hemostasis during initial operation

Coagulation disorder

7

the intercostal arteries, and the segmental pulmonary veins in lung surfaces. Breakdown of ligated or stapled major blood vessels is uncommon. Risk factors, listed in Table 7-72, include surgery for benign diseases such as bronchiectasis (bronchial artery hyperplasia), surgery in which extrapleural dissection or *parietal pleurectomy* has been required, and inadequate hemostasis during the initial operation.

Management of postoperative hemorrhage includes *replacement of blood losses;* correction of coagulation disorders if they are present; and *adequate monitoring of the patient* (Table 7-73), especially the hemodynamic status, the amount of chest tube drainage (measured every 15 minutes), the hemoglobin value, and the platelet count. Monitoring of the platelet count is particularly important because a steady decline in the number of platelets indicates *active platelet consumption* and thus active bleeding. In the event that the chest tubes have become occluded, a portable chest radiograph may show intrapleural accumulation of blood clots.

Surgical re-exploration of the patient is generally recommended if the rate of bleeding is in the range of *200 to 300 mL/h for 3 to 4 hours,* if it is *difficult to maintain a stable arterial blood pressure,* or if the *platelet count is decreasing.* If drainage appears to be slowing down and if the patient is hemodynamically stable, it is possible to wait longer before taking the patient back to surgery. In some instances, connecting the chest tubes on an underwater seal drainage system rather than on a suction system may slow active bleeding.

As a general rule, it is better to reoperate earlier rather than to expose the patient to complications such as metabolic acidosis, coagulation abnormalities, and ARDS that may be associated with multiple blood transfusions.

Management of Postoperative Complications

TABLE 7-73

KEY ELEMENTS OF THE MONITORING OF PATIENTS WHO ARE HEMORRHAGING AFTER PULMONARY RESECTION

Hemodynamic status: blood pressure and heart rate

Amount of blood loss through the chest tube (every 15 minutes)

Hourly hemoglobin and platelet count

Wound Complications

Minor Complications: Hematomas and Seromas

Superficial wound complications such as hematomas and seromas are not uncommon, but they are *seldom* the source of significant morbidity. Hematomas are due to bleeding from the skin or subcutaneous tissue; most are restricted to the incision area, although they can sometimes extend down to the pelvis. They should be treated expectantly because all will resolve spontaneously.

Wound seromas are *almost always associated with muscle-sparing incisions* where extensive subcutaneous dissection of chest wall muscles has taken place. Seromas are also common after procedures in which a muscle flap, such as the latissimus dorsi, had to be mobilized. When a seroma does occur, the diagnosis is easily made by palpating fluid underneath the skin. In such cases, the differential diagnosis must always include pleural fluid that has drained into the subcutaneous space through a partial wound dehiscence. Small seromas need no treatment, but larger ones (>100 mL) may need to be aspirated or drained by small catheters connected to Hemovac types of vacuum. If the seroma is secondary to a pleural effusion, the treatment should be tube drainage of the pleural space rather than wound drainage.

Major Complications: Dehiscence and Infection

Wound dehiscence is rare (Table 7-74), and, in general, the dehiscence is limited to the deep planes of the chest wall, with the skin remaining intact. In the context of lung resection, dehiscences are more likely to occur after pneumonectomies than after lobectomies. The majority of thoracic wound dehiscences are only partial, although large enough to let pleural air and fluid exit into the subcutaneous tissues. The diagnosis is made by asking the patient to cough and feeling the thrust of air or fluid underneath the skin.

Patients with wound dehiscences can generally be managed by draining the pleural space (tube thoracostomy away from the incision) and waiting until the site of dehiscence becomes obliterated by fibrin or granulation tissue. Seldom will a complete wound dehiscence occurring early (within 1 week of surgery) interfere with respiratory and cough mechanics and need surgical reclosure. Late dehiscences (more than 1 week postoperatively) are rarely associated with respiratory difficulties, and most can be managed by observation alone or tube drainage of the pleural space.

TABLE 7-74
FACTS ABOUT THORACIC WOUND DEHISCENCE

It is a rare complication.
It is usually limited to deep planes (skin is intact).
Most are seen after pneumonectomy.
Initial treatment is by chest tube drainage of the pleural space.
Early dehiscences associated with respiratory difficulties may need reoperation.

Wound infections are uncommon because the majority of thoracic surgical procedures are clean and uncontaminated. Superficial infections are treated by removing the skin sutures and packing the incision open with wet saline dressings. Deep infections are nearly always caused by an empyema that has drained through the incision (empyema necessitatis); the treatment of such conditions is that of the underlying empyema.

Lung Herniation

Herniation of the lung through the thoracotomy incision is always the result of wound dehiscence. It is usually recognized late during the postoperative period, often after the patient has gone home. The diagnosis is made by physical examination, and for most patients, *management should be conservative.* If the size of the hernia increases over time or if the hernia becomes symptomatic, surgical repair may be indicated.

Cardiac Herniation (Table 7-75)

Cardiac herniation is an infrequently reported but catastrophic complication of pulmonary surgery. It usually arises within 24 to 48 hours of the operation in patients who had *pneumonectomy with intrapericardial ligation* of pulmonary blood vessels. Right-sided herniations lead to obstruction of caval venous return. Left-sided herniations are more likely to lead to constriction of the left ventricle by the pericardial defect, resulting in ischemia and dysfunction of the herniated myocardium. Risk factors include an *unclosed median-size pericardial defect* and the application of suction to chest tubes. It is observed with *equal frequency* after right or left pneumonectomy.

The onset of cardiac herniation is characterized by sudden and marked hypotension, tachycardia, cyanosis, and chest pain. The clinical diagnosis rests on a high index of suspicion and a chest radiograph showing complete subluxation of the heart. Left-sided herniations may present with subtle radiographic changes, often a shift to the left of the cardiac shadow in conjunction with a rounded opacity in the lower portion of the hemithorax representing the herniated apex of the left ventricle.

Most cases of cardiac herniation are preventable if the pericardial defect is closed during the initial surgery, even if this defect appears to be relatively small. Surgical methods to close such defects include primary suture reapproximation and closure with a prosthetic (Dacron) or tissue (pleura, fascia, bovine pericardium) patch graft if the defect is larger.

7

Management of Postoperative Complications

TABLE 7-75

FACTS ABOUT POST–PULMONARY RESECTION CARDIAC HERNIATION

It is a rare complication of intrapericardial pneumonectomy (median-size pericardial defect).

Right-sided herniation leads to occlusion of venous return to the heart.

Left-sided herniation leads to constriction of the left ventricle with secondary myocardial ischemia.

Onset is always sudden and characterized by marked hypotension.

Successful management requires prompt diagnosis and reoperation.

Successful management of cardiac herniation requires *prompt diagnosis and immediate reoperation.* On the right side, the heart is returned to its normal position and the pericardium is closed, usually with a patch graft. On the left side, graft closure can also be used, or the pericardium can be opened down to the diaphragm, thus eliminating the chances of cardiac strangulation. In these patients, however, chronic displacement of the heart may cause long-term diminished cardiac output and poor exercise tolerance.

Despite prompt reoperation, the mortality associated with cardiac herniation approaches 50%.

Lobe Torsion

Torsion of a remaining lobe after lobectomy is a rare complication of pulmonary resection; the most commonly involved lobe is the middle lobe. A complete oblique fissure anteriorly (between lower and middle lobes) and the narrow middle lobe hilum make this lobe more susceptible to torsion around its own pedicle *after an upper lobectomy.* Because the horizontal fissure (between middle and upper lobes) is usually fused, middle lobe torsion is almost never seen after right lower lobectomy. Lobe torsion results in obstruction of the venous return with secondary hemorrhagic necrosis of the involved lobe.

Clinically, patients with lobe torsion present with significant hemoptysis, often during the first few postoperative hours. The chest radiograph shows increased density of the involved parenchyma. Eventually, the *patient's clinical condition will deteriorate* because the infarcted lobe will undergo necrosis and secondary infection, and the bronchus will dehisce. This sequence of events is similar to what is observed in association with mesenteric vein thrombosis, in which the colon suffers from hemorrhagic necrosis.

The diagnosis of lobe torsion can be difficult to document, especially if the twisted lobe is not the middle lobe and the surgeon does not have a high index of suspicion. When the diagnosis is made, however, *the only treatment option is to reoperate* and, in most cases, *remove the involved lobe.* In some cases when the diagnosis is made early in the process, it may be possible to untwist the lobe, thus avoiding completion lobectomy.

Prophylaxis is a key element in avoidance of lobe torsion. Indeed, it is simple to prevent torsion of the middle lobe by approximating its lower border to the lower lobe in every case of right upper lobectomy. This can be done with a stapler or with two or three individual sutures.

CONCLUSION

Most complications occurring after pulmonary surgery are predictable and thus preventable if the surgeon has a clear knowledge of their pathogenesis and risk factors and is able to clinically recognize them. If they still occur, a systematic approach based on an understanding of their pathophysiologic features is likely to minimize their impact on the overall postoperative course.

SUGGESTED READINGS

Review Articles

Trastek VF, Pairolero PC, Allen MS, Deschamps C: Unusual complications of pulmonary resection. Chest Surg Clin North Am 1992;2:853-861.

Pezzella AT, Adebonojo SA, Hooker SG, et al: Complications of general thoracic surgery. Curr Probl Surg 2000;37:742-855.

Cerfolio RJ: Chest tube management after pulmonary resection. Chest Surg Clin North Am 2002;12:507-527.

Hemorrhagic Complications

Péterffy A, Henze A: Haemorrhagic complications during pulmonary resection. A retrospective review of 1428 resections with 113 haemorrhagic episodes. Scand J Thorac Cardiovasc Surg 1983;17:283-287.

Cardiac Herniation

Deiraniya AK: Cardiac herniation following intrapericardial pneumonectomy. Thorax 1974;29:545-552.

Weinlander CM, Abel MD, Piehler JM: Spontaneous herniation after pneumonectomy. Anesth Analg 1986;65:1085-1088.

Gastrointestinal Complications

Cook DJ, Fuller HD, Guyatt GH, et al: Risk factors for gastrointestinal bleeding in critically ill patients. N Engl J Med 1994;330:377-381.

Kokoska ER, Naunheim KS: Gastrointestinal complications postthoracotomy and postvagotomy. Chest Surg Clin North Am 1998;8:645-661.

Lobe Torsion

Wong PS, Goldstraw P: Pulmonary torsion: a questionnaire survey and a survey of the literature. Ann Thorac Surg 1992;54:286-288.

Cable DG, Deschamps C, Allen MS, et al: Lobar torsion after pulmonary resection: presentation and outcome. J Thorac Cardiovasc Surg 2001;122:1091-1093.

CHYLOTHORAX

Injuries to the thoracic duct are *seldom seen after elective lung surgery;* their incidence is estimated to be around 0.05%. Extensive pleural adhesions, significant local tumor extension, and, most important, radical mediastinal lymphadenectomy have been associated with increased risks for this complication.

Comprehensive management of postoperative chyle leaks demands an understanding of the *anatomy and physiology of the thoracic duct* as well as of the *metabolic, nutritional,* and *immunologic consequences* of continuous chyle depletion. It also demands an understanding of the combined aspects of medical and surgical treatment modalities, which include space drainage, dietary management, and surgical reintervention.

ANATOMY OF THE THORACIC DUCT AND MECHANISM OF INJURY DURING LUNG RESECTION

The "textbook" anatomy of the thoracic duct (see Chapter 5, "Thoracic Anatomy") is found in only 50% of individuals. In those individuals, the thoracic duct originates as the efferent vessel of the cisterna chyli in the abdomen and ascends in the posterior mediastinum through the aortic hiatus (level of T12).

In the right posterior mediastinum, the location of the thoracic duct is the *most predictable* within the thorax. It runs in front of the vertebral bodies, somewhat behind and to the right of the esophagus, to the left of the azygos vein, and to the right of the aorta (Fig. 7-6). At approximately the T4-5 intervertebral level, the duct passes from right to left and then travels upward on the *left posterior aspect of the esophagus.* At the root of the neck, the duct passes behind the carotid sheath and then arches anteriorly to enter the venous system at the junction of the left internal jugular and left subclavian veins. Patients with not so normal anatomy have anomalous and accessory lymphatic pathways communicating with the azygos and intercostal venous systems.

Chyle leaks occurring after lung resection result from an injury to the main thoracic duct or *more often to accessory lymphatic-venous connections* around the azygos vein and carina. Injuries to the main duct usually occur during procedures done in the right lower or left upper hemithoraces. Injury to the thoracic duct below the level of T5 results in a right chylothorax; injury above that level results in a left chylothorax.

DIAGNOSIS

Although it is possible to diagnose a chyle leak during operation, this diagnosis is usually difficult because lymph is a low-pressure and low-flow system. In addition, chyle is clear in fasting patients, thus making it difficult to see during surgery.

Clinical Presentation (Table 7-76)

The clinical diagnosis of chylothorax is *often delayed* until the patient has resumed oral intake. Initially, the pleural fluid draining from chest tubes is straw colored or blood stained, but as soon as the patient starts drinking or eating, this fluid will become milky white, making it easy to recognize. If the diagnosis is still in doubt, one can administer a high-fat diet followed by careful observation of pleural fluid drainage, which will rapidly increase in volume and become milky white.

Another typical clinical feature of postoperative chylothoraces is that the *amount of pleural drainage can be as high as 1500 to 2000 mL/24 h.* If the patient has no chest tube, serial radiographs may show rapid accumulation of pleural fluid with secondary contralateral displacement of mediastinal structures. This displacement will often precipitate significant hemodynamic and respiratory difficulties due to decreased venous return and compression of the residual lobe or contralateral lung, respectively.

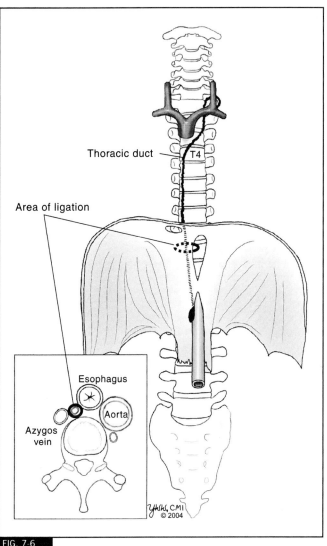

Thoracic duct — T4

Area of ligation

Esophagus

Aorta

Azygos vein

Yuki, CMI
© 2004

FIG. 7-6

Most constant position of the thoracic duct in the right lower thoracic arch. Note the position of the thoracic duct, which is posterior to the esophagus between the aorta and azygos vein.

TABLE 7-76

DIAGNOSTIC FEATURES OF CHYLOUS EFFUSION

Appearance	Commonly milky, may be serous or sanguineous in fasting patients
Odor	Odorless
Supernatant	Opalescent
Cell count	Lymphocytes predominate
Culture	Sterile
Biochemistry	Triglycerides > 110 mg/dL
	Cholesterol-to-triglyceride ratio < 1
Lipoprotein analyses	Presence of chylomicrons on electrophoresis
Ingestion of cream	Opacifies clear effusion

From Valentine VG, Raffin TA: Management of chylothorax. Chest 1992;102:586-591.

Biochemical Diagnosis (Table 7-76)

The diagnosis of chylothorax is usually confirmed by sending a pleural aspirate for biochemistry. An old but still useful analysis is to look for free microscopic fat by staining the fluid with Sudan III. Chyle has a cholesterol-to-triglyceride ratio of less than 1 and a triglyceride level that is greater than 1.24 mmol/L. Lymphocytes are the predominant cells, and a *90% lymphocyte count* is virtually diagnostic of chylothorax.

In most cases of postoperative chylothoraces, precise localization of the fistulous site is unnecessary. If it is required, however, nuclear lymphangiography with technetium Tc 99 m antimony colloid or standard bipedal contrast lymphangiography can be tried. Both techniques have limited use, and contrast lymphangiography can also be associated with significant pulmonary complications such as edema and ARDS.

CONSEQUENCES OF PROLONGED CHYLE LEAKS (TABLE 7-77)

Bearing in mind that chyle has electrolyte concentrations similar to those of plasma and that lymph flow averages 60 to 80 mL/h (it can be as high as 2 mL/minute), the *potential for extracellular fluid loss is significant;* such losses can rapidly lead to hypovolemia, hypotension, and even shock. Electrolyte imbalances are also likely to occur. Because the protein content of chyle is between 22 and 60 g/L (albumin-to-globulin ratio of 3:1), protein depletion can arise in a short time with peripheral edema due to

TABLE 7-77

CONSEQUENCES OF PROLONGED CHYLE LEAK

Pathology	Consequences
Loss of extracellular fluid	Dehydration, hypotension
	Electrolyte imbalance
Loss of protein	Hypoalbuminemia and edema
	Weight loss
Loss of lymphocytes	Immunosuppression
	Increased susceptibility to infection

hypoalbuminemia and significant weight loss. A typical feature of chylothoraces is that *patients still lose weight even if replacements appear to be adequate.*

Immunologic consequences can be severe. Decreased immunity and significant drop in the peripheral lymphocyte count (T lymphocytes) lead to a status of immunosuppression and increased susceptibility to infection.

MANAGEMENT

Conservative Management

Once the diagnosis of chylothorax has been confirmed, a trial of conservative management, at least initially, is recommended. The objectives of these measures (Table 7-78) are to drain the lymph collection, to re-expand the lung fully, to prevent dehydration, to maintain nutrition, and to minimize chyle formation.

Drainage of Lymph Collection and Promotion of Pulmonary Re-expansion

The pleural space is best drained *by way of thoracostomy tubes,* which are already in place in most patients. Thoracostomy tubes help achieve lung re-expansion while allowing accurate measurements of daily chyle production. In some cases, effective lung expansion and apposition of pleural surfaces will promote pleural symphysis, which in turn may initiate spontaneous fistula closure. If the lung is well expanded, thoracostomy tubes should be connected to an underwater seal system rather than to an active suction system.

Some surgeons have tried to stimulate adhesion formation by the intrapleural injection (through the chest tube) of talc or other products used for sclerotherapy. The result of these interventions is *unpredictable,* and talc slurry may also obstruct the thoracostomy tube.

Prevention of Dehydration and Maintenance of Nutrition

Because up to 3 liters of chyle may drain every day, large amounts of extracellular fluid and electrolytes will be lost. These losses must be monitored closely and replaced almost on an hourly basis.

The decline in total protein and albumin serum levels as well as of the body weight must also be followed closely and corrected by nutritional support as early as possible. *Parenteral nutrition is the most satisfactory method* of replacement because daily adjustments can be based on electrolyte and protein levels.

7

Management of Postoperative Complications

TABLE 7-78

GOALS OF CONSERVATIVE MANAGEMENT

Completely evacuate the collection.

Fully re-expand the lung.

Prevent dehydration.

Maintain nutrition.

Minimize chyle formation.

Minimizing Chyle Formation

Although options to minimize chyle formation include enteral feedings with low-fat diets and medium-chain triglycerides (MCT), *early implementation of parenteral feeding* is most likely to achieve resolution of the chylothorax.

The concept behind the use of MCT is that these products are absorbed directly into the portal system rather than by intestinal lymphatic vessels, thus reducing lymph formation. Unfortunately, MCT diets have had little success in reducing lymph formation, mostly because any oral intake, whether it is water, other liquids, or MCT, still stimulates chyle formation. Thus, most surgeons prefer complete *cessation of oral intake and total parenteral nutrition.* With this strategy, it is not unusual to see the amount of lymph drainage decrease by 50% or even more in the first few hours.

Somatostatin given by infusion and continued for 7 days may also reduce chyle production, although the exact mechanism of action is unknown. Experimentally, somatostatin reduces gastric and small bowel motility and inhibits gastric, pancreatic, and intestinal secretions. Analogues of somatostatin, such as octreotide, have also been tried with variable success. Other possible interventions, such as pleuroperitoneal shunting, embolization of the thoracic duct, and pleurovenous shunting, are *never used* in the management of postoperative chyle leaks.

When the chyle leak appears to have stopped, oral intake may be resumed slowly, and in this setting, MCT may be useful. Before removal of the chest tube, *thoracic duct closure must be challenged* by giving the patient a normal or a high-fat diet for 24 hours.

Surgical Treatment (Table 7-79)

Indications for Reoperation

The decision to continue with conservative management or to undertake surgical intervention must be based on the duration of fistula and *daily amount of chyle drainage,* the severity of nutritional or immunologic complications, and the nature of the operation that was done initially.

It is generally agreed that a continuing chylous leak in excess of 1000 mL/day for 7 days in a patient with complete cessation of oral intake *is an absolute indication* to undertake reoperative intervention. Reoperation should also be considered with chyle leaks greater than 500 mL/day for more than 2 weeks; in these cases, however, observation for a few extra days is safe if the patient remains in good condition and the amount of drainage appears to be decreasing. Patients with severe nutritional depletion or metabolic complications should be reoperated on early.

TABLE 7-79

INDICATIONS FOR REOPERATION

Chyle leak greater than 1000 mL/day for more than 7 days
Chyle leak greater than 500 mL/day for more than 14 days
Nutritional or metabolic complications
Should be done earlier in pneumonectomy patients

Conservative management can be done *for longer periods* after initial lobectomy because pulmonary re-expansion may fill the residual space and thus help seal the site of chyle leak. Reoperation should, on the other hand, be considered sooner in pneumonectomy patients, especially in those with a significant amount of chyle leakage.

Techniques for Closure of a Thoracic Duct Fistula

There are two currently acceptable techniques (Table 7-80) for closing a thoracic duct fistula. The first approach consists of thoracic duct ligation above the diaphragm (see Fig. 7-6). With this technique, the thoracic duct is identified and then suture ligated behind the esophagus. If the thoracic duct is not identified, mass ligature of all tissues posterior to the esophagus and between the azygos vein and the aorta just above the diaphragm is effective. Preoperative feeding of the patient with cream (300 mL of 30% cream given through nasogastric tube 3 hours before operation) will distend the duct and make it easier to locate. The advantage of this technique is that it is safe and effective in more than 95% of cases. Possible disadvantages are that the surgeon must have *clear knowledge of the local anatomy* and that, at least in theory, total interruption of lymph flow may be the source of malabsorption syndromes and lower extremity edema. In most cases, however, these complications are transient, and during a short time, new lymph channels will open up and normal lymph flow will resume.

The second technique consists of direct ligation of the site of fistula through a reopening of the previously used thoracotomy incision. Again, 30% cream is given 2 to 3 hours preoperatively so that the site of chyle leak can easily be recognized and sutured. The main disadvantage of this technique is that chyle leakage may be originating from several collaterals rather than from the main duct, thus making it more difficult to control with direct suturing. Despite this disadvantage, direct fistula ligation is effective in controlling the chyle leak in more than 90% of cases.

TABLE 7-80		
ACCEPTABLE TECHNIQUES FOR CLOSURE OF THORACIC DUCT FISTULAS		
Technique	Advantages	Disadvantages
Thoracic duct ligation	Successful in 95% of cases	Requires intimate knowledge of anatomy
	Stops flow from any possible accessory duct or abnormal lymphatic venous anastomosis	Duct may be difficult to see and one may have to do mass ligature
	Can be done by VATS techniques	May require new incision
		Completely interrupts lymph flow
Data suturing of fistula site	Successful in 90%-95% of cases	Suturing may be difficult if leak originates from multiple collaterals or accessory ducts
	Preserves anatomic integrity of thoracic duct	
	Can be done by VATS techniques	
	Thoracic duct ligation still possible if it fails	

Results

Results of surgical reintervention are good with either technique. Complication rate is low, and late sequelae are uncommon.

Role of VATS Techniques

In recent years, VATS has been used to treat postoperative chyle leaks. Under thoracoscopic vision, the site of leakage can be found and sutured or clipped, or the main duct can be identified above the diaphragm and clipped proximally and distally. If dissection of the duct is difficult because of scarred tissues, mass ligature is a satisfactory alternative. On occasion, *thoracoscopic application of fibrin glue* can be useful if the site of leakage is small.

One advantage of VATS is that it can easily be converted to an open procedure either at the same sitting or at a later date.

CONCLUSION

Postoperative chyle leak is a serious complication of pulmonary surgery because significant leakage quickly leads to loss of extracellular fluid and proteins, electrolyte imbalances, malnutrition, and immunosuppression. Ultimately, the patient will die if he or she is not treated. Because nonoperative management is successful in up to 50% of cases, it should be tried first. For chylothoraces unresponsive to conservative measures, reintervention should be considered before serious metabolic complications develop.

SUGGESTED READINGS

Review Articles

Ferguson MK, Little AG, Skinner DB: Current concepts in the management of postoperative chylothorax. Ann Thorac Surg 1985;40:542-545.

Robinson CLN: The management of chylothorax [collective review]. Ann Thorac Surg 1985;39:90-95.

Valentine VG, Raffin TA: The management of chylothorax. Chest 1992; 102:586-591.

Johnstone DW, Feins RH: Chylothorax. Chest Surg Clin North Am 1994; 4:617-628.

Paes ML, Powell H: Chylothorax: an update. Br J Hosp Med 1994; 51:482-490.

Merrigan BA, Winter DC, O'Sullivan GC: Chylothorax. Br J Surg 1997; 84:15-20.

Anatomy of Thoracic Duct

Riquet M, Le Pimpec-Barthes F, Souilamas R, Hidden G: Thoracic duct tributaries from intrathoracic organs. Ann Thorac Surg 2002;73:892-899.

Treatment of Chylothorax

Patterson GA, Todd TRJ, Delarue NC, et al: Supradiaphragmatic ligation of the thoracic duct in intractable chylous fistula. Ann Thorac Surg 1981;32:44-49.

Akaogi E, Mitsui K, Sahara Y, et al: Treatment of postoperative chylothorax with intrapleural fibrin glue. Ann Thorac Surg 1989;48:116-118.

Haniuda M, Nishimura H, Kobayashi O, et al: Management of chylothorax after pulmonary resection. J Am Coll Surg 1995;180:537-540.

Peillon C, D'Hont C, Melki J, et al: Usefulness of videothoracoscopy in the management of spontaneous and postoperation chylothorax. Surg Endosc 1999;13:1106-1109.

Wurnig PN, Hollaus PH, Ohtsuka T, et al: Thoracoscopic direct clipping of the thoracic duct for chylopericardium and chylothorax. Ann Thorac Surg 2000;70:1662-1665.

Fahimi H, Casselman FP, Mariani MA, et al: Current management of postoperative chylothorax. Ann Thorac Surg 2001;71:448-451.

Postpneumonectomy Chylothorax

Vallières E, Shamji FM, Todd TR: Postpneumonectomy chylothorax. Ann Thorac Surg 1993;55:1006-1008.

Case Series

Sarsam MAI, Rahman AN, Deiraniya AK: Postpneumonectomy chylothorax. Ann Thorac Surg 1994;57:689-690.

Cerfolio RJ, Allen MS, Deschamps C, et al: Postoperative chylothorax. J Thorac Cardiovasc Surg 1996;112:1361-1366.

Le Pimpec-Barthes F, D'Attellis N, Dujon A, et al: Chylothorax complicating pulmonary resection. Ann Thorac Surg 2002;73:1714-1719.

Shimizu K, Yoshida J, Nishimura M, et al: Treatment strategy for chylothorax after pulmonary resection and lymph node dissection for lung cancer. J Thorac Cardiovasc Surg 2002;124:499-502.

7

Management of Postoperative Complications

Management of Anastomotic Leak after Esophageal Resection

The ability to manage an esophageal leak successfully after resection is a challenging issue for both the patient and the treating team. Leaks can be effectively treated and patients put back on a satisfactory treatment path with timely decisions and patience.

The incidence of anastomotic leak after esophageal resection is 7% (0% to 30%). The incidence is higher if the anastomosis is in the neck (13%) rather than in the chest (6%). However, the mortality of a leak in the neck is 7%; it could be as high as 45% for those with a failed intrathoracic anastomosis. Other complications associated with leaks are the formation of a stricture in more than 50% of patients and the risk of formation of fistula to the airways or major vessels.

The objective of this chapter is to review the expertise necessary to treat esophageal leaks successfully.

RISK FACTORS

The integrity and viability of the anastomosis required after esophagectomy depend on a number of factors common to all gastrointestinal anastomoses and those particular to esophageal surgery (Table 8-1). Factors common to all anastomoses include malnutrition, tension on the anastomosis, and ischemia at the anastomotic site. The use of drains is a contentious issue. Anastomoses in general should be properly drained, but the drainage tube should not be left in direct contact with the anastomosis. Malnutrition is common to most patients requiring esophageal resection and is usually defined as a weight loss of more than 20% of total body weight or a serum albumin level below 3 g/dL.

The operative risk factors that have been found to be of significance in anastomotic leak after esophageal surgery are excessive blood loss and the requirement for blood transfusions, use of continuous or two-layer suture techniques rather than a stapler anastomosis, use of colon in the neck, and tumor at the resection margin. The longer the route to the neck, such as a retrosternal bypass, the more likely the anastomosis is to leak. When the stomach is used as the replacement conduit, undue stress to the anastomosis

TABLE 8-1

RISK FACTORS FOR ANASTOMOTIC LEAKAGE AFTER ESOPHAGEAL SURGERY

Anastomotic Factors	Systemic Factors	Conduit Factors
Ischemia	Malnutrition	Location of the conduit in the mediastinum
Tension	Blood loss	
Suture technique	Poor resuscitation after surgery	Use of colon
Failure to wrap the anastomosis with viable tissue		Gastric distention
Use of drains in contact with the anastomosis		
Tumor at the resection margin		

by gastric distention can lead to anastomotic leakage or dehiscence at the long staple line that is required to construct the conduit. Gastric distention is avoided by measuring residuals after clamping of the nasogastric tube when it is ready to come out and by limiting oral feeding early after the surgery. Compared with no drainage procedure, pyloroplasty or pyloromyotomy, although more effective at optimizing gastric drainage, does not seem to prevent anastomotic leakage.

Age, diabetes, chronic obstructive pulmonary disease, chemotherapy, and radiotherapy have not been shown to be risk factors for anastomotic leak after esophageal surgery.

DIAGNOSIS OF ESOPHAGEAL LEAK

The clinical presentation of patients depends on the amount of graft necrosis and contamination of the soft tissues around the anastomosis (Table 8-2). Patients can present with signs and symptoms of fulminant sepsis as early as 2 to 3 days after surgery. The toxic condition of these patients is often the result of a long necrotic conduit in the mediastinum rather than a contained collection of pus. The clinical presentation depends also on the adequacy of the drainage that has been established at the time of surgery. Patients with an anastomotic leak who have a properly drained anastomosis may show evidence of only increased drainage through the drainage tube with little or no sign of sepsis.

Small cervical leaks without graft necrosis usually become clinically evident with a cervical wound infection on days 3 to 5. Thoracic leaks can present with increased output through the drains; a poorly drained thoracic leak can present with signs and symptoms of empyema. Increased drainage through the chest tubes associated with a leak must be differentiated from a chylothorax. When the anastomosis is reinforced with omentum, the leak is often contained and small unless the entire graft is ischemic.

Patients thought to have a leak should have an evaluation of the integrity of the anastomosis. This can be done at bedside by asking the patient to swallow methylene blue or by using a contrast study with a water-soluble contrast agent swallowed by the patient or injected into the nasogastric tube. A normal study with a water-soluble agent should be completed with barium. Patients should then have a contrast-enhanced computed tomographic (CT) scan to evaluate the adequacy of drainage of the leakage.

TABLE 8-2
CLINICAL PRESENTATION OF ANASTOMOTIC LEAKAGE AFTER ESOPHAGEAL SURGERY

Type of Leak	Clinical Presentation	Etiology
Large	Fulminant sepsis	Complete graft failure
	Empyema	Partial graft failure
Small contained or well drained	Neck infection	Partial graft failure
	Usually silent	Localized anastomotic
	Increased output from the drains	dehiscence

The aim of the CT scan is detection of empyema or localized mediastinal abscesses.

The amount of the leakage is then quantified. Large leaks are those in which the contrast material is free flowing in the mediastinum and is not properly drained by the drainage tubes. Small leaks are well contained or well evacuated by the drains.

MANAGEMENT OF LEAKS

Small Contained Leaks

Small leaks are usually associated with a limited septic picture and are contained. Patients are treated by keeping them fasting by mouth, preferentially on nasogastric drainage and on jejunostomy gavage. Antibiotherapy with coverage for mouth organisms by a combination of a cephalosporin or a quinolone and clindamycin must be initiated. The swallow test is repeated 1 week after the initial study and weekly until the leak is smaller. This usually occurs within 2 weeks. The nasogastric tube can then be removed and the patient started on a clear fluid diet. As soon as the leak is reduced to a minimum size, the patient's diet is advanced to a regular diet (six small meals per day).

Patients should be started electively on a set of two or three dilation courses as early as postoperative week 2 or 3 to prevent the high likelihood of stricture development.

Large Leaks

Large or uncontained leaks on the swallow test require a more aggressive management. The viability of the graft must be assessed and suppurative collections drained. All patients should have a CT scan with administration of an intravenous contrast agent to look for the graft vascular blush and an undrained collection. Patients should also have endoscopy for assessment of the viability of the anastomosis.

Fulminant sepsis is treated with mediastinal drainage and débridement of all necrotic tissues. If there is evidence of complete graft necrosis, the graft must be taken down, the ischemic graft resected, and an exclusion system established. This consists of a cervical esophagocutaneous spit fistula and tube drainage of any residual viable graft in the abdomen. Because patients are usually very sick, a reconstruction should not be contemplated until they have completely recovered. This period is usually no less than 3 to 6 months. Antibiotherapy is continued parenterally for a period of about 10 days or until all symptoms of gross sepsis have resolved. Long-term (4 weeks) enteral antibiotherapy is continued for patients who develop empyema or mediastinal abscesses.

Incomplete graft failures are more common. When patients are taken to the operating room, the wound and the anastomosis must be explored directly in the neck or by endoscopy when the anastomosis is in the chest. If the leak appears to be small and the graft viable, simple packing in the neck and proper drainage in the chest combined with systemic antibiotic therapy and enteral nutrition will heal the leak. In the neck, saliva can be diverted into an ileostomy appliance to protect the skin around the incision from excoriation.

Larger defects of the anastomosis are due to local ischemia of the most distal part of the graft. In these cases, the residual viable graft can be preserved. The ischemic segment is resected, and if the degree of contamination is minimal and the residual graft is sufficiently mobile, a new anastomosis is created. If an immediate repair is not possible and the ischemic segment is long, the residual viable graft should be repositioned in the abdomen to be used at a later time when the patient has healed from the insult of the leak.

RECONSTRUCTION OF A FAILED ANASTOMOSIS

When graft reconstruction is planned after the patient has recuperated from complete graft failure, the posterior mediastinal route is usually not usable anymore and one has to be prepared to use a longer anterior mediastinal or rarely a subcutaneous route. If the grafts, stomach or colon, are not long enough to reach the residual esophagus, the graft can be elongated with a tube graft fashioned from a pectoralis major musculocutaneous flap or a free jejunal graft. The entire esophagus can be replaced with a supercharged jejunal conduit. It is absolutely necessary to adhere to strict tissue preservation techniques because a third repair is usually impossible.

CONCLUSION

Esophageal leak is a devastating complication. All measures must be used to prevent it by judicious preparation of the patient and the anastomotic site. Minor leaks are treated with nasogastric tube suctioning, local drainage, and jejunostomy enteral feeding. Large leaks require assessment of the viability of the graft by endoscopy and wound exploration. On occasion, the graft must be taken down and delayed reconstruction with an alternative organ undertaken when the patient has recovered.

SUGGESTED READINGS

Review Article

Urschel JD: Esophagogastrostomy anastomotic leaks complicating esophagectomy: a review. Am J Surg 1995;169:634-640.

Risk Factors

Lam TC, Fok M, Cheng SW, Wong J: Anastomotic complications after esophagectomy for cancer. A comparison of neck and chest anastomosis. J Thorac Cardiovasc Surg 1992;104:395-400.

Valverde A, Hay JM, Fingerhut A, et al: Manual versus mechanical esophagogastric anastomosis after resection for carcinoma: a controlled trial. Surgery 1996;120:476-483.

Craig SR, Walker WS, Cameron EWJ, Wightman AJA: A prospective randomized study comparing stapled with hand-sewn oesophagogastric anastomosis. J R Coll Edinb 1996;41:17-19.

Beitler AL, Urschel JD: Comparison of stapled and hand-sewn esophagogastric anastomosis. Am J Surg 1998;175:337-340.

Rindani R, Martin CJ, Cox MR: Transhiatal versus Ivor-Lewis oesophagectomy: is there a difference? Aust N Z J Surg 1999; 69:187-194.

Hulscher JBF, Tijssen JGP, Obertop H, van Lanschot JBB: Transthoracic versus transhiatal resection for carcinoma of the esophagus: a meta-analysis. Ann Thorac Surg 2001;72:306-313.

Diagnosis

Sauvanet A, Baltar J, Le Mee J, Belghiti J: Diagnosis and conservative management of intrathoracic leakage after oesophagectomy. Br J Surg 1998;85:1446-1449.

Tanomkiat W, Galassi W: Barium sulfate as contrast medium for evaluation of postoperative anastomotic leaks. Acta Radiol 2000;41:482-485.

Case Series

Lorentz T, Fok M, Wong J: Anastomotic leakage after resection and bypass for esophageal cancer: lessons learned from the past. World J Surg 1989;13:472-477.

Patil PK, Patel SG, Mistry RC, et al: Cancer of the esophagus: esophagogastric anastomotic leak—a retrospective study of predisposing factors. J Surg Oncol 1992;49:163-167.

Dewar L, Gelfand G, Finley RJ, et al: Factors affecting cervical anastomotic leak and stricture formation following esophagogastrectomy and gastric tube interposition. Am J Surg 1992;163:484-489.

Karl RC, Schreiber R, Boulware D, et al: Factors affecting morbidity, mortality, and survival in patients undergoing Ivor-Lewis esophagogastrectomy. Ann Surg 2000;231:635-643.

Griffin SM, Lamb PJ, Dresner SM, et al: Diagnosis and management of a mediastinal leak following radical oesophagectomy. Br J Surg 2001;88:1346-1351.

Blewett CJ, Miller JD, Young JEM, et al: Anastomotic leaks after esophagectomy for esophageal cancer: a comparison of thoracic and cervical anastomoses. Ann Thorac Cardiovasc Surg 2001;7:75-78.

Orringer MB, Marshall B, Iannettoni MD: Transhiatal esophagectomy for treatment of benign and malignant esophageal disease. World J Surg 2001;25:196-103.

Follow-up and Late Surgical Complications

Whether systematic follow-up benefits patients who have had resectional surgery for lung cancer *is still questionable,* at least in studies that have addressed this question. There is, however, some evidence that patients who have no symptoms at the time of recurrent disease (recurrence discovered at routine follow-up visit) are more likely to survive longer than those who have symptoms. On occasion, second primary tumors will also be detected at an earlier stage, and solitary metastases will be more amenable to aggressive multimodality treatments.

From the surgeon's point of view, follow-up clinics enable her or him to evaluate treatment strategies and to diagnose late complications related to the initial operation. Although these late events are uncommon and, for the most part, *seldom life-threatening,* they can still lead to chronicity and prolonged disabilities.

FOLLOW-UP AFTER RESECTION OF LUNG CANCER

General Objectives of Cancer Surveillance Programs (Table 9-1)

Approximately 60% of patients with completely resected lung cancers will recur within 5 years of surgery, either locoregionally or at a distance. Patients who survive 5 years after the initial surgery also have a 6% *to 10% chance for development of a second primary lung cancer,* especially if they have not stopped smoking. For these individuals, early detection of disease may translate into *earlier initiation of therapy* and *improvement of outcomes* such as survival. Similarly, patients with early-discovered solitary sites of distant metastasis, such as those occurring in the brain or the contralateral lung, are more likely to benefit from multimodality treatment including surgical resection.

For patients, secondary benefits include easier accessibility to specialized services, such as antismoking clinics, and rehabilitation programs that may not otherwise be accessible. If necessary, patients can be seen rapidly by other medical specialists such as oncologists, chest physicians, and palliative care physicians. Patients may finally benefit psychologically from a *close relationship* with their surgeon and oncology nurses. All of those benefits are difficult to measure accurately, but they often are important to the patient and the patient's relatives.

For the surgeon, one potential benefit is the possibility of evaluating the advantages and disadvantages of specific operations as well as their long-term results. Indeed, any surgeon who simply performs pulmonary resections and never follows up patients cannot learn from successes and errors. Another most important aspect of post-resection follow-up is that it provides the surgeon with opportunities to *teach the house staff* including residents and nurses about disease processes, operations, complications, and results.

TABLE 9-1	

POTENTIAL BENEFITS OF FOLLOW-UP

For the patient
Early diagnosis and early treatment of local recurrences or second primary tumors
Multimodality therapy for early-discovered solitary distant metastases
Specialized interventions available only at structured follow-up clinics
Closer relationship with surgeon and oncology nurses

For the surgeon
Evaluation of potential benefits and disadvantages of procedures
Evaluation of treatment strategies in the long term
Opportunity to teach house staff

Frequency (Table 9-2) **of Follow-up and Who Should Do It**

The first postoperative visit should be within 1 month of hospital discharge, and its *main purpose is to diagnose complications* that may have arisen after the patient left the hospital. Visits are then scheduled every 3 months for 2 years, every 6 months for 3 years, and on an annual basis after 5 years. The National Comprehensive Cancer Network recommends monitoring, including a history and physical examination, every 4 months for the first 2 years and then every 6 months for the next 3 years. A chest radiograph is obtained at each visit during this period. These proposed schedules are based on the knowledge that *most cancer recurrences* will occur within 2 years of surgery.

For systematic follow-up to be rewarding, the system must be able to detect patients who are missing their prearranged visit. In such cases, a phone call must automatically be made to inquire as to why the patient was unable to attend the clinic. This is an important step if one hopes to diagnose recurrences or new primaries at an early and still potentially treatable stage.

Follow-ups should *ideally* be done (Table 9-3) by surgeons because they know the patient best. In several cases, however, especially if the patient is older or noncompliant or if he or she lives far away from the surgical center, they can be done by chest physicians, family practitioners, or even well-trained nurse practitioners. Follow-up by family physicians is *less expensive* than that performed by thoracic surgeons, and for these economic reasons, patients may be offered this option.

TABLE 9-2	

SUGGESTED SURVEILLANCE AFTER RESECTION OF NON–SMALL CELL LUNG CANCER

First visit within 1 month of surgery
Every 3-4 months for 2 years
Every 6 months for the following 3 years
Annually after 5 years

TABLE 9-3	
WHO SHOULD DO THE FOLLOW-UP	
Best done by surgical team	
Can be done by experienced chest physicians or family practitioners	
Can probably be done by well-trained nurse practitioners	

Follow-up Guidelines

Routine Procedures

All patients should have a careful clinical history, a limited regional physical examination, and a standard chest radiograph. Signs and symptoms suggesting local recurrences are listed in Table 9-4; among them, *hemoptysis, weight loss,* and *fatigue* are the most important. Radiographic signs suggesting recurrences (Table 9-5) include the demonstration of new pulmonary densities or the presence of a pleural effusion not shown before. In many cases, *serial comparison of chest films* will detect subtle changes that may not otherwise be obvious. This is the case, for instance, of hemoclips that have been used during the operation and may have become distracted or displaced over time by local recurrent disease.

Other tests often done at follow-up visits include liver function studies and hematologic blood work.

Screening Studies

The value of specific screening studies such as sputum cytology, bronchoscopy, and spiral computed tomography (CT) is still controversial. At present, these examinations *do not appear to be helpful* or cost-effective in the follow-up of resected lung cancer patients.

Sputum Cytology and Bronchoscopy. Although there are no reports of systematic surveillance of lung cancer–resected patients by sputum cytology, large studies of unresected but high-risk patients have shown that early diagnosis by cytology screening *is not beneficial* in terms of decreasing the number of cancer-related deaths. Similarly, the available biomarkers for lung

9

Follow-up and Late Surgical Complications

TABLE 9-4	
SIGNS AND SYMPTOMS SUGGESTING A LOCOREGIONAL RECURRENCE	

Clinical symptoms
Hemoptysis or new cough
Chest pain not present before
Hoarseness not present before
Weight loss, fatigue, anorexia

Physical signs
Palpable cervical nodes
Superior vena cava obstruction

TABLE 9-5

RADIOGRAPHIC SIGNS SUGGESTING A LOCOREGIONAL RECURRENCE

New pulmonary lesion or atelectasis
New pleural effusion
Widening of mediastinum
Displacement of hemoclips that had been in stable position before
Elevation of hemidiaphragm

cancer (immunostaining of sputum cytology specimen) *are not specific* (a positive test result means that the patient has lung cancer) *or sensitive* (a negative test result means that the patient has no tumor) *enough* to justify their routine use.

Screening patients by flexible bronchoscopy has enormous disadvantages in terms of costs as well as human and physical resources.

Spiral CT. Currently, there are insufficient data to recommend systematic follow-up by chest CT scan. The main criticism of screening CT scans is that the test is unable to discriminate benign from malignant nodules, especially in the case of small nodules. Indeed, this inability is likely to be *magnified in postoperative patients,* in whom inflammatory and fibrotic reactions as well as reorientation of anatomy are always present.

LATE SURGICAL COMPLICATIONS

Infections and Space Complications

Persistent Spaces after Lobectomies or Lesser Resections

Persistent pleural air spaces after lobectomies or lesser resections are common, and for many years, they were thought to lead inevitably to infection if left untreated. This is not the case, however, and after lung cancer surgery, *most such residual spaces are not infected* and should be observed until their complete resolution. Investigation by thoracentesis or other means is not indicated and may in fact be contraindicated to avoid the risks of infecting a previously sterile space.

However, if systemic or local symptoms of infection develop or if the space is enlarging, appropriate diagnostic measures and therapy should be instituted promptly (see Chapter 7, "Prolonged Air Leaks and Space Problems").

Persistent Spaces after Pneumonectomy

On average, *filling of the residual space after pneumonectomy* requires 3 to 4 weeks to take place. Initially, the space fills up with serosanguineous fluid and plasma, which gradually becomes organized to completely obliterate the space. This phenomenon is aided by the ipsilateral shift of mediastinal structures, elevation of the hemidiaphragm, approximation of the ribs, and negative intrapleural pressure.

TABLE 9-6

PATHOGENESIS OF LATE POSTPNEUMONECTOMY EMPYEMAS

Secondary to late bronchopleural or esophagopleural fistulas
Contamination of space during initial operation
Seeding through hematogenous route
Direct spread from chest wall or intra-abdominal infection

On occasion, the pneumonectomy space will never become obliterated (postpneumonectomy thorax). Classically, these patients are asymptomatic and they have no demonstrable bronchopleural fistula. Management should be conservative because the majority of such patients will either reaccumulate pleural fluid at a later date or maintain an empty space without further complications.

Late-onset empyemas are empyemas diagnosed 6 months or more after pneumonectomy in patients who had an otherwise uneventful postoperative course. Possible pathogenetic mechanisms are listed in Table 9-6. In the absence of a fistula, the most likely mechanism is that *the pleural space was contaminated during the initial surgery* and bacteria lay dormant in small pockets or loculations of fluid. The clinical features associated with late-onset empyemas vary greatly and can be nonspecific. Often, patients will have only mild symptoms of infection, and the clinical picture will be primarily that of cough, increased dyspnea and chest pain, and fatigue. Management of such complications has been discussed previously (see Chapter 7, "Empyema and Bronchopleural Fistula").

Late Esophagopleural Fistula (Table 9-7)

Late esophagopleural fistulas after pulmonary resection are uncommon events that are difficult to diagnose and often overlooked.

They occur predominantly on the right side. The most common site of fistula formation is immediately below the carina, probably because the esophageal blood supply is segmental and *often deficient* in that location. Possible etiologic factors include cancer recurrence; esophageal wall necrosis due to radiotherapy; and the presence of pathologic nodes, such

(Margin tab: 9 — Follow-up and Late Surgical Complications)

TABLE 9-7

KNOWN FACTS ABOUT LATE POST–PULMONARY RESECTION
ESOPHAGOPLEURAL FISTULA

Most are on the right side, and the site of fistula is below the carina.
The majority occur after pneumonectomy.
Nearly all are related to recurrent cancer or radiotherapy.
Diagnosis can be difficult and requires a high index of suspicion.
Management must be individualized.
Only palliative therapy should be offered to patients with recurrent
    cancer and esophagopleural fistula.

as tuberculous nodes adjacent to the esophageal wall. In most cases, the esophagus was probably made vulnerable by having been devascularized or traumatized during the initial operation.

Clinical features are those of an empyema, and patients may present with varying degrees of toxicity, fever, dyspnea, and chest pain. Contrast-enhanced esophagography and esophagoscopy will document the diagnosis, locate the site of the fistula, and help estimate its size.

Management must be individualized. The patient's condition and oncologic status and the specific characteristics of the fistula must be considered. If, for instance, the esophagopleural fistula is secondary to recurrent carcinoma, only palliative therapy should be offered.

Late Bronchial Complications Other Than Fistula

Bronchial Stump Granulomas

Granulations at the bronchial suture line are almost always caused by highly reactive suture material such as silk. They have become uncommon because most surgeons now use staple closure for bronchi. These granulations can still occur, however, and they are almost always related to relative ischemia or impaired healing of the bronchus.

Patients with bronchial stump granulomas nearly always complain of a dry irritative cough, sometimes with hemoptysis. The diagnosis is made at bronchoscopy.

Sustained relief of symptoms will be obtained by *endoscopic removal of exposed sutures.*

Long Stump Syndromes

Long stump syndromes are *uncommon* and mostly seen after left pneumonectomy or right lower and middle lobectomies. The clinical presentation is usually that of recurring infection, chronic purulent bronchorrhea, and hemoptysis. At bronchoscopy, the stump is markedly inflamed, and suture granulomas are often present.

Management is usually conservative with respiratory hygiene, postural physiotherapy, and antibiotics when necessary. The stump may *occasionally* have to be re-resected.

CONCLUSION

Follow-up after resection of lung cancer should be directed toward the early identification of patients with recurrent disease in the hope that such early diagnosis will translate into better outcome. In all cases, follow-up requires a *simple, consistent,* and *cost-efficient* clinical protocol.

SUGGESTED READINGS

Editorial

Hiebert CA: The "cured" lung cancer patient: is follow-up by the surgeon worthwhile? Ann Thorac Surg 1995;60:1557-1558.

Follow-up after Resection for Lung Cancer

Walsh GL, O'Connor M, Willis KM, et al: Is follow-up of lung cancer patients after resection medically indicated and cost-effective? Ann Thorac Surg 1995;60:1563-1570.

Naunheim KS, Virgo KS, Coplin MA, Johnson FE: Clinical surveillance testing after lung cancer operations. Ann Thorac Surg 1995;60: 1612-1616.

Virgo KS, McKirgan LW, Caputo MCA: Post-treatment management options for patients with lung cancer. Ann Surg 1995;222:700-710.

Virgo KS, Naunheim KS, McKirgan LW, et al: Cost of patient follow-up after potentially curative lung cancer treatment. J Thorac Cardiovasc Surg 1996;112:356-363.

Younes RN, Gross JL, Deheinzelin D: Follow-up in lung cancer. How often and for what purpose? Chest 1999;115:1494-1499.

Westeel V, Choma D, Clement F, et al: Relevance of an intensive postoperative follow-up after surgery for non–small cell lung cancer. Ann Thorac Surg 2000;70:1185-1190.

Gilbert S, Reid KR, Lam MY, Petsikas D: Who should follow up lung cancer patients after operation? Ann Thorac Surg 2000;69: 1696-1700.

Egermann V, Jaeggi K, Habicht JM, et al: Regular follow-up after curative resection of nonsmall cell lung cancer: a real benefit for patients? Eur Respir J 2002;19:464-468.

Lamont JP, Karuda JT, Smith D, et al: Systematic postoperative radiologic follow-up in patients with non–small cell lung cancer for detecting second primary lung cancer in stage IA. Arch Surg 2002;137: 935-939.

Saunders M, Sculier JP, Ball D, et al: Consensus: the follow-up of the treated patient. Lung Cancer 2003;42:S17-S19.

Colice GL, Rubins J, Unger M: Follow-up and surveillance of the lung cancer patient following curative-intent therapy. Chest 2003;123: 272s-283s.

Esophagopleural Fistula

Takaro T, Walkup HE, Okano T: Esophagopleural fistula as a complication of thoracic surgery. A collective review. J Thorac Cardiovasc Surg 1960;40:179-193.

Symes JM, Page AJF, Flavell G: Esophagopleural fistula: a late complication after pneumonectomy. J Thorac Cardiovasc Surg 1972;63:783-786.

Van Den Bosch JMM, Swierenga J, Gelissen HJ, Laros CD: Postpneumonectomy oesophagopleural fistula. Thorax 1980;35:865-868.

Postoperative Spaces

Barker WL, Langston HT, Naffah P: Postresectional thoracic spaces. Ann Thorac Surg 1966;2:299-310.

9

Follow-up and Late Surgical Complications

Late Empyema

Kerr WF: Late-onset post-pneumonectomy empyema. Thorax 1977;32: 149-154.

Other

Handy JR, Child AI, Grunkemeier GL, et al: Hospital readmission after pulmonary resection: prevalence, patterns, and predisposing characteristics. Ann Thorac Surg 2001;72:1855-1860.

Principles of Pleural Drainage and Suction Systems

CLOSED DRAINAGE AND SUCTION SYSTEM

The first attempts to drain the pleural space with a tube are credited to Playfair and Hewett, who at the end of the 19th century reported on an underwater seal drainage system for the management of empyemas. Since then, the concept of pleural space drainage has *evolved considerably,* not only because of better understanding of pleural space anatomy and physiology but also because of improved technology, commercialization of drainage systems, and changing needs of surgeons.

Tube thoracostomy is considered a minor surgical procedure. It can be lifesaving, but it can also result in considerable morbidity if the operator *does not have adequate knowledge* of chest wall and pleural space anatomy or if he or she *does not have a clear understanding* of the technique to be used for tube insertion.

Despite the claims of many manufacturers, no currently available drainage system is perfect or has complete versatility so that it can be adapted to every pathologic condition of the pleural space. Each system has desirable features, but each also has its own set of deficiencies. Overall, drainage systems must be able to *evacuate* air or fluid completely from the pleural cavity, to *collapse and obliterate* residual spaces, and to ensure *complete re-expansion* of the lung. They must be able to meet the physiologic and therapeutic needs of the patient, and their design must be straightforward so that their functioning can be thoroughly understood by the entire surgical team.

TUBE DRAINAGE

Anatomic Considerations

A thorough knowledge of the anatomy of the intercostal space is important not only to avoid injury to neurovascular structures within the space but also to direct the tube properly in the desired location. The larger neurovascular structures that may be at risk during tube insertion are in the *subcostal groove at the inferior border of each rib* (see Chapter 5, "Thoracic Anatomy"). On occasion, smaller accessory intercostal vessels will also course along the superior border of the rib. In general, bleeding from an intercostal artery can be avoided by staying as close as possible to the superior border of the lower rib in the chosen interspace.

Precise knowledge of *pleural reflections and pleural space boundaries* is also necessary if one is to avoid perforation of the peritoneal cavity and possible trauma to organs in the upper abdomen. Laterally, the costal reflection of the pleura passes obliquely across the eighth rib in the midclavicular line and the tenth rib in the midaxillary line. Under abnormal conditions, such as those with increased negative pressure in the pleural space, the dome of the hemidiaphragm may be as high as the fourth interspace.

Indications (Table 10-1) **and Contraindications**

In patients with *spontaneous pneumothorax,* tube drainage is the treatment of choice. In both tension pneumothorax and open pneumothorax, it can be lifesaving. In blunt trauma, pneumothoraces should be drained unless they are small, asymptomatic, and nonprogressive.

Patients with *traumatic hemothoraces* often require tube drainage to monitor the rate of bleeding, to re-expand the lung, and to prevent chronic lung entrapment. Frank empyemas always require pleural space drainage.

Malignant pleural effusions should be drained if they are recurrent and symptomatic or if chemical pleurodesis is contemplated. Most chylothoraces should also be drained.

There are virtually no contraindications to tube drainage, although one has to be cautious when inserting a chest tube in a patient with a bleeding disorder or in a patient receiving anticoagulants. Another relative contraindication is the presence of pleural adhesions or of a giant bulla, where there may be danger of perforating it.

Tube Thoracostomy

Chest Tubes

Most chest tubes currently used in the United States are *made of Silastic.* They have multiple side holes, a radiopaque stripe, and outer diameters ranging from 6 Fr (pediatric) to 40 Fr gauge. These tubes are firm yet pliable; they induce minimal skin or pleural reaction, and they are inexpensive. Most chest tubes are straight; although curved tubes are available and mostly used for postoperative drainage.

In patients with pneumothoraces, smaller tubes (20 to 24 Fr) are sufficient. For patients with hemothoraces, malignant effusions, or empyemas, larger tubes (28 to 40 Fr) are recommended because the fluid being drained tends to occlude smaller tubes.

TABLE 10-1

POSSIBLE INDICATIONS FOR TUBE DRAINAGE

Air in the pleural space (pneumothorax)
    Spontaneous pneumothorax
    Open or tension pneumothorax
    Traumatic pneumothorax
    Iatrogenic pneumothorax
Blood in the pleural space (hemothorax)
Abnormal fluid in the pleural space (pleural effusion)
Pus in the pleural space
    Parapneumonic effusions
    Frank empyemas
Chyle in the pleural space (chylothorax)

TABLE 10-2

ADVANTAGES OF INSERTING CHEST TUBES OVER ANTERIOR OR MIDAXILLARY LINE

Less visible scar (versus anterior insertion)
No muscles to traverse during insertion
More comfortable and less restrictive for patient
Positioning at apex is easier

Preoperative Management

In all cases, the *exact site of the collection* being drained should be well documented through the use of imaging modalities. Patients *should be informed* about the technique because fearful and anxious patients can immensely complicate the procedure. Light sedation and thorough explanations will often reassure the patient and alleviate some of this anxiety.

Site of Insertion

The *ideal site of insertion* is the third or fourth intercostal space in the anterior or midaxillary line, immediately behind the pectoralis major fold (Table 10-2). In this location, the scar is hardly visible, and during insertion, there are no muscles other than the intercostals to traverse. It is *more comfortable for the patient* and less restrictive for such activities as eating, sleeping, and receiving chest physiotherapy. Proper positioning at the apex is easier because the tube has a natural tendency to slide upward along the curve of the lateral chest wall.

Anterior insertion (second space, midclavicular line) *is seldom used* because it necessitates dissection through the pectoralis major muscle, which may be painful and cause hemorrhage. It may leave a highly visible scar.

Insertion Technique (Table 10-3)

Most chest tubes are inserted under local anesthesia. *The parietal pleura* and rib periosteum should be infiltrated generously, and the effect of the local anesthetic will often be improved if one waits a few minutes before

TABLE 10-3

TECHNIQUE OF CHEST TUBE INSERTION (10 STEPS)

1. The exact site of collection is documented with computed tomography and ultrasonography.
2. Inform the patient about the technique.
3. The ideal site is the third or fourth interspace, anterior or midaxillary line.
4. Proper cleaning of skin is performed with antiseptic solution.
5. The parietal pleura is generously infiltrated with local anesthetic.
6. Skin incision is made one space below the interspace to be used.
7. Blunt dissection with a Kelly clamp is carried over superior border of rib.
8. Inspect with index finger.
9. Insert the tube.
10. Secure the tube to the skin around it, and control its position with portable radiography.

Principles of Pleural Drainage and Suction Systems

10

incising the skin. Aspiration of air or fluid through a needle and syringe is used to confirm the proper location of the drainage site.

The skin incision is made one space below the interspace to be used, and blunt dissection with a curved Kelly clamp is carried *over the superior border of the rib* (Fig. 10-1). This dissection creates a tunnel within

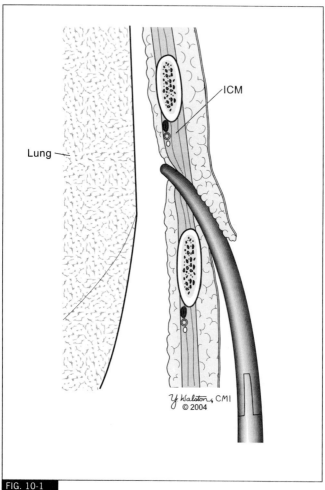

ICM

Lung

Y. Walston, CMI
© 2004

FIG. 10-1
Blunt dissection through intercostal muscles (ICM) with a curved Kelly clamp. Note the upward diagonal tunnel and the dissection, which is carried out over the superior border of the rib. *(Modified with permission from Miller KS, Sahn SA: Chest tubes. Indications, technique, management and complications. Chest 1987;91:258-264.)*

intercostal muscles and parietal pleura through which the tube can simply be advanced in its proper position. Often, the pleural space will first be inspected with the index finger to confirm that the parietal pleura has been penetrated and to avoid injuries to the underlying lung.

When the tube is in place, air condensation is easily noted over the walls of the catheter with each expiration. To prevent its dislodgment, *the tube should be sutured to the skin* around it with heavy silk sutures.

An alternative technique of insertion is the trocar method. The technique is simple, but because the trocar is a sharp-tipped metal rod and because it is often introduced forcefully in the pleural space, there is *increased risk* of injury to the underlying lung or any other intrathoracic structure.

Connecting Tubing

The best tube connectors are made of plastic and have serrated ends. It is most important that these connectors have a *large internal diameter* ($1/4$ inch, 6 mm) and that their ends *not be tapered* so that the flow of hemorrhagic fluids is not impaired. When more than one chest tube is required, the tubes can be connected to the same drainage system through a Y connector. Taping the ends of the connector to the connecting tubing aids in preventing accidental separation at the site.

Connecting tubes are made of either clear plastic or latex. They are usually 5 to 6 feet long with an internal diameter of 12 mm. Plastic tubes have the advantage of water-clear transparency so that the fluctuation of fluid can easily be observed. With latex tubing, samples of drainage fluid can be directly obtained from the tube through a No. 18 or 20 needle.

Tube Management (Table 10-4)

A chest radiograph should always be obtained immediately after tube insertion so that lung re-expansion and tube position can be assessed. Thereafter, daily chest radiographs should be done for as long as the chest tube is in place. Careful monitoring of the *nature and volume of fluid drainage* is recommended until after the tube has been removed.

Drainage tubes should not be allowed to hang as dependent loops because fluids and clots accumulating in the tubing increase the resistance

10

Principles of Pleural Drainage and Suction Systems

TABLE 10-4

PRINCIPLES OF TUBE MANAGEMENT

Monitoring
    Daily chest radiographs
    Nature and volume of air leak and fluid drainage
Tubes should almost never be clamped
Functional status of the tube determined by observation of fluid oscillation
    in tubing
Maintenance of patency
    Milking and stripping
    Irrigation not recommended
Avoidance of dependent loops
Airtightness of the system

of the system. Tubes should *almost never be clamped* other than to rule out an air leak or to change a bottle or connecting tube. Clamping during transportation of the patient, especially if the patient has an air leak, can be catastrophic because of potential lung collapse or tension pneumothorax. If a chest tube becomes accidentally disconnected from the drainage system, *it should simply be reconnected* without previous clamping.

When the functional status of the tube is in question, *observation of fluid oscillation* in the water seal or in the tubing is important. Oscillations that are synchronous with respiratory movements (tidaling) indicate tube patency. If there are no oscillations, the tube may be obstructed, or this may result from complete re-expansion of the lung. Increased oscillations are a sign of high negative intrapleural pressures, often associated with atelectasis or incomplete lung re-expansion.

Airtightness of the system should be assessed on a daily basis. If it is questionable, sequential clamping of each of the components of the system may unveil a defect in the tubing or drainage system, which should be corrected immediately. Whether a chest tube should be milked or stripped to dislodge clots or debris and to maintain patency is controversial because several studies have shown that chest tubes remain patent with or without it.

Irrigation of the chest tube with saline or fibrinolytic agents *is not recommended* because each manipulation increases the risk of contamination of the pleural space. If the tube becomes occluded, it is best to remove it and install another one if necessary.

Tube Removal

Chest tubes can be removed when there is *no longer fluctuation* in the fluid column of the tube (indicating complete lung re-expansion or tube occlusion), when daily fluid drainage is *minimal* (<100 mL in 24 hours), and when the *air leak has stopped* for more than 24 hours. Many surgeons favor clamping the tube for 12 to 24 hours before removal, especially if an air leak has been persistent for several days and is still questionable.

Chest tubes should be removed at end-inspiration to decrease the chances of air entry at the drainage site. Removal should be carried out by two people, one swiftly pulling out the tube while the other one ties down a ligature.

Probably *the most common technique* used to seal the thoracostomy incision at the time of tube removal is the tying down of a U stitch across the wound as the tube is withdrawn. Other methods involve the use of petroleum jelly (Vaseline) gauze, skin staples, or adhesives to cover the wound. A chest radiograph should be obtained 12 to 24 hours after tube removal for observation of possible reaccumulation of air.

Complications (Table 10-5)

In general, *complications are minimal* when the procedure is indicated, well planned, and done with care and when the operator has experience with the technique and is familiar with the anatomy of the intercostal and pleural spaces.

TABLE 10-5

POSSIBLE COMPLICATIONS OF TUBE THORACOSTOMY

Misplacement of the chest tube
    Tube in soft tissues of chest wall
    Tube in the wrong pleural space
    Injury to intrathoracic structure: lung, diaphragm
    Abdominal placement of the chest tube and injury to intra-abdominal organs
Hemorrhage
    Cutaneous
    Intercostal arteries
    Injury to superior or inferior vena cava, heart
Surgical emphysema
Re-expansion pulmonary edema
Intercostal neuralgia and thoracostomy lung herniation
Miscellaneous rare complications
    Horner syndrome
    Diaphragmatic paralysis
    Necrotizing fasciitis
    Chylothorax

10

Misplacement of Tubes

An effort should always be made to avoid misplacement of chest tubes; obviously, a chest tube inserted in the wrong pleural space is likely to have *catastrophic consequences.* The last side hole of the tube must be well inside the pleural space because if the tube is not advanced far enough, it may cause a false air leak or the development of surgical emphysema or have physiologic consequences similar to those associated with an open pneumothorax. Similar problems can result from inadequate suturing of the tube, accidental pullback, or loosening of the skin after prolonged drainage. A tube advanced too far in can press against the parietal pleura, causing chest or shoulder pain.

The lung is at risk of being injured during tube insertion. This is related to preexisting lung disease, pleural adhesions, presence of a large bulla, and use of a trocar catheter.

Diaphragmatic and intra-abdominal injuries are more likely to occur *when the hemidiaphragm is elevated,* such as in obese individuals, in patients with diaphragmatic palsy, or after pneumonectomy. Although every organ in the upper abdomen is at risk under those circumstances, the spleen, liver, and stomach are most often injured. The majority of these injuries *can be prevented* by high placement of the tube and finger exploration of the pleural space before tube insertion.

Hemorrhage

Intercostal artery injury is uncommon and is often related to tube placement close to the inferior border of the rib. It usually occurs *in older patients* whose intercostal arteries are more tortuous. The internal mammary artery can be at risk of injury when the site of tube insertion is anterior in the parasternal area. Massive hemorrhage can be secondary to injury to one of the cavae or to the heart. These complications are fortunately rare and *almost always due to forceful trocar insertion* of the chest tube. If this type of penetration occurs, one *should never remove the tube* at bedside but rather clamp it and bring the patient to the operating room for immediate repair.

Surgical Emphysema

Surgical emphysema can occur shortly after tube insertion or during the following days. It is always secondary to *inadequate drainage of the pleural space* as air reaches the subcutaneous tissues through the perforated pleura at the site of thoracotomy. The problem may be due to improper location of the tube in the pleural space, as is seen when pleural adhesions are numerous; to occlusion of the tube or of the connecting tubes; to a large air leak with inadequate absorption by the drainage unit; or to accidental tube pullback in the soft tissues of the chest wall.

When any of these occurs, the drainage system and thoracostomy site should first be thoroughly checked. If the whole system is airtight and the tube is functioning, the level of suction should be increased. If this does not solve the problem, the tube should be pulled back *or another tube inserted.*

Re-expansion Pulmonary Edema

Re-expansion pulmonary edema is a rare but potentially lethal complication. It occurs when air or fluid is evacuated too rapidly in a patient with lung collapse that has persisted for longer than 3 days. Possible factors implicated in the pathogenesis include increased pulmonary vascular permeability, airway obstruction, loss of surfactant, and pulmonary artery pressure changes. Although this complication can be fatal, the edema is usually self-limited and will resolve during a period of a few days. To prevent its occurrence, the lung *should not be allowed to re-expand too quickly* by clamping the chest tube intermittently.

DRAINAGE SYSTEMS (TABLE 10-6)

Passive Drainage Systems

Passive drainage systems provide *one-way drainage* that allows the outflow of gas or fluid during expiration but prevents its return into the pleural space during inspiration. These systems are often sufficient to evacuate the pleural space because the positive pressure that prevails during expiration or cough forces out both air and fluid.

The most basic of these systems is the *Heimlich one-way flutter valve*, which consists of a piece of rubber tubing, one end of which is compressed and retains its flattened shape. Several authors have shown that outpatient management of individuals with spontaneous pneumothoraces with this device is safe, efficient, and economical. If one of these commercially made valves is not available in an emergency situation, a *homemade system* can be fashioned by attaching a surgical glove at the end of the chest tube and puncturing the end of any of its fingers.

TABLE 10-6

DRAINAGE SYSTEMS

Passive drainage systems
One-way flutter valves (Heimlich valves)
Thoracic vent
Portex ambulatory chest drainage systems
Pleur$_x$ catheters
Portable chest draining devices
Homemade emergency one-way valves
Underwater seal units
    One-bottle units
    Two-bottle units

Active drainage systems
Three-bottle units
    Homemade systems
    Disposable commercially available units
    Units with dry suction
    High-pressure systems (Emerson pumps)
Balanced drainage system
Pleuroperitoneal catheter

10

Modified urinary collecting bags can be used for prolonged drainage, as are commercially available portable one-way flutter valve drainage bags (Fig. 10-2). These bags make ambulatory management of patients with moderate to large pleural fluid drainage less troublesome. An indwelling pleural catheter* can also be used for the management of malignant pleural effusions.

With the *underwater seal system,* water acts as a seal to prevent airflow from going back up the drain during inspiration. This system employs both the mechanics of respiration (positive expiratory pressure) and gravity to bring about drainage. As air or fluids are evacuated, the pleural surfaces are brought together and the intrapleural pressure becomes negative again. A vent is used to provide for the escape of air from the drainage bottle into the atmosphere.

Because the use of a one-bottle unit may be limited by the mounting level of fluid in the bottle, a *two-bottle system* can be fashioned (Fig. 10-3) by interposing a collection bottle, which traps fluids and passes air onward, thereby ensuring that the underwater seal is kept at a fixed and constant level.

Active Drainage Systems

Active drainage by the use of *continuous suction* is often necessary to achieve and maintain complete re-expansion of the lung and apposition of the pleural surfaces. This is particularly important when the amount of air leakage exceeds the underwater seal capacity of the system or when the

---

*Pleur$_x$ pleural catheter, Scientific Medics, Denver Biomaterials Inc., Golden, Colo.

Principles of Pleural Drainage and Suction Systems

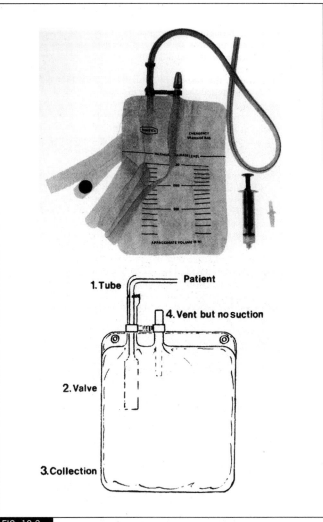

FIG. 10-2

Ambulatory chest drainage system (Portex Ltd., Hythe, Kent, UK) that incorporates a "nonstick" vertically oriented flutter valve device within a drainage bag. *(From McManus K, Spence G, McGuigan J: Outpatient chest tubes. Ann Thorac Surg 1998;66:290-300.)*

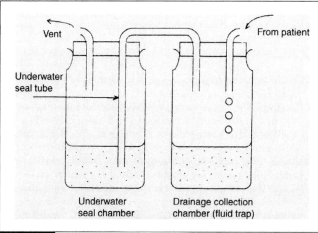

FIG. 10-3

Two-bottle system. *(From Kam AC, O'Brien M, Kam PC: Pleural drainage systems. Anesthesia 1993;48:154-161.)*

underlying lung is noncompliant and generating high negative intrapleural pressures exceeding the maximum negative pressure of the unit. Most authors recommend active suction with *negative pressures in the neighborhood of –20 cm H₂O*.

Three-Bottle Units

Most commercially available active drainage systems are three-bottle units (Fig. 10-4), the third bottle being used for suction control. When a built-in wall suction is used as vacuum (unregulated vacuum), this third bottle regulates the amount of suction applied throughout the entire system. Bubbling in the suction-control bottle indicates that the suction source is applying the correct amount of negative pressure, usually –15 to –20 cm H₂O. The advantage of the three-bottle system resides in its safety because *high suction pressures can never be reached.* Its main deficiency is that it may provide inadequate airflow in the event of a large air leak.

Disposable units with the same three-bottle suction drainage principles are now used in most institutions. These units are compact, light, and easy to assemble and operate, and most are *relatively expensive.*

High-Volume Systems

When high suction is desirable to achieve effective evacuation of the pleural space, high-volume systems such as the *Emerson pump** can be used. These are capable of reaching negative pressures on the order of –60 cm H₂O with

---

*J.H. Emerson Co., Cambridge, Mass.

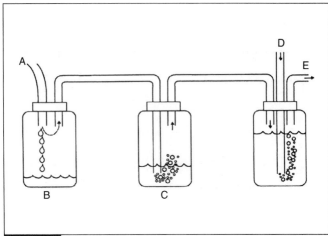

FIG. 10-4

Three-bottle unit in which the third bottle is used to regulate the amount of suction applied through the entire system. **A,** From the patient. **B,** Collecting bottle. **C,** Water seal. **D,** Vent tube. **E,** To wall suction.

airflows of more than 20 L/min. One has to remember, however, that *too much suction* may potentially increase the magnitude of an air leak, may encourage air steal that may lead to hypoxia, or may unexpectedly trap lung parenchyma in chest tube holes.

Pleuroperitoneal Shunt

The pleuroperitoneal shunt is a single-unit medical-grade silicone conduit consisting of a *unidirectionally valved pumping chamber* located between fenestrated pleural and peritoneal catheters. Manual compression of the shunt is required 150 to 200 times per day, and each compression transports about 1.5 mL of fluid from the pleural space to the peritoneum. The technique of pumping is neither painful nor difficult to master.

Malignant pleural effusions and chylothoraces are two of the most common indications for pleuroperitoneal shunting. Potential disadvantages of the technique are the cost of the device, the need for manual pumping, the contamination of the peritoneum by malignant cells, and the possible occlusion of the conduit.

CONCLUSION

Adequate knowledge of intercostal space and pleural anatomy is a prerequisite for the safe application of techniques of pleural drainage. These techniques may look simple, but they are fraught with the potential for complications that may convert what ought to be a small procedure into an unexpectedly more serious one. Fortunately, most errors can be avoided by adherence to sound anatomic and physiologic principles.

SUGGESTED READINGS

Review Articles

Von Hepple A: Chest Tubes and Chest Bottles. Springfield, Ill, Charles C Thomas, 1970.

Munnell ER, Thomas EK: Current concepts in thoracic drainage systems. Ann Thorac Surg 1975;19:261-268.

Richards V: Procedures in family practice. Tube thoracostomy. J Fam Pract 1978;6:629-635.

McFadden PM, Jones JW: Tube thoracostomy: anatomical considerations, overview of complications, and a proposed technique to avoid complications. Milit Med 1985;150:681-685.

Dalbec DL, Krome RL: Thoracostomy. Emerg Med Clin North Am 1986;4:441-457.

Julian JS, Pennell TC: A review of the basics of closed thoracic drainage. N C Med J 1987;48:127-131.

Miller KS, Sahn SA: Chest tubes. Indications, technique, management and complications. Chest 1987;91:258-264.

Symbas PN: Chest drainage tubes. Surg Clin North Am 1989;69:41-46.

Munnell ER: Thoracic drainage [collective review]. Ann Thorac Surg 1997;63:1497-1502.

Technique

Guyton SW, Paull DL, Anderson RP: Introducer insertion of minithoracostomy tubes. Am J Surg 1988;155:693-696.

Parmar JM: How to insert a chest drain. Br J Hosp Med 1989;40:231-233.

Riquet M, Chehab A, Souilamas R, et al: Elective drainage of the apical chest by posterior approach. Ann Thorac Surg 1998;66:1824-1825.

Historical Papers

Roe BB: Physiologic principles of drainage of the pleural space with special reference to high flow, high vacuum suction. Am J Surg 1958;96:246-253.

Anatomy of the Intercostal Space

Moore KL: Clinically Oriented Anatomy, 2nd ed. Baltimore, Williams & Wilkins, 1985.

Complications of Tube Drainage

Robinson G, Brodman R: Going down the tube. Ann Thorac Surg 1980;31:400-401.

Mahfood S, Hix WR, Aaron BL, et al: Reexpansion pulmonary edema. Current review. Ann Thorac Surg 1988;45:340-345.

Outpatient Management

Ponn RB, Silverman HJ, Federico JA: Outpatient chest tube management. Ann Thorac Surg 1997;64:1437-1440.

Lodi R, Stefani A: A new portable chest drainage device. Ann Thorac Surg 2000;69:998-1001.

PRINCIPLES OF OPEN DRAINAGE

As stated by Dr. Willard A. Fry, open drainage is an *old-fashioned operation* for *old-fashioned diseases.* It is usually accomplished with rib resection "involving" two to four ribs. Whereas it once was one of the most common operative procedures in thoracic surgery, it is currently used infrequently because other means of therapy, such as video-assisted thoracoscopic surgical (VATS) débridement, have rendered it of limited use.

In general, open drainage is indicated for the following:

1. patients with postpneumonectomy empyema where the surgeon wants adequate and dependent drainage of the space;
2. patients with chronic organizing empyemas where long-term drainage appears necessary;
3. patients too debilitated to undergo decortication or other major procedures.

Despite these few indications, the procedure of open drainage should be in the surgical repertoire of every surgeon performing thoracic surgical procedures.

INDICATIONS

In 1935, Eloesser described *a technique of open drainage* that became known as the Eloesser flap. This flap was designed to act as a tubeless one-way valve to drain chronic pleural, often tuberculous, effusions. The procedure consisted of making a U-shaped skin incision, resecting a segment of rib over the most dependent portion of the space, suturing the skin flaps to the pleura, and suturing the remaining edges of skin together. The only aspect of Eloesser's operation that still applies today is the concept of providing *adequate drainage of an empyema cavity with an epithelialized stoma.*

Although open thoracic window is a simple and well-tolerated procedure, the indications for it are few (Table 10-7). It is a valuable option for treating patients with *chronic empyemas when long-term or permanent drainage* is indicated or seems to be necessary. Open thoracic window also is indicated for patients who have chronic empyemas and who are too debilitated to undergo a major operation, such as decortication. The procedure is a good option for the drainage of postpneumonectomy empyemas with or without bronchopleural fistula (Clagett procedure), and it can also be of value in patients *who do not understand* or *will not cooperate* and who have a reasonably large cavity, especially patients with underlying lung disease. Another indication may be for patients who are waiting for a more radical procedure and in whom a period of rehabilitation and correction of nutritional deficiencies may be necessary or indicated.

TABLE 10-7
POSSIBLE INDICATIONS FOR OPEN DRAINAGE
Chronic empyema (stage of organization)
Patients waiting for a more radical procedure
Patients with no response to conventional therapy
Patients too debilitated for major thoracic procedures
Expectation of long-term drainage
Patients who do not understand or will not cooperate
Postpneumonectomy empyema

TECHNIQUE

Operative Procedure (Table 10-8)

Although open thoracic window is *usually performed under general anesthesia,* some authors believe that local anesthesia is as well if not more suited for these patients (often elderly) who are in poor general condition. If a bronchopleural fistula is documented or suspected, a double-lumen endotracheal tube should be used. The site of incision *must be planned carefully* by reviewing chest radiographs and a thoracic computed tomographic scan. Ultrasonographic localization of the empyema cavity and marking of the disease's extent may also be helpful.

Different incisions have been described: U-shaped (Eloesser), inverted U–shaped (Symbas), H-shaped, and triradiate. Whatever incision is preferred, the window should be placed at the most dependent portion of the empyema cavity. We prefer the *H-shaped incision* (Fig. 10-5) (10 to 12 cm long) because it allows larger skin flaps that can be used to marsupialize the undersurface of the window. Musculocutaneous flaps are then raised away from the ribs, and *15-cm segments* of two or three ribs are resected along with the intercostal muscles, neurovascular bundles, and underlying parietal pleura. It is important that an adequate number and length of ribs be resected because as maturation occurs, the skin opening can contract down quickly to half of the original size, leaving an inadequate aperture for drainage.

TABLE 10-8
TECHNIQUE OF OPEN THORACIC WINDOW
Usually performed under general anesthesia
Double-lumen tube if bronchopleural fistula is documented or suspected
Site of incision planned by reviewing computed tomographic scan
H-shaped skin incision
Musculocutaneous flaps are raised away from the ribs
15-cm segments of 2 or 3 ribs are resected
Cavity is débrided
Flaps are turned inside the window and sutured to parietal pleura edges
Tight packing with petroleum jelly gauzes

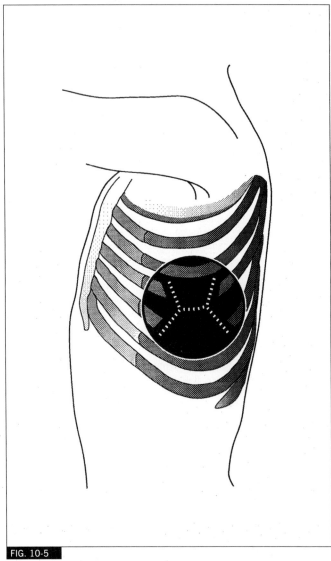

FIG. 10-5
Open thoracic window; outline of H-shaped incision.

The cavity is drained and débrided, avoiding disruption of the visceral pleura and parietal adhesions that surround the cavity. The flaps are then turned into the window and sutured to the parietal pleura edges with interrupted heavy absorbable sutures (Fig. 10-6). The cavity is tightly packed with petroleum jelly gauzes, which is preferred over loose packing because it may prevent postoperative oozing or, in some cases, important bleeding. Petroleum jelly gauzes are also easier and relatively painless to remove for the first few dressing changes.

Postoperative Care

Dressings should be changed *at least daily* or more often if needed at the beginning, and these dressing changes can be done at bedside with little or no sedatives. Because the initial viewing of the surgical site can be frightening, *the surgeon should address the issue* in advance with the patient and his or her relatives.

After a few days of dressing changes, loose packing with lightly moist (saline) dressings can be used because they provide better débridement and have a better resorption potential than do petroleum jelly gauzes. Other products, such as povidone-iodine (Betadine) 2:1 and Dakin solution ($\frac{1}{32}$), can be used to irrigate the cavity or to moisten the gauzes used to pack the cavity. In general, the mechanical débridement afforded by the gauzes is more important than the solution used to moisten the dressing. For large spaces, gauzes can be tied to each other to ensure that no gauze is forgotten inside the space. Sometimes the patient may have to be re-examined in the operating room for a complete inspection and débridement of the cavity or for revision of the stoma if the skin opening has contracted too much. Once the patient is mobile, he or she can get into a shower or bath, and if a hose and nozzle are available, the cavity can be irrigated with ordinary tap water. After several weeks, the skin sutures used for marsupialization can be removed.

Follow-up and Results

Adequate drainage of the empyema and local control of the infection are usually achieved with an open thoracic window. The systemic signs and symptoms of sepsis subside rapidly, and the procedure is surprisingly *well tolerated* despite the inconveniences of daily care.

In time, many of these thoracic windows will be obliterated and re-epithelialized completely, leaving only an indentation over the chest wall. This contraction can be appreciated by visually inspecting the space and by recording radiologic measurements or the number of milliliters of saline that is necessary to fill the space.

In most patients, however, the cavity is *too large to expect spontaneous obliteration,* and surgical closure must be performed at a later stage, depending on the status of the cavity and the patient. If the overall condition of the patient is poor, if the cavity is not clean, or if there is evidence of disseminated carcinoma, surgical closure should not be performed (Table 10-9). The presence of bronchoalveolar fistulas or of

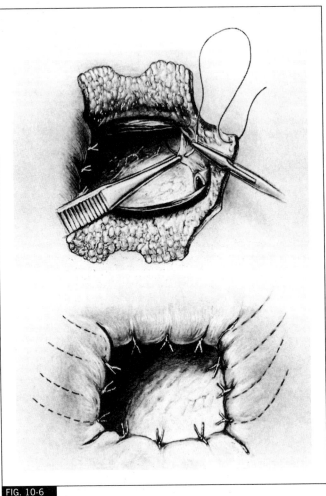

FIG. 10-6

Creation of an epithelialized track by suturing the edge of skin flap to the edge of parietal pleura. *(From Hurvitz RJ, Tucker BL: The Eloesser flap: past and present. J Thorac Cardiovasc Surg 1986;92:958-961.)*

small bronchopleural fistulas is not a contraindication to closure because these can be handled at the same time as the window closure.

To achieve proper closure, the residual space must be obliterated, preferably through the use of muscle transfer. Notably, some patients live with an open thoracic window for several years or for the rest of their lives,

TABLE 10-9

CONTRAINDICATIONS TO CLOSURE OF OPEN WINDOW THORACOSTOMY

Large bronchopleural or esophagopleural fistulas
Poor general condition
Evidence of metastatic or locally recurrent carcinoma
Cavity not clean
Patient's refusal

thereby avoiding the need for a second major surgical procedure. These patients have *adjusted* to a lifestyle of daily dressing changes that are often performed by the spouse, who is an important participant in the management of these individuals.

CLAGETT PROCEDURE

The Clagett procedure is a two-stage operation designed for the treatment of postpneumonectomy empyema. The first stage is open drainage of the postpneumonectomy empyema cavity, which is then irrigated daily for 6 to 8 weeks. During the second stage, the edges of the thoracic window are excised, the cavity is filled with saline solution that contains antibiotics, and the wound is closed in layers.

CONCLUSION

Overall, open thoracic window is worthwhile in selected cases of empyema that occur in sick and elderly patients. It has the potential to control severe life-threatening septic conditions rapidly, but its main drawback is the prolonged conservative treatment period that is required before healing and obliteration spontaneously occur. Indeed, in some cases, a second procedure may be necessary to ensure that the space is obliterated.

SUGGESTED READINGS

Review Articles

Somers J, Faber LP: Historical developments in the management of empyema. Chest Surg Clin North Am 1996;6:403-418.

Miller JI Jr.: The history of surgery of empyema, thoracoplasty, Eloesser flap, and muscle flap transposition. Chest Surg Clin North Am 2000;10:45-53.

Historical Papers

Eloesser L: An operation for tuberculous empyema. Surg Gynecol Obstet 1935;60:1096-1097.

Fry WA: Open drainage. In Pearson FG, Cooper JD, Deslauriers J, et al: Thoracic Surgery, 2nd ed. Philadelphia, Churchill Livingstone, 2002:1300-1307.

Clagett OT, Geraci JE: A procedure for the management of postpneumonectomy empyema. J Thorac Cardiovasc Surg 1963;45:141-145.

Case Series

Symbas PN, Nugent JT, Abbott OA, et al: Nontuberculous pleural empyema in adults. The role of a modified Eloesser procedure in its management. Ann Thorac Surg 1971;12:69-78.

Weissberg D: Empyema and bronchopleural fistula. Experience with open window thoracostomy. Chest 1982;82:447-450.

Smolle-Jüttner F, Beuster W, Pinter H, et al: Open-window thoracostomy in pleural empyema. Eur J Cardiothorac Surg 1992;6:635-638.

Ali SM, Siddiqui AA, McLaughlin JS: Open drainage of massive tuberculous empyema with progressive reexpansion of the lung: an old concept revisited. Ann Thorac Surg 1996;62:218-224.

Garcia-Yuste M, Ramos G, Duque JL, et al: Open-window thoracostomy and thoracomyoplasty to manage chronic pleural empyema. Ann Thorac Surg 1998;65:818-822.

Thourani VH, Lancaster RT, Mansour KA, Miller JI: Twenty-six years of experience with the modified Eloesser flap. Ann Thorac Surg 2003;76:401-406.

Special Challenges in Thoracic Surgery

MANAGEMENT OF THE PATIENT WITH MASSIVE HEMOPTYSIS

Massive hemoptysis has been defined as hemorrhage from the tracheobronchial tree in *excess of 600 mL over a 24-hour period.* It is a significant clinical problem because of the asphyxiation that may result from acute flooding of the lungs. Indeed, massive hemoptysis *is often defined* by the threat to life it poses rather than by the actual rate of bleeding.

Massive hemoptysis is usually associated with infectious conditions of the lung, such as tuberculosis, bronchiectasis, abscesses, and aspergillomas. In more than 90% to 95% of cases, the hemorrhage originates from *systemic arteries,* both bronchial and nonbronchial; in 5% to 10% of patients, it arises from the pulmonary artery, usually a Rasmussen aneurysm associated with old tuberculosis.

Treatment objectives are to *prevent asphyxiation* of the patient, to *stop the hemorrhage,* and to *prevent its recurrence.* Although previous experiences indicated that early surgery might offer a reduced mortality compared with conservative management, it is currently recommended that control of the hemorrhage be gained by *noninvasive techniques* such as embolization before an operation is considered. Surgical resection should almost never be carried out until the patient has stopped bleeding and has clinically stabilized.

DEFINITIONS AND TERMINOLOGY (TABLE 11-1)

Although the exact definition of major airway hemorrhage has never been agreed on, two categories of patients can clearly be identified by the rate of hemoptysis.

Quantitatively, patients whose rate of bleeding is *in excess of 600 mL* in a 24-hour period are defined as having *massive hemoptysis.* This definition is based on earlier retrospective studies that reported higher mortality rates when the hemoptysis was in excess of 600 mL over a 24-hour period. Patients with *exsanguinating hemoptysis* have a rate of bleeding of 150 mL or more per hour or cough up 300 to 400 mL of blood in one expectoration.

Qualitatively, patients with poor lung function are at significant risk of complications or even death with smaller amounts of blood spilling in their bronchial tree.

COMMON CAUSES OF HEMOPTYSIS

Origin of the Bleeding (Table 11-2)

Most episodes of massive hemoptysis occur in patients with known chronic inflammatory diseases of the bronchi or lung. In more than 90% of these individuals, *the bleeding is systemic* and originates from dilated bronchial

DEFINITIONS OF MASSIVE HEMOPTYSIS

Massive hemoptysis
600 mL or more per 24 hours

Exsanguinating hemoptysis
150 mL or more in 1 hour
300-400 mL or more in one expectoration

arteries in the vicinity of the lesion or from collaterals supplied by intercostal, internal mammary, subclavian, and axillary arteries.

In approximately 5% to 10% of cases, the hemoptysis arises from the pulmonary arterial system. This can be observed in *chronic tuberculous lesions,* in which pulmonary artery branches in the vicinity of the lesion have become dilated or even aneurysmal *(Rasmussen aneurysm)* from high-flow shunts between pulmonary and bronchial circulations. Pulmonary artery hemorrhaging can also be a consequence of radiation therapy; the necrotic tumor being irradiated ulcerates directly into an adjacent pulmonary artery branch.

Etiology of the Bleeding

Massive hemoptysis is usually associated with *benign suppurative pulmonary parenchymal diseases,* and tuberculosis accounts for the majority of cases. In those patients, hemoptysis is mainly associated with inactive disease presenting in the forms of cavitary, bronchiectatic, or destroyed lung residuals. Overall, significant hemoptysis will occur in 1% to 5% of tuberculous patients.

Most aspergillomas are located in the upper lobes, where they develop in chronic tuberculous cavities or long-standing sarcoidosis. The bleeding is systemic from bronchial arteries or collaterals from the intercostals or axillary arteries reaching the lung through pleural adhesions.

Massive hemoptysis can originate from calcified nodes eroding through the bronchus and bronchial arteries, a condition called *broncholithiasis*. In most cases, broncholithiasis is the end result of previous tuberculosis or histoplasmosis.

ORIGIN OF HEMOPTYSIS

Systemic blood (90%-95%)
Dilated and fragile bronchial arteries
Ulcerated nonbronchial arteries in vicinity of lesion
    Intercostal arteries
    Internal mammary arteries
    Branches from subclavian or axillary arteries

Pulmonary artery blood (5%-10%)
Rasmussen aneurysm in vicinity of chronic tuberculous lesions
Lung cancer eroding directly in adjacent central pulmonary artery branch

Lung abscesses are an infrequent cause of massive hemoptysis, and when it occurs, the bleeding is secondary to the local necrotizing effect of the primary infection. Patients with bronchiectasis often have hemoptysis, but hemorrhaging is seldom significant (see later, "Management of Patients with Suppurative Lung Disease"). Cystic fibrosis patients bleed because of dilated and fragile bronchial arteries and lung abscesses.

Characteristically, lung cancer patients present with *small amounts of hemoptysis* related to simple neoplastic mucosal ulcerations. Massive hemoptysis is nearly always the result of a central tumor's eroding into the pulmonary artery or aorta.

Trauma-related massive hemoptysis is unusual and generally associated with tracheobronchial ruptures. In those cases, the bleeding originates from *torn bronchial arteries* at the site of disruption. Among the iatrogenic causes of massive hemoptysis, those related to tracheotomy are of particular interest because they are usually fatal. In such patients, the hemoptysis is secondary to erosion of the innominate artery, either by the main body of the cannula or by its tip through the anterior tracheal wall. Rarely, massive hemoptysis will be secondary to catheter-induced (Swan-Ganz) pulmonary artery perforations or to endobronchial biopsies during the course of diagnostic bronchoscopy.

Other unusual causes of massive hemoptysis are listed in Table 11-3, and these should be ruled out before definitive therapy is planned. Patients with mitral stenosis or coagulopathies, for instance, should be identified because they can be successfully managed by simple drug therapies.

TABLE 11-3
COMMON CAUSES OF MASSIVE HEMOPTYSIS

Infections
Mycobacterial: active or inactive tuberculosis
Fungal: aspergilloma
Bacterial: bronchiectasis, lung abscess, necrotizing pneumonia, cystic fibrosis
Broncholithiasis

Neoplastic
Bronchogenic carcinomas

Traumatic and iatrogenic
External trauma (penetrating and blunt)
Iatrogenic trauma: tracheal surgery, tracheotomy, bronchoscopy,
    Swan-Ganz catheterization

Cardiovascular
Pulmonary venous hypertension due to mitral stenosis
Vascular malformations of pulmonary artery or vein
Primary pulmonary hypertension

Others
Coagulopathies
Pulmonary diseases: necrotizing angiitis, granulomatosis, sarcoidosis, cystic fibrosis

11

Special Challenges in Thoracic Surgery

TABLE 11-4

CHARACTERISTICS OF HEMOPTYSIS AND HEMATEMESIS

	Hemoptysis	Hematemesis
Previous history	Positive for respiratory illness	Positive for upper gastrointestinal symptoms
Symptoms	Coughing often precedes bleeding	Nausea and vomiting often precede bleeding
Color of the blood	Usually bright red and will stay that color for several days	Usually brownish or dark red due to oxidation and mixture with gastric contents (food particles)
Appearance of the blood	Frothy because it contains air	Not frothy
Biochemistry	Alkaline reaction	Acid reaction

DIAGNOSIS

Clinical Features

Epistaxis and bleeding from the gums (stomatitis, gingivitis) as well as hematemesis (Table 11-4) *can easily be confused* with hemoptysis. These must be ruled out in a patient with active bleeding.

The clinical history should include a recording of the approximate amount of blood loss and duration of hemoptysis, of possible previous similar episodes, and of the presence of other symptoms such as chest pain. One must finally inquire about the patient's being anticoagulated or having a prior history of hemorrhagic disorder or heart disease.

Interestingly, some patients *are able* to determine the side of the bleeding because they have a sensation of heaviness or tickling on that side.

Diagnostic Studies

The *chest radiograph* is an important diagnostic tool because it can often identify the cause and source of the hemoptysis. It may show localized pulmonary infiltrations, cavitations, masses, or other abnormalities indicating the likely source of bleeding. In 20% to 40% of cases, however, initial radiographs will be interpreted as normal, and *computed tomographic (CT) scanning* with contrast material will be necessary to improve the radiologic diagnostic yield. CT scan can show bronchiectasis, small tumors, or arteriovenous malformations not visible on plain chest radiographs. It can also provide better definitions of masses or cavities not clearly outlined previously. Except for life-threatening situations, CT should be performed before bronchoscopic exploration.

Bronchoscopy (Table 11-5) should be the next step in the evaluation of patients with hemoptysis. Indeed, bronchoscopy done during active bleeding or within 48 hours of the beginning of the episode significantly increases the likelihood of identifying the bleeding site. One important aspect of early bronchoscopy is that it can at least lateralize (right or left) the source of bleeding.

What type of bronchoscope should be used and where the examination should be done remain controversial. Two obvious advantages of flexible bronchoscopy are, first, that it can be done at bedside and, second, that

---

TABLE 11-5

BRONCHOSCOPY DURING MASSIVE OR LIFE-THREATENING HEMOPTYSIS

Flexible bronchoscopy
Best for moderate hemoptysis
Can easily be done by most physicians
Should be done in intensive care environment
Better view of distal segmental bronchi

Rigid bronchoscopy
Best for life-threatening hemoptysis
Need experienced endoscopist to be useful
Done in operating room under general anesthesia
Most effective means of suctioning
Allows use of bronchial blocking balloons to isolate bleeding lung
Provides better control of airway and possible means for ventilation

---

most clinicians are familiar with the technology. Fiberoptic bronchoscopy also allows visualization of more peripheral portions (segmental bronchi) of the bronchial tree. In the setting of massive hemoptysis, fiberoptic bronchoscopy should always be done in an intensive care environment where the airway can be secured should the rate of bleeding increase during the procedure.

When the hemorrhage is life-threatening (100 to 150 mL/h), the most valuable instrument to locate the site of bleeding or at least to lateralize the bleeding *is the rigid bronchoscope.* The procedure must be done in the operating room under general anesthesia by an experienced endoscopist. The main advantage of the rigid bronchoscope (over fiberoptic) is its wide conduit, which allows ventilation, suctioning of blood, and excellent visualization of central airways. The rigid bronchoscope also allows the passage of balloon-bearing catheters that may be used to tamponade the site of bleeding and prevent spilling of blood in the normal lung.

When bronchoscopy fails to localize the source of bleeding, systematic bilateral arteriographic examination of the bronchial and pulmonary arteries can be done. This examination may demonstrate active bleeding or show indirect signs of a bleeding vessel (Table 11-6).

MANAGEMENT

The management of a patient with massive or life-threatening hemoptysis includes general measures and medical therapy, specific interventions to gain interim control of the bleeding site, and definitive treatment of the cause of hemoptysis.

TABLE 11-6

INDIRECT ANGIOGRAPHIC SIGNS INDICATING POSSIBLE SOURCE
OF HEMOPTYSIS

Parenchymal hypervascularity
Vascular hyperplasia, tortuosity, irregularities
Bronchopulmonary shunting
Aneurysm formation

Initial Management of Massive Hemoptysis (Table 11-7)

Patients with massive hemoptysis should be cared for *in an intensive care unit.* For most of them, however, the hemoptysis is not immediately life-threatening, and one has some time to initiate conservative measures and to document the source and cause of hemoptysis.

Conservative management includes complete bed rest (upright position) in a quiet room and around-the-clock medications *to suppress cough without abolishing it* (codeine every 3 or 4 hours) and to relieve anxiety. Intravenous large-spectrum antibiotics must also be given because most episodes of massive hemoptysis are associated with an acute respiratory infection even when symptoms cannot be documented by clinical history.

Careful inquiry may provide clues to the cause of hemoptysis. Patients with bronchiectasis often have a history of chronic suppuration; those with tuberculosis may have clear-cut knowledge of their previous disease. Review of chest radiographs and CT scans is helpful, but the chest radiograph will often be entirely normal or show only abnormalities that are not necessarily related to hemoptysis. Bronchoscopy done while the bleeding is still active *is the single most important diagnostic study.* It will nearly always lateralize the source of bleeding and, in close to 90% of cases, localize it to a specific lobe or segment.

Obvious causes of bleeding, such as coagulation disorders, should be treated with specific measures, and blood should be transfused when necessary. If the oxygen saturation is less than 90%, supplemental oxygen should be given.

Initial Management During Life-Threatening Hemoptysis

In this situation, the hemoptysis is exsanguinating. The primary objectives of management are to *stop ongoing bleeding,* to *prevent asphyxiation,* to *stabilize the patient,* and ultimately to prepare the patient for specific treatment.

TABLE 11-7

INITIAL MANAGEMENT OF MASSIVE HEMOPTYSIS

Conservative measures to stop the bleeding
Complete bed rest (upright position)
Cough suppressants (codeine given around the clock)
Anxiolytic drugs (given around the clock)
Intravenous antibiotics (large spectrum)
Oxygen
Intensive care environment

General work-up
Clinical history
Blood work, coagulation studies, electrocardiography

Specific work-up to localize site of bleeding
Chest radiography, CT scanning
Bronchoscopy
Angiography

The most valuable diagnostic procedure is *rigid bronchoscopy,* which again should be carried out in the operating room with the assistance of an anesthetist. Once control of the airway has been achieved, the site of bleeding can at least be lateralized and a Fogarty catheter advanced into the bleeding bronchus. The balloon can then be inflated to occlude the airway, isolate the contralateral lung, and provide some extra time to plan further management strategies. Alternatively, a double-lumen tube can be inserted to allow separate ventilation of the nonbleeding lung.

Interim Control of the Bleeding

In the majority of patients with either massive or life-threatening hemoptysis, bronchial artery embolization or endobronchial therapeutic interventions will successfully achieve interim control of the bleeding. Because these techniques are highly successful, *emergency surgery is almost never required.* Indeed, surgical therapy during active bleeding carries substantially *higher mortality and morbidity* rates compared with elective pulmonary resections (Table 11-8). This is related to hemodynamic instability at the time of operation as well as to spillage of blood in the dependent lung. In addition, the performance of pulmonary resection in poorly prepared patients often with inadequate pulmonary reserve is an important risk factor for postoperative morbidity.

Bronchial Artery Embolization

Bronchial artery embolization is currently considered the *most effective method* to obtain immediate control of bleeding. Overall, the bleeding vessel can successfully be embolized and the hemoptysis stopped in up to 90% to 95% of patients. Because these high success rates are directly related to the experience of the operator, it is recommended that within a community or city, all bronchial artery embolization be done by the same group of interventional radiologists.

The technique involves retrograde introduction of suitable catheters into the bronchial arteries supplying the pathologic lung and embolization of those arteries with embolization material. If no active bleeding artery is identified during the examination, *blind embolization* of the bronchial arteries most likely responsible for causing the bleeding should be done.

A potential complication of bronchial artery embolization is spinal cord damage by inadvertent injection of contrast medium or coils into the spinal artery sometimes arising from a bronchial or a high intercostal artery.

TABLE 11-8

REASONS TO AVOID SURGERY IN PATIENTS WITH ACTIVE HEMOPTYSIS

Interim control can nearly always be obtained by conservative measures
High mortality rates associated with
    Ongoing bleeding and hemodynamic instability
    Spillage of blood in dependent lung
Higher mortality rates associated with inadequate preparation in patients
    with poor cardiopulmonary function

11

Special Challenges in Thoracic Surgery

Fortunately, this complication is rare (<1%) if the operator is experienced with the technique. Another disadvantage of bronchial artery embolization is that it is seldom a definitive procedure. Bleeding is likely to recur weeks or months later because of recanalization of embolized arteries or because of ongoing active disease and formation of new collaterals.

Endobronchial Therapeutic Interventions

Most of these techniques are available to control life-threatening hemoptysis and are done through the rigid bronchoscope. Again, the purpose of these interventions is to gain time for restoration of clinical stability. If the bleeding site is identified, packing material can be applied directly to the site, or the bleeding can be controlled by local tamponade with a balloon-type catheter. This catheter is secured in the airway for a period of 24 hours and then removed under control of fiberoptic bronchoscopy.

Additional measures that can occasionally be useful include endobronchial lavage with ice-cold saline and endobronchial infusion of thrombin or fibrinogen solutions.

Definitive Treatment

Pulmonary resection is the most definitive way of controlling the hemoptysis and preventing its recurrence. In most cases, however, it should be delayed until active bleeding has stopped, the patient is clinically stable, and the lungs have cleared of blood clots, usually 2 to 3 weeks after the acute episode. Ultimately, the indication for surgery is based on having an anatomically circumscribed lesion, the high likelihood that the lesion will rebleed, and the ability of the patient to withstand the type of resection likely to be required (see Chapter 2, "Assessment of Pulmonary Reserve").

CONCLUSION

Patients presenting with massive hemoptysis should initially be treated conservatively. In this setting, an experienced interventional radiologist should be part of the team because bronchial artery embolization will provide interim control of the hemoptysis in nearly all patients. Emergency surgery should be avoided because it yields significant morbidity and mortality.

SUGGESTED READINGS

Review Articles

Jones DK, Davies RJ: Massive hemoptysis. Medical management will usually arrest the bleeding. Br Med J 1990;300:889-890.

Wedzicha JA, Pearson MC: Management of massive haemoptysis. Respir Med 1990;84:9-12.

Thompson AB, Teschler H, Rennard SI: Pathogenesis, evaluation, and therapy for massive hemoptysis. Clin Chest Med 1992;13:69-82.

Stoller JK: Diagnosis and management of massive hemoptysis: a review. Respir Care 1992;37:564-581.

Cahill BC, Ingbar DH: Massive hemoptysis. Assessment and management. Clin Chest Med 1994;15:147-168.

Patel U, Pattison CW, Raphael M: Management of massive haemoptysis. Review. Br J Hosp Med 1994;52:74-78.

Colice GL: Hemoptysis. Three questions that can direct management. Postgrad Med 1996;100:227-236.

Marshall TJ, Flower CD, Jackson JE: The role of radiology in the investigation and management of patients with haemoptysis. Clin Radiol 1996;51:391-400.

Sarbit J, Lien DC: Hemoptysis: diagnosis and management. Prairie Med J 1996;66:59-63.

Jean-Baptiste E: Clinical assessment and management of massive hemoptysis. Crit Care Med 2000;28:1642-1647.

Haponik EF, Fein A, Chin R: Managing life-threatening hemoptysis. Has anything really changed? Chest 2000;118:1431-1435.

Karmy-Jones R, Cuschieri J, Vallières E: Role of bronchoscopy in massive hemoptysis. Chest Surg Clin North Am 2001;11:873-906.

Embolization

Katoh O, Kishikawa T, Yamada H, et al: Recurrent bleeding after arterial embolization in patients with hemoptysis. Chest 1990;97:541-546.

Lampmann LE, Tjan TG: Embolization therapy in haemoptysis. Eur J Radiol 1994;18:15-19.

Marshall TJ, Jackson JE: Vascular intervention in the thorax: bronchial artery embolization for haemoptysis. Eur Radiol 1997;7:1221-1227.

Mal H, Rullon I, Mellot F, et al: Immediate and long-term results of bronchial artery embolization for life-threatening hemoptysis. Chest 1999;115:996-1001.

White RI Jr.: Bronchial artery embolotherapy for control of acute hemoptysis. Analysis of outcome. Chest 1999;115:912-915.

Swanson KL, Johnson M, Prakash UB, et al: Bronchial artery embolization. Experience with 54 patients. Chest 2002;121:789-795.

Goh PYT, Lin M, Teo N, Wong DES: Embolization for hemoptysis: a six-year review. Cardiovasc Intervent Radiol 2002;25:17-25.

Investigation

Saumench J, Escarrabill J, Padró L, et al: Value of fiberoptic bronchoscopy and angiography for diagnosis of the bleeding site in hemoptysis. Ann Thorac Surg 1989;48:272-274.

Millar AB, Boothroyd AE, Edwards D, Hetzel MR: The role of computed tomography (CT) in the investigation of unexplained haemoptysis. Respir Med 1992;86:39-44.

McGuinness G, Beacher JR, Harkin TJ, et al: Hemoptysis: prospective high-resolution CT/bronchoscopic correlation. Chest 1994;105:1155-1162.

Poe RH, Israel RH, Marin MG, et al: Utility of fiberoptic bronchoscopy in patients with hemoptysis and a nonlocalizing chest roentgenogram. Chest 1998;92:70-75.

Dweik RA, Stoller JK: Role of bronchoscopy in massive hemoptysis. Clin Chest Med 1999;20:89-105.

Case Series

Corey R, Hla KM: Major and massive hemoptysis: reassessment of conservative management. Am J Med Sci 1987;294:301-309.

Santiago S, Tobias J, Williams AJ: A reappraisal of the causes of hemoptysis. Arch Intern Med 1991;151:2449-2451.

Knott-Craig CJ, Oostuizen JG, Rossouw G, et al: Management and prognosis of massive hemoptysis. Recent experience with 120 patients. J Thorac Cardiovasc Surg 1993;105:394-397.

Hirshberg B, Biran I, Glazer M, Kramer MR: Hemoptysis: etiology, evaluation, and outcome in a tertiary referral hospital. Chest 1997;112: 440-444.

Lee TW, Wan S, Choy DK, et al: Management of massive hemoptysis: a single institution experience. Ann Thorac Cardiovasc Surg 2000;6: 232-235.

Endo S, Otani SI, Saito N, et al: Management of massive hemoptysis in a thoracic surgical unit. Eur J Cardiothorac Surg 2003;23: 467-472.

Ong TH, Eng P: Massive hemoptysis requiring intensive care. Intensive Care Med 2003;29:317-320.

Other

Weber F: Catamenial hemoptysis. Ann Thorac Surg 2001;72:1750-1751.

Surgery

Jougon J, Ballester M, Delcambre F, et al: Massive hemoptysis: what place for medical and surgical treatment. Eur J Cardiothorac Surg 2002; 22:345-351.

Ayed A: Pulmonary resection for massive hemoptysis of benign etiology. Eur J Cardiothorac Surg 2003;24:689-693.

Hemoptysis and Lung Cancer

Panos RJ, Barr LF, Walsh TJ, Silverman HJ: Factors associated with fatal hemoptysis in cancer patients. Chest 1988;94:1008-1013.

MANAGEMENT OF THE PATIENT WITH A PARAPNEUMONIC EFFUSION OR EMPYEMA

Parapneumonic effusions occur in about 50% to 60% of patients hospitalized with bacterial pneumonia. Some of these effusions will resolve without treatment other than that of the underlying pneumonia, whereas others must be drained. Unfortunately, clinical approaches and criteria to determine which parapneumonic effusions must be drained and the best method for draining them often vary from surgeon to surgeon and from center to center.

Empyema thoracis is defined as a purulent pleural effusion. The infection usually *originates from the lung,* although it may have entered the pleural space through the chest wall or from sources below the diaphragm or in the mediastinum. Management depends on the *cause of the empyema* and its clinical stage, the *state of the underlying lung,* the presence or absence of a bronchopleural fistula, and the patient's clinical and nutritional status.

Although clinical practice guidelines on the medical and surgical treatment of empyemas are available, the management of these patients often has to be individualized.

TERMINOLOGY

The American Thoracic Society recognizes three distinct stages in the formation of an empyema (see Chapter 3, "Assessment of the Patient with a Pleural Disorder") indicative of disease progression in the pleural space. In daily clinical practice, however, management is based on two distinct phases of evolution: an acute process and an organizing phase.

Acute Phase

Early in the disease process, the pleural membranes are edematous and discharge a thin exudative fluid called a parapneumonic effusion. With *early and vigorous treatment of the underlying pneumonia,* most of these effusions will remain uninfected, and they will generally be associated with a good outcome. At this very early stage, the volume of pleural fluid is minimal, and the effusion is free flowing on lateral decubitus films.

If the disease process is allowed to continue, large amounts of fibrin will be deposited mostly over the parietal pleura; the amount of pleural fluid will also increase significantly, and it will become loculated. When the host reaction is eventually overwhelmed by the number and virulence of the inoculum, the pleural fluid becomes turbid or frankly purulent (fibrinopurulent phase). If left undrained, these collections are associated with poor outcomes even if the pleura is still relatively intact and the lung can still be re-expanded.

Pleural effusions occurring early in the parapneumonic process are often called *uncomplicated* because they are likely to resolve without tube drainage. By contrast, those occurring during the fibrinopurulent phase are called *complicated* because they will require surgical drainage.

Organization Phase

Within 3 to 4 weeks or sometimes sooner, organization begins with massive ingrowth of fibroblasts and formation of collagen fibers over both parietal and visceral pleura. The lung, which at this stage is virtually functionless, is imprisoned within a thick fibrous peel and can no longer expand with tube drainage.

CATEGORIZING RISK FOR POOR OUTCOME

The real difficulty in the management of patients with parapneumonic effusions is to be able to distinguish *between a noncomplicated, noninfected effusion and a complicated one* in which an empyema is

Special Challenges in Thoracic Surgery

11

pending or already present. Evaluating the risk for poor outcome and categorizing it (Table 11-9) are therefore important and should be based on three variables: *pleural space anatomy, pleural fluid bacteriology,* and *pleural fluid chemistry.* The presence of clinical symptoms such as fever, chest pain, or systemic toxicity is less important because these can be related to the underlying pneumonia as much as to the secondary pleural effusion.

Standard chest radiographs are useful, at least initially, to document the pleural effusion and to determine if the collection is *free flowing or loculated* (decubitus films). CT scanning is used to assess the underlying lung as well as to determine the presence or absence of loculations, thickened parietal pleura, or trapped lung. Ultrasonography is perhaps *the best imaging technique* to demonstrate septations and loculations.

Ultrasonography is also the preferred method for guiding thoracentesis, especially when diaphragmatic position cannot be clearly ascertained on chest radiographs. Aspirates should be sent for cytology, biochemical analysis, Gram stain, and aerobic and anaerobic studies including bacterial sensitivity tests. The best chemistry test is the pH, and pleural effusions with low fluid pH (<7.2) may represent an indication for tube drainage, especially if the effusion is large (half or more of the hemithorax). Low glucose concentration (<60 mg/dL) and high lactate dehydrogenase contents (>1000 U/L) may also indicate an impending empyema. Repeated thoracentesis *should be considered* if the effusion enlarges or if the patient's clinical condition deteriorates.

The *gross appearance and odor* of pleural fluid are often significant items of information. Thin fluid may respond to selective antibiotherapy of the pneumonia, whereas fluid with positive bacteriologic results or frank

TABLE 11-9

CATEGORIZING RISK IN PATIENTS WITH PARAPNEUMONIC EFFUSIONS

Pleural Space Anatomy (Imaging)	Pleural Fluid Bacteriology (Thoracentesis)	Pleural Fluid Chemistry (Thoracentesis)	Risk of Poor Outcome	Drainage
Minimal flowing effusion (<10 mm) on lateral decubitus film	Unknown	Unknown	Very low	No
Small to moderate free-flowing effusion (>10 mm and <½ hemithorax)	Negative Gram stain and culture	pH ≥ 7.20	Low	No
Larger free-flowing effusion (≥½ hemithorax), loculated effusion, or effusion with thickened parietal pleura	Positive Gram stain or culture	pH < 7.20	Moderate	Yes
	Frank pus	pH < 7.0	High	Yes

pus requires formal surgical drainage. Negative pleural cultures can be due to inadequate culture techniques or to prior effective antibiotherapy.

Organized empyemas are best documented by CT scanning, which shows separated, thickened visceral and parietal pleurae as well as compressed and *trapped lung*.

MANAGEMENT

Empyema management depends on the clinical stage of disease and patient's clinical status.

Acute Phase (Fig. 11-1)

In patients with acute parapneumonic effusions, the estimated risk for poor outcome (Table 11-9) *forms the basis* for determining whether the effusion should be drained. Patients with very low or low risk of poor outcome do not require drainage because the effusion will most likely disappear with the resolution of the pneumonia. In those patients, treatment primarily consists of antibiotic therapy with or without repeated thoracentesis.

In patients with high or very high risk of poor outcome, removal of contaminated pleural fluid or of pus by closed pleural drainage is mandatory. Early drainage results in *improved survival, shortened hospital stay,* and *reduced need for second intervention*.

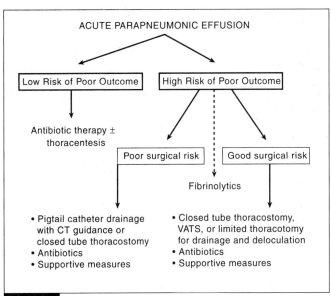

FIG. 11-1

Suggested algorithm for managing parapneumonic effusions during the acute phase. VATS, video-assisted thoracoscopic surgery.

11

Special Challenges in Thoracic Surgery

Drainage

In patients with poor surgical risk, drainage can be accomplished by *closed tube thoracostomy* or through the use of image-guided (CT or ultrasonography) percutaneous catheters. This latter technique is very useful although it is often considered to be an interim step before a subsequent procedure may result in more definitive treatment of the empyema. Overall, success rates ranging from 70% to 90% have been reported with the use of pigtail catheters. If pleural drainage is accomplished by closed tube thoracostomy, a 24 to 28 Fr thoracotomy tube is typically used, and it should be connected to an active suction system.

In patients with good surgical risk in whom multiple loculations are likely to impede chest tube drainage and in patients in whom closed thoracostomy has failed, video-assisted thoracoscopic surgery (VATS) techniques are optimal to *evacuate the pus,* to *disrupt loculations,* to *remove fibrin,* to *re-expand the lung,* and to *position one or two chest tubes* in the dependent portions of the space. Because it is minimally invasive, VATS can also be done in critically ill patients or in rescue situations when incomplete resolution of the empyema or only partial lung re-expansion has been achieved with tube drainage. A limited thoracotomy approach can also be used with the same objectives.

Once the empyema process has resolved, the tubes can be removed when the amount of drainage is low (<50 mL/day) and when the pleural space is obliterated by full lung re-expansion. This is likely to have occurred when there are *no up-and-down movements of fluid* in the tubing (fluid oscillations) or when no pneumothorax develops if the tube is opened to atmospheric pressure.

Open drainage *has no role* in the management of acute parapneumonic effusions or empyemas.

Intrapleural Fibrinolytic Therapy

Fibrinolytic therapy may sometimes be an acceptable approach for management of patients with moderate risk of poor outcome (see Table 11-9). Fibrinolytic agents are used to *break up fibrin strands* that may have developed between visceral and parietal pleurae, thus preventing lung re-expansion.

The most commonly used fibrinolytic agent is streptokinase, which is given through the chest tube daily for 3 days (250,000 units in 100 mL of saline with a 2-hour dwell time). Adverse effects include *chest pain and fever;* temperature can be as high as 40°C. Anaphylaxis and major hemorrhage are extremely rare events.

Antibiotics and Supportive Measures (Table 11-10)

Several factors, such as the pathogen involved and the immune status of the host, determine the response to antibiotics. Initially, and while awaiting the results of antibiotic susceptibility, a *semisynthetic penicillin such as clindamycin* should be given if the empyema has been acquired in the community or if the Gram staining reveals clusters of gram-positive

TABLE 11-10	
PRINCIPLES OF MANAGEMENT OF ACUTE EMPYEMAS	

Closed tube drainage
Appropriate antibiotics
Intrapleural fibrinolytic agents
Supportive measures: respiratory care, nutrition
Treatment of comorbid conditions
Treatment of underlying cause of empyema

cocci *(Staphylococcus aureus)*. Antibiotics are then continued intravenously for 1 to 2 weeks and orally for an additional 2 weeks.

Other supportive measures, such as respiratory care with therapy for associated respiratory infection and obstructive pulmonary disease and maintenance of nutrition, are essential for the successful management of early empyemas. Because nearly 50% to 60% of patients have a major associated medical illness, it is also imperative that *these conditions be recognized and appropriately managed.*

Organization Phase

Usual causes of chronicity include a delay in diagnosis, inadequate antibiotic therapy, improper drainage during the acute phase, continued reinfection (such as that which occurs with a bronchopleural fistula or lung abscess), presence of a foreign body, and presence of a specific infection (such as tuberculosis or fungal infection). In 1896, Paget wrote, "One might add a score of cases to show that an unhealed empyema is, as a rule, the direct result of the patient's neglect, or of the surgeon's delay, or of inadequate and useless surgery; but our business now is to inquire how we may most safely cure it." When the empyema has reached this stage, *simple forms of therapy including VATS are ineffective* because of the thick peel encasing the lung.

Treatment in Poor-Risk Patients: Open Thoracic Window (Open Drainage)

In poor-risk and elderly debilitated patients, adequate drainage of the empyema can be achieved by the creation *of an open thoracic window* (see Chapter 10) (Fig. 11-2). The procedure is relatively minor, but it should be done *only when sufficient adhesions have formed* to prevent an open pneumothorax. The advantages of open thoracic window are that the cavity can easily be irrigated and cleaned and that dressings can be changed daily on an outpatient basis.

Given time, some of these windows will close spontaneously, either by filling of the space with granulomatous tissue or through re-epithelialization from the skin flaps. In other cases, the window may have to be left open permanently, or it may be closed at a later stage with a muscle transplant (space filling) on a pedicle.

Treatment in Good-Risk Patients with a Normal Lung: Decortication

Decortication, which is defined as the removal of a constricting peel over the lung, is the best treatment option for *patients at good surgical risk with a*

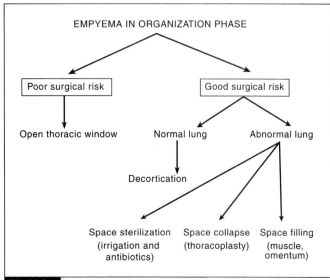

FIG. 11-2

Suggested algorithm for management of patients with empyemas during the organization phase.

normal underlying lung. Success rates depend on an intact visceral pleura (peel is dissected free from visceral pleura), meticulous surgical technique, *a lung that can expand,* and, most important, *a space that can be completely obliterated* by pulmonary re-expansion. The timing of decortication is still somewhat controversial, although most authors believe that it is best to wait 3 months or more after the diagnosis of chronic empyema has been made.

By contrast to decortication, "empyemectomy" refers to the complete excision of the empyema and of its contents without entering it. The rationale behind this procedure is that if both visceral and parietal peels are excised together, one can avoid contaminating either the thoracotomy wound or the free pleural space. Empyemectomy is usually reserved *for small and loculated empyemas.*

Treatment in Good-Risk Patients with an Abnormal Lung

In these individuals, pretreatment investigation will suggest that even with proper decortication, there will be insufficient pulmonary tissue to obliterate the space. This may be due to intrinsic disease or to fibrosis secondary to the long-standing effect of the empyema.

Space Sterilization. In some of these individuals, *the space can be sterilized through chest tube irrigation and systemic antibiotic therapy.*

The tubes, which can be inserted under videothoracoscopic guidance, are used for continuous irrigation (50 to 100 mL/h) of an antiseptic solution (Dakin$^1/_{32}$). Irrigations are continued for 2 to 3 weeks or until cultures done on 3 consecutive days are negative. Specific antibiotics must also be given for a period of 4 to 6 weeks.

With newer antibiotics, which have better penetrance of the pleura, injected spaces can be sterilized in 50% to 70% of patients who do not have an associated bronchopleural fistula.

Space Collapse (Thoracoplasty). The concept of resecting ribs to remove the skeletal support of the chest wall, thus decreasing the size of chronic spaces and promoting their obliteration, dates to the end of the 19th century. During the past years, however, thoracoplasties *have lost much of their popularity* because they are considered to be mutilating, poorly tolerated by patients, and associated with significant long-term sequelae. In addition, most modern surgeons have never seen one of these procedures done. The procedure, which involves the extramuscular-periosteal resection of five or six ribs (preserving the first rib), is, however, useful for the treatment of *chronically infected apical spaces*.

Space Filling (Muscle Transposition). Since transposition of muscle flaps on pedicles was first reported early in the 20th century, it has been used extensively in therapy for chronically infected spaces. Muscle selection is based not only on its availability but also on the location, size, and shape of the empyema space. The blood supply, innervation, and bulk of the muscle must be preserved, and the transposed muscle must fill the entire space because empyema is likely to recur if a residual space is left. The thoracic muscles *most commonly* used are the latissimus dorsi and the pectoralis major.

Chronic spaces can also be filled with omentum mobilized from the abdomen and advanced in the pleural space through a diaphragmatic opening.

Supportive Measures

Supportive measures for the treatment of patients with chronic empyemas are essentially the same as those described in the management of patients seen during the acute phase of the process. In chronic empyemas, however, special attention must be given to *maintenance of nutrition,* and this often has to be done through enteral feedings (feeding tube or jejunostomy).

SPECIAL PROBLEMS

Empyema in Children (Table 11-11)

Most empyemas that occur in children are complications of upper or lower respiratory tract infections. As in adults, the pathologic response is divided into acute and chronic phases. The principles of therapy are based on appropriate selection of antibiotics, drainage of the pleural space, and maintenance of lung expansion.

TABLE 11-11

PRINCIPLES OF TREATMENT OF EMPYEMAS IN CHILDREN
Early deloculation in patients with anaerobic empyemas or empyemas due to beta-hemolytic streptococci or *Haemophilus influenzae*
Tube drainage in patients with *Staphylococcus aureus* or other gram-positive organisms
Early decortication during organization phase
Avoidance of open thoracic window

In children, the bacteriologic findings of empyema are particularly important because they affect the speed and severity of loculations that may develop in the space. Anaerobic effusions, for instance, loculate quickly. Staphylococcal effusions are often fibrinoid deposits with little actual pleural fluid. These are amenable to treatment by tube drainage alone, whereas anaerobic empyemas or empyemas caused by beta-hemolytic streptococci or *Haemophilus influenzae* may require early deloculation for complete re-expansion of the lung and excellent long-term results.

Another factor that may alter treatment strategies in children is the degree of lung trapping, as documented by CT scanning. When the empyema is organized, *decortication should be carried out early* because lung growth and function may be permanently adversely affected. In children, there is also *little role for open thoracic windows* because both failure rates and late sequelae are common.

In children, the most important objectives of therapy are to re-expand the trapped lung, to restore mobility of the chest wall and diaphragm, to return lung function to normal, and to eliminate complications associated with chronicity.

Empyema in Immunocompromised Patients

Immunocompromised patients are at high risk for infectious complications. These include not only patients with AIDS and transplant recipients but also patients with long-term steroid use, patients with malignant neoplasms, malnourished patients, patients with congenital or acquired immunoglobulin deficiencies, postoperative patients, and others. The treatment of empyema in patients with human immunodeficiency virus (HIV) infection is similar to that described for patients with non-HIV infections. Early closed tube drainage, specific antibiotics, and intrapleural enzymes should be part of treatment in these individuals. In general, patients with empyema and HIV infection require *longer hospitalization and have more prolonged air leaks* than do patients who are not infected with HIV. Often, the patient has not been previously diagnosed with HIV infection when the diagnosis of empyema is made.

CONCLUSION

Empyema thoracis has been a major medical concern throughout recorded medical history. During the past 2 decades, however, management has been influenced by the recognition of new and more virulent pathogens and by the *increasing number of immunologically compromised patients.* Fortunately, new antibiotics have contributed to major advances in therapy, as has early drainage by thoracoscopic techniques.

Although the overall mortality rate associated with empyema still ranges between 5% and 10%, most deaths occur in elderly patients or from conditions that predispose patients to the empyema rather than from the empyema itself.

SUGGESTED READINGS

Review Articles

Light RW: Parapneumonic effusions and empyema. Clin Chest Med 1985;6:55-62.

Magovern CJ, Rusch VW: Parapneumonic and post-traumatic pleural space infections. Chest Surg Clin North Am 1994;4:561-582.

Bryant RE, Salmon CJ: Pleural empyema [state-of-the-art clinical article]. Clin Infect Dis 1996;22:747-764.

Lee-Chiong TL, Matthay RA: Current diagnostic methods of medical management of thoracic empyemas. Chest Surg Clin North Am 1996;6:419-438.

Teixeira LR, Villarino MA: Antibiotic treatment of patients with pneumonia and pleural effusion. Curr Opin Pulm Med 1998;4:230-234.

Colice GL, Curtis A, Deslauriers J, et al: Medical and surgical treatment of parapneumonic effusions. An evidence-based guideline. Chest 2000;118:1158-1171.

de Hoyos A, Sundaresan S: Thoracic empyema. Surg Clin North Am 2002;82:643-671.

Investigation

Himelman RB, Callen PW: The prognostic value of loculations in parapneumonic pleural effusions. Chest 1986;90:852-856.

Waite RJ, Carbonneau RJ, Balikian JP, et al: Parietal pleural changes in empyema: appearances at CT. Radiology 1990;175:145-150.

Treatment Modalities

LeMense GP, Strange C, Sahn SA: Empyema thoracis. Therapeutic management and outcome. Chest 1995;107:1532-1537.

Thourani VH, Brady KM, Mansour KA, et al: Evaluation of treatment modalities for thoracic empyema: a cost-effectiveness analysis. Ann Thorac Surg 1998;66:1121-1127.

Treatment—Drainage

Stavas J, van Sonnenberg E, Casola G, Wittich GR: Percutaneous drainage of infected and noninfected thoracic fluid collections. J Thorac Imaging 1987;2:80-87.

Moulton JS: Image-guided management of complicated pleural fluid collections. Radiol Clin North Am 2000;38:345-374.

Treatment—Thoracoscopic

MacKinlay TA, Lyons GA, Chimondeguy DJ, et al: VATS débridement versus thoracotomy in the treatment of loculated postpneumonia empyema. Ann Thorac Surg 1996;61:1626-1630.

Wait MA, Sharma S, Hohn J, Dal Nogare A: A randomized trial of empyema therapy. Chest 1997;111:1548-1551.

Striffeler H, Gugger M, Hof VI, et al: Video-assisted thoracoscopic surgery for fibrinopurulent pleural empyema in 67 patients. Ann Thorac Surg 1998;65:319-323.

Roberts JR: Minimally invasive surgery in the treatment of empyema: intraoperative decision making. Ann Thorac Surg 2003;76: 225-230.

Treatment—Fibrinolytics

Laisaar T, Püttsepp E, Laisaar V: Early administration of intrapleural streptokinase in the treatment of multiloculated pleural effusions and pleural empyemas. Thorac Cardiovasc Surg 1996;44:252-256.

Chronic Empyema

Rzyman W, Skokoswki J, Romanowicz G, et al: Decortication in chronic pleural empyema—effect on lung function. Eur J Cardiothorac Surg 2002;21:502-507.

MANAGEMENT OF THE PATIENT WITH PRIMARY OR SECONDARY PNEUMOTHORAX

Primary spontaneous pneumothorax occurs in young people *without clinically apparent underlying lung disease.* In these patients, it is generally agreed that the first episode can be managed by observation alone or by intercostal tube drainage. If the pneumothorax recurs or if there is a persistent air leak, further measures are necessary; these involve operative closure of the site of air leakage, usually a ruptured bleb, and obliteration of the pleural space (pleurodesis). At present, the relative merits of the VATS approach versus those of the limited axillary incision *are still debated,* although the results appear to be similar in terms of morbidity and prevention of further recurrences.

The problems associated with pneumothoraces secondary to chronic obstructive pulmonary disease (COPD) are different *because all of these patients are older,* and they often have significant associated comorbidities. In addition, pneumothoraces are poorly tolerated in individuals with limited pulmonary reserve. In such cases, early surgery, often at the time of the first episode, and use of VATS approaches are recommended if the patient presents with an acceptable operative risk.

MANAGEMENT OF THE PATIENT WITH PRIMARY SPONTANEOUS PNEUMOTHORAX

Epidemiology

A spontaneous pneumothorax is called primary when it occurs in apparently healthy individuals, usually young men aged 15 to 40 years (Table 11-12). Radiographic signs of lung disease are absent, although apical blebs can be identified on CT scanning. In general, patients present with *sudden chest pain whose severity correlates well with the degree of lung collapse* (see Chapter 3, "Assessment of the Patient with a Pleural Disorder"). Life-threatening complications are rare, and recurrences develop in 10% to 15% of patients after a first episode. Most of these recurrences are seen within 2 years of the initial episode, and the majority are ipsilateral. In general, the occurrence of primary spontaneous pneumothorax bears no relationship with exercise.

Management

Uncomplicated First Episode

Asymptomatic patients with small pneumothoraces (<20%) can be treated expectantly. Air resorption from a sealed off spontaneous pneumothorax *is estimated to be in the range of 1.25% per volume of the radiographic lung per 24 hours* (50 to 70 mL/day). Outpatient management requires observation until follow-up films show stable or resolving pneumothorax and resolution of symptoms. Patients must be carefully instructed about the potential hazards for development of a tension pneumothorax or other complications. Follow-up should be done within 24 to 48 hours.

Conventional tube thoracostomy is the *standard method* of treatment for large primary spontaneous pneumothoraces (more than 20% of magnitude) and for patients with significant symptoms. Small-caliber (8 or 9 Fr) chest tubes can be used, and with a flutter valve (Heimlich valve), patients do not require hospitalization. The use of these valves is safe, efficient, and reliable. Chest tubes are removed after the air leak has

TABLE 11-12

DIFFERENCES BETWEEN PRIMARY AND SECONDARY PNEUMOTHORACES

	Primary	Secondary to COPD
Age	15-40 years	>40 years
Sex	Predominantly male	Predominantly male
Body features	Tall and thin	Barrel chest
Smoking habit	Often present	Usually present
Main symptom	Chest pain	Dyspnea
Significant complications	Rare	Can be life-threatening
Radiographs (standard, CT scan)	No evidence of pulmonary disease	Evidence of COPD
Chances of recurrence after first episode	10%	30%-50%
Chances of recurrence after second episode	50%	>80%

stopped for 24 to 48 hours and the affected lung has remained expanded. Tube clamping before removal is not recommended.

If lung expansion cannot be obtained with a Heimlich valve, a larger thoracostomy tube may have to be inserted. It should be connected to an active drainage system (see Chapter 10, "Closed Drainage and Suction System"). In those cases, it is preferable to admit the patient to the hospital.

Complicated First Episode (Table 11-13)

Surgery is usually indicated at the time of the first episode if the pneumothorax is complicated by tension, prolonged air leak, incomplete lung re-expansion, or hemopneumothorax.

Tension Pneumothorax. When a tension pneumothorax develops, a positive intrapleural pressure is created because *the air accumulated in the pleural space cannot flow back into* the bronchial tree. With each inspiration, more air is brought into the pleural space, thus increasing pressure and tension over the lungs and mediastinum and decreasing venous return and cardiac output. In such cases, immediate decompression of the pleural space is imperative. Once the lung is expanded with tube thoracostomy, these patients should be considered for surgery even if the episode was not life-threatening.

Persistent Air Leak and Incomplete Lung Re-expansion. Most air leaks related to primary spontaneous pneumothorax seal within 24 to 48 hours of tube drainage, and only 3% to 5% of patients will have a persistent fistula beyond 4 to 5 days. In such cases, however, it is *unlikely* that the site of fistula will heal on its own, and these patients should be evaluated for surgery. Operation may also become necessary in patients whose lung does not re-expand (despite adequate drainage) because of adhesions, visceral pleural membrane, or significant air leakage.

Hemopneumothorax. Spontaneous hemopneumothorax is a well-documented entity that occurs in about 5% of primary pneumothoraces. The bleeding, which can be severe, results *from a torn adhesion between parietal and visceral pleurae*. Because the vessels contained in adhesions have thin walls, they are unable to retract after disruption and thus will bleed actively in the empty pleural space. Surgery may be required for definitive control of the bleeding site or for the prevention of late complications of hemothoraces, such as empyemas and fibrothoraces.

TABLE 11-13

POSSIBLE INDICATIONS FOR SURGERY DURING A FIRST EPISODE OF PRIMARY SPONTANEOUS PNEUMOTHORAX

Tension pneumothorax
Prolonged air leak (>5 days)
Incomplete lung re-expansion
Hemopneumothorax

TABLE 11-14

PRINCIPLES OF SURGERY IN THE TREATMENT OF RECURRENT SPONTANEOUS PNEUMOTHORAX

Resection of blebs
Wedge resection
Suture or staple closure

Pleurodesis
Parietal pleurectomy
Mechanical pleural abrasion
Introduction of chemical irritants: talc, autologous blood

Recurrences

Recurrence is the most common indication for surgery. Operation is generally recommended at the time of the first recurrence.

Principles of Surgery (Table 11-14)

Surgery involves closure of the air leak, resection of apical blebs, and obliteration of the pleural space (pleurodesis).

Virtually all surgeons agree that the blebs, which are nearly always located at the apex, *should be resected* even when no obvious lesion has been identified (blind apical stapling).

Another goal of surgery is to stimulate the formation of dense and permanent adhesions between the lung and endothoracic fascia, thus preventing further pneumothoraces. This can be accomplished *by apical parietal pleurectomy or by mechanical abrasion of the pleura* (with dry gauze sticks), a technique that has the advantage of preserving the extrapleural plane. Both procedures result in effective pleurodesis with recurrence rates of the pneumothorax below 5%.

Pleurodesis can also be achieved through pleural space instillation of chemical irritants such as talc, bleomycin, and even autologous blood. These agents can be instilled at the time of operation or at bedside through the chest tube. However, *the high failure rates* associated with chemical pleurodesis and the *possibility of significant adverse effects* make these techniques unsuitable for use in young patients with primary spontaneous pneumothoraces. In addition, surgeons are generally concerned about the use of chemical pleurodesis in young patients who have the potential for developing late toxicities.

Surgical Approaches

The operation can be done *through an axillary incision or with VATS techniques.* The axillary incision is vertical and located behind the posterior border of the pectoralis major. It measures 5 to 6 cm in length, and the pleural space is entered through the third interspace. *Blebs are stapled and excised under direct vision,* and the parietal pleura is stripped from the endothoracic fascia over the upper third of the thorax (apical pleurectomy). A single chest tube is left for 72 hours postoperatively. Cosmetic and long-term results are excellent; reported recurrence rates are in the range of 1% to 2%.

VATS potentially has the advantages of reduction of postoperative pain, shorter hospital stay, and speedier recovery. In most series, however, the incidence of further recurrences after operation is higher than what has been reported after transaxillary pleurectomy. Several surgeons now recommend a hybrid approach with the combination of a small axillary incision with one thoracoscopic port incision for a video camera.

Special Therapeutic Considerations

Simultaneous bilateral pneumothoraces are uncommon, but when they occur, this should be followed by definitive surgery at least on one side. The same principle of management applies to patients who have suffered nonsynchronous bilateral pneumothoraces.

Pneumothoraces during pregnancy are relatively rare and usually seen during the third trimester. Difficulties in management are due to increased oxygen demand, fear of teratogenic effects of radiographs, inadequate fetal oxygenation, and a general consensus that one must avoid general anesthesia. Under such circumstances, tube thoracostomy should be considered the treatment of choice; chest radiographs should be avoided, especially during the first trimester. If surgery is required, a VATS approach should be considered. If the patient is near term, *every effort should be made to delay surgery until early in the postpartum period*.

Patients at risk for development of pneumothoraces in relation to their occupation, such as flight personnel and scuba divers, may be treated by surgery at the time of the first episode. Similarly, patients living in isolated areas or patients who travel frequently, especially those with evidence of bullae on chest radiographs, may also be candidates for early surgery.

TABLE 11-15

COMMON CAUSES OF SECONDARY PNEUMOTHORAX

Airway disease
    Chronic obstructive lung disease
    Asthma
    Cystic fibrosis
Interstitial lung disease
    Sarcoidosis
    Pulmonary fibrosis
    Lymphangioleiomyomatosis
Infectious lung disease
    Mycobacterial disease (*Mycobacterium tuberculosis,* mycobacteria other than
        tubercle bacilli)
    Pneumocystis carinii infections (AIDS)
    Bacterial infections (necrotizing pneumonias, lung abscess)
Neoplastic lung disease
    Primary or secondary lung cancer
Endometriosis (catamenial pneumothorax)
Connective tissue disease
    Rheumatoid arthritis
    Scleroderma

MANAGEMENT OF THE PATIENT WITH SECONDARY SPONTANEOUS PNEUMOTHORAX

Epidemiology

A spontaneous pneumothorax is termed secondary if it occurs in the setting of an underlying pulmonary disease (Table 11-15). Most of these patients are men older than 45 years, and they have *documented or clinically apparent lung disease.*

The most common disorder related to secondary pneumothorax is COPD (Table 11-12). Because of *limited pulmonary reserve, these patients often show little tolerance for even a small pneumothorax;* not uncommonly, they present with acute respiratory distress, hypoxia, hypercapnia, and respiratory acidosis. Chances of recurrence are much higher in this group (30% to 50%) than in patients with primary spontaneous pneumothoraces.

Pneumothoraces can be seen in about 10% of patients with cystic fibrosis. Because pneumothoraces usually occur in patients with advanced disease (severe airflow obstruction, chronic infections), they can be associated with life-threatening situations.

In AIDS patients, there is also a high incidence of secondary pneumothoraces related to the rupture of subpleural apical air spaces filled with *Pneumocystis carinii* organisms. AIDS patients have an *increased incidence of synchronous bilateral pneumothoraces, bronchopleural fistulas, and recurrences.* Secondary pneumothoraces are also commonly associated with metastatic sarcomas to the lung.

Management

Pneumothorax Secondary to COPD

Most patients should initially be treated with tube thoracostomy because even small pneumothoraces are poorly tolerated. If the pleural space is adequately drained, the lung will re-expand, the patient will stabilize, and treatment options can be further evaluated.

Because of the significant incidence of prolonged air leaks, high risks of recurrence, and potential lethality of this condition, surgical intervention should be considered *at the time of first occurrence.* The emergence of videothoracoscopy has considerably changed the magnitude of operation, which can now be done with low operative morbidity or mortality even in high-risk cases. Although the procedure must be individualized for each patient and based on the extent of disease as documented by CT scan, staple resection of bullae, closure of the site of air leak, and subtotal parietal pleurectomy are the best surgical options. If the site of air leak cannot be found or if the lung is diffusely emphysematous (vanishing lung syndrome), it is best to avoid the resection of lung tissue; one should carry out only a parietal pleurectomy, pleural abrasion, or talc (powder form) insufflation.

If the operative risk is considered too significant or even prohibitive, management consists of prolonged tube drainage with or without bedside administration of talc slurry (2 to 5 g diluted in 50 to 250 mL of normal saline) or of other sclerosants through the chest tube.

Pneumothorax Secondary to Cystic Fibrosis

In this group of patients, the possibility of subsequent lung transplantation has to be considered before a decision is made about operation. Small pneumothoraces can be observed on an outpatient basis; larger or symptomatic ones should be drained. In cases of recurrence or persistent air leakage for more than 7 days, thoracoscopic surgical intervention with lung resection and limited parietal pleurectomy is recommended. In patients with severe respiratory failure, bedside instillation of talc slurry should be considered.

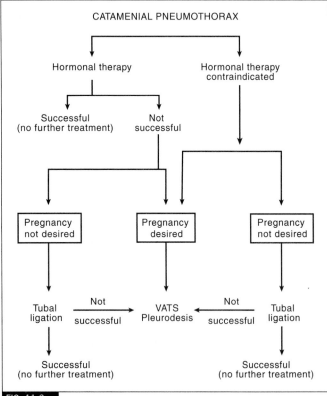

FIG. 11-3

Proposed treatment algorithm for catamenial pneumothorax. VATS, video-assisted thoracoscopic surgery. *(From Fleisher AB, Clement PB, Nelems B: Catamenial pneumothorax: pathophysiology and management. In Deslauriers J, Lacquet LK, eds: International Trends in General Thoracic Surgery, vol 6. St. Louis, Mosby–Year Book, 1990:132.)*

Pneumothorax Secondary to AIDS

Whenever possible, the initial management should be conservative because small pneumothoraces will sometimes resolve with observation alone.

Refractory pneumothoraces *should be drained.* The most efficient method for treatment of patients with prolonged air leaks or recurrences is videothoracoscopic resection of the diseased site and mechanical pleurodesis (parietal pleurectomy or pleural abrasion). VATS talc poudrage can also be used to control the pneumothorax and associated air leak.

MANAGEMENT OF THE PATIENT WITH CATAMENIAL PNEUMOTHORAX

Pneumothoraces *occurring within 48 to 72 hours of the onset of menstruation* are called catamenial pneumothoraces. Most commonly, they are on the right side, and they may be recurrent over several years before being diagnosed. Although the exact pathogenesis of catamenial pneumothoraces is still debated, air may reach the pleural space from the cervix through congenital diaphragmatic defects, or there may be focal endometrial implants in the lung with air leakage occurring during menstruation.

Management of the first occurrence is similar to that of other types of pneumothoraces. Management of recurrences is more controversial and includes several options (Fig. 11-3), such as use of oral contraceptives or weak androgens to suppress ovulation, chemical pleurodesis, and mechanical pleurodesis.

CONCLUSION

As a general rule, spontaneous pneumothorax occurs in two basic clinical settings. The first is the sudden development of pleuritic chest pain that is characteristically seen in young healthy adults. The lesions consist of small apical bullae that rupture in the pleural space and allow the development of what is called a primary spontaneous pneumothorax. Recurrences are often multiple, and the results of pleural space obliteration with or without blebectomy are excellent.

The other setting in which spontaneous pneumothorax occurs is the older patient with underlying COPD. The treatment in this group is more critical, and *surgical intervention should be considered after a first occurrence.*

SUGGESTED READINGS

Review Articles

Miller AC, Harvey JE: Guidelines for the management of spontaneous pneumothorax. BMJ 1993;307:114-116.

Sahn SA, Heffner JE: Spontaneous pneumothorax (review article). N Engl J Med 2000;342:868-874.

Baumann MH, Strange C, Heffner JE, et al: Management of spontaneous pneumothorax. An American College of Chest Physicians Delphi Consensus Statement. Chest 2001;119:590-602.

Special Challenges in Thoracic Surgery

11

Ng CSH, Wan S, Lee TW: Video-assisted thoracic surgery in spontaneous pneumothorax. Can Respir J 2002;9:122-127.

Catamenial Pneumothorax

Carter EJ, Ettensohn DB: Catamenial pneumothorax. Chest 1990;98: 713-716.

Pneumothorax and AIDS

Trachiotis GD, Vricella LA, Alyono D, et al: Management of AIDS-related pneumothorax. Ann Thorac Surg 1996;62:1608-1613.

Flum DR, Steinberg SD, Bernik TR, et al: Thoracoscopy in acquired immunodeficiency syndrome. J Thorac Cardiovasc Surg 1997;114: 361-366.

Secondary Pneumothorax

Tanaka F, Itoh M, Esaki H, et al: Secondary spontaneous pneumothorax. Ann Thorac Surg 1993;55:372-376.

Waller DA, Forty J, Soni AK, et al: Videothoracoscopic operation for secondary spontaneous pneumothorax. Ann Thorac Surg 1994;57:1612-1615.

Hemopneumothorax

Tatebe S, Kanazawa H, Yamazaki Y, et al: Spontaneous hemopneumothorax. Ann Thorac Surg 1996;62:1011-1015.

Kakaris S, Athanassiadi K, Vassilikos K, Skottis I: Spontaneous hemopneumothorax: a rare but life-threatening entity. Eur J Cardiothorac Surg 2004;25:856-858.

Sakamoto K, Ohmori T, Takei H, et al: Autologous salvaged blood transfusion in spontaneous hemopneumothorax. Ann Thorac Surg 2004;78:705-707.

Management

Mercier C, Pagé A, Verdant A, et al: Outpatient management of intercostal tube drainage in spontaneous pneumothorax. Ann Thorac Surg 1976;22:163-165.

Deslauriers J, Beaulieu M, Després JP, et al: Transaxillary pleurectomy for treatment of spontaneous pneumothorax. Ann Thorac Surg 1980;30:569-574.

So S, Yu DYC: Catheter drainage of spontaneous pneumothorax: suction or no suction, early or late removal? Thorax 1982;37:46-48.

Noppen M, Alexander P, Driesen P, et al: Manual aspiration versus chest tube drainage in first episodes of primary spontaneous pneumothorax. A multicenter, prospective, randomized pilot study. Am J Respir Crit Care Med 2002;165:1240-1244.

Pneumothorax and Thoracoscopy

Kim KH, Kim HK, Han JY, et al: Transaxillary minithoracotomy versus video-assisted thoracic surgery for spontaneous pneumothorax. Ann Thorac Surg 1996;61:1510-1512.

Massard G, Thomas P, Wihlm JM: Minimally invasive management for first and recurrent pneumothorax. Ann Thorac Surg 1998;66:592-599.

Liu HP, Yim APC, Izzat MB, et al: Thoracoscopic surgery for spontaneous pneumothorax. World J Surg 1999;23:1133-1136.

Hatz RA, Kaps MF, Meimarakis G, et al: Long-term results after video-assisted thoracoscopic surgery for first-time and recurrent spontaneous pneumothorax. Ann Thorac Surg 2000;70:253-257.

Chan P, Clarke P, Daniel FJ, et al: Efficacy study of video-assisted thoracoscopic surgery pleurodesis for spontaneous pneumothorax. Ann Thorac Surg 2001;71:452-454.

Hyland MJ, Ashrafi AS, Crepeau A, Mehran RJ: Is video-assisted thoracoscopic surgery superior to limited axillary thoracotomy in the management of spontaneous pneumothorax? Can Respir J 2001;8:339-343.

Cardillo G, Facciolo F, Regal M, et al: Recurrences following videothoracoscopic treatment of primary spontaneous pneumothorax: the role of redo-videothoracoscopy. Eur J Cardiothorac Surg 2001;19:396-399.

Wu YC, Lu MS, Yeh CH, et al: Justifying video-assisted thoracic surgery for spontaneous hemopneumothorax. Chest 2002;122:1844-1847.

Chen JS, Hsu HH, Kuo SW, et al: Needlescopic versus conventional video-assisted thoracic surgery for primary spontaneous pneumothorax: a comparative study. Ann Thorac Surg 2003;75:1080-1085.

Freixinet JL, Canalis E, Julia G, et al: Axillary thoracotomy versus videothoracoscopy for the treatment of primary spontaneous pneumothorax. Ann Thorac Surg 2004;78:417-420.

Talc Poudrage

Milanez RC, Vargas FS, Filomeno LB, et al: Intrapleural talc for the prevention of recurrent pneumothorax. Chest 1994;106:1162-1165.

Tschopp JM, Boutin C, Astoul P, et al: Talcage by medical thoracoscopy for primary spontaneous pneumothorax is more cost-effective than drainage: a randomised study. Eur Respir J 2002;20:1003-1009.

Case Series

Vernejoux JM, Raherison C, Combe P, et al: Spontaneous pneumothorax: pragmatic management and long-term outcome. Respir Med 2001;95:857-862.

Other

Noppen M, Alexander P, Driesen P, et al: Quantification of the size of primary spontaneous pneumothorax: accuracy of the Light Index. Respiration 2001;68:396-399.

MANAGEMENT OF THE PATIENT WITH SUPERIOR VENA CAVA OBSTRUCTION

The superior vena cava (SVC) originates from the confluence of both brachiocephalic veins behind the first right costal cartilage. It is located in the right anterosuperior mediastinum and returns the blood from the upper half of the body into the right atrium. When partial or total obstruction of the SVC precludes normal venous return, *venous stasis develops in the neck and*

11

Special Challenges in Thoracic Surgery

upper extremities, the magnitude of which is related to the rate of progression and extent of obstruction as well as to the adequacy of collateral circulation.

Although SVC obstruction is associated with malignant neoplasms most of the time, it is important to establish a specific histologic diagnosis so that treatment can be individualized and optimized. Unfortunately, most patients with SVC obstruction can only benefit from palliative treatment, and currently the *most effective palliation* is offered by endovascular stenting.

PATHOPHYSIOLOGIC CONSIDERATIONS

Normal Anatomy of Superior Vena Cava

The SVC is formed by the union of the right and left brachiocephalic veins behind the first costal cartilage. It descends anterolateral and to the right of the trachea to join the right atrium posteriorly. It is a thin-walled low-pressure vascular structure with an average length of 7 cm and a diameter of 2 cm. The distal 2 cm of the SVC is within the pericardium, and it is relatively fixed as it enters the pericardial reflection.

The azygos vein is *the only collateral* that enters the SVC. The junction between azygos vein and SVC is above the right main pulmonary artery and anterior to the right main bronchus.

Types and Causes of Obstruction (Table 11-16)

Benign Processes

SVC obstruction secondary to benign intrathoracic processes occurs in approximately *5% to 10% of all patients.* Thrombosis of the SVC and subclavian vein is not uncommon and can be related to indwelling catheters used for chemotherapy or intravenous hyperalimentation or to pacemaker electrodes.

Goiters originating in the neck and extending down into the mediastinum (retrosternal goiters) are the most common benign mediastinal masses that may cause SVC obstruction, usually by external compression at the junction between the innominate vein and the SVC.

TABLE 11-16
TYPES AND CAUSES OF SUPERIOR VENA CAVA OBSTRUCTION

Benign processes (5%-10%)
Thrombosis secondary to indwelling catheter
Extrinsic compression
    Benign mediastinal tumors: goiters, teratomas, aortic aneurysms
    Chronic mediastinitis: histoplasmosis, post–radiation therapy, fibrosis, idiopathic
    Others (rare): trauma, hemomediastinum, acute mediastinitis
Benign tumors of SVC

Malignant processes (90%-95%)
Extrinsic compression
    Malignant mediastinal cancers: thymomas, germ cell tumors, sarcomas
    Malignant lymph nodes: lung cancer, metastatic cancer from other sites
    Lymphomas
Direct invasion by lung cancer in right upper lobe
Malignant tumors of SVC

Aortic aneurysms and benign teratomas can also cause SVC obstruction, but these types of compression are seldom encountered.

Most cases of fibrosing chronic mediastinitis are secondary to *histoplasmosis* and are characterized by a fibrotic reaction (mediastinal fibrosis) that slowly narrows down the SVC lumen, the main pulmonary artery, and the trachea and main bronchi. Radiation fibrosis is an unusual cause of SVC obstruction because most patients with malignant neoplasms treated by mediastinal radiation therapy have limited survival.

Malignant Processes

SVC syndrome is secondary to a malignant tumor in more than 90% of patients. Lung cancer is by far the most common cause of obstruction. In the majority of such cases, the obstruction is due to an *extrinsic compression of the vein by metastatic mediastinal nodes* with or without superimposed thrombosis. *Lymphomas* presenting either as solitary anterior mediastinal masses or as diffuse nodal disease in the middle mediastinum are the second most common group of malignant neoplasms associated with obstruction of the SVC. Other metastatic tumors occasionally associated with SVC syndrome are carcinomas of the breast, colon, kidney, and testis.

On occasion, primary malignant tumors (rare) of the SVC or extrinsic compression by primary anterior and middle mediastinal tumors such as thymomas, germ cell tumors, and sarcomas (see Chapter 3, "Assessment of the Patient with a Mediastinal Mass") will also be the cause of SVC obstruction. Direct invasion by primary lung tumors located in the anterior segment of the right upper lobe can cause partial or complete blockage of the SVC.

Collateral Pathways (Table 11-17)

Several pathways of collateral venous return from the upper body to the heart are present in patients with SVC obstruction.

The first and most important pathway *is the azygos vein system,* which is used when the obstruction is distal to the junction between azygos vein and SVC (Fig. 11-4). With this system, the blood is redirected into the inferior vena cava through the azygos and hemiazygos veins (retrograde flow) and their interconnecting veins and the lumbar veins.

If the obstruction is proximal to the entrance of the azygos vein, the collateral venous pathway from the neck is through the *superior intercostal vein* (Fig. 11-5). If the obstruction involves both azygos vein and SVC,

TABLE 11-17

MAIN COLLATERAL VENOUS PATHWAYS IN SUPERIOR VENA CAVA OBSTRUCTION

Site of Obstruction	Collateral Venous Pathway
Obstruction of SVC distal to junction between azygos vein and SVC	Azygos and hemiazygos veins
	Communicating lumbar veins (Fig. 11-4)
Obstruction of SVC proximal to junction between azygos vein and SVC	Superior intercostal vein (Fig. 11-5)
Obstruction of SVC and azygos vein	Internal mammary system connecting with epigastric veins and external iliac veins

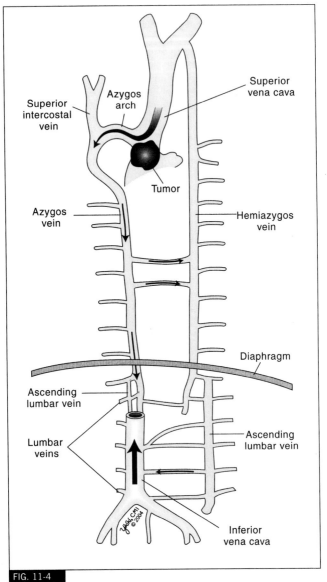

FIG. 11-4

Collateral pathways through lumbar veins when SVC obstruction is distal to junction between azygos vein and SVC.

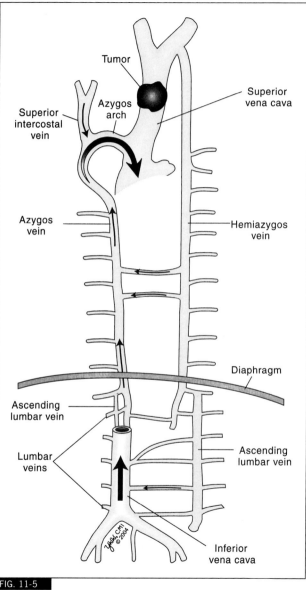

FIG. 11-5

Collateral pathway through superior intercostal vein when SVC obstruction is proximal to junction between azygos vein and SVC.

TABLE 11-18
FACTORS IMPLICATED IN CLINICAL PRESENTATION OF SUPERIOR VENA CAVA SYNDROME
Rate of progression of syndrome (rapid or slow progression)
Adequacy of collateral circulation
Extent of obstruction (partial, complete)
Anatomic relationship between obstruction and azygos venous system
Nature of underlying process (benign, malignant)

alternative collateral venous pathways are through the internal mammary veins, epigastric veins, and inferior vena cava by way of the external iliac veins.

All of these collateral venous pathways *are interconnected* and eventually redirect venous blood from the upper body into the inferior vena cava.

CLINICAL FEATURES

In general, the magnitude and severity of clinical features are proportional (Table 11-18) to the *rate of progression of the obstruction* (rapid progression or chronic duration), to the *adequacy of collateral venous pathways,* to the *extent of venous obstruction* (partial or complete), to the relationship between the *site of obstruction and the azygos vein,* and finally to the *underlying disease process* (benign or malignant) causing the obstruction.

Rapidly developing symptoms and physical signs usually indicate a malignant process; slowly developing symptoms are more likely to be associated with a benign process. Similarly, symptoms will be more significant in acute situations where there are no collaterals or when both SVC and azygos vein have become obstructed.

Typical symptoms (Table 11-19) are usually observed in patients with total obstruction. *Common features* include facial and cervical swelling, headaches, distortion of vision, dizziness when bending over, and dyspnea. Other symptoms, such as cough, stridor, and weight loss, may be related to the underlying neoplasm or to simultaneous compression of the airway more than to the SVC obstruction itself. The *main physical findings* associated with SVC syndrome (Table 11-20) are dilated veins and sometimes edema over the neck, anterior chest wall, and upper extremities; cyanotic or flushed skin over these same areas; and periorbital edema.

TABLE 11-19
COMMON SYMPTOMS ASSOCIATED WITH SUPERIOR VENA CAVA SYNDROME
Cervical and facial swelling
Distorted vision
Headaches
Dizziness when bending over
Cough and dyspnea

TABLE 11-20

COMMON PHYSICAL SIGNS ASSOCIATED WITH SUPERIOR VENA CAVA SYNDROME

Venous distention and cyanotic skin over neck, anterior chest wall, and upper extremities

Cervical and facial swelling

Periorbital edema

Symptoms of laryngeal edema, such as respiratory distress and stridor, and those related to cerebral edema, such as alteration in mental status, stupor, and convulsions, are uncommon and observed only in *acute obstructions.* This would be the case, for instance, of severe crush thoracic injuries causing a marked increase in SVC pressure. Patients suffering from this syndrome called *traumatic asphyxia* often have a moribund appearance with craniofacial cyanosis, edema, petechiae, subconjunctival hemorrhage, and periorbital bruising. Other than those few cases, severe cerebral manifestations of SVC syndrome such as blindness, convulsion, or others are extremely unusual. As a rule, death is *almost never* directly related to SVC syndrome.

DIAGNOSIS

Anatomic Diagnosis

The diagnosis of SVC obstruction can often be made by clinical history and physical examination alone. Chest radiographs are usually abnormal; they may show diffuse widening of the superior mediastinum, hilar or mediastinal masses, a malignant neoplasm in the right upper lobe, or a pleural effusion that is present in up to 25% of cases. In the absence of other visible abnormalities, the presence of *calcified nodes in the mediastinum* is suggestive of mediastinal fibrosis, especially if the patient's symptoms have been slowly progressive for a period of months or years.

Contrast-enhanced thoracic CT scan is the imaging procedure of choice to demonstrate the anatomy of the lesion including size, location (mediastinum, lung), site of compression, and relationship with surrounding structures. CT is also useful to document *the presence or absence of an intramural thrombus,* to document the patency of the azygos system, and to determine the choice of the best approach for biopsy. Magnetic resonance imaging (MRI) may be used to demonstrate vessel patency or to delineate contacts between mediastinal tumors and SVC.

Histologic Diagnosis

In patients with known malignant disease such as lung cancer, for instance, it is appropriate to assume that the SVC obstruction is related to the original malignant neoplasm, and there is no need for further diagnostic work-up. For all other patients, *tissue diagnosis must be obtained* because both treatment strategies and prognosis can be greatly affected by the nature of the underlying tumor. Fortunately, there is, in most cases, enough time to carry out these additional investigations without risk to the patient.

NONINVASIVE DIAGNOSTIC TECHNIQUES USEFUL IN PATIENTS WITH SUPERIOR VENA CAVA OBSTRUCTION

Technique	Usefulness
Serum level of tumor markers	Germ cell tumors
Fine-needle biopsy of supraclavicular nodes	Lymphomas, lung cancer
Fine-needle biopsy of mediastinal masses	Lymphomas, thymomas, germ cell tumors
Fine-needle biopsy of lung masses	Lung cancer
Bronchoscopy	Lung cancer

Noninvasive Techniques (Table 11-21)

In some cases, the diagnosis of germ cell tumors can be made by increased serum level of tumor markers, such as carcinoembryonic antigen, alpha-fetoprotein, or human chorionic gonadotropin β (see Chapter 3, "Assessment of the Patient with a Mediastinal Mass"). In other patients, fine-needle biopsy of *palpable cervical nodes* will yield the correct tissue diagnosis at minimal risk of morbidity. In many cases, bronchoscopy will document the presence of an endobronchial tumor, which can be sampled, again at low risk to the patient. If the lesion is accessible, the diagnosis can be obtained by CT-guided fine-needle biopsy.

Invasive Techniques (Table 11-22)

Most invasive diagnostic techniques are done under general anesthesia. They are indicated either when the diagnosis is completely unknown or when a known diagnosis of germ cell tumor or lymphoma needs further *characterization*.

Such procedures include open peripheral node biopsy, usually in the supraclavicular area; cervical mediastinoscopy for patients with widened mediastinum; and anterior mediastinotomy for patients with primary malignant anterior mediastinal tumors. Formal thoracotomy should be *avoided* because the incision may produce disruption of collateral venous pathways and worsening of symptoms. In such cases, it is best to carry out a videothoracoscopic procedure rather than a formal thoracotomy.

Complications of Invasive Diagnostic Procedures

In general, invasive diagnostic procedures are associated with few complications when they are done by experienced teams including

INVASIVE DIAGNOSTIC TECHNIQUES USEFUL IN PATIENTS WITH SUPERIOR VENA CAVA OBSTRUCTION

Technique	Usefulness
Open supraclavicular node biopsy	Lung cancer, lymphomas
Mediastinoscopy	Lung cancer, nodal metastasis from other primary tumors, lymphomas
Anterior mediastinotomy	Anterior mediastinal tumors: lymphomas, thymomas, germ cell tumors, sarcomas

a knowledgeable anesthetist (see Chapter 5, "Principles of Anesthesia for the Patient with an Anterior Mediastinal Mass") and surgeon.

Uncontrollable bleeding due to venous engorgement can potentially occur, but it is uncommon if the operation is done with care and biopsy samples are confined to abnormal tissues. Worsening of laryngeal edema is a potential adverse effect that can be avoided by meticulous anesthetic technique. On occasion, it may be useful to prepare the patient for a general anesthetic with diuretics and steroids.

MANAGEMENT

Initial Treatment and General Measures

Initial treatment of the patient with SVC obstruction generally includes *elevation of the head and upper extremities* to promote gravitational venous drainage, *diuretics* to reduce peripheral edema and cardiac output, and *oxygen supplementation*. Systemic steroids can be added to decrease laryngeal and cerebral edema or to reduce the inflammatory reaction related to radiation therapy. Systemic anticoagulation is generally *not indicated*.

Management Directed at Underlying Cause

In the past, standard therapy for all patients with SVC obstruction was empirical radiation therapy. This was done on the assumption that SVC obstruction was related to malignant tumors in more than 90% of cases and that among those tumors, lung cancer was the most common.

There were *many disadvantages* to this approach (Table 11-23), not the least being that after the mediastinum had been irradiated, it became virtually impossible to obtain tissue for diagnosis. Other disadvantages included a remission usually not seen before 3 to 4 weeks after the beginning of treatments, a distinct possibility that the symptoms would get worse early on because of interstitial edema, and a recurrence of the SVC syndrome in 60% to 80% of individuals. Patients with SVC obstruction due to a benign process, such as those with mediastinal fibrosis, could obviously be *made worse* by empirical radiotherapy.

Because of such potentially significant adverse effects, radiotherapy is currently reserved for patients with acute and symptomatic SVC obstruction in whom there is a high probability of a malignant disease–related syndrome. In those cases, radiation is directed at the mediastinum, and the total dose delivered ranges from 50 to 60 Gy.

11

Special Challenges in Thoracic Surgery

TABLE 11-23

POSSIBLE DISADVANTAGES OF EMPIRICAL RADIOTHERAPY IN PATIENTS WITH SUPERIOR VENA CAVA OBSTRUCTION

Impossibility of obtaining a diagnosis after the mediastinum has been irradiated

Remission usually not seen for 3-4 weeks after beginning of treatment

Possibility of transient increase in severity of symptoms

Recurrence rate of obstruction in the range of 60%-80%

Patients with benign process can be aggravated

TABLE 11-24

POTENTIAL ADVANTAGES OF ENDOVASCULAR STENTING

Immediate remission of symptoms (24-48 h)
Effective in >90% of cases
Prolonged duration of response
Presence of a stent makes it easier to start chemotherapy or radiation therapy
Low recurrence rate of SVC obstruction
Simple, safe, and minimally invasive technique
Well tolerated by most patients

For most other patients, however, an *accurate histologic diagnosis must be established* before treatment is started, thus increasing the likelihood of a good result in terms of tumor control, relief of SVC syndrome, and outcome. In some patients, such as those with locoregional small cell lung cancer or those with lymphomas, chemotherapy, radiotherapy, or a combination of both can be effective and sometimes even curative. In patients with non–small cell lung cancer, objective responses to chemoradiation are lower than in those with small cell lung cancer (20% to 40% compared with 70%) and recurrence rates are higher, but anticancer therapy should still be offered and forms the basis of initial treatment.

Symptomatic Treatment: Endovascular Stenting

The use of endovascular stents to achieve SVC patency has now become *an accepted option* in the management of patients with SVC obstruction. It is a particularly interesting option in patients with severe symptoms, such as stridor, dyspnea, or signs of encephalopathy; in patients in whom the clinician wants to gain time to document the diagnosis; and in patients expected to have transient worsening of symptoms early during the course of radiation therapy or chemotherapy. Stenting can also be useful in patients with recurrent SVC obstruction after initial successful treatment and in those with SVC syndrome related to benign disease processes.

The potential advantages of endovascular stenting are listed in Table 11-24. Most important, endovascular stents achieve *early permeability of the SVC* (24 to 48 hours) and remission of symptoms in the majority of patients, and they offer prolonged remission of symptoms with few complications.

Although there are several possible complications associated with endovascular stenting (Table 11-25), such events *are rare* if the operator is experienced with the technique. Heart failure due to sudden increase

---

TABLE 11-25

POSSIBLE COMPLICATIONS RELATED TO ENDOVASCULAR STENTING

Perforation of SVC wall during insertion
Heart failure due to sudden increase in venous return after stent placement
Stent misplacement, migration, or occlusion
Stent failure in 10%-12% of cases due to thrombosis

in venous return after stent placement can be prevented by diuresis of the patient before the procedure. Stent migration is uncommon with the use of newer models of self-expanding metallic stents, which have greater endovascular adhesion.

The stents (diameters of 10 to 16 mm) are introduced percutaneously (local anesthesia) through a catheter. They are advanced to the site of obstruction (high-resolution fluoroscopic control), where they are released from the catheter, and they self-expand to their original diameter. Within a few weeks, they become incorporated into the vascular wall.

Contraindications to stent insertion include patients unable to lie flat, patients with long-standing total venous occlusion, and patients with congestive heart failure.

Indications for Surgery

Surgery is *seldom indicated in SVC obstruction* because most patients have advanced disease and limited life expectancy.

Curative Operations (Table 11-26)

Indications for curative operations include the resection of benign mediastinal masses (goiter, teratoma, aortic aneurysm) abutting the vena cava or of selected cases of right upper lobe bronchogenic carcinomas extending directly into the SVC wall. Most of these surgeries are done through a right posterolateral thoracotomy or median sternotomy. They may involve (especially in lung cancer cases) partial resection of the SVC with primary suturing or complete circumferential resection and reconstruction with autologous material (pericardial tube, spiral vein graft) or prosthetic polytetrafluoroethylene grafts.

Palliative Bypass

Palliative surgical bypass may be indicated for patients with benign diseases such as fibrosing mediastinitis. In such cases, however, the procedure should be done only after *prolonged periods of observation* because over time, the collateral circulation may have become so efficient that there is no need for an operation.

Venous reconstruction is usually done with spiral saphenous autogenous vein grafts implanted between the left innominate vein and right atrial appendage. In most cases, prolonged relief of SVC syndrome will be observed, and long-term patency (up to more than 15 years) of the graft is the rule.

CONCLUSION

Most cases of SVC obstruction are related to a malignant etiology and as such are associated with the patient's limited survival. On the basis

11

Special Challenges in Thoracic Surgery

TABLE 11-26
POTENTIAL INDICATIONS FOR CURATIVE SURGERY IN PATIENTS WITH SUPERIOR VENA CAVA OBSTRUCTION
Benign mediastinal masses abutting the SVC
Selected cases of right upper lobe tumors extending directly into the SVC
Selected cases of primary benign SVC tumors (hemangioendothelioma)

of the nature and cause of the obstruction, chemoradiation therapy
and endovascular stenting can both be used as early therapy.

SUGGESTED READINGS

Review Articles

Parish JM, Marschke RF, Dines DE, Lee RE: Etiologic consideration in
superior vena caval syndrome. Mayo Clin Proc 1981;56:407-413.

Ahmann FR: A reassessment of the clinical implications of the superior
vena caval syndrome. J Clin Oncol 1984;2:961-968.

Baker GL, Barnes HJ: Superior vena cava syndrome: etiology, diagnosis,
and treatment. Am J Crit Care 1992;1:54-64.

Escalante CP: Causes and management of superior vena cava syndrome.
Oncology (Huntingt) 1993;7:61-77.

Rowell NP, Gleeson FV: Steroids, radiotherapy, chemotherapy and stents
for superior vena caval obstruction in carcinoma of the bronchus:
a systematic review. Clin Oncol 2002;14:338-351.

Diagnosis of Superior Vena Cava Syndrome

Little AG, Golomb HM, Ferguson MK, et al: Malignant superior vena cava
obstruction reconsidered: the role of diagnostic surgical intervention.
Ann Thorac Surg 1985;40:285-288.

Jahangiri M, Goldstraw P: The role of mediastinoscopy in superior vena
caval obstruction. Ann Thorac Surg 1995;59:453-455.

Porte H, Metois D, Finzi L, et al: Superior vena cava syndrome of
malignant origin. Which surgical procedure for which diagnosis?
Eur J Cardiothorac Surg 2000;17:384-388.

Stenting

Shah R, Sabanathan S, Lowe RA, Mearns AJ: Stenting in malignant obstruction of superior vena cava. J Thorac Cardiovasc Surg 1996;112:335-430.

Hochrein J, Bashore TM, O'Laughlin MP, Harrison JK: Percutaneous
stenting of superior vena cava syndrome: a case report and review
of the literature. Am J Med 1998;104:78-84.

Smayra T, Otal P, Chabbert V, et al: Long-term results of endovascular
stent placement in the superior caval venous system. Cardiovasc
Intervent Radiol 2001;24:388-394.

García-Mónaco R, Bertoni H, Pallota G, et al: Use of self-expanding vascular
endoprostheses in superior vena cava syndrome. Eur J Cardiothorac Surg
2003;24:208-211.

Urruticoechea A, Mesia R, Dominguez J, et al: Treatment of malignant
superior vena cava syndrome by endovascular stent insertion. Experience
on 52 patients with lung cancer. Lung Cancer 2004;43:209-214.

Surgery of Superior Vena Cava Syndrome

Doty DB, Doty JR, Jones KW: Bypass of superior vena cava. Fifteen years'
experience with spiral vein graft for obstruction of superior vena cava
caused by benign disease. J Thorac Cardiovasc Surg 1990;99:889-896.

Thomas P, Magnan PE, Moulin G, et al: Extended operation for lung cancer
    invading the superior vena cava. Eur J Cardiothorac Surg 1994;8:
    177-182.

Case Series

Chen JC, Bongard F, Klein SR: A contemporary perspective on superior
    vena cava syndrome. Am J Surg 1990;160:207-211.
Yellin A, Rosen A, Reichert N, Lieberman Y: Superior vena cava syndrome.
    The myth—the facts. Am Rev Respir Dis 1990;141:1114-1118.

MANAGEMENT OF THE PATIENT WITH A PANCOAST TUMOR

In 1932, Henry Pancoast reported on seven patients with clinical
symptoms peculiar to malignancies located in the superior sulcus of the
lung. At that time, these tumors were considered to be inoperable, and
they were almost universally fatal. In 1961, Shaw and Paulson showed,
however, that Pancoast tumors could indeed be completely resected with a
hope for cure. Their strategy of preoperative irradiation followed by
resection through a high posterior approach became the standard of care
until recently. Over the past 15 years, the Shaw-Paulson approach has
been revisited, and a variety of alternative strategies such as resection
through the neck and induction chemoradiation have been proposed.
Despite the introduction of these new concepts, the oncologic precepts of
en bloc resection of involved adjacent structures combined, at minimum,
with lobectomy have stood the test of time.

TERMINOLOGY

A tumor of the superior pulmonary sulcus (Table 11-27) is usually a lung
cancer posteriorly located at the apex of the chest. It causes a clinical
syndrome called the Pancoast syndrome, which is characterized by
shoulder pain radiating down the arm, and Horner syndrome, caused by
involvement of the stellate ganglion. The tumor is often small and located
near the neck of the first two ribs.

   According to the TNM terminology, Pancoast tumors have the *T3
descriptor* if the invasion is limited to the chest wall (ribs) and the *T4
descriptor* if they invade the brachial plexus, subclavian vessels, and
vertebral bodies. Although the T4 descriptor usually defines tumors that

TABLE 11-27
CHARACTERISTICS OF SUPERIOR SULCUS TUMORS
Small homogeneous shadow at the apex of the chest
Posterior location near the neck of the first two ribs
Mostly lung cancers
Clinical syndrome characterized by shoulder pain and Horner syndrome

TABLE 11-28

CLINICAL PRESENTATION OF SUPERIOR SULCUS TUMORS

Symptoms often attributed to benign musculoskeletal disorder

Initial symptom is usually shoulder pain (steady and severe)

Pain may radiate down the arm (T1)

Pain may extend down the ulnar surface of forearm (C8)

Weakness and atrophy of hand muscles

Horner syndrome (stellate ganglion)

Respiratory symptoms in only 10% of patients

are technically unresectable, resection is still possible in selected patients with tumors invading the lower trunk of the brachial plexus (C8-T1) or the subclavian blood vessels.

CLINICAL PRESENTATION (TABLE 11-28)

Even if the clinical presentation is nearly always characteristic, the diagnosis of Pancoast tumor is often delayed by several months or even years because the *pain is wrongly attributed* to benign musculoskeletal disorders such as arthritis, bursitis of shoulder, or psychiatric illness. Such delays are more likely to occur in younger patients whose chest radiographs were initially interpreted as being normal.

The most common symptom associated with Pancoast tumors is shoulder pain, which is the result of local invasion of the brachial plexus, first and second ribs, and sometimes adjacent vertebral bodies. The pain is usually *steady and severe,* and it may radiate down the arm in the distribution of the ulnar nerve (involvement of T1). Indeed, the pain may be so severe that the patient has to support the elbow *to reduce tension* on the shoulder and upper arm. Weakness and atrophy of hand muscles may eventually develop, and if the tumor extends to the sympathetic chain and stellate ganglion, Horner syndrome is also likely to develop. Respiratory symptoms, such as cough and hemoptysis, are uncommon and seen in only 10% of patients.

DIAGNOSIS AND STAGING (TABLE 11-29)

The diagnosis of Pancoast tumor is first suspected when radiographs of the shoulder or neck are obtained to investigate the cause of shoulder pain. These radiographs may show a *small apical density* located posteriorly against the mediastinum or a unilateral *apical cap* of more than 5 mm in thickness. Because Pancoast tumors are mostly peripheral, bronchoscopy

TABLE 11-29

CLINICAL STAGING OF PANCOAST TUMORS

Tumor Evaluation	Best Test
T status	CT scan, MRI
N status	Mediastinoscopy, ultrasonography of the neck, and possible needle biopsy
M status	Imaging of brain, bone scan
	Positron emission tomography scan

is generally normal, and the diagnosis is obtained by fine *needle biopsy* through the supraclavicular area or posterior cervical triangle.

Whereas CT is useful to determine tumor characteristics and status of mediastinal nodes, MRI is more sensitive to demonstrate bone involvement (first and second ribs, spine), extension into the spinal canal, or invasion of subclavian blood vessels and brachial plexus.

Mediastinoscopy should be done in *every case presumed to be operable* because N2 disease predicts poor long-term survival and generally indicates inoperability. Similarly, supraclavicular ultrasonographic examination can demonstrate pathologic nodes, which should also be sampled by needle biopsy.

All patients, even those without symptoms, must have *extrathoracic staging,* ideally with imaging of the brain (CT, MRI) and positron emission tomography scan.

SURGICAL TREATMENT

Selection of Patients for Surgery

Although deep rib involvement is associated with decreased survival, it does not contraindicate surgical resection. Involvement of the vertebral bodies or subclavian blood vessels is also not a contraindication to surgery, but resection of these structures must be done by experienced surgeons who possess secure knowledge of the anatomy of the lower neck and thoracic inlet. These extensive resections should preferably be done by multidisciplinary teams of surgeons, including thoracic surgeons, neurosurgeons, and orthopedic surgeons.

If involved, the subclavian vein can simply be ligated; the subclavian artery can be resected and reconstructed. The advent of surgeons with large experiences in spinal surgery is now allowing *partial or total vertebrectomy* in selected patients. Involvement of the intervertebral foramina or spinal canal is a contraindication to surgery, but invasion of the C8-T1 nerve root is not a contraindication even if patients can expect some degree of postoperative disability.

Patients with N2 disease *should not* have surgery, especially if the N2 status has been documented at mediastinoscopy. Ipsilateral supraclavicular nodal involvement (N3 disease) is also considered a contraindication to surgery, although some reports are now suggesting that in superior sulcus tumors, metastasis to supraclavicular or prescalenic nodes occurs transpleurally and thus represents a situation that is similar to N1 disease in patients with non-Pancoast tumors.

Induction Therapies

The strategy of preoperative radiation (30 to 35 cGy in 3 weeks) followed 3 weeks later by surgical resection has been the standard of care since the early 1960s. The purpose of preoperative radiation is to *shrink the tumor,* making complete resection easier to perform. Another objective of preoperative radiation is to *control pain,* thus having patients come to operation in better overall condition.

TABLE 11-30

POSTERIOR SHAW-PAULSON APPROACH

Advantages
Ideal for posterior tumors
Excellent exposure to posterior chest wall including vertebral bodies and nerve roots
Most surgeons familiar with posterolateral approaches

Disadvantages
Not ideal for anterior tumors or tumors extending into the neck
Vascular involvement difficult to deal with
Major mobilization necessary before extent of disease and resectability fully assessed

Recently published phase 2 clinical trials are now suggesting that preoperative chemoradiotherapy (cisplatin and etoposide plus 45 cGy during 5 weeks) is associated with higher complete response rates, higher complete resection rates, and improved disease-free survival.

Surgical Approaches

Posterior Shaw-Paulson Approach (Table 11-30)

This approach is still the preferred one to deal with posteriorly placed apical tumors involving ribs or vertebrae. A generous posterolateral thoracotomy is made with its upper limit at the level of the C7 spinous process (Fig. 11-6). Once the scapula is elevated, resection involves en bloc removal of the upper two to four ribs with or without transverse processes of vertebrae, removal of the involved roots of the lower brachial plexus (usually T1), and an upper lobectomy. Depending on the amount of chest wall removed, reconstruction with a prosthetic mesh may or may not be necessary.

One of the disadvantages (Table 11-30) of this approach is that *major mobilization of the chest wall is necessary* before the extent of disease and resectability can be fully assessed.

Anterior Dartevelle Approach

This approach (see Fig. 5-16) is preferred for *anteriorly placed tumors* thought to involve the subclavian vessels (Table 11-31). The incision is made along the anterior border of the sternocleidomastoid muscles and extends in a curved fashion laterally beneath the clavicle toward the deltopectoral groove. The medial half of the clavicle is excised, thus exposing the internal jugular and subclavian veins, which are divided. Once the subclavian artery and brachial plexus are exposed, the entire resection can be accomplished, including en bloc upper lobectomy after the first two ribs have been removed. When the posterior ribs or vertebral bodies are involved, a combined anterior and posterior approach may be required.

A limitation of the anterior approach is the excision of the medial half of the clavicle, which sometimes causes postoperative deformities including long-term shoulder immobility. As a solution to this problem, some authors advocate a transmanubrial approach, which has the advantage of leaving

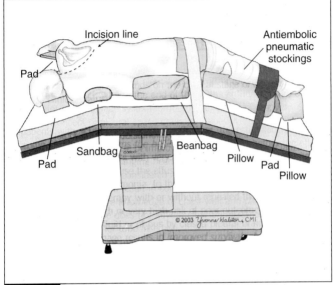

FIG. 11-6

High posterior thoracotomy. Incision extends along the tip of scapula, midway between the posterior edge of scapula and spinous processes, up to level of C7.

the clavicle–manubrial joint intact while still providing excellent exposure for the operation.

Hemi-clamshell Approach (Korst and Burt Approach)

In some patients, a standard *hemi-clamshell incision* (see Fig. 5-18) can be used in conjunction with a sternomastoid incision. The sternotomy is carried down to the third interspace before the anterior thoracotomy is completed.

TABLE 11-31

ANTERIOR DARTEVELLE APPROACH

Advantages
Ideal for anterior tumors
Excellent exposure to subclavian vessels and brachial plexus

Disadvantages
Sometimes necessary to make a separate posterior incision to complete the operation
Excision of medial half of clavicle may lead to postsurgical deformities
Most thoracic surgeons are not familiar with anatomy of the neck

With this approach, the clavicle need not be resected to expose the underlying vessels, but a combined approach may be required if the tumor is located posteriorly.

Surgical Principles and Extended Operations

When tumors involve the C7 nerve root, aggressive approaches may include the removal of this nerve root together with the lower trunk of the brachial plexus. Unfortunately, removal of the C7 nerve root is likely to result in a *deformity called the intrinsic-minus hand*. This deformity of the hand, however, can be improved by appropriate tendon transfers performed at a later date.

Tumors invading the subclavian artery can be freed by dissection through the subadventitial plane. If the artery is invaded beyond the adventitia, resection of the involved segment and *end-to-end anastomosis* should be considered. If a graft is required for reconstruction, a No. 6 or 8 ring polytetrafluoroethylene graft may be used.

When cancellous bone in the vertebral body of C7, T1, or T2 is involved, en bloc resection including vertebrectomy can be done. Recent advances in instrumentation are now allowing more complete resections.

In most series, pulmonary resections less than lobectomies (limited resections) have yielded poorer long-term results.

Complications of Surgery

Resection of superior sulcus tumors is generally well tolerated from the respiratory standpoint because the chest wall defect is beneath the scapula and the large muscles of the back.

Most patients will have a Horner syndrome, which is of little consequence, but patients and relatives should be warned about this problem before the operation. If the Horner syndrome persists or becomes a real disability, patients should be referred to an *ophthalmologist,* who can correct the situation through a relatively minor procedure.

Ulnar nerve function is only partially affected by the division of the T1 nerve root (Table 11-32). Inclusion of the C8 nerve root results in a potentially more debilitating situation, although it is generally well tolerated and patients are likely to improve with physiotherapy over a period of a few months. A more serious disability is that of decreased function of the intrinsic muscles of the hand, making prehension or writing difficult. Again, patients must be told about these potential disabilities.

TABLE 11-32
POSSIBLE NEUROLOGIC SEQUELAE AFTER RESECTION OF PANCOAST TUMORS

Structure Excised	Deficit
Stellate ganglion	Horner syndrome
T1 nerve root	Minimal sensory deficit
C8-T1 nerve roots	Sensory deficit of ulnar distribution
	Deficit of motor function of intrinsic muscles of hand
C7-C8-T1 nerve roots	Intrinsic-minus hand
Entry in dural sheath	Spinal fluid leak, meningitis

If resection of vertebral bodies is necessary, entry into the dural sheaths can occur. In those cases, spinal fluid leaks should be looked for intraoperatively. If it is found, the site of the leak should be repaired.

Vascular complications are unusual. If they occur, they can lead to significant morbidity.

Results

In patients whose T3 Pancoast tumors are completely resected and in whom mediastinal nodes are negative, the 5-year survival is in the range of 35% to 40%. The value of surgery in the management of T4 tumors remains a question not completely answered.

Resection of Pancoast tumors to relieve pain (palliative resection), knowing that resection is incomplete, *is generally not helpful*.

CONCLUSION

The surgical technique for resection of a superior pulmonary sulcus tumor usually involves removal of the first three ribs, portions of the first three dorsal vertebrae (transverse processes), lower trunk of the brachial plexus (C8-T1), and portion of the stellate ganglion together with an upper lobectomy. The surgeon doing these operations must have thorough knowledge of the anatomy of the thoracic inlet, and a *multidisciplinary approach* is recommended. With complete resection, up to 40% of superior sulcus tumors can be cured.

SUGGESTED READINGS

Historical Articles

Pancoast HK: Superior pulmonary sulcus tumors. Tumor characterized by pain, Horner's syndrome, destruction of bone and atrophy of hand muscles. JAMA 1932;99:1391-1396.

Teixeira JP: Concerning the Pancoast tumor: what is the superior pulmonary sulcus? Ann Thorac Surg 1983;35:577-578.

Shaw RR: Pancoast's tumor. Ann Thorac Surg 1984;37:343-344.

Review Articles

Johnson DE, Goldberg M: Management of carcinoma of the superior pulmonary sulcus. Oncology (Huntingt) 1997;11:781-786.

Arcasoy SM, Jett JR: Superior pulmonary sulcus tumors and Pancoast's syndrome. N Engl J Med 1997;337:1370-1376.

Jones DR, Detterbeck FC: Pancoast tumors of the lung. Curr Opin Pulm Med 1998;4:191-197.

Patterson GA: Approaching the apical sulcus tumor: patient selection and approach strategies. Proceedings of the 32nd Postgraduate Program of the Society of Thoracic Surgeons, 1999:22-24.

Komaki R, Putnam JB, Walsh G, et al: The management of superior sulcus tumors. Semin Surg Oncol 2000;18:152-164.

Vallières E, Karmy-Jones R, Mulligan MS: Pancoast tumors. Curr Probl Surg 2001;38:306-376.

11

Ginsberg RJ: Surgical approaches to the superior sulcus lesion. AATS Symposium on General Thoracic Surgery, 2002.

Detterbeck FC: Changes in the treatment of Pancoast tumors. Ann Thorac Surg 2003;75:1990-1997.

Shahian DM: Contemporary management of superior pulmonary sulcus (Pancoast) lung tumors. Curr Opin Pulm Med 2003;9:327-331.

Kraut MJ, Vallières E, Thomas CR Jr.: Pancoast (superior sulcus) neo-plasms. Curr Probl Cancer 2003;27:81-104.

Pitz CC, de la Rivière AB, van Swieten HA, et al: Surgical treatment of Pancoast tumours. Eur J Cardiothorac Surg 2004;26:202-208.

Investigation

Heelan RT, Demas BE, Caravelli JF, et al: Superior sulcus tumors: CT and MR imaging. Radiology 1989;170:637-641.

Sihoe AD, Lee TW, Ahuja AT, Yim AP: Should cervical ultrasonography be a routine staging investigation for lung cancer patients with impalpable cervical lymph nodes? Eur J Cardiothorac Surg 2004;25:486-491.

Induction Treatment

Shaw RR, Paulson DL, Kee JL Jr.: Treatment of the superior sulcus tumor by irradiation followed by resection. Ann Surg 1961;154:29-40.

Suntharalingam M, Sonett JR, Haas ML, et al: The use of concurrent chemotherapy with high-dose radiation before surgical resection in patients presenting with apical sulcus tumors. Cancer J 2000;6:365-371.

Rusch VW, Giroux DJ, Kraut MJ: Induction chemoradiation and surgical resection for non–small cell lung carcinomas of the superior sulcus: initial results of Southwest Oncology Group Trial 9416 (Intergroup Trial 0160). J Thorac Cardiovasc Surg 2001;121:472-483.

Surgery

Grunenwald D, Spaggiari L: Transmanubrial osteomuscular sparing approach for apical chest tumors. Ann Thorac Surg 1997;63:563-566.

Korst RJ, Burt ME: Cervicothoracic tumors: results of resection by the "hemi-clamshell" approach. J Thorac Cardiovasc Surg 1998;15:286-295.

Gandhi S, Walsh GL, Komaki R, et al: A multidisciplinary surgical approach to superior sulcus tumors with vertebral invasion. Ann Thorac Surg 1999;68:1778-1785.

Dartevelle P, Macchiarini P: Surgical management of superior sulcus tumors. Oncologist 1999;4:398-407.

Fadel E, Missenard G, Chapelier A, et al: En bloc resection of non–small cell lung cancer invading the thoracic inlet and intervertebral foramina. J Thorac Cardiovasc Surg 2002;123:676-685.

Case Series

Attar S, Krasna MJ, Sonett JR, et al: Superior sulcus (Pancoast) tumor: experience with 105 patients. Ann Thorac Surg 1998;66:193-198.

Hagan MP, Choi NC, Mathisen DJ, et al: Superior sulcus lung tumors: impact of local control on survival. J Thorac Cardiovasc Surg 1999;117:1086-1094.

Rusch VW, Parekh KR, Leon L, et al: Factors determining outcome after surgical resection of T3 and T4 lung cancers of the superior sulcus. J Thorac Cardiovasc Surg 2000;119:1147-1153.

Martinod E, D'Audiffret A, Thomas P, et al: Management of superior sulcus tumors: experience with 139 cases treated by surgical resection. Ann Thorac Surg 2002;73:1534-1540.

Pfannschmidt J, Kugler C, Muley T, et al: Non–small-cell superior sulcus tumor: results of en bloc resection in fifty-six patients. Thorac Cardiovasc Surg 2003;51:332-337.

11

Special Challenges in Thoracic Surgery

MANAGEMENT OF THE PATIENT WITH SUPPURATIVE LUNG DISEASE

From the time of Laennec's description of the disease (1819) to the discovery of antibiotics, bronchiectasis was considered a morbid condition associated with high mortality rates mostly from respiratory failure and cor pulmonale. With the advent of specific antibiotics and effective treatment of pulmonary infection in childhood, however, the incidence and surgical significance of the disease have decreased considerably even if bronchiectasis still constitutes a *significant public health problem* in developing countries.

Primary lung abscesses are localized pulmonary suppurations with necrosis. They are commonly related to aspiration, and most occur in dependent portions of the lung. Although their management is essentially medical, every thoracic surgeon must be familiar with the indications for surgical intervention including those related to complications of the abscess, such as *bronchopleural fistula, empyema, and hemorrhage.*

BRONCHIECTASIS

Terminology

Bronchiectasis is defined as permanent bronchial dilatations with *nonreversible destruction* of their walls. This definition differentiates true bronchiectasis from functional bronchiectasis, which is expected to revert to normal once control of the infection has been achieved.

In the context of clinical practice, there are two types of bronchiectasis in which pathogenesis, management, and prognosis differ considerably (Table 11-33). *Localized bronchiectasis* is usually the result of childhood pneumonia; it often has a benign course characterized by recurrent infection, always in the same anatomic territory. On the contrary, diffuse bronchiectasis is often related to immune deficiencies, is bilateral, and may lead to death from respiratory failure and cor pulmonale.

TABLE 11-33

LOCALIZED AND DIFFUSE BRONCHIECTASIS

	Localized Bronchiectasis	Diffuse Bronchiectasis
Anatomy	Confined to one site distal to segmental, lobar, or main bronchus	Multisegmental, multilobar, and often bilateral
Clinical signs	Repeated infections characterized by fever, cough, purulent sputum, and sometimes chest pain and hemoptysis	Chronic infection, daily purulent bronchorrhea, sinusitis Rhonchi always present Clubbing common in advanced disease
Imaging	Localized pneumonic infiltrate Loss of volume Localized dilatation on CT	Diffuse disease predominantly in lung bases
Bronchoscopy	Must be done to rule out foreign body or tumor	Must be done for culture and sensitivity of secretions
Spirometry	Often normal	Mixed obstruction and destruction with decreased Pao_2
Management	Surgery for repeated infections, hemoptysis	Surgery seldom indicated
Prognosis	Good	Poor with eventual hypoxemia, pulmonary hypertension, and cor pulmonale

Pathology and Classification

Bronchiectasis predominates at the level of the second to the sixth bronchial divisions and often affects *the most dependent portions* of the lung. Overall, one third of bronchiectases are unilateral and affect a single lobe, one third are unilateral but affect more than one lobe, and one third are bilateral. The "middle lobe syndrome" consists of a small atelectatic lobe, usually due to extrinsic bronchial compression secondary to enlarged nodes.

In the most commonly used classification (Table 11-34), bronchiectasis is divided into a *cylindrical variety,* in which the dilated bronchi maintain a regular outline until they reach the junction with smaller airways; a *varicose pattern,* in which dilated bronchi have irregular contours similar to those of varicose veins; and a more severe form of *cystic or saccular bronchiectasis,* in which there are cystic dilatations of bronchi and air-fluid levels are often noted.

Gross examination of bronchiectatic lungs shows dilatation of bronchi, which are filled with suppurative thick yellow-green pus. In general,

TABLE 11-34

ANATOMIC CLASSIFICATION OF BRONCHIECTASIS (REID CLASSIFICATION)

Cylindrical	Dilated bronchi maintain regular outlines until they reach smaller airways
Varicose	Dilated bronchi have irregular contours similar to varicose veins
Saccular	Cystic dilatations with air-fluid levels

the distal lung is atelectatic and has signs of chronic pneumonitis and fibrosis. Bronchiectasis nearly always has associated bronchial artery hyperplasia.

Pathophysiology and Pathogenesis

The occurrence of bronchiectasis is associated with a *wide spectrum of causative factors,* often interacting together and leading to retention of secretions, bronchial obstruction, infection, and secondary damage to the bronchial mucosa and lung (Table 11-35). In general terms, pathogenicity includes host factors (often congenital and familial) and factors related to acquired disease processes. Bronchiectasis related to congenital factors is more likely to be diffuse, whereas that related to infection is more likely to be localized.

Most cases of bronchiectasis are acquired and result from prior bacterial or viral pneumonia (pertussis, measles, influenza). Indeed, a *single severe pneumonia* or repeated moderate infections can lead to retention of secretions and destruction of the bronchial wall. In such cases, the specific nature of the infection is not nearly as important as the bronchial obstruction, prolonged infection, and delayed resolution.

Bronchial obstruction from endobronchial lesions, external compression, or repeated aspiration from the esophagus or more commonly from nasal accessory sinuses can cause retention of secretions, secondary infection, and bronchiectasis.

Host factors are uncommon causes of bronchiectasis, although it is likely that in many cases, *immunodeficiency is present but cannot be adequately documented* by laboratory testing. Bronchiectasis is strongly associated with primary ciliary dyskinesia, cystic fibrosis, and immunoglobulin deficiencies (see Table 11-35). Patients with Kartagener syndrome have sinusitis, situs inversus, bronchiectasis, decreased serum levels of immunoglobulin A, and abnormal ciliary motility.

TABLE 11-35

PATHOGENESIS OF BRONCHIECTASIS

Acquired factors
  Infection (60%)
    Bacterial, viral
    Tuberculosis
  Obstruction (15%)
    Intrinsic: foreign bodies, aspiration
    Extrinsic: enlarged nodes
Host factors (15%)
  Congenital ciliary defects (primary ciliary dyskinesia)
  Kartagener syndrome
  Cystic fibrosis
  Immunoglobulin deficiencies
  Alpha$_1$-antitrypsin deficiencies
Unknown factors (10%)

Diagnosis

The clinical presentation of bronchiectasis is variable and depends on the *pathogenesis of disease* and whether the condition is *localized or diffuse* (see Table 11-33). The hallmark of bronchiectasis is, however, that of *chronic cough, bronchial suppuration, and purulent bronchorrhea,* which in some cases can amount to as much as 100 to 200 mL/day. Patients often present with a history of *recurrent febrile episodes* or recurrent pneumonia with or without hemoptysis (seldom life-threatening). Clinical signs of denutrition and cor pulmonale are uncommon and indicate advanced disease. Complaints of chronic sinusitis, repeated infections at other sites, or a family history of similar disorders may be helpful in identifying host-related factors.

CT scanning is currently the best imaging technique to establish the presence, severity, and distribution of bronchiectasis. Although CT can be done during an acute infectious episode, the final decision regarding presence or absence of "true" bronchiectasis should be based only on imaging done at least 6 to 8 weeks after resolution of the infection. Other important tests include bronchoscopy to rule out a foreign body or a tumor, bacteriology of bronchial secretions, sweat test for cystic fibrosis, CT scanning of the sinuses, and simple immunologic work-up.

Pulmonary function studies are usually normal in patients with localized bronchiectasis but often show evidence of airway obstruction in patients with diffuse bronchiectasis.

Management

Medical Management

For nearly all patients with bronchiectasis, the *initial treatment should be conservative* (Table 11-36). This includes infection control, bronchodilatation, and active physical therapy. In general, antibiotics tend to reduce the amount of sputum, and bronchodilators tend to reduce mucosal edema and bronchospasm. Other measures that are part of medical management include breathing exercises and reduction of exposure to irritants such as tobacco smoke.

Perhaps one of the most important aspects of medical management is aggressive treatment of associated conditions such as chronic sinusitis, gastroesophageal reflux, and immunoglobulin deficiencies.

Surgical Treatment

Patients who are candidates for surgical resection must fulfill the criteria listed in Table 11-37. They must have *localized and symptomatic disease,*

TABLE 11-36

OBJECTIVES OF CONSERVATIVE TREATMENT

Elimination of underlying cause if it is reversible

Treatment of associated and contributing disorders (sinusitis, gastroesophageal reflux)

Control of infection by antibiotics

Improved clearance of secretions (physical therapy, postural drainage)

Reversal of airflow limitation by bronchodilators

TABLE 11-37
NECESSARY CRITERIA FOR SURGICAL RESECTION OF BRONCHIECTASIS
Localized bronchiectasis documented by CT scanning
Adequate pulmonary reserve to tolerate proposed resection
Irreversible process
Significant symptoms, such as chronic productive cough, repeated hemoptysis, recurring pneumonia
Failure to improve after adequate trial of medical management

continued productive cough, repeated or significant hemoptysis, or *recurring episodes of pneumonia* always involving the same bronchiectatic lobe.

Surgery is seldom indicated in patients with multisegmental disease (Table 11-38). In this group, patients who may yet benefit from operation are those with symptomatic bronchiectasis that is unresponsive to conservative management and can be completely resected; those with hemoptysis that cannot be controlled or recurs after bronchial artery embolization; and those in whom there is a need for palliation and the most involved lobes or segments are resected to improve symptoms. In such highly selected patients, *limited resections of targeted segments* may achieve lasting symptomatic improvement. Surgical resection of bronchiectasis in patients with cystic fibrosis or in patients with primary ciliary dyskinesia is seldom indicated.

As a rule, the objective of surgery is to remove all diseased segments while preserving normal lung. Patients must be actively prepared by specific antibiotics given at least 48 hours before operation and by active physical therapy. For the surgeon, it is imperative to preoperatively determine the extent of resection likely to be required because it may be difficult at operation to judge which segments are involved and which are not.

During surgery, a double-lumen tube should always be used to avoid contaminating contralateral lobes. Technical difficulties may arise from dense adhesions, hyperplastic nodes around the pulmonary artery and its branches, and incomplete fissures. Bronchial artery hyperplasia is always present, and, although it may be the source of bleeding, it provides additional blood supply to the bronchial stump, thus lowering the chances of postoperative bronchopleural fistulas (versus pulmonary resection done for lung cancer).

TABLE 11-38
POSSIBLE INDICATIONS FOR SURGERY IN PATIENTS WITH MULTISEGMENTAL BRONCHIECTASIS
Bronchiectasis that is symptomatic and unresponsive to medical treatment
Recurring hemoptysis
Complete resection is possible
Need for palliation in which the most involved segments are resected to improve symptoms

11

Special Challenges in Thoracic Surgery

Prognostic factors for good surgical results include *cylindrical type of bronchiectasis, absence of sinusitis,* and *complete resection of disease.*

LUNG ABSCESS

Lung abscesses are necrotizing infections of the lung usually consecutive to aspiration of oropharyngeal material. Less frequently, they are related to the evolution of pneumonia or to local endobronchial processes such as bronchogenic carcinomas.

Classification and Pathogenesis

Lung abscesses are usually classified into primary or secondary based on their pathogenesis (Table 11-39).

Primary lung abscesses include those *related to aspiration* (gastrointestinal contents or pharyngeal secretions) and those that may have occurred as a result of *necrotizing pneumonia.* Indeed, aspiration of infected oropharyngeal secretions is the main reason why most lung abscesses occur in the dependent portions of the lung (Figs. 11-7 and 11-8), such as the posterior segment of the right upper lobe and the superior segments of both lower lobes. Predisposing factors (Table 11-40) include impaired level of consciousness (suppressed cough reflex); poor oral hygiene (increased bacterial load); esophageal disorders; and decreased host defenses, such as seen in association with steroid therapy, diabetes, and malnutrition.

Although aspiration was long considered the only cause of primary lung abscesses, recent information suggests that an increasing number of such abscesses are due *to necrotizing pneumonia* caused by virulent organisms like *Klebsiella pneumoniae* and *S. aureus* or to opportunistic infections in immunosuppressed patients.

Secondary lung abscesses are those due to infection of preexisting lesions (cysts, pneumatocele, bullae) and those related to obstructing endobronchial tumors or foreign bodies. Lung abscesses may also be secondary to pulmonary extension of an infection in an adjacent space, such as the mediastinum, pleural space, or subphrenic space, or it can occur as a consequence of trauma. *Infrequently,* multiple lung abscesses will be secondary to septic embolization originating from distant sites.

TABLE 11-39
ETIOLOGIC CLASSIFICATION OF LUNG ABSCESSES

Primary lung abscesses
Aspiration of gastrointestinal contents or oropharyngeal secretions
Necrotizing pulmonary infections
Opportunistic infections

Secondary lung abscesses
Preexisting cavity (tuberculosis, cysts)
Complication of bronchial obstruction (cancer, foreign body)
Extension of adjacent suppurative infection (mediastinum, pleura, subphrenic)
Trauma
Septic emboli

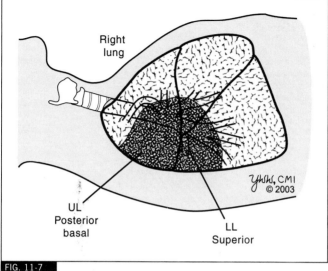

FIG. 11-7

Aspiration in the right lung in supine position. UL, upper lobe; LL, lower lobe.

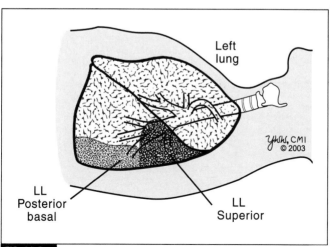

FIG. 11-8

Aspiration in the left lung in supine position. LL, lower lobe.

FACTORS PREDISPOSING TO ASPIRATION-RELATED LUNG ABSCESSES

Increased risk of aspiration
    Impaired level of consciousness (general anesthesia, drugs, alcohol, stroke)
    Esophageal disorders (achalasia, Zenker diverticulum)
Increased bacterial load
    Poor oral hygiene (gingivodental sepsis)
Decreased host defenses
    Preexisting pulmonary disease
    Immunosuppression (steroid therapy, chemotherapy, organ transplantation)
    Systemic conditions (malnutrition, diabetes)

Bacteriology (Table 11-41)

Bacteria isolated from lung abscesses always reflect their underlying pathogenesis. In lung abscesses due to aspiration, for instance, gram-positive cocci and anaerobic gram-negative bacilli can be isolated from both the site of orodental infection and the lung abscess. Primary lung abscesses due to necrotizing pneumonia are colonized by a variety of organisms including *Streptococcus* species, *S. aureus,* and *K. pneumoniae.*

Diagnosis

The diagnosis of lung abscess is usually based on clinical history and radiographic findings.

Although the symptoms can be variable, patients typically complain of *cough and fever* (insidious onset), sometimes associated with pleuritic chest pain. Once cavitation has occurred, most patients will *expectorate* large amounts of foul and purulent sputum. Hemoptysis may occur at any time and varies from blood-streaked sputum (more common) to massive hemorrhage (rare).

The diagnosis of lung abscess, the determination of its specific location, and its differentiation from a loculated empyema can be *established by imaging techniques.* Posteroanterior and lateral chest radiographs will usually show a thin-walled cavitary lesion with an air-fluid level often in a dependent portion of the lung. A peripherally loculated or interlobar empyema may be mistaken for a lung abscess, but CT findings will in most cases differentiate between the two entities. A lung abscess in the periphery of the lung *typically forms an acute angle* with the chest wall, whereas a

TABLE 11-41

MOST COMMON BACTERIOLOGY OF LUNG ABSCESSES

Lung abscess due to aspiration
    Aerobic gram-positive cocci: *Streptococcus pneumoniae, Staphylococcus aureus*
    Anaerobic gram-negative bacilli: *Fusobacterium, Bacteroides*
    Anaerobic gram-positive cocci: *Peptostreptococcus, Peptococcus*
Lung abscess secondary to pneumonia
    Streptococcus species, *Staphylococcus aureus, Klebsiella pneumoniae, Haemophilus influenzae*

loculated empyema *forms an obtuse angle.* In the fissure, an empyema has a fusiform shape; a lung abscess is nearly always round. CT scan is also helpful in differentiating a primary lung abscess from cavitations secondary to carcinomas, infected bullae or cyst, and less common lesions (such as tuberculosis, fungal infections, and Wegener granulomatosis).

Bronchoscopy *should always be done* to rule out an obstructing endobronchial lesion or foreign body and to obtain specimens for culture. In most cases, however, better specimens are obtained through the use of techniques bypassing possible contamination from upper airways. In the past, transtracheal aspiration was used to obtain such specimens, but it is now recommended that the specimen be sampled directly from the abscess cavity by needle aspiration (ultrasound or CT guidance). The technique is well tolerated, has few complications, obtains samples uncontaminated by upper respiratory tract flora, and *has a yield* of *more than 90%* in identifying the causative bacteria.

Natural History of Primary Lung Abscesses (Fig. 11-9)

In most cases of appropriately treated primary lung abscesses, *resolution takes place without sequelae.* The patient evacuates the contents of the abscess through expectoration, the cavity collapses, and the lung re-expands. On occasion, the abscess will be complicated by rupturing in the pleural space and causing empyema and bronchopleural fistula; by bleeding massively due to erosion into adjacent blood vessels; or by generating systemic sepsis, which is more likely to occur in older and immunosuppressed patients.

Incomplete resolution of the abscess *may finally lead to chronicity.* In such cases, the abscess has a thick wall that prevents cavity collapse even when surgical drainage has been provided.

Management

The main consideration involved in the management of lung abscesses is the use of appropriate antibiotics for an extended period of time.

Medical Management

Current therapy for lung abscesses is largely medical. The objectives are to destroy the bacterial flora, to drain and obliterate the cavity, to treat comorbidities and predisposing conditions, and to maintain the anabolic state of the patient.

In most cases of aspiration-related lung abscesses, *high-dose penicillin* (up to 20 million units per day) is the drug of choice because it is effective against gram-positive aerobes and most anaerobic organisms. In recent years, however, *clindamycin* (600 mg intravenously every 6 hours) and a third-generation cephalosporin have become better drugs, mostly because of penicillin-resistant anaerobic species. Although the length of therapy is dictated by the clinical and radiographic responses, intravenous antibiotics should be administered until the patient is no longer toxic; at that point, it can be changed to an oral regimen of equal efficacy.

Drainage *is just as important as antibiotics in the treatment of lung abscesses.* Because most abscesses communicate with the bronchial tree,

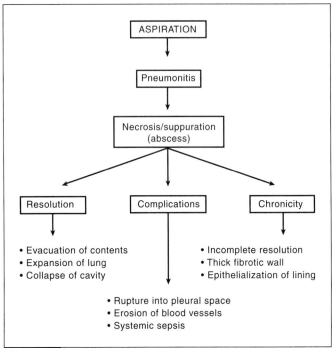

FIG. 11-9

Natural history of primary lung abscess. *(Modified with permission from Delarue NC, Pearson FG, Nelems JM, Cooper JD: Lung abscess: surgical implications. Can J Surg 1980;23:297-302).*

adequate drainage occurs spontaneously and is promoted by physiotherapy and postural maneuvers. If the abscess does not drain internally, it can be drained by bronchoscopic techniques with use of brush forceps and specially designed catheters or more often by the *insertion under CT guidance of percutaneous pigtail catheters.* All of these techniques are associated with low morbidity, are well tolerated by the patient, and have a high cure rate. If catheter drainage fails to evacuate the abscess, alternative techniques including insertion of a chest tube directly in the abscess cavity should be looked at and tried.

Supportive therapies include *maintenance of nutrition* and treatment of associated comorbidities, such as gingivodental sepsis and diabetes.

Clinical improvement is evidenced by a decrease in sputum production, improvement in the general condition of the patient, resolution of fever, and radiologic evidence of decreasing infiltrates and cavitation.

TABLE 11-42
INDICATIONS FOR SURGICAL INTERVENTION IN PRIMARY LUNG ABSCESSES
Complications of the abscess such as empyema, hemorrhage
Unsuccessful medical management after 6-8 weeks of intensive treatment
Persistence of a thick-walled chronic abscess
Suspected malignant neoplasm

Surgical Treatment

Surgical treatment is *seldom indicated during the acute phase of primary lung abscesses* other than to treat complications of the abscess (Table 11-42). Chronicity of the abscess, lack of response to medical therapy, and suspicion of or inability to rule out cavitary lung cancer are also possible indications for surgical intervention. In general, cavities that persist with no or minimal improvement after a period of 6 to 8 weeks of adequate therapy should be operated on.

When operating on patients with lung abscesses, important surgical considerations include the use of a double-lumen tube to protect the contralateral lung and avoidance of intraoperative spillage of pus to prevent postoperative empyemas. Because of this latter consideration, extrapleural lobectomy is often preferred over more limited resections of the abscess.

LUNG ABSCESS IN IMMUNOCOMPROMISED PATIENTS

Immunocompromised patients include patients with malignant neoplasms, those who are receiving chemotherapeutic or immunosuppressive agents, those with HIV infection, and those who have undergone organ transplantation. Because all of these patients have an altered immune function, not only are they more susceptible to pulmonary infection, but the spectrum of disease is also different from that observed in immunocompetent individuals.

The characteristics of patients with immunosuppression and lung infections are listed in Table 11-43. In immunocompromised patients, bacterial pneumonia is *more likely to progress* to lung abscess; the pathogens involved are often multiple, including opportunistic organisms such as fungi. Potential association with known risk factors such as gingivitis and alcohol use is generally lacking.

TABLE 11-43
CHARACTERISTICS OF IMMUNOCOMPROMISED PATIENTS WITH LUNG INFECTION
Bacterial pneumonia more likely to progress to lung abscess
Pathogens involved often multiple and may include opportunistic organisms
Potential association with known risk factors not present
Multiple sites (lobes) often involved
Longer antibiotic treatment required
Worse prognosis (higher recurrence rate and death rate)

Longer courses of antibiotherapy are required, especially if the patient is neutropenic. The overall outcome is worse than in immunocompetent patients, with significantly higher recurrence rates of the abscess and higher death rates.

LUNG GANGRENE

Lung gangrene is a rare entity that can complicate severe lung infection. It is caused by *vascular thrombosis* of pulmonary arteries and veins in an area of severe infection. Eventually, these thromboses will cause devitalization of the lung, ischemic necrosis, and secondary anaerobic infection. Predisposing and important contributing factors include alcohol abuse and immunosuppression.

Various pathogens such as *K. pneumoniae,* Friedländer bacillus, and *Aspergillus* (invasive aspergillosis) have been found to be causative agents. Invasive aspergillosis, for instance, produces a necrotizing bronchopneumonia that leads to thrombosis, hemorrhage, and secondary gangrene.

The radiographic features of lung gangrene are characteristic of this disease. They show *rapid progression from consolidation to cavitation* with simultaneous appearance of an intracavitary mass due to large amounts of gangrenous lung that partially accumulate in the cavity.

The recognition of lung gangrene is important because it must be promptly treated by surgical resection of all necrotic tissues.

CONCLUSION

With improvements in health care and availability of more potent antibiotics, the prevalence of bronchiectasis *has decreased significantly* in industrialized countries, and most patients can be successfully treated by conservative measures. Similarly, most patients with lung abscesses can be treated conservatively with specific antibiotics and in some cases external drainage of the abscess.

SUGGESTED READINGS

Bronchiectasis

Brooke Nicotra M, Rivera M, Dale AM, et al: Clinical, pathophysiologic, and microbiologic characterization of bronchiectasis in an aging cohort. Chest 1995;108:955-961.

Smit HJ, Schreurs JM, Van den Bosch JM, Westermann CJ: Is resection of bronchiectasis beneficial in patients with primary ciliary dyskinesia? Chest 1996;109:1541-1544.

Agasthian T, Deschamps C, Trastek VF, et al: Surgical management of bronchiectasis. Ann Thorac Surg 1996;62:976-980.

Prieto D, Bernardo J, Matos MJ, et al: Surgery for bronchiectasis. Eur J Cardiothorac Surg 2001;20:19-24.

Fujimoto T, Hillejan L, Stamatis G: Current strategy for surgical management of bronchiectasis. Ann Thorac Surg 2001;72:1711-1715.

Kutlay H, Cangir AK, Enön S, et al: Surgical treatment in bronchiectasis: analysis of 166 patients. Eur J Cardiothorac Surg 2002;21: 634-637.

Mazières J, Murris M, Didier A, et al: Limited operation for severe multisegmental bilateral bronchiectasis. Ann Thorac Surg 2003;75: 382-387.

Lung Abscess

Bartlett JG, Gorbach SL, Tally FP, Finegold SM: Bacteriology and treatment of primary lung abscess. Am Rev Respir Dis 1974;109:510-518.

Estrera AS, Platt MR, Mills LJ, Shaw RR: Primary lung abscess. J Thorac Cardiovasc Surg 1980;79:275-282.

Delarue NC, Pearson FG, Nelems JM, Cooper JD: Lung abscess: surgical implications. Can J Surg 1980;23:297-301.

Hagan JL, Hardy JD: Lung abscess revisited. Ann Surg 1983;197:755-762.

Pohlson EC, McNamara JJ, Char C, Kurata L: Lung abscess: a changing pattern of the disease. Am J Surg 1985;150:97-101.

Rice TW, Ginsberg RJ, Todd TRJ: Tube drainage of lung abscesses. Ann Thorac Surg 1987;44:356-359.

Wiedemann HP, Rice TW: Lung abscess and empyema. Semin Thorac Cardiovasc Surg 1995;7:119-128.

Hammond JM, Potgieter PD, Hanslo D, et al: The etiology and antimicrobial susceptibility patterns of microorganisms in acute community-acquired lung abscess. Chest 1995;108:937-941.

Furman AC, Jacobs J, Sepkowitz KA: Lung abscess in patients with AIDS. Clin Infect Dis 1996;22:81-85.

Hirshberg B, Sklair-Levi M, Nir-Paz R, et al: Factors predicting mortality of patients with lung abscess. Chest 1999;115:746-750.

Tseng YL, Wu MH, Lin MY, et al: Surgery for lung abscess in immunocompetent and immunocompromised children. J Pediatr Surg 2001;36:470-473.

Mansharamani N, Balachandran D, Delaney D, et al: Lung abscess in adults: clinical comparisons of immunocompromised to non-immunocompromised patients. Respir Med 2002;96:178-185.

Lung Gangrene

Refaely Y, Weissberg D: Gangrene of the lung: treatment in two stages. Ann Thorac Surg 1997;64:970-974.

MANAGEMENT OF THE PATIENT WITH MALIGNANT PLEURAL EFFUSION

A pleural effusion containing malignant cells is called a malignant pleural effusion. Pathologic substantiation of such an entity can be obtained by simple techniques such as thoracentesis and percutaneous pleural biopsy or by thoracoscopic examination, which has a diagnostic yield of more than 95%.

11

Special Challenges in Thoracic Surgery

TABLE 11-44
CHARACTERISTICS OF MALIGNANT PLEURAL EFFUSIONS
Diagnosis based on finding malignant cells in effusion
Cumulative result of increased capillary permeability and impaired lymphatic drainage
Two thirds of malignant effusions are accounted for by lung cancer,
breast cancer, lymphoma
Site of primary lesion remains unknown in 15% of patients

A malignant pleural effusion is always a sign of advanced disease, and this must be kept in mind while selecting treatment. Indeed, expedient and effective palliation of dyspnea should be the main objective of therapy, especially in patients with tumors unlikely to respond to systemic therapy.

Bedside chemical pleurodesis is an excellent option to control the reaccumulation of fluid, to alleviate symptoms of pain and dyspnea, and to improve the quality of life.

TERMINOLOGY AND PATHOGENESIS

Malignant Pleural Effusions (Table 11-44)

Malignant pleural effusions result from the cumulative effects of increased capillary permeability secondary to tumor implants on pleural surfaces *(increased fluid production)* and impaired fluid resorption due to tumor invasion of the pleural-mediastinal lymphatics *(lymphatic obstruction)*. Direct invasion of the parietal pleura by lung cancer or less commonly by primary pleural tumors is yet another mechanism that can increase fluid production. Through a combination of each of these mechanisms, several liters of fluid can accumulate in the pleural space, causing lung (ipsilateral and contralateral) as well as mediastinal (vena cava) compression.

Although nearly all forms of malignant disease can be the cause of malignant pleural effusions, approximately two thirds of these effusions are accounted for by *lung cancer, breast cancer, and lymphomas*. In approximately 15% of patients, the site of the primary lesion is unknown.

Paramalignant Pleural Effusions (Table 11-45)

Paramalignant pleural effusions are cancer-related effusions in *which no malignant cells are found*. In lung cancer, the significance of such effusions (usually related to bronchial obstruction) is that patients can still undergo complete and curative resection of the tumor. Other typical

TABLE 11-45
CHARACTERISTICS OF PARAMALIGNANT PLEURAL EFFUSIONS
No malignant cells in effusion
Develop because of local or systemic effects of tumor or complications of therapy
Majority accounted for by lung cancer
Do not affect operability of lung cancer

examples of paramalignant effusions are those due to prior mediastinal radiotherapy and those secondary to trapped lung or hypoalbuminemia.

DIAGNOSIS (TABLE 11-46)

The clinical setting in which an effusion occurs helps determine its possible cause (see Chapter 3, "Assessment of the Patient with a Pleural Disorder"). A lung cancer patient with N2 disease who develops a pleural effusion, for instance, is likely to have a malignant effusion. Similarly, a woman who develops an effusion months or years after treatment of a breast cancer is also likely to have a malignant effusion.

Approximately half of malignant pleural effusions are diagnosed by one fluid cytologic analysis; a second and third thoracentesis increase the incidence of positive findings to 65% to 70%. *Videothoracoscopy* with direct pleural biopsy has an accuracy of more than 95%, and as such, *it is the most definitive diagnostic technique.*

In most cases of malignant effusion due to pleural metastasis from a primary at a distant site, the histology of the tumor can be determined by biopsy. The exact site of the primary may be difficult to document, however, unless the patient is symptomatic or already has a known primary in another system.

MANAGEMENT OF PATIENTS WITH MALIGNANT PLEURAL EFFUSIONS

The treatment of patients with initial or recurrent malignant pleural effusions can be complex. Given the limited survival of most of these individuals, it must provide expedient and effective relief of symptoms, minimize hospitalization time, and improve quality of life.

Treatment of Underlying Malignant Disease

If the malignant neoplasm responsible for the effusion is likely to be sensitive to systemic chemotherapy, *such therapy should be tried first.* This is the case, for example, of patients with breast carcinomas, small cell lung cancer, lymphomas, or ovarian carcinomas. Treatment of the primary tumor may be effective in eliminating the effusion and avoiding further therapy.

Palliative Treatment of Malignant Effusions

When the tumor is unlikely to be responsive to systemic therapy, as in patients with non–small cell lung cancer, palliative treatment should be considered.

TABLE 11-46
DIAGNOSIS OF MALIGNANT PLEURAL EFFUSIONS
Clinical setting is important in determining possible etiology
50% are diagnosed by one fluid cytologic analysis
70% are diagnosed by a combination of thoracentesis and closed pleural biopsy
95% are diagnosed by videothoracoscopic examination
Most hemorrhagic effusions are malignant

Repeated Thoracentesis (Table 11-47)

Although thoracentesis provides fast and satisfactory relief of symptoms in the majority of patients, *it is ineffective to prevent reaccumulation* of pleural fluid. Thus, it is not a suitable option for long-term management even if the procedure can easily be done in an outpatient setting and requires minimal equipment. This approach often results in the patient's increased anxiety and discomfort in addition to repeatedly exposing him or her to the risks and complications of the technique, such as pneumothoraces and empyemas.

Repeated thoracentesis can, however, be offered to patients in need of immediate relief because of *acute respiratory distress,* to terminal patients whose survival is expected to *be less than 1 month,* and to patients with slowly reaccumulating effusions.

Chemical Pleurodesis

The objective of chemical pleurodesis is to produce adhesions between visceral and parietal pleurae, thus obliterating the potential pleural space.

Indications and Prerequisites (Table 11-48). The presence of *significant symptoms,* such as dyspnea and chest pain, *that are clearly related to the effusion* is the main indication for chemical pleurodesis. This symptom-effusion relationship is best documented by removing 1.5 to 2.0 liters of fluid and assessing its effect on breathlessness. If the dyspnea does not improve, other possible causes, such as bronchial obstruction or lymphangitic carcinomatosis, must be considered before proceeding with pleurodesis.

Another prerequisite for successful pleurodesis is radiologic evidence that the *underlying lung can re-expand* and is not trapped by a fibrous or neoplastic peel lying on its visceral surface. This is often best documented by inserting a chest tube, evacuating the pleural fluid, and obtaining a chest radiograph, which will demonstrate whether the lung can re-expand.

Patients selected for pleurodesis must finally have an effusion that is recurrent, and the recurrence must correlate with symptoms. One possible

---

TABLE 11-47

ADVANTAGES AND DISADVANTAGES OF REPEATED THORACENTESIS

Advantages
Provides immediate relief of respiratory distress
Good option for terminal patients with survival expected to be less than 1-2 months
Good option for patients with slowly reaccumulating fluid

Disadvantages
Ineffective to prevent reaccumulation of fluid
Results in the patient's increased anxiety and discomfort
Repeated hospital or clinic visits
Repeated exposure to risks and complications of procedure
    (pneumothorax, empyema, loculation)
May predispose to development of fibrous peel, limiting re-expansion

TABLE 11-48

INDICATIONS FOR AND CONTRAINDICATIONS OF CHEMICAL PLEURODESIS FOR MANAGEMENT OF MALIGNANT PLEURAL EFFUSIONS

Indications
Tumor unlikely to be responsive to systemic therapy
Effusion must be symptomatic (dyspnea, pain)
Symptoms must be clearly related to effusion
Should be evidence of complete re-expansion of underlying lung
Pleural effusion must be recurrent

Contraindications
Patients with limited life span
Patients with incomplete re-expansion of underlying lung

exception is the patient who lives far from the treatment center and in whom the effusion has a high likelihood of recurring.

Chemical pleurodesis is contraindicated in patients with limited life span (<30 days) and in patients with incomplete re-expansion of the underlying lung.

Chemicals Used for Pleurodesis. The list of chemicals that can produce pleurodesis is long, but the selection is made easy by practical considerations of *availability, cost, effectiveness, comfort of the patient, and incidence of side effects.* Currently, the agents most commonly used are talc, doxycycline, and bleomycin (Table 11-49).

Talc. Talc is the oldest and most effective agent used for pleurodesis. It controls malignant pleural effusions in *more than 90% of patients,* and short-term morbidity appears to be minimal. The most common adverse effects are transient fever and pleural pain, and both are easily controlled. Talc may be administered as a slurry through the chest tube (bedside administration), or it can be insufflated during thoracoscopy (Table 11-50).

When talc is used as a slurry, 5 g of asbestos-free purified talc is mixed with 100 mL of normal saline solution and 10 mL of 1% lidocaine to form a suspension that is instilled directly into the chest tube. Major advantages of this procedure are that it is simple and safe, that it can be done

TABLE 11-49

CHEMICALS COMMONLY USED FOR PLEURODESIS

	Talc	Doxycycline*	Bleomycin
Availability of product	Wide	Wide	Wide
Cost	Minimal	Minimal	High
Effectiveness†	>90%	50%-75%	60%-85%
Inconvenience (adverse effects)‡	++	+++ (chest pain)	++
Toxicity (morbidity)	Minimal	Minimal	Minimal

*Doxycycline is a tetracycline analogue.
†30-day success rate in controlling effusion.
‡Most common adverse effects are nausea and vomiting, pleural pain, and fever.

TABLE 11-50

TALC PLEURODESIS

	Talc Slurry (bedside)	Talc Insufflation (VATS)
Product used and technique	5 g of talc diluted in 100 mL of saline instilled in chest tube	5 g of talc insufflated with atomizer over lung and pleura
Advantages	Simplicity Performed at bedside Local anesthesia High success rate (>90%)	Complete evacuation of pleural space Multiple biopsies can be performed Homogeneous distribution over all surfaces Loculations of fluid can be broken down Visual placement of chest tubes High success rate (>90%)
Disadvantages	Occasionally associated with pneumonitis Chest tube more likely to become occluded by talc particles	Additional costs (operating room costs) General anesthesia and one-lung ventilation

at bedside, and that it is associated *with high success rates* (>90%). Disadvantages include possible transient ipsilateral pneumonitis (rare cases of adult respiratory distress syndrome have been reported) and the possibility of chest tube occlusion by clumping of the talc. The possible nonhomogeneous distribution of the slurry over the lung does not seem to have an effect on end results.

VATS talc insufflation is also an effective and popular technique. Major disadvantages are the requirement for general anesthesia and one-lung ventilation, the additional costs associated with the use of an operating room, and the fact that *most studies have shown results to be no better than when talc is given as a slurry.* One clear advantage of VATS insufflation is that biopsy of the pleura is possible for pathologic confirmation of the malignant neoplasm. Asbestos-free talc is commercially available, but it must be dry-sterilized before use. In general, 5 g is insufflated through the use of an atomizer.

Doxycycline. Doxycycline is a tetracycline analogue that has a success rate of 50% to 75% when used as a sclerosing agent. It is administered at bedside through the chest tube in a suspension that has 500 mg of doxycycline diluted in 50 to 100 mL of 0.9% saline solution. Ten to 20 mL of lidocaine 1% is often added to the solution because pleuritic pain is a common adverse effect of doxycycline pleurodesis.

Bleomycin. Bleomycin is a chemotherapy agent that has been shown to be effective for control of malignant pleural effusions in 60% to 85%

of patients. The major drawback of bleomycin is its cost, which amounts to approximately 800 dollars (US) for 60 units.

Bleomycin is given through the chest tube. The sclerosing dose is 60 units diluted in 50 to 100 mL of 0.9% saline solution.

Technique of Bedside Pleurodesis (Table 11-51). A large-bore thoracostomy tube (28 Fr or larger) should first be inserted (see Chapter 10, "Closed Drainage and Suction System") under local anesthesia and the pleural fluid evacuated, a process that should be done *slowly because re-expansion pulmonary edema* may occur, especially if the lung has been compressed for prolonged periods of time. The best way to evacuate the pleural space is to remove 200 mL hourly until the space is completely emptied. The chest tube is then connected to an *active suction system,* and a radiograph is obtained to ensure that the pleural space has indeed been emptied and that the lung has re-expanded. The actual pleurodesis is done when daily pleural drainage has been less than 200 to 300 mL/day for at least 1 or 2 days.

Before the pleurodesis is carried out (20 to 30 minutes before), the patient should be premedicated. The suspension (always prepared at the hospital pharmacy) is then *instilled into the chest tube,* which is clamped for 3 to 4 hours after the instillation. During that time, the patient is turned in different positions so that the solution can be distributed over all pleural surfaces. The chest tube is then unclamped, reconnected to an active suction system (-20 cm H_2O), and left in the patient until the daily output decreases below 3 to 5 mL/kg body weight. At such a time, the chest tube is removed.

Technique of Thoracoscopic Pleurodesis (Table 11-52). One of the prerequisites for VATS pleurodesis is the ability of the patient to tolerate a general anesthetic. The procedure is performed with selective one-lung ventilation and the patient in the lateral decubitus position. One or two access ports are used. Initially, the pleural fluid is aspirated, the space is inspected, loculations are broken down, and biopsy samples are taken; 5 g of purified talc is then insufflated with an atomizer in such a way as

11

Special Challenges in Thoracic Surgery

TABLE 11-51

TECHNIQUE OF BEDSIDE PLEURODESIS

Insert a large-bore (28 Fr) thoracostomy tube under local anesthesia.
Slowly empty the pleural space to avoid re-expansion pulmonary edema.
Once the space is emptied, the tube is connected to an active suction system.
A chest radiograph is obtained to make sure the lung is expanded.
Chemical pleurodesis is done when drainage is less than 200 to 300 mL/day.
Make sure the patient is not allergic to the chemical used or to lidocaine.
Premedicate with narcotic-benzodiazepine 30 minutes before pleurodesis.
Instill the pleurodesis solution in the chest tube.
Clamp the chest tube for 3 to 4 hours.
Turn the patient in different positions during the clamping period.
Unclamp the tube and reconnect it to an active suction system (-20 cm H_2O).
Remove the tube when daily output is below 3 to 5 mL/kg body weight.

TABLE 11-52

TECHNIQUE OF THORACOSCOPIC PLEURODESIS

Make sure that the patient can tolerate general anesthesia.
The procedure is done with selective one-lung ventilation and the patient
  in lateral decubitus position.
One or two access ports are used.
Pleural fluid is aspirated, and biopsy samples are taken.
Purified talc is insufflated to cover pleural surfaces homogeneously.
Two thoracostomy tubes are positioned under direct vision.
Tubes are connected to active suction system.
Remove tubes when daily output is below 3 to 5 mL/kg body weight.

to cover the entire pleural (visceral and parietal) surfaces. We recommend leaving *two thoracostomy tubes (28 Fr),* which are positioned under direct vision and connected to an active suction system. These tubes are removed as described with the technique of bedside pleurodesis.

Drainage by Indwelling Pleural Catheter

The use of a semipermanent pleural drain* has been described for the management of malignant pleural effusions. The catheter is inserted percutaneously (on an outpatient basis), and either the patient or a home care visiting nurse can drain the pleural space with the supplied vacuum bottle system, usually every day at the beginning. When not in use, the catheter is coiled under a dressing, thus avoiding the need to carry around a drainage system.

The main advantage (Table 11-53) of using an indwelling catheter is that the entire technique can be done on an *outpatient basis,* thus substantially reducing treatment costs. In addition, there are no adverse effects or morbidities because chemical pleurodesis is not used. Interestingly, a substantial number of patients will achieve spontaneous pleurodesis over time, and at that point, the catheter can be removed.

---

*Pleur$_x$ catheter, Scientific Medics, Denver Biomaterials Inc., Golden, Colo.

TABLE 11-53

**ADVANTAGES AND DISADVANTAGES OF DRAINAGE BY INDWELLING
PLEURAL CATHETER**

Advantages
Does not require hospitalization
No adverse effects, toxicity, or morbidity
Low cost because of no hospitalization
Effective to palliate dyspnea
Possibility of spontaneous pleurodesis

Disadvantages
May be more expensive for patient (has to pay vacuum bottle system)
Possible need for repeated drainage of the effusion

One of the disadvantages of the Pleur$_x$ catheter drainage system is the possible need for repeated drainage of the effusion if spontaneous pleurodesis does not occur. Another disadvantage is that it may become costly if the patient has to replace the vacuum bottle systems and dressing kits at her or his own expense.

Management of Refractory Malignant Pleural Effusion

In some patients, initial failure of chemical pleurodesis is the result of suboptimal technique. In such cases, a *repeated attempt at sclerosis* can be carried out with a different product or approach.

Often, however, treatment failure is related to the patient's having a trapped lung. In those individuals, dyspnea is secondary to compression of the mediastinum and contralateral lung and can thus be helped by emptying the pleural space (even if the ipsilateral lung is trapped). This can be achieved by use of a Pleur$_x$ catheter drainage system or by insertion of a *pleuroperitoneal shunt.* Open pleurectomy is seldom an option because it carries significant morbidity and mortality (6% to 10%) rates, making it difficult to justify as a palliative procedure.

Pleuroperitoneal Shunting

Because the use of pleuroperitoneal shunts requires significant participation of the patient, he or she must be in generally good physical condition, alert, intelligent, and well motivated. The principle of the pleuroperitoneal shunt is that it *transfers pleural fluid from the pleural space into the peritoneum,* where it is reabsorbed. Placement of the shunt usually requires general anesthesia; the advantages and disadvantages of the technique are listed in Table 11-54. The main disadvantages are that the patient's cooperation is needed (must pump 250 to 400 times/day [1 mL of pleural fluid is transferred each time]) and that, over time, shunt failures will occur in approximately 15% of patients. Most shunt failures require shunt removal and replacement.

CONCLUSION

Although malignant pleural effusions are a common problem in the management of cancer patients, the treatment plan is not always clear

11

Special Challenges in Thoracic Surgery

TABLE 11-54

ADVANTAGES AND DISADVANTAGES OF PLEUROPERITONEAL SHUNT FOR MALIGNANT PLEURAL EFFUSIONS

Advantages
Single intervention
Provides reliable and effective palliation of symptoms
Avoids prolonged hospitalization

Disadvantages
High cost of device
Requires general anesthesia
Requires the patient's cooperation and motivation
Late complications (15% of cases) may require shunt removal and replacement

and management often has to be individualized. In the majority of cases, however, treatment options are only palliative. In this setting, therapy should be expedient and effective, cause little discomfort, avoid prolonged hospitalization, and above all prevent recurrence of the effusion.

SUGGESTED READINGS

Review Articles

Hausheer FH, Yarbro JW: Diagnosis and treatment of malignant pleural effusion. Semin Oncol 1985;12:54-75.

LoCicero J 3rd: Thoracoscopic management of malignant pleural effusion. Ann Thorac Surg 1993;56:641-643.

Moores DW: Management of pleural effusions—benign and malignant. Postgraduate Medical Education Course. The New York Society for Thoracic Surgery, 1995.

DeCamp MM, Mentzer SJ, Swanson SJ, Sugarbaker DJ: Malignant effusive disease of the pleura and pericardium. Chest 1997;112: 291s-295s.

Sahn SA: Malignancy metastatic to the pleura. Clin Chest Med 1998;19:351-361.

Grossi F, Pennuci MC, Tixi L, et al: Management of malignant pleural effusions. Drugs 1998;55:47-58.

Antony VB: Pathogenesis of malignant pleural effusions and talc pleurodesis. Pneumologie 1999;53:493-498.

Antunes G, Neville E: Management of malignant pleural effusions. Thorax 2000;55:981-983.

Reeder LB: Malignant pleural effusions. Curr Treat Options Oncol 2001;2:93-96.

Antony VB, Loddenkemper R, Astoul P, et al: Management of malignant pleural effusions. ERS/ATS statement. Eur Respir J 2001;18: 402-419.

Putnam JB: Malignant pleural effusions. Surg Clin North Am 2002;82:867-883.

Thoracoscopy and Malignant Pleural Effusions

Yim APC, Chan ATC, Lee TW, et al: Thoracoscopic talc insufflation versus talc slurry for symptomatic malignant pleural effusion. Ann Thorac Surg 1996;62:1655-1658.

Danby CA, Adebonojo SA, Moritz DM: Video-assisted talc pleurodesis for malignant pleural effusions utilizing local anesthesia and IV sedation. Chest 1998;113:739-742.

de Campos JR, Vargas FS, de Campos Werebe E, et al: Thoracoscopy talc poudrage. A 15-year experience. Chest 2001;119:801-806.

Schulze M, Boehle AS, Kurdow R, et al: Effective treatment of malignant pleural effusion by minimal invasive thoracic surgery: thoracoscopic talc pleurodesis and pleuroperitoneal shunts in 101 patients. Ann Thorac Surg 2001;71:1809-1812.

Cardillo G, Facciolo F, Carbone L, et al: Long-term follow-up of video-assisted talc pleurodesis in malignant recurrent pleural effusions. Eur J Cardiothorac Surg 2002;21:302-306.

Chemical Pleurodesis

Sanchez-Armengol A, Rodriguez-Panadero F: Survival and talc pleurodesis in metastatic pleural carcinoma, revisited. Report of 125 cases. Chest 1993;104:1482-1485.

Walker-Renard PB, Vaughan LM, Sahn SA: Chemical pleurodesis for malignant pleural effusions. Ann Intern Med 1994;120:56-64.

Kennedy L, Rusch VW, Strange C, et al: Pleurodesis using talc slurry. Chest 1994;106:342-346.

Petrou M, Kaplan D, Goldstraw P: Management of recurrent malignant pleural effusions. The complementary role of talc pleurodesis and pleuroperitoneal shunting. Cancer 1995;75:801-805.

Zimmer PW, Hill M, Casey K, et al: Prospective randomized trial of talc slurry vs. bleomycin in pleurodesis for symptomatic malignant pleural effusions. Chest 1997;112:430-434.

Martinez-Moragon E, Aparicio J, Sanchis J, et al: Malignant pleural effusion: prognostic factors for survival and response to chemical pleurodesis in a series of 120 cases. Respiration 1998;65:108-113.

Patz EF, McAdams HP, Erasmus JJ, et al: Sclerotherapy for malignant pleural effusions. A prospective randomized trial of bleomycin vs. doxycycline with small-bore catheter drainage. Chest 1998;113:1305-1311.

Patz EF Jr.: Malignant pleural effusions. Recent advances and ambulatory sclerotherapy. Chest 1998;113:74s-77s.

Saffran L, Ost DE, Fein AM, Schiff MJ: Outpatient pleurodesis of malignant pleural effusions using a small-bore pigtail catheter. Chest 2000;118:417-421.

Parulekar W, DiPrimio G, Matzinger F, et al: Use of small-bore vs. large-bore chest tubes for treatment of malignant pleural effusions. Chest 2001;120:19-25.

Bernard A, de Dompsure RB, Hagry O, Favre JP: Early and late mortality after pleurodesis for malignant pleural effusion. Ann Thorac Surg 2002;74:213-217.

Pleuroperitoneal Shunt

Lee KA, Harvey JC, Reich H, Beattie EJ: Management of malignant pleural effusions with pleuroperitoneal shunting. J Am Coll Surg 1994;178:586-588.

Genc O, Petrou M, Ladas G, Goldstraw P: The long-term morbidity of pleuroperitoneal shunts in the management of recurrent malignant effusions. Eur J Cardiothorac Surg 2000;18:143-146.

Pleural Catheter

Putnam JB Jr., Walsh GL, Swisher SG, et al: Outpatient management of malignant pleural effusion by a chronic indwelling pleural catheter. Ann Thorac Surg 2000;69:369-375.

11

Special Challenges in Thoracic Surgery

Smart JM, Tung KT: Initial experiences with a long-term indwelling tunnelled pleural catheter for the management of malignant pleural effusion. Clin Radiol 2000;55:882-884.

Pien GW, Gant MJ, Washam CL, Sterman DH: Use of an implantable pleural catheter for trapped lung syndrome in patients with malignant pleural effusion. Chest 2001;119:1641-1646.

Others

Burrows CM, Mathews C, Colt HG: Predicting survival in patients with recurrent symptomatic malignant pleural effusions. An assessment of the prognostic values of physiologic, morphologic, and quality of life measures of extent of disease. Chest 2000;117:73-78.

Fujita A, Takabatake H, Tagaki S, Sekine K: Combination chemotherapy in patients with malignant pleural effusions from non–small cell lung cancer. Cisplatin, ifosfamide, and irinotecan with recombinant human granulocyte colony-stimulating factor support. Chest 2001;119:340-343.

MANAGEMENT OF THE PATIENT WITH CHRONIC INTERCOSTAL NEURALGIA

The concepts of post-thoracotomy pain and of its management are complex but, at the same time, fascinating. Unfortunately, chronic intercostal neuralgia is often dismissed as being unimportant, even if the pain has been persistent, recurring, and severe for several months or even years. Most surgeons find the therapy of these syndromes frustrating because in their view, the results are unsatisfactory.

Once the diagnosis of chronic intercostal neuralgia has been confirmed, treating physicians must have a systematic plan of evaluation, including ruling out recurrent neoplastic disease as the cause of pain. Indeed, they must *understand the pathophysiology* of the pain syndrome and have a *working diagnosis* if they hope to provide successful therapy. In general, management of these patients benefits from a multidisciplinary approach.

DEFINITION AND INCIDENCE

The International Association for the Study of Pain defines the post-thoracotomy pain syndrome *as pain that persists or recurs along a thoracotomy scar at least 2 months after operation.* Although its true incidence is unknown, mild chest pain without repercussion on daily life is common, with an incidence of approximately 50%. Severe disabling pain is much less common, affecting less than 5% to 10% of patients.

PATHOGENESIS AND CLINICAL FEATURES

Different causes of chronic post-thoracotomy pain syndrome have been described. In any given patient, one must distinguish *pain as a "symptom"* (somatic pain) from *pain as a "disease"* (neuropathic pain) (Table 11-55).

TABLE 11-55

PATHOGENESIS OF CHRONIC POST-THORACOTOMY PAIN SYNDROME

Pain as a "symptom" (somatic pain)
Pain related to surgical trauma to the chest wall (skin, bone, muscles)
Myofascial pain syndrome
Shoulder bursitis or tendinitis
Disease recurrence or progression
Chronic empyemas

Pain as a "disease" (neurogenic pain)
Entrapment of nerve fibers in scar tissue (intercostal neuralgia)
Intercostal neuroma
Sympathetic dystrophy

11

Special Challenges in Thoracic Surgery

Somatic chronic pain syndromes originate in the muscles or bones (ribs) of the chest wall. Unrecognized rib fractures, for instance, may be involved in the production of pain. Similarly, section of the richly innervated chest wall muscles may generate chronic musculoskeletal pain syndromes. A specific type of musculoskeletal post-thoracotomy pain known as *myofascial pain syndrome* has also been described. In these cases, patients have trigger points or localized areas in thoracic muscles, such as the serratus anterior or latissimus dorsi, that produce pain referred to distant sites on palpation.

Somatic painful conditions may also result from associated conditions such as shoulder bursitis and tendinitis. Somatic pain may finally be related to recurrent carcinoma in the chest wall or pleura. Often, these patients will *have had a pain-free interval* followed by recurrent pain usually associated with significant debility. Chronic empyemas may also present with persistent pain often associated with low-grade fever and weight loss.

When no somatic cause can be found, the chronic pain can be dealt with as a disease process. These forms of post-thoracotomy pain syndromes *are usually neurogenic in origin* (Table 11-56). The pain may result from *entrapment of intercostal nerves in the scar tissue;* in such cases, light touch produces intense radiating pain accompanied by a burning sensation if a reflex sympathetic dystrophy is associated. Typical features are those of burning, dysesthetic, and lancinating sensation over the incision. Because intercostal nerve dermatomes reach the upper abdominal wall, patients may also complain of local swelling, which is due to bulging of paralyzed or atrophied muscles. This type of pain is often aggravated by carrying heavy objects or is worse in humid and cold climatic conditions. In some individuals, pain is sufficiently severe to *become a true disability* in which depression, insomnia, and asthenia coexist.

Another cause of chronic post-thoracotomy pain *is an intercostal nerve neuroma.* A palpable mass in the wound, the loss of pinprick sensation over the skin, and pain on palpation may be helpful in establishing this diagnosis.

TABLE 11-56

SYMPTOMS CHARACTERISTIC OF NEUROPATHIC PAIN

Allodynia	Pain caused by nonpainful stimulus
Analgesia	Absence of pain in response to painful stimulus
Dysesthesia	Unpleasant abnormal sensation, occurring spontaneously or provoked
Hyperalgesia	Exaggerated response to normal pain stimulus
Hyperesthesia	Increased sensitivity to all types of stimulation
Hypoesthesia	Reduction of sensitivity to any type of stimulation
Neuralgia	Pain in the cutaneous distribution of a nerve
Paresthesia	Abnormal sensation, occurring spontaneously or provoked

Sympathetic dystrophy is uncommon, and these patients present with burning pain often associated with decreased skin temperature and increased sweating.

RISK FACTORS FOR CHRONIC POST-THORACOTOMY PAIN SYNDROME (TABLE 11-57)

Even if there is little in the way of scientific data, it is likely that *the extent of local tissue damage* during the original thoracotomy is closely related to the incidence of post-thoracotomy pain syndromes. Accordingly, minimizing soft tissue and skeletal trauma may be helpful in reducing the incidence, severity, and duration of pain. These injuries include direct intercostal nerve damage from excessive rib spreading, posterior rib fractures, and anterior costochondral separations. Whether deliberate rib resection (whole rib or

TABLE 11-57

RISK FACTORS FOR CHRONIC POSTOPERATIVE PAIN SYNDROMES
AND PROPHYLAXIS

Risk Factor	Prophylaxis
Likely involved	
Tissue damage during thoracotomy	
Excessive rib spreading	Avoid excessive rib spreading
Rib fractures	?Deliberate rib resection; slow opening of intercostal space
Tissue damage during VATS	Avoid excessive torquing of instruments during operations
	Use small instruments
Pain control during early postoperative period	Preemptive analgesia and optimal pain control early
Possibly involved	
Division of large chest wall muscles (latissimus dorsi and serratus anterior)	?Use of muscle-sparing thoracotomy
Use of pericostal sutures during closure	?Use of rib punch instrumentation for thoracotomy closure

small fragment of posterior rib) to allow rib spreading with less chance of rib fractures lowers the incidence of chronic post-thoracotomy pain syndromes is unknown. Similarly, the avoidance of division of latissimus dorsi and serratus anterior muscles *through muscle-sparing thoracotomies* (see Chapter 5) *does not* seem to affect the incidence of long-standing post-thoracotomy pain. It is generally agreed, however, that muscle-sparing incisions, whether through vertical or lateral thoracotomies, will lower the incidence of shoulder-related pain syndromes.

The technique of closure of the intercostal space may, to some extent, also be responsible for chronic pain syndromes. *Pericostal sutures, for instance, may damage intercostal nerves,* and some authors recommend the use of a "rib punch" to drill small holes in the rib, thus avoiding trauma to the intercostal nerves. Unfortunately, intercostal nerve anatomy is unpredictable so that avoidance of trauma is not always possible. In addition, intercostal nerves travel in a closed compartment formed by innermost and internal intercostal muscles so that any condition resulting in the *accumulation of blood or serum* can cause a compartment syndrome with resultant effects on the nerve.

VATS techniques do not seem to lower the incidence of chronic pain syndromes because intercostal nerve injuries as well as soft tissue and rib damage can occur from trocar incision or excessive torquing of instruments during the procedure. Indeed, chronic pain syndromes may be more common after VATS procedures when large instruments are pushed into position through small incisions. Strategic intercostal access and use of smaller diameter instruments may potentially reduce such problems.

Some authors have shown that patients are *more likely to have chronic pain syndromes if they experienced significant pain during the early postoperative period.* These findings highlight the importance of preemptive analgesia as well as of optimal pain control during the first 2 or 3 postoperative days.

CLINICAL EVALUATION

All patients presenting with chronic post-thoracotomy pain syndromes must be thoroughly evaluated by clinical history, complete physical examination, and a work-up that includes a chest radiograph, a CT scan or MRI, and a bone scan. If the cause of pain is identified as being recurrent cancer or an infectious complication, it can be appropriately treated. The use of CT scan is most important for patients whose thoracic pain has recurred after a painless interval and for patients with systemic symptoms such as weight loss. Finding no such processes is a reassurance for the patient, and it often becomes an effective therapeutic measure.

When no specific cause can be identified, it is important to obtain details about the location and severity of the pain as well as some information about precipitating factors such as movement, tactile stimulations, cough, climatic variations, and need for analgesics. A social worker or psychologist is usually involved in this part of the evaluation.

Physical examination may reveal skin or muscle changes, intense pain produced by light touching of specific areas, or even infectious or cancer complications such as fluctuating or solid masses.

MANAGEMENT

The management of patients with post-thoracotomy pain syndromes is difficult and often benefits from a systematic, integrated, and multidisciplinary approach. Indeed, in-hospital well-structured "pain clinic" can play a key role in development of an appropriate therapeutic plan. Management must be done with the understanding that pain is a *subjective symptom* and that we often lack objective evidence to explain this symptom.

Local Measures (Table 11-58)

Local measures represent first-line therapy and can be valuable. Intercostal nerve blocks by a *local anesthetic* (e.g., bupivacaine) with or without steroids can be useful for the treatment of intercostal neuropathic pain syndromes or of pain due to an identifiable musculoskeletal sequela such as a malunited rib fracture. Nerve blocks can be done paravertebrally over multiple intercostal spaces above and below the involved dermatomes or directly over the area that is painful. Although a single session of nerve blocking seldom eradicates pain on a prolonged basis, *repeated infiltrations* (at least three times) are often effective in doing so. If an intercostal neuroma is documented, a small amount of local anesthetic may be injected into it, and if pain is relieved, the procedure can be repeated with the injection of a neurolytic solution. Sympathetic dystrophy may have to be treated by paravertebral sympathetic blocks, nerve root blocks, or an epidural infusion.

Other local measures that are valuable include physical therapy to strengthen muscle tone and improve shoulder mobilization, heat massages, and ultrasound treatments. Transcutaneous electrical nerve stimulation (TENS) is also recommended, especially in the presence of *myofascial pain syndromes*. It is easy to implement and can be effective for some patients. Other simple measures that are cheap and accessible include frequent baths and showers and the application of hot and cold. On occasion, patients may be referred to private clinics for acupuncture or manipulations.

Neurolytic procedures, such as alcoholization and cryoanalgesia, and neuroablative techniques through wound exploration and nerve excision

---

TABLE 11-58

LOCAL MEASURES APPLICABLE TO THE TREATMENT OF CHRONIC PAIN SYNDROMES

Nerve blocks with local anesthetics with or without steroids
Physical therapy
Transcutaneous electrical nerve stimulation
Heat massages, ultrasound treatments
Heat and cold treatments (baths, showers)
Acupuncture, manipulations
Neurolytic and neuroablative procedures

should *almost never be attempted.* They are associated with significant risks of creating further damage and increased pain.

Systemic Drug Therapy (Table 11-59)

Somatic Pain

Somatic pain can be treated with acetaminophen and opioid analgesics. Opioids are particularly effective, but they often have side effects such as *mood alteration, constipation,* and *drug abuse.* In addition, patients may develop drug tolerance so that dosage has to be increased. In general, opioids are most useful when they are part of multifaceted strategies. Patients with a history of substance abuse are eligible for treatment, but boundaries must be set.

In general, tolerance and psychological dependency are less common with the use of long-acting opioids such as morphine continuous release (MS Contin) and oxycodone sustained release (OxyContin). The dosage of these medications should be based on the amount of short-acting opioids that the patient was taking at the time of presentation. Dosages can be decreased when opioids are given in combination with other drugs such as antidepressants or anticonvulsant medications.

Patients receiving long-acting opioids should be prescribed *stool softeners and be advised to drink large amounts of liquids* to avoid dehydration.

Nonsteroidal anti-inflammatory drugs are usually ineffective for management of chronic post-thoracotomy pain syndromes. Their use can be associated with significant side effects.

Neuropathic Pain

Tricyclic antidepressants such as amitriptyline (Elavil) are useful in patients with burning or dysesthetic neuropathic pain. They are effective at a dose lower than that required for antidepressant therapy and are often given in association with long-acting opioids. The starting dose is 10 to 25 mg at bedtime, increasing by 10 to 25 mg every 3 to 7 days to a maximum of 150 to 200 mg daily. *Maximal effectiveness is usually not seen for 2 to 3 weeks into the treatment,* and this must be discussed with patients.

11

Special Challenges in Thoracic Surgery

TABLE 11-59

DRUG MANAGEMENT OF CHRONIC POST-THORACOTOMY SYNDROMES

Somatic pain
Acetaminophen
Long-acting opioids (morphine sulfate [MS Contin], oxycodone [OxyContin])

Neuropathic pain
Tricyclic antidepressants (amitriptyline [Elavil])
Anticonvulsants (carbamazepine [Tegretol], phenytoin [Dilantin],
 gabapentin [Neurontin])
Antispasmodic (baclofen)
Corticosteroids (prednisone)

Anticonvulsants such as carbamazepine (Tegretol), phenytoin (Dilantin), and gabapentin (Neurontin) are *drugs of choice when lancinating neuropathic pain is a component.* Carbamazepine is the most commonly used anticonvulsant; the starting dose is 200 to 400 mg three times a day to a maximum of 1000 mg/day. Gabapentin (300 to 3600 mg/day) can be associated with numerous side effects, such as somnolence, dizziness, ataxia, and peripheral edema.

Baclofen (Lioresal) *is an antispasmodic* drug with weak anticonvulsant properties that has been shown to be efficacious in neuropathic pain with or without muscle spasms. The drug is started at doses of 5 mg three times a day; it can be increased every third day to a maximum of 80 mg/day. Side effects include somnolence, tiredness, and hypotension.

Corticosteroids may be indicated for patients with severe refractory neuropathic pain. Prednisone is started at doses of 5 to 10 mg twice daily (low dose). Potentially significant side effects *should be monitored*.

Other Treatments

An important treatment strategy is to encourage and support the patient in his or her return to normal daily activities. The patient must often accept some degree of pain during rehabilitation with the hope that given time, *most of it will disappear*.

Psychological counseling addresses the symptoms of depression and anxiety and teaches techniques for stress management. Patients are also instructed in cognitive and behavioral techniques to improve their interpretation of and reaction to chronic pain. These include techniques of relaxation, which often involve the spouse. Indeed, *involving the spouse* in this part of the treatment *is essential to its success.*

Patients must be reassured that their chronic pain is benign (noncancer pain) but that it may never completely disappear although its level of intensity will become easier to control as time goes by.

RESULTS OF TREATMENT

By the combination of various therapeutic approaches and use of a multidisciplinary strategy, nearly all patients with neuropathic chronic post-thoracotomy pain syndrome will be improved during a period of months. Although patients must understand that a certain level of pain is likely to persist, *significant pain relief* can be provided to more than 95% of patients.

CONCLUSION

Persistent chest wall pain is common after thoracotomy, but it is usually not severe and will disappear over time. When pain is significant and debilitating, cancer recurrence must first be ruled out; treatment should then be individualized and directed toward the likely source of pain. In all patients with neuropathic pain syndromes, physical treatments and physical rehabilitation are essential if patients are to return to normal life.

It is important for the surgeon to understand that prophylactic measures applied at the time of thoracotomy may significantly decrease the incidence of chronic post-thoracotomy pain syndromes.

SUGGESTED READINGS

Review Articles

d'Amours RH, Riegler FX, Little AG: Pathogenesis and management of persistent postthoracotomy pain. Chest Surg Clin North Am 1998;8: 703-721.

Rogers ML, Duffy JP: Surgical aspects of post-thoracotomy pain. Eur J Cardiothoracic Surg 2000;18:711-716.

Haythornthwaite JA, Benrud-Larson LM: Psychological aspects of neuropathic pain. Clin J Pain 2000;16:S101-S105.

Treatment

Roesch R, Ulrich DE: Physical therapy management in the treatment of chronic pain. Phys Ther 1980;60:53-57.

Covington EC: Anticonvulsants for neuropathic pain and detoxification. Cleve Clin J Med 1998;65(suppl 1):S1-21–S1-29; discussion S1-45–S1-47.

Guay DR: Adjunctive agents in the management of chronic pain. Pharmacotherapy 2001;21:1070-1081.

Case Series

Dajczman E, Gordon A, Kreisman H, Wolkove N: Long-term postthoracotomy pain. Chest 1991;99:270-274.

Conacher ID: Therapist and therapies for post-thoracotomy neuralgia. Pain 1992;48:409-412.

Landreneau RJ, Mack MJ, Hazelrigg SR, et al: Prevalence of chronic pain after pulmonary resection by thoracotomy or video-assisted thoracic surgery. J Thorac Cardiovasc Surg 1994;107:1079-1086.

Keller SM, Carp NZ, Levy MN, Rosen SM: Chronic postthoracotomy pain. J Cardiovasc Surg 1994;35:161-164.

Richardson J, Sabanathan S, Mearns AJ, et al: Post-thoracotomy neuralgia. Pain Clin 1994;7:87-97.

Perttunen K, Tasmuth T, Kalso E: Chronic pain after thoracic surgery: a follow-up study. Acta Anaesthesiol Scand 1999;43:563-567.

Others

Moore DC: Anatomy of the intercostal nerve: its importance during thoracic surgery. Am J Surg 1982;144:371-373.

Katz J, Jackson M, Kavanagh BP, Sandler AN: Acute pain after thoracic surgery predicts long-term post-thoracotomy pain. Clin J Pain 1996;12:50-55.

MANAGEMENT OF THE PATIENT WITH ESOPHAGEAL RUPTURE

Esophageal perforations are surgical emergencies for which early diagnosis is the most important element for good outcome. Indeed, mortality rates as high as 50% are commonly reported when treatment is delayed by more than 24 hours. Because management strategies also depend on the *site of perforation* (cervical, thoracic), the cause of perforation, the clinical presentation, and the presence or absence of comorbidities, each patient must be assessed on his or her own and treatment individualized.

In general, esophageal perforations should *be surgically explored* and the *site of perforation primarily repaired,* even if the interval from perforation to repair is longer than 24 to 48 hours. In highly selected patients with contained perforations, minimal symptoms, and absence of sepsis, however, nonoperative management can also be successful.

ETIOLOGY

Most esophageal perforations are iatrogenic and related to esophagoscopy or esophageal bougienage. They can occur in the cervical or thoracic esophagus.

Common Causes of Esophageal Perforation (Table 11-60)

The majority of esophageal perforations are related to *instrumentation of the esophagus.* Their incidence is approximately 1 in 10,000 procedures whether biopsy specimens are taken or not. The areas at greatest risk are the piriform fossa and the cervical esophagus (cricopharyngeal region), especially in patients who have associated osteophytes of the cervical spine (level of C5-6 vertebrae).

Dilatation of strictures or tumors and pneumatic dilatation for achalasia can also rupture the esophageal wall (incidence of 1% to 5% with pneumatic dilatation). Often forgotten, the placement of nasogastric tubes, Sengstaken-Blakemore tubes, and endoesophageal stenting prostheses,

---

TABLE 11-60

COMMON CAUSES OF ESOPHAGEAL RUPTURE AND THEIR RELATIVE INCIDENCE

Instrumental (50%)
  Esophagoscopy with or without biopsy
  Bougienage for strictures
  Pneumatic dilatation for achalasia
  Placement of intraesophageal tubes (nasogastric, Sengstaken-Blakemore, stents)

Traumatic (20%)
  Blunt trauma (cervical or thoracic)
  Penetrating trauma (cervical or thoracic)
  Foreign bodies (dental prosthesis, fish bones)
  Caustic injuries

Spontaneous (Boerhaave) (15%)

Postoperative (10%)
  Iatrogenic injuries from operations involving the esophagus or structures adjacent
    to the esophagus (thyroid, lung, stomach)

Neoplastic (5%)
  Spontaneous
  Post–radiation therapy

especially those of the *push-through type,* can also be the source of esophageal perforation.

Blunt cervical or thoracic traumas can cause free esophageal ruptures, but these types of injuries are uncommon when compared to post-traumatic tracheoesophageal fistulas (see next, "Management of the Adult Patient with a Tracheoesophageal Fistula"). Esophageal injuries due to penetrating neck trauma are fairly common and are often associated with great vessels and airway penetrations. Esophageal perforation can also be secondary to the *ingestion of foreign bodies,* such as fish and chicken bones, dental prostheses, and flip-top tabs from aluminum cans. Meat impaction is not in itself a cause of perforation, but treatment of late impactions by trials of endoscopic removal can lead to esophageal wall penetration. Traumatic perforation can finally be associated with the ingestion of *caustic substances.*

Spontaneous esophageal perforations (Boerhaave syndrome) are characterized by *longitudinal rents of various lengths nearly always on the left posterolateral wall of the esophagus just above the gastroesophageal junction.* The rupture is related to a sudden and rapid rise in intraesophageal pressure associated with a failure of relaxation of the upper esophageal sphincter. Although these types of perforations classically occur during the act of forceful vomiting, they can also be seen during childbirth or weightlifting. In most such patients, the underlying esophagus is normal both anatomically and physiologically.

Intraoperative iatrogenic injuries to the esophagus can occur during surgeries involving the esophagus itself or those involving a neighboring structure, such as the thyroid gland, the stomach, or the lung. Most reported cases of esophageal trauma during pulmonary resection have been associated with pneumonectomy and extensive mediastinal node dissection.

Other less common causes of esophageal perforation are those related to esophageal carcinomas, which can either rupture primarily or rupture during or after radiation therapy.

Etiology by Site of Perforation (Table 11-61)

Perforation of the Cervical Esophagus

Most pharyngeal or cervical esophagus perforations are secondary to instrumentation, especially the use of the *rigid esophagoscope.* They can

11

Special Challenges in Thoracic Surgery

TABLE 11-61	
COMMON CAUSES BY SITE OF PERFORATION	
Site of Perforation	**Most Common Cause**
Cervical esophagus	Esophagoscopy
	Foreign bodies
	Penetrating trauma
Thoracic esophagus	Dilatation of stricture, achalasia
	Stent placement
	Spontaneous (Boerhaave)
	Operative iatrogenic

also result from swallowing of foreign bodies, particularly in mentally disturbed individuals. In the remaining patients, cervical esophageal rupture is the result of stab or gunshot wounds; such injuries are often discovered at the time of surgical exploration.

Perforation of the Thoracic Esophagus

Most perforations of the thoracic esophagus also result from *instrumentation,* including the use of bougies to dilate strictures and of pneumatic dilatation for the treatment of achalasia. Areas of the thoracic esophagus at risk of perforation during esophagoscopy are the distal esophagus just proximal to the gastroesophageal junction and the segment of esophagus located over the left main bronchus.

Other causes include perforations during the placement of endoluminal stents and those related to *intraoperative injuries,* such as may occur during mediastinoscopy (nodal biopsy in subcarinal space), pneumonectomy, extensive mediastinal nodal dissection (electrocautery injuries), or operations for gastroesophageal reflux. Spontaneous perforations *always occur* in the thoracic esophagus above the diaphragm (80% to 90%) or more proximally in the lower third of the thoracic esophagus (10% to 20%).

CONSEQUENCES OF ESOPHAGEAL PERFORATIONS

The immediate consequences of esophageal perforations depend on the site of perforation (cervical, thoracic) and its cause. Eventually, however, the infectious process initiated by soft tissue contamination from the esophagus will *reach the mediastinum* through retrovisceral spaces (Fig. 11-10). In the end, this spread of infection will result in a *diffuse necrotizing mediastinitis,* which, if left untreated, will almost invariably lead to systemic sepsis, multiorgan failure, and death.

When the cervical esophagus is ruptured, soft tissue contamination is from saliva and oropharyngeal flora. Because most such perforations are secondary to instrumentation and occur in fasting patients, the extent of contamination tends to be initially limited. The compact nature of the cervical tissue planes also tends to prevent wide dissemination of the infection and local soft tissue abscesses will often form before the infection reaches the mediastinum.

In perforations of the thoracic esophagus, the mediastinitis occurs at an early stage not only because the intrathoracic esophagus is *located within the posterior mediastinum* but also because the esophagus is surrounded by loose areolar tissues that are unable to contain the spread of infection. This phenomenon is even worse in spontaneous perforations, in which violent vomiting, which classically occurs on a full stomach, will forcefully eject the gastric contents directly into the mediastinum or even the pleural space. When the integrity of the mediastinal pleura is lost, pneumothoraces and empyemas will occur, often bilaterally.

DIAGNOSIS (TABLE 11-62)

The early diagnosis of esophageal rupture can be difficult to make because the clinical findings are often nonspecific. Acute pain over the area of

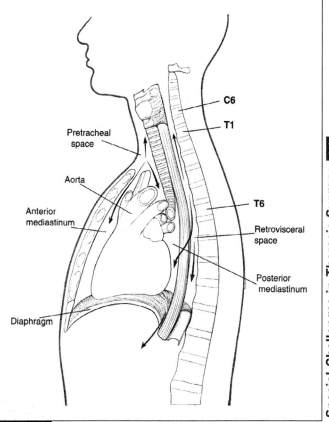

FIG. 11-10

Diagram showing pathways for spread of infection to mediastinum and pleural spaces after esophageal perforation. *(Courtesy of Doctor Stanley C. Fell.)*

TABLE 11-62

FACTS ABOUT THE DIAGNOSIS OF ESOPHAGEAL PERFORATION

Early diagnosis can be difficult.

Delayed detection results in higher morbidity and mortality.

Acute pain in the area of perforation is the most common symptom.

Initial neck or chest radiographs are often interpreted as normal in perforation of the cervical esophagus.

Contrast study with Gastrografin has abnormal findings in 90% of cases.

perforation is probably the *most common clinical finding* (90% of patients), followed by *fever* and *local subcutaneous crepitation* (subcutaneous emphysema). The presence of these symptoms in a patient with a prior history of instrumentation or forceful vomiting should definitely suggest the possibility of esophageal perforation.

Plain radiographs of the chest or neck can confirm the clinical suspicion of perforation by showing *air in the mediastinum or prevertebral spaces,* although these initial films are often interpreted as being normal. Contrast study of the esophagus with water-soluble solutions such as Gastrografin will have abnormal findings *in 90% of cases*. If the patient is already intubated or is uncooperative or very ill, the contrast material can be introduced in a nasogastric tube positioned above the presumed site of perforation. If the Gastrografin study shows no perforation but the diagnosis is still likely, a barium swallow examination (standing or supine) might show the tear. Barium should be used with some caution, however, because it can initiate an intense mediastinal reaction with secondary fibrosis.

If, at the end, the diagnosis remains in doubt, flexible esophageal endoscopy should be done, even if small perforations can be missed or the procedure may extend an initially small tear into a longer one. Many surgeons also believe that even if the diagnosis of esophageal perforation has been made by esophagography, endoscopic evaluation should always be carried out to directly visualize the nature and extent of the injury as well as to determine the presence or absence of esophageal disorders such as peptic strictures or carcinomas.

CT scanning is useful to rule out other processes, such as aortic dissections, that may also present with chest pain as well as to determine the extent of mediastinal contamination.

Clinical Features and Diagnosis of Perforation of Cervical Esophagus

Instrumental cervical perforations are characterized by *cervical pain, neck stiffness, and cervical swelling* due to the presence of subcutaneous emphysema. In penetrating injuries, the clinical picture may be highlighted by signs of associated airway injury (75% of patients), such as respiratory distress and obvious air leakage from the wound, or by signs of great vessel injury, such as massive hemorrhage. Fever and leukocytosis develop rapidly, and the radiograph may show air in the prevertebral space extending up to the neck and down to the posterior mediastinum. In most cases, the diagnosis is easily confirmed by Gastrografin study.

Clinical Features and Diagnosis of Perforation of Thoracic Esophagus

Patients with Boerhaave syndrome nearly always present with the *classic history* of having ingested a large meal, followed by forceful vomiting, chest pain (usually retrosternal), and dyspnea. In many cases, however, this history will be obtained from relatives because the patient is in shock, is in severe pain, is intubated, or has received large amounts of narcotics. Even initially, chest radiographs are usually abnormal; they may show air and widening of the mediastinum, pneumothoraces, and unilateral (left > right) or bilateral pleural effusions. Despite such apparently typical findings, the diagnosis is delayed by 12 hours *in more than 80% of patients,* mostly because the initial symptoms are wrongly interpreted as being due to a myocardial infarct, aortic dissection, perforated peptic ulcer, or other conditions.

In virtually every case, the site of esophageal leakage can accurately be identified by Gastrografin contrast swallow study. If the patient has a pleural effusion, thoracentesis will show a cloudy or even purulent exudate with high amylase content derived from saliva. Indeed, this feature is almost pathognomonic of esophageal perforation.

Differences in clinical features between patients with perforation of the cervical esophagus and those with perforation of the thoracic esophagus are listed in Table 11-63. Overall, the most significant and important difference is that *systemic symptoms* including fever, sepsis, hemodynamic instability, and shock are a *lot more common* with perforations of the thoracic esophagus.

The typical feature of intramural esophageal perforation (Mallory-Weiss syndrome) on contrast swallow study is a thin linear extravasation of contrast substance parallel to the esophageal lumen without actual extravasation in the mediastinum.

MANAGEMENT

The management of esophageal ruptures continues to evolve. Most surgeons now recommend primary closure of the site of perforation even in cases in which the diagnosis has been made several days after the event. Similarly, many surgeons advocate a trial of nonoperative management if the leak is contained and the patient has minimal symptoms, especially in the context of instrumental perforations. Improvements in techniques of nutrition, both enteral and parenteral, as well as the introduction of better antibiotics to control sepsis of oropharyngeal origin have also helped reduce morbidity and mortality.

TABLE 11-63

CLINICAL DIFFERENCES IN PERFORATIONS OF THE CERVICAL
AND THORACIC ESOPHAGUS

	Cervical Esophagus	Thoracic Esophagus
Clinical features		
Pain	+	+++
Crepitation over neck (subcutaneous emphysema)	+++	+
Systemic symptoms	+	++++
Radiographic features		
Mediastinal emphysema	0/+	+++
Deep cervical emphysema	++	++
Pneumothorax/pleural effusion	0	+++

Scale: 0, none; +, mild; ++, moderate; +++, severe; ++++, very severe.

TABLE 11-64
OBJECTIVES OF TREATMENT IN PATIENTS WITH ESOPHAGEAL PERFORATION
Drain the infected spaces*
Prevent further contamination by repairing the site of rupture
Restore esophageal continuity
Re-expand the lung
Prevent gastroesophageal reflux
Maintain nutritional support
Maintain ventilatory support
Give appropriate and specific antibiotics
*Retroesophageal cervical, posterior mediastinum, right or left pleural spaces.

In management of patients with esophageal perforations, the primary objectives of therapy (Table 11-64) are to drain the infected spaces, to prevent further contamination of those spaces, and to restore normal esophageal continuity. Secondary objectives are to maintain adequate hydration and nutrition throughout the ordeal and to provide the patient with specific antibiotherapy.

Cervical Perforation

Once cervical esophageal perforation is suspected, oral intake must cease, nasogastric suction is commenced, and antibiotics for oral flora contamination are given parenterally. When the diagnosis is confirmed, surgical exploration (Table 11-65) should be carried out without delay.

The operation is done through a *neck incision* extending along the anterior border of the sternocleidomastoid muscle. If the site of perforation is identified, it is primarily repaired with absorbable sutures. If it cannot be located, the retroesophageal prevertebral space is developed downward to the posterior mediastinum, allowing copious irrigations of the entire area and insertion of two soft suction drains (Fig. 11-11). In some cases of late diagnosis and significant tissue necrosis, the wound can be packed and left open until the leak has sealed and the local tissues granulate. In patients with penetrating trauma and associated airway injury, a pedicle flap of omohyoid or strap muscle should be interposed between the two sites of repair.

Oral intake is withheld until cervical drainage has ceased or until the leak has sealed or the fistula output is minimal as documented by contrast

TABLE 11-65
OPERATIVE APPROACH TO CERVICAL ESOPHAGEAL PERFORATION
Oblique incision along anterior border of sternocleidomastoid muscle on the side of perforation
Lateral retraction of carotid sheath and sternocleidomastoid muscle and medial retraction of trachea
If perforation is seen, repair with absorbable suture*
Bluntly develop the prevertebral space and insert two soft suction drains
*Primary repair is not a requirement for successful treatment.

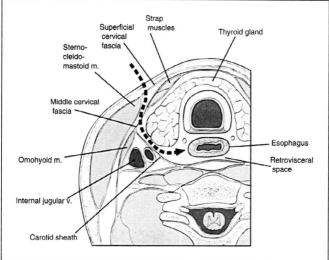

FIG. 11-11

Operative technique for cervical mediastinal drainage. *(Courtesy of Doctor Stanley C. Fell.)*

swallow study. In some cases when chronicity is expected, the insertion of *gastrostomy and feeding jejunostomy tubes* should be strongly considered. Intravenous antibiotics are continued for at least 1 week after cervical drainage has stopped.

Thoracic Perforation

Because delays in instituting treatment of perforations of the thoracic esophagus are associated with significant morbidity and mortality, bringing the patient to operation *must be a top priority* once the diagnosis is confirmed. The "golden period" for closure of thoracic esophageal perforations is the first 24 hours. Preoperative supportive measures such as hydration, administration of intravenous antibiotics, nasogastric intubation, and tube thoracostomy when a pleural effusion is present must be done expeditiously because prolonged attempts at resuscitation are generally counterproductive.

Upper and middle third thoracic perforations are best approached through a right fourth or fifth intercostal space thoracotomy; lower third perforations are best approached through a left sixth or seventh space posterolateral thoracotomy. Several options (Table 11-66) are available to the surgeon.

Direct Primary Repair of the Perforation

This approach is preferred even in treatment of esophageal leaks diagnosed more than 24 hours after the event.

TABLE 11-66

SURGICAL MANAGEMENT OF PERFORATIONS OF INTRATHORACIC ESOPHAGUS

Surgical Option	Comment
Primary repair	Preferred technique
	Still possible even with delays in diagnosis > 24 hours
	Site of repair must be reinforced with healthy vascularized tissue
Primary repair and correction of underlying condition	Perforation usually diagnosed early and commonly occurs in fasting patients
	Short strictures can be dilated, closed, and covered with fundoplication
	Long strictures may need resection
	Perforations due to pneumatic dilatation are managed by two-layer closure and myotomy
	Perforations due to carcinomas can be treated by resection if cancer is low stage and mediastinal soilage is limited
Exclusion and division (Urschel technique)	Seldom required
	Commits patient to second major procedure
	Reserved for patients with extensive esophageal destruction
T-tube drainage (Abbott technique)	Seldom required
	May be useful in cases of late perforations with extensive esophageal necrosis
	Involves closure of perforation around a large-bore Silastic T tube
Resection and reconstruction	Can be considered in cases of instrumental perforation of carcinomas or long strictures
	Reconstruction best deferred until patient's condition has improved

The technique of primary repair (Table 11-67) involves elevation of the esophagus, identification of the site of perforation, *longitudinal incision of the muscle layer to visualize the entire length of the mucosal defect,* trimming of the mucosal edges, removal of necrotic debris, and two-layer closure of the defect. The site of closure should *always be reinforced* with healthy vascularized tissues, most commonly thickened parietal pleura (Grillo flap), pedicled intercostal musculopleural flap (Fig. 11-12), pericardial fat, strip of pedicled diaphragm, or even omentum and gastric fundus (Thal patch). The repair is then checked for tightness by pulling the nasogastric tube back above the suture line and gently injecting air or methylene blue mixed with saline into the tube. The operation is completed by saline irrigation of the pleural space, wide opening of the mediastinal pleura up to the aortic arch, débridement of the mediastinum, and insertion of two or three thoracostomy tubes. In all cases, the ipsilateral lung must also be completely freed and decorticated to ensure its full re-expansion. After closure of the thoracotomy incision, the patient is repositioned supine,

TABLE 11-67

TECHNIQUE OF PRIMARY CLOSURE OF THORACIC ESOPHAGEAL PERFORATIONS

Ipsilateral posterolateral thoracotomy

Elevation of esophagus and location of esophageal defect

Longitudinal incision of esophageal muscle to ensure that entire length of defect is visualized

Two-layer closure reinforced with healthy vascularized tissue

Wide débridement of mediastinum and decortication of lung

Insertion of 2 or 3 thoracostomy tubes

Gastrostomy and feeding jejunostomy should strongly be considered

and drainage gastrostomy (to prevent reflux) and feeding jejunostomy are performed.

Late perforations can be treated in the same fashion, although the operation is likely to be technically more difficult because of the inflammatory reaction that is present in both the pleural space and mediastinum. In such cases, it is even more important to incise the esophageal muscle wall longitudinally to expose the full length of the mucosal tear, which may have retracted well beyond the visible site of perforation. If primary mucosal closure appears not to be possible, a pedicled intercostal musculopleural flap can be sutured down to the edges of the tear in such a way as to completely buttress the defect.

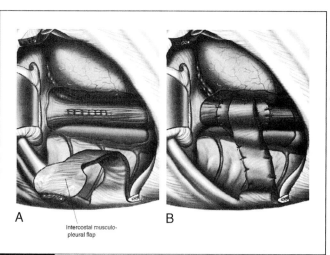

FIG. 11-12

A, Two-layer closure of site of perforation. **B,** Buttressing the site of perforation with pedicled musculopleural flap. *(Courtesy of Doctor Stanley C. Fell.)*

Primary Repair and Correction of Underlying Condition

Esophageal perforations may occur in patients undergoing esophagoscopy or instrumentation for such esophageal disorders as peptic strictures and achalasia. Ruptures occurring in this subset of patients are usually diagnosed early in addition to occurring in fasting patients with less contamination of the mediastinum and pleural spaces. In these patients the preexisting esophageal disorder may require definitive correction, which can be done concomitantly with the repair of the perforation.

Benign strictures can be dilated and then closed transversely and reinforced with a fundoplication, which is used as an antireflux procedure. Perforations in the context of esophageal shortening or long strictures are better managed by esophageal resection mostly because healing of a perforation proximal to a stricture is unlikely. Perforations resulting from pneumatic dilatation for achalasia are best managed by *two-layer closure and performance of a myotomy on the opposite wall* of the esophagus. A partial fundoplication can be added to reinforce the repair and prevent reflux.

In cases of esophageal carcinomas perforated during diagnostic endoscopy, immediate esophagectomy should be considered, especially if the tumor is low stage and mediastinal soilage is limited. Reconstruction of esophageal continuity may be either immediate or staged, depending on the condition of the patient.

Exclusion and Diversion (Urschel Technique)

Esophageal exclusion and diversion are seldom indicated. Not only do they commit the patient to a later difficult reconstruction, but the feasability of primary repair obviates the need for this procedure. In general, this approach is reserved for patients with extensive esophageal damage in whom no other options are acceptable.

The operation involves creation of a loop (in continuity) or end-cervical esophagostomy (total diversion), division and suture of the gastroesophageal junction, and gastrostomy.

T-Tube Drainage (Abbott Technique)

This technique involves ipsilateral thoracotomy and closure of the perforation around a large-bore Silastic T tube. The distal vertical limb of the T tube traverses the gastroesophageal junction; the horizontal limb exits the chest wall and thus creates a controlled esophagocutaneous fistula. A nasogastric tube is then passed through the T-tube lumen into the stomach.

T-tube drainage may be indicated in *cases of late perforation* where there is extensive mucosal necrosis at the site of perforation and where the success of primary repair is doubtful.

Resection and Reconstruction

Esophagectomy is an option in patients with early-stage carcinomas, in those with long peptic strictures, and in patients with overwhelming sepsis when successful management by other means is considered unlikely. The resection can be performed through the transthoracic or transhiatal route.

Reconstruction is best deferred until the patient's condition has improved, usually several months after the event.

Postoperative Recovery (Table 11-68)

Nearly all patients recovering from the repair of intrathoracic esophageal ruptures require *mechanical ventilation* for variable periods. Mechanical ventilation ensures adequate oxygenation during the recovery period and helps maintain maximal lung expansion. Once the patient has stabilized both hemodynamically and from the septic condition and has met criteria for extubation (see Chapter 7, "Mechanical Ventilation for the Surgeon"), he or she can be weaned off the respirator.

Maintenance of nutrition is essential for a positive anabolic balance to be regained, which will facilitate healing and recovery from sepsis. This is best accomplished through the insertion of a feeding jejunostomy tube at the time of the initial repair. Feedings can be started almost immediately after the operation. We recommend keeping the jejunostomy tube in place until one is absolutely certain that the leak has healed and that the patient will require no further interventions. Many patients will in fact go home with their jejunostomy tube still in place.

Specific antibiotherapy based on culture of mediastinal and pleural space samples must be maintained for several weeks postoperatively. In patients with significant mediastinitis, infectious disease specialists should always be consulted for the selection of antibiotics and duration of treatment. The spectrum of antibiotherapy often has to be modified during the postoperative period, especially if residual septic foci have become colonized with resistant or opportunistic organisms.

Oral feedings should be withheld until an esophagogram with aqueous contrast material has demonstrated esophageal wall integrity. If extravasation of contrast material persists (observed in 15% to 20% of cases), patients should be given nothing by mouth until another examination done 7 to 10 days later shows that the site of perforation has completely healed. Such postoperative fistulas are *usually not clinically significant,* and *the majority will heal spontaneously.*

11

Special Challenges in Thoracic Surgery

TABLE 11-68

POSTOPERATIVE CARE OF PATIENTS WITH THORACIC ESOPHAGEAL PERFORATION

Mechanical ventilation is mandatory during the early postoperative period.
Maintain adequate nutrition through feeding jejunostomy tube.
Maintain specific antibiotics for prolonged periods.
Withhold oral feedings until the esophagogram has shown integrity
    of the esophageal wall.
Never remove the chest tubes until there is no further esophageal leakage
    and the pleural space is obliterated.
Remove the chest tubes in a gradual fashion.
If residual spaces are demonstrated, drain them with pigtail catheters
    inserted under CT guidance.

One of the most important aspects of the postoperative care of patients with intrathoracic esophageal ruptures is the maintenance of adequate pleural space and mediastinum drainage. This part of the treatment starts during the operation when the mediastinum and pleural space are thoroughly débrided and all necrotic and alimentary debris is removed. These spaces are then drained by *two or three thoracostomy tubes.* The first tube is positioned near the repair, the second one along the posterior mediastinum, and if necessary a third one more anteriorly in the pleural space. All three tubes are connected to active suction systems and should not be removed until the surgeon is certain that there is no further esophageal leakage and that the pleural space is absolutely obliterated. At that point, we recommend pulling the tubes out in a gradual fashion as described in "Management of the Patient with a Parapneumonic Effusion or Empyema." If an undrained collection or space is identified during the postoperative period, drainage can easily be accomplished through the use of *pigtail catheters* inserted under CT guidance.

Other items of importance during the postoperative period include active chest physiotherapy, prophylaxis against deep vein thrombosis, and use of the gastrostomy tube inserted at the time of operation to prevent gastroesophageal reflux.

NONOPERATIVE MANAGEMENT

Minor perforations, especially limited ones related to instrumentation, can be treated *nonoperatively* if they are contained within the mediastinum and if they drain spontaneously back into the esophagus (Table 11-69). Patients must also have minimal or no local symptoms and show no signs of systemic sepsis.

Conservative treatment consists of withholding oral feedings for 8 to 10 days, providing nutritional support parenterally or enterally (Keofeed tube in jejunum), and giving broad-spectrum antibiotics for at least 10 to 14 days. Small pleural or mediastinal collections can be drained through CT-directed drainage catheters.

Failure to show signs of clinical stability or of improvement should quickly prompt reconsideration for operative therapy.

RESULTS AND OUTCOME (TABLE 11-70)

The recognized factors for good outcome in patients with esophageal ruptures are listed in Table 11-70. Patients with contained perforations and minimal soilage of adjacent cavities do well, and this is the reason why

TABLE 11-69
CRITERIA FOR NONOPERATIVE MANAGEMENT OF ESOPHAGEAL PERFORATIONS
Contained perforation within the mediastinum
Collection drains back into the esophagus
Minimal or no local symptoms
Minimal or no systemic sepsis

TABLE 11-70
FACTORS PREDICTIVE OF GOOD OUTCOME IN PATIENTS WITH ESOPHAGEAL PERFORATION
Younger age
Iatrogenic and instrumental perforation (versus spontaneous)
Cervical perforation (versus thoracic)
Contained perforation (versus noncontained)
Early diagnosis within 24 hours (versus late diagnosis > 24 hours)
Buttressing of suture line (versus nonbuttressed repair)

many physicians advocate nonoperative therapy in such individuals. Similarly, the mortality of cervical perforations is lower than that of thoracic perforations (6% versus 30%) because cervical perforations are often diagnosed early and are contained within the neck, whereas thoracic perforations are usually associated with extensive contamination of the mediastinum and of one or both pleural spaces.

All published information also shows that early diagnosis and management favorably affect the outcome. Both morbidity and mortality increase significantly when the diagnosis is made more than 24 hours after the perforation. Finally, buttressing the suture line, especially if the perforation is intrathoracic, appears to decrease the mortality.

CONCLUSION

Despite significant advances in diagnostic methods and supportive therapy, mortality rates for esophageal rupture are still high, especially in patients for whom diagnosis and therapy are delayed. The main issues in treatment of such patients are adequate control of sepsis, construction of a protected dehiscence-proof repair, and maintenance of fluid and nutritional requirements.

SUGGESTED READINGS

Review Articles

Henderson JAM, Peloquin AJM: Boerhaave revisited: spontaneous esophageal perforation as a diagnostic masquerader. Am J Med 1989;86:559-567.

Pillay SP, Ward M, Cowen A, Pollard E: Esophageal ruptures and perforations—a review. Med J Aust 1989;150:246-252.

Jones WG, Ginsberg RJ: Esophageal perforation: a continuing challenge. Ann Thorac Surg 1992;53:534-543.

Bjerke HS: Boerhaave's syndrome and barogenic injuries of the esophagus. Chest Surg Clin North Am 1994;4:819-825.

Cooper JD: Management strategies for esophageal perforation. Proceedings of the 9th Annual Contemporary Cardiothoracic Surgery Course, St. Louis, Sept 2000.

Brinster CJ, Singhal S, Lee L, et al: Evolving options in the management of esophageal perforation. Ann Thorac Surg 2004;77;1475-1483.

11

Special Challenges in Thoracic Surgery

Esophageal Trauma

Cohn HE, Hubbard A, Patton G: Management of esophageal injuries. Ann Thorac Surg 1989;48:309-314.

Weiman DS, Walker WA, Brosnan KM, et al: Noniatrogenic esophageal trauma. Ann Thorac Surg 1995;59:845-850.

Treatment

Orringer MB, Stirling MC: Esophagectomy for esophageal disruption. Ann Thorac Surg 1990;49:35-43.

Salo JA, Isolauri JO, Heikkilä LJ, et al: Management of delayed esophageal perforation with mediastinal sepsis. Esophagectomy or primary repair? J Thorac Cardiovasc Surg 1993;106:1088-1091.

Ohri SK, Liakakos TA, Pathi V, et al: Primary repair of iatrogenic thoracic esophageal perforation and Boerhaave's syndrome. Ann Thorac Surg 1993;55:603-606.

Whyte RI, Iannettoni MD, Orringer MB: Intrathoracic esophageal perforation. The merit of primary repair. J Thorac Cardiovasc Surg 1995;109:140-146.

Wright CD, Mathisen DJ, Wain JC, et al: Reinforced primary repair of thoracic esophageal perforation. Ann Thorac Surg 1995;60:245-249.

Wang N, Razzouk AJ, Safavi A, et al: Delayed primary repair of intrathoracic esophageal perforation: is it safe? J Thorac Cardiovasc Surg 1996;111: 114-122.

Gupta NM: Emergency transhiatal esophagectomy for instrumental perforation of an obstructed thoracic esophagus. Br J Surg 1996;83:1007-1009.

Bufkin BL, Miller JI, Mansour KA: Esophageal perforation: emphasis on management. Ann Thorac Surg 1996;61:1447-1452.

Iannettoni MD, Vlessis AA, Whyte RI, Orringer MB: Functional outcome after surgical treatment of esophageal perforation. Ann Thorac Surg 1997;64:1606-1610.

Altorjay Á, Kiss J, Vörös A, Szirányi E: The role of esophagectomy in the management of esophageal perforations. Ann Thorac Surg 1998;65:1433-1436.

Muir AD, White JJ, McGuigan JA, et al: Treatment and outcome of oesophageal perforation in a tertiary referral center. Eur J Cardiothorac Surg 2003;23:799-804.

Jougon J, McBride T, Delcambre F, et al: Primary esophageal repair for Boerhaave's syndrome whatever the free interval between perforation and treatment. Eur J Cardiothorac Surg 2004;25:475-479.

Case Series

Michel L, Grillo HC, Malt RA: Operative and nonoperative management of esophageal perforations. Ann Surg 1981;194:57-63.

Bladergroen MR, Lowe JE, Postlethwait RW: Diagnosis and recommended management of esophageal perforation and rupture. Ann Thorac Surg 1986;42:235-239.

Nesbitt JC, Sawyers JL: Surgical management of esophageal perforation. Am Surg 1987;53:183-191.

Pate JW, Walker WA, Cole FH, et al: Spontaneous rupture of the esophagus: a 30-year experience. Ann Thorac Surg 1989;47:689-692.

Attar S, Hankins JR, Suter CM, et al: Esophageal perforation: a therapeutic challenge. Ann Thorac Surg 1990;50:45-51.

White RK, Morris DM: Diagnosis and management of esophageal perforations. Am Surg 1992;58:112-119.

Lawrence DR, Moxon RE, Fountain SW, et al: Iatrogenic oesophageal perforations: a clinical review. Ann R Coll Surg Engl 1998;80:115-118.

Tomaselli F, Maier A, Pinter H, Smolle-Jüttner F: Management of iatrogenous esophagus perforation. Thorac Cardiovasc Surg 2002;50:168-173.

Port JL, Kent MS, Korst RJ, et al: Thoracic esophageal perforations: a decade of experience. Ann Thorac Surg 2003;75:1071-1074.

MANAGEMENT OF THE ADULT PATIENT WITH A TRACHEOESOPHAGEAL FISTULA

Despite the anatomic proximity of the tracheobronchial tree and esophagus, abnormal communications between these two structures are uncommon. In the adult population, they are mostly due to malignant neoplasms of the esophagus or are secondary to mechanical ventilation or external trauma.

Malignant tracheoesophageal fistulas (TEFs) are preterminal events that most commonly occur in patients with carcinoma of the esophagus. Although treatment options depend on several factors, including the overall condition of the patient, the general objective is palliative.

Postintubation TEFs are due to a combination of pressure on the tracheal mucosa from a cuffed endotracheal tube and pressure on the esophageal mucosa from a rigid nasogastric tube. Management is difficult, especially *for patients in whom mechanical ventilation is still required* because under those circumstances, any attempt to close the fistula surgically is almost certain to fail.

Most post-traumatic TEFs are secondary to blunt thoracic injuries. They can occur in the upper neck, where they are associated with cricoid cartilage fractures, or near the carina, where they are secondary to a tear of the membranous trachea with partial disruption of the esophageal wall. Most of these patients are best treated by direct surgical repair.

MALIGNANT TRACHEOESOPHAGEAL FISTULA

Malignant TEFs occur *more frequently* during the course of carcinoma of the esophagus (5% of patients with esophageal cancer will eventually develop a malignant TEF) than that of lung cancer (incidence < 1%). However, the much higher incidence of lung cancer in North America makes this cause more prevalent.

Epidemiology (Table 11-71), **Pathophysiology, and Natural History**

Overall, 75% to 80% of malignant TEFs are related to carcinoma of the esophagus, 15% to 20% to bronchogenic carcinomas, and less than 5% to other tumors such as thyroid or laryngeal cancers or lymphomas. The trachea is *the most common site of fistulization (>50%);* the left and right main stem bronchi are the site of communication in approximately 20% of cases each. In less than 10% of patients will fistulization occur with the lung parenchyma.

The most common mechanisms responsible for fistulization are direct tumor invasion of the airway, devascularization and necrosis due to radiation therapy, and local trauma due to instrumentation (biopsy, dilatation) or surgical resection.

Patient's impairment and symptoms relate to continuous aspiration of esophageal contents (saliva, food) in the tracheobronchial tree, pulmonary suppuration in dependent lobes and segments, and malnutrition. If left untreated, most malignant TEFs will lead to death within 2 to 3 months of having been diagnosed.

Diagnosis and Investigation

Patients with malignant TEFs can present with symptoms directly attributable to the fistula, to pulmonary complications arising from aspiration, or to the underlying esophageal or lung tumor. Two typical clinical features attributable to the fistula are violent coughing while swallowing and expectoration of sputum mixed with food. Common symptoms associated with malignant TEF are listed in Table 11-72.

A variety of imaging modalities, such as contrast esophagography (preferably with dilute barium) and CT scan, can *adequately demonstrate* the fistula track in patients with malignant TEF. CT can also show the underlying carcinoma and its local extension as well as the complications, such as pneumonia and lung abscesses, that may have arisen because of aspiration. Endoscopy *should always be part of treatment planning,* especially if one wants to determine the feasibility of inserting an endoprosthesis.

TABLE 11-71

EPIDEMIOLOGY OF MALIGNANT TRACHEOESOPHAGEAL FISTULAS

Primary tumor
Esophageal cancer: 75%-80% of cases
Lung cancer: 15%-20% of cases
Others: <1% of cases

Site of fistula
Trachea and carina: 50%
Main bronchi: 20%-25%
Peripheral lung: <10%

TABLE 11-72

MOST COMMON SYMPTOMS ASSOCIATED WITH MALIGNANT TRACHEOESOPHAGEAL FISTULAS

Symptom	Prevalence
Cough	>50%
Aspiration	35%–40%
Fever	25%
Dysphagia	20%

Management

For most patients, treatment objectives (Table 11-73) include mechanical interruption of the fistula to prevent aspiration, restoration of esophageal continuity to allow more normal deglutition, and avoidance of external venting of esophagus and stomach to provide greater comfort. Ultimately, the objectives are *to shorten the duration of hospitalization* and *improve the quality of life.*

Intubation and Stenting

Intubation and stenting of an obstructing esophageal tumor with TEF will occlude the fistula, prevent ongoing airway contamination, and restore orogastric continuity. In general, stenting is possible when there is a shelf of tumor capable of supporting the upper end of the stent; push-through intubations are preferred to pull-through intubations.

Successful fistula occlusion can be achieved with relatively *minimal morbidity* in more than 90% of patients. Potential complications include increasing the size of the TEF due to stent manipulations, stent migration in up to 25% of patients, and stent occlusion. Despite these potential drawbacks most patients with malignant TEF should be treated primarily with self-expanding metal stents.

Bypass Procedures

Because bypass procedures are fraught with high complication and mortality rates, they should be done only in the most fit individuals who have a *relatively long life expectancy.* The whole stomach is generally used as a replacement organ, the proximal esophagus is closed, and adequate drainage of the distal esophagus is achieved by a standard Roux-en-Y loop of jejunum.

11

Special Challenges in Thoracic Surgery

TABLE 11-73

TREATMENT GOALS IN PATIENTS WITH MALIGNANT TEF

Mechanical interruption of fistula

Restoration of esophageal continuity

Avoidance of external venting of esophagus and stomach

Esophageal Exclusion Alone

The creation of a cervical esophagostomy and gastrostomy as a method to exclude the esophagus can relieve the chronic pulmonary sepsis due to aspiration, but this procedure carries significant morbidity and is associated with poor quality of life. For these reasons, *it is seldom recommended.*

BENIGN ACQUIRED TRACHEOESOPHAGEAL FISTULAS

TEFs secondary to benign processes are rare but pose difficult management problems. They are generally divided into those associated with mechanical ventilation and those that are not (Table 11-74).

Etiology and Pathogenesis

In patients being mechanically ventilated, *direct pressure necrosis* by high-pressure cuffs of endotracheal or tracheotomy tubes can result in *full-thickness ulceration* of the posterior membranous trachea with secondary perforation into the adjacent esophagus that lies against the rigid spine. In such cases, the presence of a *nasogastric tube* appears to provide a fixed point for ulcerations. The typical patient who develops a postintubation TEF (Table 11-75) is also nutritionally depleted, has required high peak inspiratory pressure and high positive end-expiratory pressure, and often has been receiving systemic steroid therapy. Ultimately, the most important predisposing factors are tracheostomy tube cuffs that have been overinflated for long periods of time and prolonged mechanical ventilation. Most TEFs secondary to percutaneous tracheostomies are the result of technical complications related to accidental perforation of the membranous trachea with either the dilator or the tracheostomy tube itself (see Chapter 7, "Mechanical Ventilation for the Surgeon").

TABLE 11-74
COMMON CAUSES OF BENIGN ACQUIRED TRACHEOESOPHAGEAL FISTULAS

TEF associated with cuffed tubes and mechanical ventilation
TEF not associated with cuffed tubes and mechanical ventilation
    Trauma
        Penetrating or blunt cervical and thoracic trauma
        Instrumental trauma, esophageal dilatation, biopsy, laser therapy
        Operative trauma: lung or esophageal resection, tracheostomy,
            anterior spine fusion
        Chemical or burn-induced traumas
        Foreign bodies
    Mediastinal infection
        Tuberculosis
        Mycosis: histoplasmosis, actinomycosis
        AIDS
    Others
        Perforation of Barrett ulcer

TABLE 11-75

FACTORS PREDISPOSING TO TRACHEOESOPHAGEAL FISTULA
DUE TO CUFFED ENDOTRACHEAL OR TRACHEOSTOMY TUBES

Hyperinflation of tube cuffs
High-pressure cuffs
Constant movement of the tube with each mechanical inspiration
Presence of rigid nasogastric tube in esophagus
Nutritional depletion
Systemic steroid therapy
Patient requires high Paw and high positive end-expiratory pressure
Patient requires prolonged mechanical ventilation

Post-traumatic TEFs may develop in the *upper neck,* where they
result from impaction of fractured cricoid or thyroid cartilages through
the pharyngeal mucosa. Post-traumatic TEFs may also occur *at or near the
carina,* where they are secondary to a tear in the membranous trachea
associated with contusion and partial disruption of the adjacent esophageal
wall. Over a period of a few days after the trauma, ischemic necrosis and
fistulization will occur.

Post-traumatic TEFs may also be secondary to erosion through the
esophageal wall of a foreign body (such as an endoesophageal prosthesis),
corrosive injuries of the esophagus, and iatrogenic instrumental or operative
trauma (Table 11-74).

Most postinflammatory TEFs are due to tuberculosis of the subcarinal
nodes. In such cases, fistulization may occur between the proximal right
main bronchus and the esophagus in association with a traction diverticulum
of the esophagus.

Diagnosis and Management of TEF due to Cuffed Tubes and Mechanical Ventilation

TEFs are rare but serious complications of cuffed tracheostomy tubes with
assisted ventilation. Indeed, one of the *most difficult challenges* in the
practice of thoracic surgery is that of a patient with a TEF for whom
continued assisted ventilation with a cuffed endotracheal tube or
tracheostomy tube is still deemed necessary.

Diagnosis (Table 11-76)

In most patients, clinical features of a TEF will become *manifest while the
patient is still being ventilated.* Such features include a sudden increase in
the amount of tracheal secretions, increased difficulties in maintaining
ventilatory parameters, a large air leak around a hyperinflated cuffed tube,
and gastric dilatation. If the patient is being fed, feedings may be suctioned
off the tracheobronchial tree.

The diagnosis is best confirmed by bronchoscopy, which will also
define the size of the fistula and its exact location, especially in relation to
the cricoid cartilage.

TABLE 11-76

DIAGNOSIS OF TRACHEOESOPHAGEAL FISTULA IN PATIENTS BEING VENTILATED

Increase in amount of tracheal secretions
Increased difficulties in ventilating patient
Large inspiratory air leaks
Gastric dilatation
Feedings will appear in airway
Anatomic diagnosis best confirmed by bronchoscopy

Management of Patients Still Requiring Mechanical Ventilation

Management of patients still requiring mechanical ventilation is difficult because tracheal *anastomotic breakdown is likely to occur* if surgical repair is attempted. Not only will the endotracheal tube traumatize the anastomosis and interfere with its vascular supply, but also such patients are usually seriously ill with respiratory and other problems, thus increasing the likelihood of significant morbidity.

In selected patients, exclusion and diversion of the esophagus above and below the fistula may be a satisfactory option, with the understanding that this option commits the patient to multiple later reconstructive operations. As suggested by Dr. F. G. Pearson, distal esophageal stapling, a relatively simple procedure that can be done by laparoscopic approach, will *prevent continuation of airway contamination* by gastric contents. A double layer of staples, without division of the esophagus, does not devascularize any part of the esophageal wall, and the esophageal lumen will reopen spontaneously and completely within a few months. This maneuver will provide *many weeks of airway protection,* allowing delay of definitive repair until the patient has been weaned off the respirator.

Other maneuvers that can be useful include repositioning a low-pressure cuffed tracheostomy tube below the level of the TEF and installing both a draining gastrostomy and a feeding jejunostomy. Such repositioning of the tracheostomy tube may, however, increase the size of the fistula rather than solve the problem. On occasion, high-frequency ventilation may be of benefit.

Management of Patients Who Can Be Weaned Off the Respirator

Definitive repair is most easily and effectively achieved if the patient has recovered sufficiently to be weaned off the respirator and extubated altogether.

The technique of repair (Table 11-77) usually requires a *cervical incision only.* The fistula is first identified and the esophageal side is divided. The esophageal defect is then closed (two-layer closure), with particular care taken to close the mucosal defect with closely spaced interrupted sutures. A pedicled strap muscle flap is then applied over the esophageal closure.

In most cases, there is associated severe damage to the trachea throughout its circumference, and this should be managed like any other tracheal defect and stenosis. Indeed, segmental resection of the damaged segment with primary anastomosis is usually required.

TABLE 11-77

PRINCIPLES OF SURGICAL REPAIR OF TRACHEOESOPHAGEAL FISTULA
DUE TO CUFFED TUBES

Most can be done through cervical incision
Identify site of TEF (may be difficult)
Divide esophageal side of fistula and use two-layer closure of defect
Apply pedicled strap muscle flap over closure
Segmental resection of damaged trachea usually necessary
Primary end-to-end anastomosis of trachea if resection is necessary

---

Diagnosis and Management of TEF Secondary to Blunt Thoracic Trauma

The diagnosis of post-traumatic TEF is *often delayed* by days or weeks either because the patient has a tracheotomy that masks the symptoms or because several days are required for a communication between distal trachea and esophagus to mature. In addition, many of these patients have severe associated injuries, including neurologic, that will delay the diagnosis.

Because all patients with a TEF related to blunt laryngeal trauma have an *associated subglottic stricture,* the clinical features are more often related to the stricture than to the TEF. Bronchoscopy and esophagoscopy should always be done to visualize the orifice of the fistula and to plan the repair, which again should be delayed until the patient is off the respirator and pulmonary sepsis and malnutrition have been corrected. The surgical approach is through a cervical collar incision; the operation involves *division of the fistula, closure of the esophageal defect,* and *subglottic resection* of the larynx and upper trachea.

Patients with distal post-traumatic TEF may have symptoms for weeks or even months before a clinician with a high index of suspicion documents the diagnosis. Classically, patients have bouts of coughing seconds after swallowing, chronic productive cough, and sometimes dysphagia. Whereas standard chest radiographs may be normal or show basal lung infiltrations, bronchiectasis, or pleural effusions, the definitive diagnosis can be established by contrast esophagography. Surgical repair is best done through a right posterolateral thoracotomy. Once the fistula has been identified, it is divided, and both esophageal and tracheal defects are closed. *Interposition of well-vascularized tissue* such as pleura, pericardium, or intercostal muscle between the suture lines is highly recommended.

CONGENITAL RESPIRATORY-ESOPHAGEAL FISTULA IN THE ADULT

Although the majority of congenital TEFs without esophageal atresia are diagnosed in infancy, several cases presenting in adulthood have been reported. These delayed presentations may be due (Table 11-78) to late rupture of a membrane covering the site of fistula, to a proximal fold of esophageal mucosa acting as a flap valve and covering the site of fistula, to the angle between fistula and esophagus that allows it to close during swallowing, or to the general upward direction of the fistula from esophagus to bronchus. In addition, the diagnosis may have been delayed

TABLE 11-78

POSSIBLE EXPLANATIONS AS TO WHY CONGENITAL TRACHEOESOPHAGEAL FISTULA MAY ONLY BE DIAGNOSED IN THE ADULT

Membrane covering the site of fistula eventually ruptures
Proximal fold of esophageal mucosa acts as a flap valve
Angle between site of fistula and esophagus allows the fistula
to close during swallowing
General upward direction of fistula from esophagus to airway
Physician does not suspect the diagnosis
May be difficult to demonstrate by barium swallow examination

simply because the clinician did not entertain this possibility or because it may take several swallows of barium and several belching maneuvers to distend and radiologically demonstrate these usually very small fistulas.

Clinically, patients with congenital TEF complain of coughing spasms after drinking and suffer from recurrent pulmonary infections. A definitive diagnosis can be made by *barium swallow examination* or by instilling methylene blue into the esophagus while performing bronchoscopy.

Surgical treatment is always indicated because the natural history of these fistulas is that significant suppurative respiratory complications, such as bronchiectasis and lung abscesses, will eventually develop. The procedure involves division of the fistula, closure of both the esophageal and tracheal sides of the track, and interposition of viable tissue between the two suture lines.

BRONCHOESOPHAGEAL FISTULAS

The majority of bronchoesophageal fistulas seen in the adult population are the result of locally advanced malignant neoplasms, such as lung or esophageal cancers; in many cases, fistulization will have occurred as a result of radiation therapy. These patients have limited survival, and their treatment should be palliative.

Benign bronchoesophageal fistulas are extremely uncommon; most are *post-traumatic* or are due to *primary mediastinal inflammation,* such as seen in association with histoplasmosis or tuberculosis. Tuberculosis causes caseation necrosis of mediastinal lymph nodes and abscess formation, and this may be followed by erosion and eventual rupture into the esophagus and trachea. Tuberculosis and histoplasmosis can also cause mediastinal fibrosis with secondary traction diverticula of the esophagus, which can rupture in the adjacent bronchi.

The diagnosis of bronchoesophageal fistula should be suspected in any patient who presents with cough associated with swallowing, repeated pulmonary infections, or adult-onset asthma. The presence of a fistula can be confirmed by barium esophagography, CT of the mediastinum, or bronchoscopy.

Even in relatively asymptomatic patients and in patients with small fistulas, management should be surgical. The operation involves dissection of the fistula through an ipsilateral posterolateral thoracotomy, division of the fistula track, individual closure of the bronchial (one-layer closure) and esophageal (two-layer closure) sides of the bronchoesophageal fistula, and interposition of viable tissue between the two suture lines.

CONCLUSION

TEFs are rare clinical conditions associated with severe debilitation in both the patient with an underlying malignant neoplasm and the one in whom the fistula is secondary to a benign process. TEFs secondary to mechanical ventilation are particularly serious problems with significant in-hospital mortality. In all cases in which surgical correction of a TEF is contemplated, attempts must be made to wean the patient off the respirator before proceeding with the operation.

11

SUGGESTED READINGS

Review Articles

Pearson FG: Post-intubation tracheo-esophageal fistula. Proceedings of the University of Toronto thoracic surgery refresher course. Toronto, June 1976.

Goldberg M: Management of malignant tracheoesophageal fistula. Proceedings of the University of Toronto thoracic surgery refresher course, Toronto, June 1979.

Duranceau A, Jamieson GG: Malignant tracheoesophageal fistula. Ann Thorac Surg 1984;37:346-354.

Dartevelle P, Macchiarini P: Management of acquired tracheoesophageal fistula. Chest Surg Clin North Am 1996;6:819-836.

Couraud L, Ballester MJ, Delaisement C: Acquired tracheoesophageal fistula and its management. Semin Thorac Cardiovasc Surg 1996;8:392-399.

Benign Tracheoesophageal Fistula

Thomas AN: The diagnosis and treatment of tracheoesophageal fistula caused by cuffed tracheal tubes. J Thorac Cardiovasc Surg 1973;65:612-619.

Grillo HC, Moncure AC, McEnany MT: Repair of inflammatory tracheoesophageal fistula. Ann Thorac Surg 1976;22:112-119.

Hilgenberg AD, Grillo HC: Acquired nonmalignant tracheoesophageal fistula. J Thorac Cardiovasc Surg 1983;85:492-498.

Gerzić Z, Rakić S, Randjelović T: Acquired benign esophagorespiratory fistula: report of 16 consecutive cases. Ann Thorac Surg 1990;50:724-727.

Mathisen DJ, Grillo HC, Wain JC, Hilgenberg AD: Management of acquired nonmalignant tracheoesophageal fistula. Ann Thorac Surg 1991;52:759-765.

Azoulay D, Regnard JF, Magdeleinat P, et al: Congenital respiratory-esophageal fistula in the adult. Report of nine cases and review of the literature. J Thorac Cardiovasc Surg 1992;104:381-384.

Macchiarini P, Verhoye JP, Chapelier A, et al: Evaluation and outcome of different surgical techniques for postintubation tracheoesophageal fistulas. J Thorac Cardiovasc Surg 2000;119:268-276.

Special Challenges in Thoracic Surgery

Wolf M, Yellin A, Talmi YP, et al: Acquired tracheoesophageal fistula in critically ill patients. Ann Otol Rhinol Laryngol 2000;109:731-735.

Oliaro A, Rena O, Papalia E, et al: Surgical management of acquired non-malignant tracheoesophageal fistulas. J Cardiovasc Surg 2001;42: 257-260.

Zacharias J, Genc O, Goldstraw P: Congenital tracheoesophageal fistulas presenting in adults. Presentation of two cases and a synopsis of the literature. J Thorac Cardiovasc Surg 2004;128:316-318.

Fiala P, Černohorský S, Čermák J, et al: Tracheal stenosis complicated with tracheoesophageal fistula. Eur J Cardiothorac Surg 2004;25:127-130.

Bronchoesophageal Fistula

Braimbridge MV, Keith HI: Esophago-bronchial fistula in the adult. Thorax 1965;20:226-233.

Spalding AR, Burney DP, Richie RE: Acquired benign bronchoesophageal fistulas in the adult. Ann Thorac Surg 1979;28:378-383.

Rämö OJ, Salo JA, Mattila SP: Congenital bronchoesophageal fistula in the adult. Ann Thorac Surg 1995;59:887-890.

Lazopoulos G, Kotoulas C, Lioulias A: Congenital bronchoesophageal fistula in the adult. Eur J Cardiothorac Surg 1999;16:667-669.

Mangi AA, Gaissert HA, Wright CD, et al: Benign bronchoesophageal fistula in the adult. Ann Thorac Surg 2002;73:911-915.

Malignant Tracheoesophageal Fistula

Burt M, Diehl W, Martini N, et al: Malignant esophagorespiratory fistula: management options and survival. Ann Thorac Surg 1991;52:1222-1229.

Albes JM, Schäfers HJ, Gebel M, Ross UH: Tracheal stenting for malignant tracheoesophageal fistula. Ann Thorac Surg 1994;57:1263-1266.

Kotsis L, Zubovits K, Vadász P: Management of malignant tracheo-esophageal fistulas with a cuffed funnel tube. Ann Thorac Surg 1997;64:355-358.

Meunier B, Stasik C, Raoul JL, et al: Gastric bypass for malignant esophagotracheal fistula. A series of 21 cases. Eur J Cardiothorac Surg 1998;13:184-189.

Stents

Low DE, Kozarek RA: Comparison of conventional and wide mesh expandable prosthesis and surgical by-pass in patients with malignant esophagorespiratory fistulas. Ann Thorac Surg 1998;65:919-923.

Case Series

Gudovsky LM, Koroleva NS, Biryukov YB, et al: Tracheoesophageal fistulas. Ann Thorac Surg 1993;55:868-875.

Other

Low DE: Keeping an open mind while restoring esophageal patency in patients with cancer and esophagorespiratory fistula. Ann Thorac Surg 1996;62:961-962.

MANAGEMENT OF THE PATIENT WITH EMPHYSEMA

Pulmonary bullae are defined as *emphysematous spaces larger than 1 cm in diameter* usually demarcated from surrounding lung by curved hairline shadows. In general, they are considered nonsurgical entities other than for the management of specific complications, such as pneumothoraces and infections. When resection of a bulla is done to reduce dyspnea and improve pulmonary function, the best results are obtained in patients with large bullae in whom *compression of potentially functional surrounding lung* can be demonstrated.

Lung volume reduction surgery (LVRS) was developed as a means of surgical treatment for diffuse nonbullous emphysema. The rationale for surgery is similar to that of bullectomy since the procedure involves the surgical excision of nonfunctional distended air spaces thought to interfere with function of the surrounding more normal lung.

Results of follow-up studies indicate that in selected patients, both bullectomy and LVRS may improve quality of life and pulmonary function.

TERMINOLOGY AND CLASSIFICATION OF AIR SPACE DISORDERS

Emphysema

Emphysema is characterized by an abnormal increase in the size of air spaces distal to the terminal bronchiole. From an anatomic standpoint, the classification of emphysema is based on the portion of acinus involved (Table 11-79 and Fig. 11-13), an acinus being a unit of bronchopulmonary tissue distal to a terminal bronchiole.

Centriacinar emphysema (proximal) develops in the proximal portion of the acinus and is associated with inflammatory destruction of the respiratory bronchioles (Fig. 11-13*A*). It is most common in the upper lung fields and is related to smoking.

11

Special Challenges in Thoracic Surgery

TABLE 11-79

CLASSIFICATION OF EMPHYSEMA

Centriacinar emphysema (centrilobular, proximal)
  Proximal portion of acini
  Most common in upper lung fields
  Associated with smoking
Panacinar emphysema (panlobular)
  All portions of acini
  Distributed throughout lung fields
  Associated with alpha$_1$-antitrypsin deficiencies
Paraseptal emphysema (distal)
  Distal part of acini
  Most common at apices
  Associated with formation of blebs and pneumothoraces

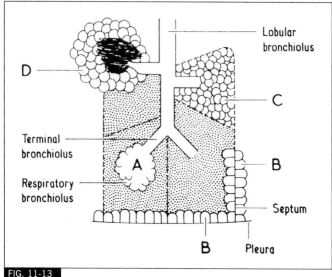

FIG. 11-13

Schematic showing various forms of emphysema. **A,** Centriacinar emphysema.
B, Periacinar or paraseptal emphysema. **C,** Panacinar emphysema. **D,** Irregular (scan)
emphysema. *(Courtesy of Dr. Edward E. Gaensler.)*

In panacinar emphysema, *all portions of the acinus are uniformly destroyed,* and because of that, it is often called diffuse emphysema (Fig. 11-13C). Progressive destruction of lung tissue results in enlargement of air spaces, and ultimately, little remains other than the supporting framework of vessels, septa, and bronchi. This variety of emphysema is commonly associated with alpha$_1$-antitrypsin deficiencies.

Paraseptal or distal emphysema results from *disruption of subpleural alveoli* and thus involves the distal part of the acinus, ducts, and alveoli (Fig. 11-13B). These tiny disruptions tend to coalesce into larger air spaces called *blebs,* and eventually they can form *large subpleural bullae.* This particular type of emphysema can be associated with spontaneous pneumothoraces; it is often confined to the apices of the lungs.

Blebs and Bullae

A bleb is a *subpleural collection of air* caused by ruptured alveoli. The outer wall of a bleb is made of visceral pleura, and the underlying lung is normal. Blebs are small and peripheral, and most are located at the lung apices.

TABLE 11-80

CLASSIFICATION OF BULLOUS EMPHYSEMA

Group I bullae
20% of all cases
Underlying lung relatively normal
Well demarcated from surrounding lung
Bullae are often located at lung apices

Group II bullae
80% of all cases
Underlying lung has severe emphysema
Poorly demarcated from surrounding lung
Bullae are often multiple and bilateral

Bullae are air-filled spaces within the lung parenchyma that can be associated with any variety of emphysema. Their walls are made of destroyed lung, and they are trabeculated by remnants of alveolar septa. Multiple small bronchial communications often are apparent at the base of any bulla.

In the context of clinical practice, bullous emphysema is often classified according to the *presence or absence of significant emphysema in the nonbullous lung* (Table 11-80). *Group I bullae* (20% of all cases) are well demarcated from surrounding lung, are usually located at the apex, and typically have a narrow base of implantation. The underlying lung is relatively normal. *Group II bullae* are seen in approximately 80% of patients, and initially at least, they are simply a local exaggeration of diffuse panacinar emphysema. These bullae are often multiple and bilateral, and the underlying lung is emphysematous. *Giant bullae* are bullae that occupy one third or more of the volume of one hemithorax.

An alternative method of classifying bullous emphysema is depicted in Table 11-81.

Other Types of Emphysema

There are two additional varieties of emphysema that are pertinent to the thoracic surgeon. The first one, called *compensatory emphysema,* represents hyperinflation of a portion of lung to fill a hemithorax. Compensatory emphysema

TABLE 11-81

CLASSIFICATION OF BULLOUS EMPHYSEMA ACCORDING TO DEVRIES AND WOLFE

Group	Bullae	Underlying Lung
I	Large, single	Normal
II	Multiple	Normal
III	Multiple	Diffuse emphysema
IV	Multiple	Other lung diseases

From DeVries WC, Wolfe WG: The management of spontaneous pneumothorax and bullous emphysema. Surg Clin North Am 1980;60:851.

Special Challenges in Thoracic Surgery

11

is usually associated with atelectasis or resectional surgery. This is not true emphysema because destruction of the acinus has not occurred.

Air space enlargement associated with pulmonary fibrosis is common but bears little clinical significance. *Cicatricial emphysema* (Fig. 11-13D) is associated with scarred tuberculosis and honeycomb lung with chronic inflammatory diseases.

SURGERY FOR BULLOUS EMPHYSEMA

Among all procedures that have ever been recommended for the surgical management of COPD, the only operation that has stood the test of time is bullectomy, in which *distended air spaces are resected* to allow the re-expansion of potentially functional adjacent lung.

Rationale and Indications

Surgery for Complications of the Bulla

Surgery may be indicated for spontaneous secondary pneumothorax, a potentially dangerous event because of further reduction in pulmonary function in already compromised patients. Secondary pneumothoraces are also associated with prolonged air leaks and significant risks of recurrences. *True infection of bullae is unusual,* and most bullae containing an air-fluid level are only the site of an inflammatory reaction secondary to pneumonitis in the surrounding lung. Surgery is not indicated for this problem alone because eventual fluid resorption may be associated with significant shrinkage and resolution of the bulla (autobullectomy). On occasion, *chest pain* related to overdistention of the bulla during exercise may be the sole indication for bullectomy.

Preventive surgery, defined as the *resection of asymptomatic bullae,* is legitimate when the bulla occupies half or more of the hemithorax, compresses normal lung, or has enlarged during a period of years. This is done with the belief that most of these large bullae will ultimately lead to serious complications. It is also assumed that function is unlikely to return to normal if the lung adjacent to such large bullae has been compressed for prolonged periods of time.

Surgery for Dyspnea

A most common belief is that large bullae act as *space-occupying lesions* and that removal of such lesions will improve elastic recoil, airflow, and gas exchange in compressed lung areas. It is also thought that bullectomy will restore normal diaphragmatic configuration, strength, and contractility as well as improve chest wall mechanics. If patients are well selected for operation, these physiologic benefits are likely to translate into subjective improvement in dyspnea.

Selection for Surgery

The main determinants of successful outcome after bullectomy are the size of the bulla, the condition of the rest of the lung, and the evidence of compression. Indeed, the best results are obtained in patients with large bullae in whom there is evidence of compression of a significant volume of potentially functional surrounding lung (Table 11-82).

CT scanning is the best imaging technique to delineate the anatomy of bullous lung disease, and as a rule, the best results are obtained with the *resection of giant bullae.* The observation that a bulla has enlarged over time is pertinent, especially if this enlargement is associated with concomitant worsening in dyspnea.

Isotope scans can determine the function of a bulla with respect to ventilation and perfusion. The demonstration that the bulla to be resected is underperfused compared with adjacent lung improves the likelihood of a good outcome after bullectomy.

One other important step in the preoperative investigation of patients with bullous lung disease is to demonstrate that a given bulla *compresses adjacent lung and prevents its expansion*. Most compression signs (Table 11-83) can

TABLE 11-82

SELECTION OF PATIENTS FOR BULLECTOMY (PATIENT'S CLINICAL PROFILE)

Area of Investigation	Best Technique	Most Suitable for Surgery	Least Suitable for Surgery
Anatomy of bullous disease	CT scan	Large (>50% hemithorax) bulla	Multiple, small, and bilateral bullae
		Enlargement over time	No enlargement over time
Function of bulla	Isotope scans	Nonventilated, nonperfused bulla	Ventilated and perfused bulla
Compression	Standard radiographs, CT scan, angiography	High index (3 or more signs or compression)	Low index (less than 3 signs of compression)
Status of compressed lung	Isotopic scans, CT scan	Good capillary filling	Poor capillary filling
		Good washout of xenon (ventilation)	Retention of xenon
Severity of emphysema	Pulmonary function studies, exercise testing	Minimal or moderate COPD $FEV_1 > 50\%$ predicted Resting $Pco_2 <45$	Severe COPD $FEV_1 < 35\%$ predicted Significant desaturation during exercise Resting $Pco_2 >50$
Clinical features	Clinical history, cardiac evaluation, nutritional status	Young age Normal heart No weight loss Smoking cessation	Older age Cor pulmonale Significant weight loss No smoking cessation

TABLE 11-83

RADIOLOGIC SIGNS OF COMPRESSION

Vascular crowding in parenchyma adjacent to bulla
Arcuate displacement of blood vessels in periphery of bulla
Displacement of hilum
Mediastinal displacement
Anterior mediastinal herniation of the lung
Displacement of lung fissures

be appreciated on standard chest radiographs or CT scan, and it has been shown that the presence of three or more of these indices of compression correlates well with good results after bullectomy.

Although it is difficult to predict, *the potential for re-expansion and function of the compressed lung* can be estimated through isotopic studies of regional lung function and CT scanning. Adequacy of perfusion in the compressed lung demonstrated by dense peripheral capillary filling observed on contrast-enhanced CT and dynamic ventilation estimated by the amount of xenon Xe-133 washout during the first minute are good indicators of perfusion/ventilation efficiency and good predictors of postoperative improvement.

In general, results of bullectomy are poor in patients with severe COPD. It has been shown that patients with an FEV_1 greater than 50% of predicted values *gain most benefit* from bullectomy, whereas those with an FEV_1 lower than 35% of predicted value *do poorly* after surgery. Patients with significant desaturation during exercise (<90%) also do poorly in addition to having increased chances of postoperative morbidity.

Virtually all patients with bullous lung disease have a history of smoking, and smoking cessation improves the chances for a good outcome. Older patients with clinical evidence of chronic bronchitis, cor pulmonale, or significant weight loss have a higher surgical risk and a lower chance of good outcome.

The best way to decide whether patients are good candidates for bullectomy is to establish their clinical profile according to the six criteria listed in Table 11-82 and determine if they are most or least suitable for surgery.

Operative Approaches and Procedures

There is general agreement that the operative strategy should be to remove the bulla while *preserving all potentially functioning lung tissue* (Table 11-84). Lobectomy, for instance, is seldom indicated because functional lung is often present at the hilum of the lobe, although the surgeon may believe that the entire lobe is destroyed. Preoperatively, all patients must have *active preparation* including rehabilitation, specific drug treatment to relieve airway obstruction, smoking cessation, and, if possible, discontinuation of steroid therapy.

The technique of anesthesia must take into account the abnormal physiology of the emphysematous lung, and the surgeon must be present during induction in the event of a pneumothorax that may need quick

---

TABLE 11-84

GROUND RULES FOR SUCCESSFUL BULLECTOMY

Selectivity for operation

Active preparation: rehabilitation, specific drug treatment, smoking cessation, discontinuation of steroid therapy

Surgeon in operating room during induction

Thoracic epidural catheter inserted before beginning of operation

Use of double-lumen tube

Video-assisted or limited axillary approaches

Stapler resection of bullae

Reinforcement of staple lines with pericardial strips or covering of lung surfaces with glues

Associated subtotal parietal pleurectomy

Adequate drainage of pleural space by two chest tubes

Early extubation

Optimal postoperative pain control (epidural narcotic injection)

Aggressive chest physiotherapy postoperatively

---

decompression. A *thoracic epidural catheter* should also be inserted before the beginning of surgery because continuous administration of epidural narcotics during the operation will decrease the need for intravenous medication or other anesthetic agents (see Chapter 6). Patients should be ventilated with a *double-lumen tube* so that the lung being operated on can be collapsed.

Most operations for bullous lung disease are currently done by VATS or limited ancillary incisions because these approaches are associated with lower morbidity. Once the bulla has been identified and its base demarcated, it is deflated and simply excised by multiple applications of the Endo-GIA stapler.

In patients with multiple bullae, it is important to *tailor the resection* so that there will be enough remaining lung to fill the space. Air leaks can be minimized by reinforcing the staple lines with pericardial strips or by covering the lung surfaces with biologic or artificial glues. A *subtotal parietal pleurectomy* is usually added to the procedure, and two drainage tubes are left in the pleural space. The purpose of the pleurectomy is to create an *inflammatory surface* to which the lung can adhere, thus minimizing the occurrence of prolonged air leaks.

External Drainage of a Bulla

External drainage of a bulla is a *useful technique* for patients considered to be at high risk for major surgery. The procedure can be done under local anesthesia and does not preclude later bullectomy. In most cases, however, external drainage is done under *general anesthesia*. The bulla is intubated with a large Foley catheter (32 Fr) that is held in place by purse-string sutures inserted in the bulla wall (Brompton technique). Postoperatively, the Foley catheter is connected to an underwater seal drainage system; it can be removed 8 to 10 days later, irrespective of residual air leakage.

With the development of VATS techniques, however, external drainage of bullae is now infrequently done.

Postoperative Care

Once the operation is completed, *assisted ventilation must be discontinued as soon as the patient is awake;* most are extubated in the operating room. Adequate postoperative care includes optimal pain control (epidural narcotics), aggressive chest physiotherapy, early ambulation, and drug treatment when required.

In general, morbidity after bullectomy relates to delayed expansion of the lung, prolonged air leaks, and pleuropulmonary infections. Respiratory failure is uncommon because with proper selection of patients, pulmonary function is expected to improve with the removal of giant bullae.

LUNG VOLUME REDUCTION SURGERY FOR NONBULLOUS EMPHYSEMA

LVRS has been advocated for dyspneic patients with severe emphysema and diffuse hyperinflation.

Rationale for Surgery (Table 11-85)

The main objective of LVRS is to remove redundant air spaces thought to interfere with hyperinflated but more functional adjacent lung tissue. This will *improve elastic recoil in the remaining lung,* which in turn will increase radial traction on terminal bronchioles, allowing them to remain open throughout the respiratory cycle. Another objective of LVRS is to improve the mechanical efficiency of important respiratory muscles, such as the diaphragm, the intercostals (chest wall mechanics), and even the scalenes, by correcting the hyperinflation that places such muscles at a disadvantageous position for adequate function.

Two additional objectives can be achieved by surgery. Surgery might *improve nutritional status and oxygenation,* and these improvements are likely to translate into better respiratory function. LVRS can finally *lower the high expiratory intrathoracic pressures* observed in patients with severe emphysema, thus facilitating venous return and improving cardiac contractility and performance (increased cardiac output).

TABLE 11-85

RATIONALE FOR LUNG VOLUME REDUCTION SURGERY IN DIFFUSE EMPHYSEMA

Remove redundant and nonfunctioning lung tissue

Improve elastic recoil in remaining lung

Increase radial traction around terminal bronchioles, thus improving expiratory airflow

Improve efficiency of respiratory muscles, such as the diaphragm, the intercostals, and the scalenes

Improve nutritional status

Improve arterial hypoxemia

Improve hemodynamics

Selection for Surgery

Although selection criteria may vary, important prerequisites (Table 11-86) are the presence of *severe airway obstruction* with FEV_1 decreased to 20% to 35% of predicted value, *severe hyperinflation* with total lung capacity greater than 130% of predicted, and *heterogeneity of disease* where nonfunctional target areas can be identified on CT. In addition, the patient must have *stopped smoking* for at least 6 months preoperatively and must be able to complete a rehabilitation program.

Criteria used in most institutions to exclude patients for surgery are given in Table 11-87. Most of these criteria do not represent absolute contraindications to LVRS, and none taken by itself is an absolute exclusionary criterion. It is rather the presence of *several risk factors* for poor outcome that is a contraindication for the procedure. Currently, only 25% to 40% of patients considered for LVRS will eventually have the operation.

Operative Approaches and Procedures

At most institutions, pulmonary rehabilitation is the norm before LVRS is performed. It is believed that such programs will improve strength and aerobic conditioning of patients, *making surgery less morbid* and postoperative recovery faster.

Access to the lung for LVRS may be obtained by median sternotomy or by VATS. The essential advantage of sternotomy is that it achieves maximum benefit at one operation with minimum morbidity. When conditions are favorable, however, VATS may offer comparable results with lower morbidity. In general, bilateral procedures, whether they are done by

---

TABLE 11-86
BEST PROFILE FOR LUNG VOLUME REDUCTION SURGERY

Clinical guidelines
End-stage emphysema refractory to medical treatment
Significant dyspnea at rest or at minimal activity
Minimal corticosteroids (<10 mg daily)
Ability to complete rehabilitation program of 6-10 weeks
Age < 70 years and no significant comorbidity
High motivation and acceptance of operative risk
Abstinence of cigarette smoking for at least 6 months preoperatively
Satisfactory nutritional status

Physiologic and morphologic guidelines
Severe airflow limitation (FEV_1 20%-35% of predicted)
Hyperinflation (total lung capacity > 130% of predicted)
$Paco_2$ < 55 mm Hg; diffusing capacity of the lung for carbon monoxide > 20% of predicted
Pulmonary artery pressure < 35 mm Hg (mean)
Heterogeneous distribution of disease
Potential for ventilation and perfusion of residual lung

TABLE 11-87

WORSE PROFILE FOR LUNG VOLUME REDUCTION SURGERY

Clinical guidelines
Bronchitic symptoms or asthma
Age > 70 years
Severe cachexia or obesity
Previous pleurodesis or thoracotomy
Severe left ventricular dysfunction or coronary artery disease
Acquired thoracic deformity
Alcohol dependency

Physiologic and morphologic guidelines
Homogeneous distribution of disease
Inability of residual lung to ventilate and perfuse
$Paco_2$ > 55 mm Hg
Pulmonary hypertension (mean > 35 mm Hg)
Diffusing capacity of the lung for carbon monoxide < 20% of predicted
Ventilator dependency

---

sternotomy or by bilateral VATS approaches, are associated with better results than unilateral reductions are.

The operative technique involves *staple resection of 20% to 30% of the volume of each lung,* target areas having been identified preoperatively by CT scanning or $\dot{V}/\dot{Q}$ isotopic scans. For most patients with emphysema related to smoking, these target areas will be in the upper lobes (Fig. 11-14). With use of single-lung ventilation alternatively on each side (worse lung done first), hyperinflated areas are resected; prolonged air leaks can somewhat be prevented by reinforcing the staple lines with bovine pericardial strips or other material. If an air space is likely to be a problem, a *pleural tent* can be made by dissecting the parietal pleura off the chest wall, thus reducing the boundaries of the pleural space.

Nd:YAG Contact Laser Treatment

Neodymium:yttrium-aluminum-garnet (Nd:YAG) contact laser contracts and shrinks emphysematous areas of the lung. To date, however, most studies have shown that this technique is associated with prolonged air leaks, fewer benefits, and *shorter lasting improvements* in lung function and dyspnea.

Postoperative Care

Postoperative management of LVRS patients is the same as that described for patients undergoing bullectomy (Table 11-88). All patients are extubated immediately after completion of the procedure. Patients usually have one or two chest tubes in each pleural space, and at least initially, these tubes are under suction. Within 24 hours, however, these tubes can

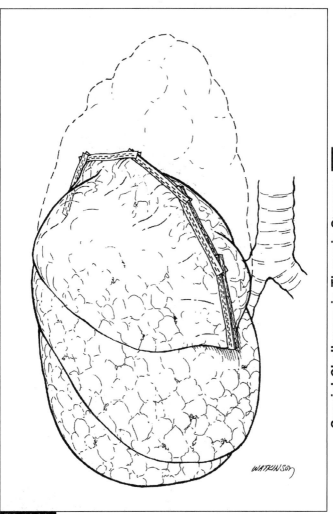

FIG. 11-14

A continuous staple line is used to excise the upper half to two thirds of the upper lobe. The excision begins at the medial aspect of the lobe and is directed upward, over the top, and down the back side at a 45-degree angle to the sagittal plane.
(From Cooper JD: Lung volume reduction for severe emphysema. Chest Surg Clin North Am 1995;5:815).

TABLE 11-88
POSTOPERATIVE MANAGEMENT
Early extubation
Chest tubes in each pleural space
Active respiratory care
Adequate pain control

be placed under water seal drainage, which tends to reduce the severity of air leaks. The use of a Heimlich valve may also facilitate earlier hospital discharge. Adequate pain control is essential for the patient's cooperation and early ambulation; postoperative morbidity usually relates to pulmonary insufficiency, lung infection, or cardiac events.

LUNG TRANSPLANTATION (TABLE 11-89)

The experience of institutions performing both LVRS and lung transplantation suggests that 30% to 50% of patients with advanced disease are concerned with both procedures. Sometimes, LVRS is done to improve the quality of life of patients on a waiting list for transplantation, and on occasion, it may delay transplantation.

In general, patients with an FEV_1 of 20% to 30% of predicted and *heterogeneous patterns of disease* should have LVRS. Patients with an FEV_1 lower than 20% and *homogeneous pattern* are better suited for transplantation.

CONCLUSION

As a rule, surgery for emphysema should be considered palliative if one excludes lung transplantation. It can, however, offer significant benefits in rigorously selected patients who have exhausted other more conservative treatment options.

In addition to rigorous selection, keys to good postoperative outcome include proper understanding of the abnormal physiology related to emphysema, meticulous anesthetic and surgical techniques, and optimal postoperative care.

TABLE 11-89
TRANSPLANTATION AND EMPHYSEMA
30% to 50% of patients with end-stage emphysema are concerned with both LVRS and transplantation
Better operation for patients with $FEV_1 < 20\%$ of predicted
Better operation for patients with homogeneous disease

SUGGESTED READINGS

Review Articles

Gaensler EA, Jederlinic PJ, FitzGerald MX: Patient work-up for bullectomy. J Thorac Imaging 1986;1:75-93.

Klingman RR, Angelillo VA, DeMeester TR: Cystic and bullous lung disease. Ann Thorac Surg 1991;52:576-580.

Cooper JD, Patterson GA: Lung-volume reduction surgery for severe emphysema. Chest Surg Clin North Am 1995;5:815-831.

Todd TR: The preoperative selection of patients for emphysema surgery. Eur J Cardiothorac Surg 1999;16(suppl):s51-s56.

Marchand E, Gayan-Ramirez G, Delyn P, Decramer M: Physiological basis of improvement after lung volume reduction surgery for severe emphysema: where are we? Eur Respir J 1999;13:686-696.

Shrager JB, Kaiser LR, Edelman JD: Lung volume reduction surgery. Curr Probl Surg 2000;37:257-317.

Stirling GR, Babidge WJ, Peacock MJ, et al: Lung volume reduction surgery in emphysema: a systematic review. Ann Thorac Surg 2001;72:641-648.

Koebe HG, Kugler C, Dienemann H: Evidence-based medicine: lung volume reduction surgery. Thorac Cardiovasc Surg 2002;50:315-322.

Gelb AF, McKenna RJ: Lung volume reduction surgery for emphysema: the pros and cons. J Respir Dis 2002;23:475-481.

Gelb AF, McKenna RJ: Lung volume reduction surgery update. Chest 2003;123:975-977.

Deslauriers J, Leblanc P: Emphysema of the lung and lung volume reduction operations. In Shields TW, Locicero J III, Ponn RB, Rusch VW (eds): General Thoracic Surgery, 6th ed, Vol 2. Philadelphia, Lippincott Williams & Wilkins, 2004:1187-1219.

Deslauriers J, Gregoire J, Leblanc D: Bullous and bleb diseases of the lung. In Shields TW, Locicero J III, Ponn RB, Rusch VW (eds): General Thoracic Surgery, 6th ed, Vol 2. Philadelphia, Lippincott Williams & Wilkins, 2004:1168-1187.

Bulla—Surgical Technique

Shaw SS, Goldstraw P: Surgical treatment of bullous emphysema: experience with the Brompton technique. Ann Thorac Surg 1994;58:1452-1456.

Divisi D, Battaglia C, Di Francescantonio W, et al: Giant bullous emphysema resection by VATS. Analysis of laser and stapler techniques. Eur J Cardiothorac Surg 2002;22:990-994.

Bulla—Case Series

Brochard L, Piquet J, Baldeyrou P, et al: Evaluation de l'efficacité du traitement chirurgical de l'emphysème pan-lobulaire. Rev Mal Resp 1986;4:187-194.

Connolly JE, Wilson A: The current status of surgery for bullous emphysema. J Thorac Cardiovasc Surg 1989;97:351-361.

O'Donnell DE, Webb KA, Bertley JC, et al: Mechanisms of relief of exertional breathlessness following unilateral bullectomy and lung volume reduction surgery in emphysema. Chest 1996;110:18-27.

De Giacomo T, Rendina EA, Venuta F, et al: Bullectomy is comparable to lung volume reduction in patients with end-stage emphysema. Eur J Cardiothorac Surg 2002;22:357-362.

Lung Volume Reduction Surgery—Technique

Cooper JD: Technique to reduce air leaks after resection of emphysematous lung. Ann Thorac Surg 1994;57:1038-1039.

Lung Volume Reduction Surgery—Results

McKenna RJ, Brenner M, Fischel RJ, et al: Patient selection criteria for lung volume reduction surgery. J Thorac Cardiovasc Surg 1997;114:957-967.

Weder W, Thurnheer R, Stammberger U, et al: Radiologic emphysema morphology is associated with outcome after surgical lung volume reduction. Ann Thorac Surg 1997;64:313-320.

Zenati M, Keenan RJ, Courcoulas AP, Griffith BP: Lung volume reduction or lung transplantation for end-stage pulmonary emphysema? Eur J Cardiothorac Surg 1998;14:27-32.

Maki DD, Miller WT Jr., Aronchick JM, et al: Advanced emphysema: preoperative chest radiographic findings as predictors of outcome following lung volume reduction surgery. Radiology 1999;212:49-55.

Pompeo E, Marino M, Nofroni I, et al: Reduction pneumoplasty versus respiratory rehabilitation in severe emphysema: a randomized study. Ann Thorac Surg 2000;70:948-954.

Bloch KE, Georgescu CL, Russi EW, Weder W: Gain and subsequent loss of lung function after lung volume reduction surgery in cases of severe emphysema with different morphologic patterns. J Thorac Cardiovasc Surg 2002;123:845-854.

Fujimoto T, Teschler H, Hillejan L, et al: Long-term results of lung volume reduction surgery. Eur J Cardiothorac Surg 2002;21:483-488.

Ciccone AM, Meyers BF, Guthrie TJ, et al: Long-term outcome of bilateral lung volume reduction in 250 consecutive patients with emphysema. J Thorac Cardiovasc Surg 2003;125:513-525.

Yusen RD, Lefrak SS, Gierada DS, et al: A prospective evaluation of lung volume reduction surgery in 200 consecutive patients. Chest 2003;123:1026-1037.

National Emphysema Treatment Trial Research Group: A randomized trial comparing lung volume-reduction surgery with medical therapy for severe emphysema. N Engl J Med 2003;348:2059-2073.

Iwasaki A, Yosinaga Y, Kawahara K, Shirakusa T: Evaluation of lung volume reduction surgery (LVRS) based on long-term survival rate analysis. Thorac Cardiovasc Surg 2003;51:277-282.

Chest Trauma

The spectrum of blunt chest injuries ranges from isolated rib fractures to complex tracheobronchial disruptions and exsanguinating cardiovascular ruptures. Overall, 25% of all trauma deaths are the direct result of chest injuries, which are also a contributing factor in an additional 25%.

The first few hours after the injury are critical not only to document the extent of injuries but also to initiate resuscitation. In this context, it is important to remember that 85% to 90% of blunt chest injuries can be managed with little more than thoracostomy or endotracheal tubes. Emergency department thoracotomy is required in less than 1% to 2% of patients with blunt thoracic trauma.

MECHANISMS AND PATHOPHYSIOLOGY OF INJURY IN BLUNT CHEST TRAUMA (TABLE 12-1)

Most blunt traumas are due to motor vehicle accidents, followed by falls from a height, assaults, and sports crushing injuries. Because the immediate management of these victims is often related to a *proper understanding of the mechanism of injury,* such mechanisms must be known by surgeons and indeed by all physicians working in resuscitation rooms.

Direct impact over the chest wall may result in rib fractures, flail chest, and lung and cardiac contusions. *Forceful anteroposterior compression* increases the transverse diameter of the thoracic cavity and may lead to tracheobronchial tears; in these cases, the negative intrapleural pressure pulls the lungs away from the fixed carina, and main bronchial disruption may occur. In head-on car accidents, the unrestrained occupant

TABLE 12-1
COMMON MECHANISMS OF INJURY IN BLUNT CHEST TRAUMA

Mechanism of Injury	Possible Consequence
Direct impact over thorax	Rib fracture, flail chest, lung and cardiac contusion
Direct impact over hyperextended neck (dashboard injury)	Laryngotracheal injury
Direct impact with closed glottis	Bronchial disruption
Rapid deceleration	Aortic or bronchial rupture
Vertical deceleration (falling from a height)	Aortic rupture
Spinal flexion injuries	Rupture of thoracic duct
Sudden rise in intra-abdominal pressure	Diaphragmatic rupture

(no seat belt) may be thrust forward, and the *direct impact of the steering wheel or the dashboard* over the hyperextended neck may cause significant laryngotracheal injuries.

Rapid deceleration results in shearing forces on the airway and aorta and may thus contribute to the high incidence of bronchial or aortic ruptures observed in motor vehicle accidents. *Vertical deceleration,* such as falling from a height, may be associated with ruptures of the ascending aorta; *longitudinal deceleration* is more likely to result in aortic ruptures distal to the aortopulmonary ligament. Spinal flexion injuries may result in rupture of the thoracic duct (rare injury).

A blunt impact to the chest occurring with a closed glottis often produces a sudden rise in airway pressure that may contribute to tracheobronchial disruptions. Similarly, a *rapid increase in intra-abdominal pressure* may be a precursor of diaphragmatic rupture.

Blunt forces associated with blast exposure can cause significant injuries to gas-containing structures, such as the lungs, intestine, and eardrums.

Blunt chest trauma has the potential for unique consequences because its pathophysiology involves the close relationship between the rigid chest wall and the underlying heart and lungs. Respiratory failure, for instance, may result from the cumulative effects of the loss of integrity of the chest wall (flail chest), interference with pleural mechanics by blood (hemothorax) or air (pneumothorax), interruption of the airway, and *ventilation/perfusion mismatches* due to lung contusion or atelectasis with secondary pneumonia.

INITIAL EVALUATION AND MANAGEMENT

Patient's Clinical History (Table 12-2)

The process of obtaining a clinical history and details about the accident often begins with the first message about a trauma victim's being brought to the hospital. Important information to be obtained includes the *mechanism and time of injury* and, in patients who fell from a height, the height of the fall and the surface on which the patient landed.

Certain forms of trauma are associated with specific types of thoracic injuries. A head-on collision impact with bent steering wheel may, for instance, suggest substantial trauma to the upper airway (larynx, cervical trachea), chest wall, lungs, and myocardium. If a seat belt was not worn, the patient is likely to have continued to move forward after the car has stopped and thus have more severe injuries. Rapid deceleration may suggest avulsion of anatomic structures fixed in the mediastinum, such as the tracheobronchial bifurcation or aortic isthmus.

The *trauma victim's age* is also an important consideration. Children have more elastic ribs than adults do and thus are less exposed to rib fractures, even when they are involved in major blunt trauma. Blunt aortic ruptures, for example, almost always occur without rib fractures in children.

TABLE 12-2

IMPORTANCE OF OBTAINING A GOOD CLINICAL HISTORY IN ASSESSMENT OF
BLUNT CHEST TRAUMA VICTIMS

Patients involved in motor vehicle accident
Time of injury relative to arrival in hospital
Type of impact (head-on collision or side impact)
Patient's location within vehicle (front, back, driver)
Approximate vehicle speed
Ejection from vehicle
Death of another occupant of vehicle
Was the trauma victim wearing a seat belt?

Patients involved in fall from a height
Height of fall
Surface on which patient landed

The opposite is true with elderly or osteoporotic patients, in whom multiple rib fractures can result from relatively minor injuries.

Physical Examination (ABC) (Table 12-3)

Physical examination must be done according to the *Advanced Trauma Life Support guidelines,* and one must be able to determine within a short time if the patient's life is immediately threatened. If it is not, physical examination must be carried out in a systematic fashion. *Airway, breathing, and circulation (ABC)* constitute the priorities of both the initial assessment and management.

TABLE 12-3

IMPORTANCE OF PHYSICAL EXAMINATION IN ASSESSMENT OF BLUNT CHEST
TRAUMA VICTIMS

Area of Examination	Important Clinical Signs	Possible Injury
Airway	Tachypnea, stridor	Airway obstruction or disruption
		Inhalation of a foreign body
Breathing	Abnormal chest wall movements	Flail chest
	Use of accessory muscles of respiration	Severe lung contusion
	Absence of breath sounds	Respiratory failure
		Pneumothoraces, hemothoraces
Circulation	Low blood pressure, tachycardia	Significant hemorrhage
Cervical spine	Pain in back of neck	Fracture-dislocation
Intracranial	Immobility or altered state of consciousness	Head injury

Airway and Breathing (AB)

The top priority in the initial management of patients with severe blunt thoracic traumas is to *establish an airway*. One must therefore look for clinical signs of airway obstruction (or disruption), such as a patient's struggling for air, tachypnea, stridor, hoarseness, or the presence of subcutaneous emphysema. Massive hemoptysis (>500 mL) may suggest a major bronchial rupture.

The chest must be exposed by removing the patient's clothes or by cutting them down. One must carefully observe chest wall movements, which may reveal a *flail segment* (paradoxical movements), diminished movements of one hemithorax or both hemithoraces, or use of accessory respiratory muscles, all signs of impending respiratory failure. Palpation may reveal *crepitation* from fractured ribs or subcutaneous emphysema. Auscultation of both lung fields will document the presence or absence of breath sounds.

Circulation (C)

Initial assessment of the circulatory status is done through the *recording of vital signs* (blood pressure, heart rate), which must be obtained immediately on admission and compared with those obtained in the field. The hemodynamic response to ongoing resuscitation maneuvers must also be monitored frequently. *Profound hypotension* generally indicates severe blood loss, whereas *intact peripheral pulses and well-perfused extremities* imply a normovolemic status.

Other Features of Initial Physical Examination

Because many patients with severe blunt thoracic injuries also have head injuries or fractures of the cervical spine, these must be looked for during the initial evaluation. Cervical spine fractures or dislocations may be suggested by the mechanism of injury involved in the trauma or by *severe pain* in the back of the neck. If these are suspected, *manual cervical spine alignment* must be maintained throughout the initial resuscitation and evaluation. Patients who are immobile, difficult to rouse, or totally unconscious must be suspected of having an intracranial injury.

Diagnostic Procedures

Other than in moribund patients, portable chest radiographs *should always be obtained in the resuscitation room*. Unfortunately, many trauma patients cannot have standard erect radiographs, so the clinician must rely on supine anteroposterior views.

Diagnostic clues that may be present on these initial radiographs and may be indicative of severe underlying intrathoracic injuries are listed in Table 12-4. The combination of upper rib fractures and widened mediastinum may, for example, raise the possibility of aortic trauma; a pneumomediastinum may signal an airway rupture, while an *elevated hemidiaphragm* should raise the possibility of diaphragmatic rupture.

TABLE 12-4

CLUES ON INITIAL PORTABLE CHEST RADIOGRAPH THAT MAY INDICATE SEVERE INTRATHORACIC INJURY

Finding	Possible Injury
Chest wall	
Fracture of upper ribs (1-2)	Aortic rupture, tracheobronchial disruption
Multiple rib fractures	Flail chest
Mediastinum	
Widened mediastinum (>8 cm at level of origin of left subclavian artery)	Aortic rupture
Pneumomediastinum	Airway disruption
Pleural space	
Pneumothorax	Bronchial rupture, lung laceration
Massive hemothorax	Major blood vessel laceration or rupture
Elevated hemidiaphragm	Diaphragmatic rupture
Lungs	
Opacification of lung fields	Lung contusion
Heart	
Widened cardiac silhouette	Cardiac injury, tamponade
Spine	
Misalignment of vertebral bodies	Fracture

Misalignment of vertebral bodies (cervical, thoracic) should be looked for as it may provide the first clue about a *possible spinal fracture*. The initial radiograph may finally be useful to determine the position of the various indwelling tubes (endotracheal, thoracostomy) that may have been inserted. The structures most commonly involved in major blunt thoracic traumas are listed in Table 12-5.

During the resuscitation, blood should be sent for blood gas analysis, complete blood work (hematologic and biochemical), and crossmatch. Blood gas analysis is particularly useful because it provides insight into the quality of gas exchange and possible indication for mechanical ventilation. An electrocardiogram should be obtained because the recording may suggest severe myocardial contusion or pericardial tamponade.

TABLE 12-5

ORGANS MOST COMMONLY INVOLVED IN SEVERE BLUNT THORACIC TRAUMA

Organ	Incidence
Chest wall	70%
Lungs	20%-25%
Heart	10%
Diaphragm	5%
Aorta	3%-4%

TABLE 12-6

CAUSES OF LIFE-THREATENING INJURIES IN BLUNT CHEST TRAUMA

Airway obstruction
    Blood, foreign body, secretions
    Laryngotracheal disruption
Respiratory failure
    Flail chest, severe lung contusion
    Tension pneumothorax
    Tracheobronchial disruption
Massive intrathoracic hemorrhage
    Hemothoraces
    Rupture of major blood vessel
Cardiac failure
    Severe cardiac contusion, tamponade
    Rupture of cardiac valve apparatus

Once the patient has been stabilized, the more definitive investigation of specific intrathoracic injuries can proceed through the use of imaging modalities such as computed tomographic (CT) scanning, angiography, and ultrasonography or endoscopic techniques such as bronchoscopy.

ROLE OF THORACIC SURGEON IN IMMEDIATE STABILIZATION OF PATIENT WITH LIFE-THREATENING THORACIC INJURIES
(TABLE 12-6)

In addition to being part of the resuscitation team, the thoracic surgeon's role in the emergency department is to recognize and treat those thoracic injuries that are an immediate threat to life. These include airway obstruction, respiratory failure, hemorrhage, and cardiac tamponade.

Airway Obstruction

The first priority is to secure the airway, which may have become obstructed by blood, secretions, or foreign bodies such as teeth or dentures (Table 12-7). This can often be done by *simple maneuvers,* such as hand removal of foreign bodies, suctioning of secretions, lifting the jaw anteriorly (lifts up the epiglottis and brings it forward), and use of nasopharyngeal or oropharyngeal airway tubes.

Ultimately, endotracheal intubation is the *best method of airway control.* It can be done through the nose or over a flexible bronchoscope if a cervical spine injury is suspected. Repeated attempts at intubation should, however, be avoided because they may exacerbate mucosal injuries or transform a partial airway disruption into a complete one. In such cases, *emergency tracheostomy* should be performed quickly and without hesitation. One must avoid excessive neck manipulations until a cervical spine fracture has definitely been ruled out.

TABLE 12-7

CAUSES OF UPPER AIRWAY OBSTRUCTION IN BLUNT TRAUMA

Common causes
Blood, secretions
Foreign body

Uncommon causes
Severe maxillofacial injury
Laryngotracheal rupture

Respiratory Failure

Acute and life-threatening respiratory failure can be caused by *severe lung contusion, flail chest, tension pneumothorax, tracheobronchial rupture,* or a combination of these injuries.

Pulmonary contusion is often associated with multiple rib fractures or flail chest. In severe cases, respiratory failure can develop quickly as it relates to multiple factors including the flail segment, severe pain, lung damage with alveolar hemorrhage and interstitial edema, and reflex diaphragmatic paralysis (see Chapter 12, "Management of Rib Fractures and Flail Chest"). If initial supportive care consisting of oxygen supplementation, pain control, and chest physiotherapy including suctioning does not relieve the problem, intubation and mechanical ventilation may become necessary.

Tension pneumothoraces are caused by a *valvular mechanism* that allows air to enter the pleural space during inspiration but prevents its escape during expiration. Eventually, the positive pleural pressure will cause mediastinal displacement, compression of the opposite lung, and distortion in venae cavae with secondary decrease in venous return and cardiac output. Immediate treatment involves *space decompression* either with a needle attached to a water seal or with thoracostomy tube drainage.

Most tracheobronchial ruptures occur *within 2.5 cm of the carina,* and the most common injury is a *complete avulsion of the right main bronchus* off the trachea. Because associated injuries are common, most such patients do not reach the hospital alive. If they do, however, early diagnosis is possible, and most tears can be successfully repaired with preservation of lung tissue (see Chapter 12, "Management of the Patient with Possible Airway Trauma").

Massive Hemorrhage

Massive intrathoracic hemorrhage is usually the consequence of major thoracic vascular injuries. Unfortunately, most patients with such injuries do not reach the hospital alive. If they do, however, it is because the *rupture was contained* either by the adventitia of the blood vessel or by the mediastinal pleura. In such patients, early resuscitation must aim at

12

Chest Trauma

TABLE 12-8

POSSIBLE INDICATIONS FOR EMERGENCY THORACOTOMY IN PATIENTS WITH BLUNT THORACIC TRAUMA

Hemorrhage
  Initial blood loss > 1200 mL
  Continued tube drainage > 300 mL/h
  Hemodynamically unstable patient
Tracheobronchial disruption with open communication with pleural space
Documented or probable rupture of major intrathoracic blood vessel

---

keeping the arterial blood pressure no higher than 70 to 80 mm Hg because higher levels may result in completion of the rupture before repair can be performed. The aorta will rupture within 24 hours of trauma in *25% of initial survivors,* and the risk of delayed rupture declines in an exponential fashion thereafter.

In all cases of hemothoraces, a large-bore chest tube should be used to evacuate the pleural space. Thoracotomy (Table 12-8) may be indicated for an initial tube thoracostomy blood loss greater than 1200 mL, continued drainage greater than 300 mL/h, or a hemodynamically unstable patient. Videothoracoscopic examination is sometimes useful, especially if the amount of bleeding is between 1000 and 1500 mL or if the surgeon has doubts about the indication for formal thoracotomy. Radiologic signs possibly associated with aortic or other large vessel injury are listed in Table 12-9.

TABLE 12-9

RADIOLOGIC SIGNS POSSIBLY ASSOCIATED WITH AORTIC INJURY SECONDARY TO BLUNT TRAUMA

Best signs
  Widened mediastinum (>8 cm)
  Blurred aortic knob
Deviation of structures
  Depression of left main bronchus
  Deviation of esophagus or nasogastric tube to the right
  Deviation of trachea or endotracheal tube to the right
Obliteration
  Loss of paraspinous stripe
  Obliteration of aortopulmonary window
Associated findings
  Massive hemothorax (left)
  First rib fracture
  Left apical cap (apical hemothorax)

From Jackimczyk K: Blunt chest trauma. Emerg Med Clin North Am 1993;11:81-96, with permission.

Circulatory Failure

Failure to maintain adequate vital signs despite optimal management may be due to circulatory failure secondary to blunt injury of the heart and pericardium. Most of these injuries are associated with *motor vehicle accidents* in which the heart is compressed between sternum (steering wheel) and spine or a deceleration force throws the heart forward against the sternum.

Although myocardial contusion is probably common in severe thoracic blunt injuries (20% of patients in autopsy series), the lesion may be difficult to confirm because there are no standard diagnostic criteria. Most of these injuries may cause transient decrease in cardiac output, which will resolve rapidly.

Pericardial tamponade is rare after blunt chest trauma, but it can occur in association with myocardial laceration or even heart rupture (usually right ventricle) suffered in head-on automobile accidents. The diagnosis is clinically suggested by *profound hypotension and rise in central venous pressure* (evidenced by distended neck veins) and confirmed by echocardiography or pericardiocentesis. In such cases, release of the tamponade is a true emergency but should preferably be done in the operating room. Small pericardial effusions secondary to myocardial contusions are of no clinical or physiologic consequence.

Valvular lesions secondary to blunt trauma are *uncommon* in patients who reach the hospital alive. The spectrum of injury ranges from papillary muscle rupture to leaflet laceration or disruption (more commonly aortic valve), and on occasion, the clinical symptoms at presentation will be those of cardiogenic shock or fulminating pulmonary edema secondary to mitral regurgitation. In general, it is best to delay surgical repair until the patient has sufficiently recovered from the trauma because the operation implies the use of heparin.

Commotio cordis is a rare entity in which a ventricular arrhythmia is precipitated by low-energy and low-velocity blows to the chest often suffered in the context of sporting activities. Only 15% of patients will survive the event through prompt cardiopulmonary resuscitation and defibrillation.

MANAGEMENT OF PATIENTS INITIALLY UNRESPONSIVE TO RESUSCITATION MEASURES: INDICATIONS FOR EMERGENCY DEPARTMENT THORACOTOMY (TABLE 12-10)

Other than in the most unusual circumstance, emergency department thoracotomy is of *extremely limited benefit* in blunt trauma victims. One possible indication is the patient who is about to sustain a cardiac arrest as a result of cardiac tamponade. In these individuals, decompression of the pericardium may be lifesaving, although hemorrhage may recur once the tamponade effect of blood has been released and the pericardium has been decompressed. On occasion, thoracotomy may also be indicated for internal cardiac massage and treatment in patients who have suffered a witnessed cardiac arrest in the emergency department.

12

Chest Trauma

TABLE 12-10

POSSIBLE INDICATIONS FOR EMERGENCY DEPARTMENT THORACOTOMY
IN BLUNT TRAUMA VICTIMS

Cardiac arrest as a result of tamponade

Witnessed cardiac arrest in emergency department

CONCLUSION

Because the chest is involved in about one third of blunt traumas, optimal management often requires the expertise of a thoracic surgeon. Fortunately, the majority of thoracic trauma can be managed nonoperatively with careful resuscitation and simple diagnostic and therapeutic maneuvers.

SUGGESTED READINGS

Review Articles

Hiebert CA: Thoracicoabdominal trauma: a plan for initial management. Can J Surg 1975;18:335-337.

Lewis FR: Thoracic trauma. Surg Clin North Am 1982;62:97-104.

Mattox KL, Allen MK: Emergency department treatment of chest injuries. Emerg Med Clin North Am 1984;2:783-798.

Cooper C, Militello P: The multi-injured patient: the Maryland shock trauma protocol approach. Semin Thorac Cardiovasc Surg 1992;4:163-167.

Feliciano DV: The diagnostic and therapeutic approach to chest trauma. Semin Thorac Cardiovasc Surg 1992;4:156-162.

McSwain NE Jr.: Blunt and penetrating chest injuries. World J Surg 1992;16:924-929.

Jackimczyk K: Blunt chest trauma. Emerg Med Clin North Am 1993;11:81-95.

Samson L, Cordeau MP: Chest trauma: practical radiologic signs. Can J Diagn 1999;16:133-140.

Shapiro MB, Jenkins DH, Schwab CW, Rotondo MF: Damage control: collective review. J Trauma 2000;49:969-978.

Karmy-Jones R, Jurkovich GJ: Blunt chest trauma. Curr Probl Surg 2004;41:205-380.

Cardiovascular Blunt Trauma

Maron BJ, Gohman TE, Kyle SB, et al: Clinical profile and spectrum of commotio cordis. JAMA 2002;287:1142-1146.

Blunt Trauma in Children

Dowd MD, Krug S: Pediatric blunt cardiac injury: epidemiology, clinical features, and diagnosis. J Trauma 1996;40:61-67.

Ceran S, Sunam GS, Aribas OK, et al: Chest trauma in children. Eur J Cardiothorac Surg 2002;21:57-59.

Balci AE, Kazez A, Eren S, et al: Blunt trauma in children: review of 137 cases. Eur J Cardiothorac Surg 2004;26:387-392.

Blunt Trauma in Elderly

Shorr RM, Rodriguez A, Indeck MC, et al: Blunt chest trauma in the elderly. J Trauma 1989;29:234-237.

Tube Thoracostomy and Blunt Trauma

Meyer DM, Jessen ME, Wait MA, Estrera AS: Early evacuation of traumatic retained hemothoraces using thoracoscopy: a prospective, randomized trial. Ann Thorac Surg 1997;64:1396-1401.

Bailey RC: Complications of tube thoracostomy in trauma. J Accid Emerg Med 2000;17:111-114.

Luchette FA, Barrie PS, Oswanski MF, et al: Practice management guidelines for prophylactic antibiotic use in tube thoracostomy for traumatic hemopneumothorax: the EAST Practice Management Guidelines Work Group. J Trauma 2000;48:753-757.

Deneuville M: Morbidity of percutaneous tube thoracostomy in trauma patients. Eur J Cardiothorac Surg 2002;22:673-678.

Thoracotomy and Blunt Trauma

Rhee PM, Acosta J, Bridgeman A, et al: Survival after emergency department thoracotomy: review of published data from the past 25 years. J Am Coll Surg 2000;190:288-298.

Grove CA, Lemmon G, Anderson G, McCarthy M: Emergency thoracotomy: appropriate use in the resuscitation of trauma patients. Am Surg 2002;68:313-317.

Athanasiou T, Krasopoulos G, Nambiar P, et al: Emergency thoracotomy in the pre-hospital setting: a procedure requiring clarification. Eur J Cardiothorac Surg 2004;26:377-386.

Airway Management and Blunt Trauma

Karch SB, Lewis T, Young S, et al: Field intubation of trauma patients: complications, indications, and outcomes. Am J Emerg Med 1996;14:617-619.

Bulger EM, Copass MK, Maier RV, et al: An analysis of advanced prehospital airway management. J Emerg Med 2002;23:183-189.

Ben-Nun A, Altman E, Best LAE: Emergency percutaneous tracheostomy in trauma patients: an early experience. Ann Thorac Surg 2004;77: 1045-1047.

Case Series

Shorr RM, Crittenden M, Indeck M, et al: Blunt thoracic trauma. Analysis of 515 patients. Ann Surg 1987;206:200-205.

Peterson RJ, Tepas JJ, Edwards FH, et al: Pediatric and adult thoracic trauma: age-related impact on presentation and outcome. Ann Thorac Surg 1994;58:14-18.

Other

Dulchavsky SA, Schwarz KL, Kirkpatrick AW, et al: Prospective evaluation of thoracic ultrasound in the detection of pneumothorax. J Trauma 2001;50:201-205.

INITIAL MANAGEMENT OF THE PATIENT WITH PENETRATING TRAUMA

Penetrating chest wounds are among the most challenging problems in the practice of thoracic surgery. In urban centers, they are usually caused by low-velocity missiles (handguns); in war zones, bomb fragments and high-velocity missiles are the main sources of injury. Although less frequent, industrial accidents or high-speed motor vehicle accidents can also be associated with penetrating chest injuries such as open pneumothoraces.

Survival of penetrating trauma victims depends on the type of weapon that was used, the location of the injury, the on-site recognition and early management of critical lesions, and most important, the *prompt referral to major trauma centers* where systematic evaluation and treatment can be carried out by skilled personnel including experienced thoracic surgeons. Whereas most patients reaching the hospital alive can be successfully managed conservatively, approximately 15% to 20% of penetrating trauma victims will require emergency or immediate thoracotomy.

EPIDEMIOLOGY

Incidence and General Considerations

In large industrial centers, penetrating injuries to the chest are *about two to three times more common* than penetrating wounds to the abdomen, and most are located over the anterior chest wall (left > right). The type of weapon used reflects the circumstances of the aggression as well as the availability of specific weapons. Knife wounds, for instance, are frequently encountered in street gang fighting; guns are often fired during robberies, altercations, or "crimes of passion."

Although the exact ratio of trauma due to gunshot versus stab wounds is difficult to determine, *firearm injuries are generally considered to be more common* than stab wounds in North American urban centers.

Pathophysiology and Mechanism of Injury

The amount of tissue destruction suffered during traumatic penetration of the chest depends on the type of weapon used as well as the *velocity and mass of the missile* in cases of firearm injuries (Table 12-11). Stab wounds and low-velocity missiles (<300 m/sec) from handguns have low-impact kinetic energy that generally causes no major tissue destruction beyond the trajectory of the missile. By contrast, high-velocity missiles (750 to 850 m/sec), such as those coming off automatic rifles or machine guns, have high-impact energy that creates an *explosion-like effect causing laceration and cavitation* of tissues adjacent to the missile's trajectory (collateral damage). Such high-impact energy weapons also produce *secondary missiles,* such as rib fragments, that can add to the magnitude of the injury. Shrapnel are *projected missiles* coming off bombs, mines, or grenades. They have various sizes, weight, and speed as well as *unpredictable* paths in living tissues.

TABLE 12-11

MAGNITUDE OF INJURY IN PENETRATING TRAUMAS

The magnitude of injury is proportional to the kinetic energy involved:

$$F = M \times V$$

F   Force of kinetic energy involved
M   Mass (weight) of impacting object
V   Velocity (or acceleration) of impacting object

In high-velocity injuries, the extent of tissue damage also relates to the *range of shooting* and *characteristics of the tissue being injured*. Short-range shots (<5 meters) from shotguns, for instance, cause more massive tissue destruction than long-range shots do. Compact tissues such as those of chest wall muscles often absorb increased kinetic energy so that patients hit by high-velocity missiles may suffer significant cardiac or pulmonary contusion without the missile's having actually penetrated the pleural space (Fig. 12-1).

Injuries by Location (Table 12-12)

Although the chest wall is penetrated in 100% of cases, rib flexibility may have diverted the missile away from the pleural space. In such cases, broken ribs may have caused injury to intercostal pedicles (intercostal arteries) or even to the lung with secondary hemothoraces or pneumothoraces or both. Patients wearing bulletproof vests can also experience fractured ribs or *high kinetic energy–related pulmonary contusion* when they are hit by high-velocity missiles.

If the penetration reaches the parietal pleura, 90% of patients will have a lung injury and 50% to 60% will have a pneumohemothorax. Other possible intrathoracic visceral injuries include those to the diaphragm (20% to 30%) and to the heart and great vessels (10%). Penetrating trauma to the airway or esophagus is unusual.

In many cases of lower chest wounds, associated intra-abdominal injuries will have occurred through *penetration of the diaphragm*. The most commonly injured organs are the liver (20%), the stomach (8%), the small and large bowel, and the kidneys.

ASSESSMENT OF THE PATIENT WITH PENETRATING CHEST INJURY

Initial Assessment

The initial assessment of the patient with penetrating chest trauma must include a brief recording of the nature of the incident. The length of the blade in cases of knife wounds, the *caliber of the firearm* and range of shooting, the position of the victim during the injury, and what happened afterward (Did the patient fall out of a window?) are all helpful pieces of information.

Vital signs should immediately be recorded, and if the patient is in cardiac arrest or imminent cardiac arrest, he or she may need immediate

12

Chest Trauma

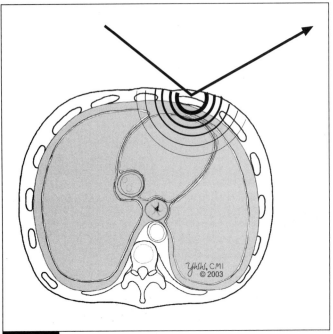

FIG. 12-1

High-velocity missiles ricocheting from the chest wall can potentially cause significant cardiac or pulmonary contusion.

emergency department thoracotomy without further investigation.
The adequacy of airway and ventilation must also be determined, and if possible, *mechanical ventilation should be avoided* to prevent expulsion of air into the pulmonary veins with subsequent air embolism.

For the missile's trajectory to be assessed, the sites of entrance and exit wounds should be looked for, remembering that bullet trajectories are not

TABLE 12-12

COMMONLY INJURED THORACIC STRUCTURES IN PENETRATING TRAUMA

Structure	Incidence
Chest wall	100%
Lung	90%
Diaphragm	20%-30%
Heart and great vessels	10%
Airway	<5%
Esophagus	<2%

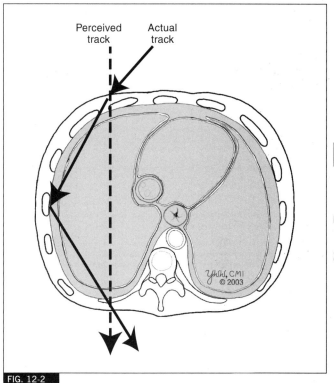

FIG. 12-2

Altered trajectory of a missile because of ricochet over the chest wall. Note that high-velocity missiles can create an explosion-like effect within the pleural space.

always in a straight line from entrance to exit (Fig. 12-2) and that several shots may have been fired. On occasion, cautious digital exploration may be of some value in assessing the direction of a knife track. If there is an open pneumothorax with sucking wound, temporary closure of the defect can be accomplished by covering it with a plastic sheet taped over three sides. If the patient's condition has stabilized, signs and symptoms of specific injuries can then be sought and a portable chest radiograph obtained.

An elevated central venous pressure (distended neck veins) in the presence of a low or decreasing arterial pressure should raise the possibility of cardiac penetration with *pericardial tamponade.* Central entrance wounds *in the parasternal area* with either hemorrhagic shock or cardiac tamponade are also suggestive of cardiac or great vessel injuries.

Wounds in the clavicular area should raise the possibility of thoracic inlet vascular injury, especially if the patient has diminished or absent upper extremity pulses. Diaphragmatic and intra-abdominal injuries must be considered with any stab wound below the nipples anteriorly or at the same level in the flank or back and with gunshot wounds in the lower chest. In such cases, abdominal examination is often nonspecific, but some patients with perforated abdominal viscera may have guarding or rebound tenderness. The presence of subcutaneous emphysema in the chest or neck is a sign of pneumothorax and most likely of lung injury.

Initial chest radiographs are useful to demonstrate pneumothoraces, hemothoraces, and mediastinal widening. In the absence of an exit wound, these radiographs may also delineate the location of the bullet in relation to mediastinal structures.

Other Investigations (Table 12-13)

In stable patients, CT scanning, angiography, and two-dimensional echocardiography often provide complete diagnostic evaluation without surgical exploration of the chest.

Angiography is useful to demonstrate vascular injuries, although *contrast-enhanced helical CT scanning* has now been shown to be an effective and more readily available technique for diagnosis of such injuries. Two-dimensional echocardiography can be done to rule out or to document the presence of blood in the pericardium. Diagnostic videothoracoscopy or subxiphoid pericardial window can be used in patients with possible penetrating cardiac wounds.

TABLE 12-13
USEFUL DIAGNOSTIC TECHNIQUES IN PATIENTS WITH PENETRATING CHEST TRAUMA*

Technique	Usefulness
CT scanning	Trajectory and location of missiles
	Diagnosis of mediastinal lesions (blood vessels, heart, esophagus)
	Assessment of severity of lung contusion
Angiography	Laceration of innominate, subclavian, carotid arteries
Two-dimensional echocardiography or transesophageal echocardiography	Diagnosis of hemopericardium
Subxiphoid pericardial window	Diagnosis of hemopericardium
Videothoracoscopy	Diagnosis of diaphragmatic or cardiac injuries
Laparoscopy	Diagnosis of diaphragmatic injury and of associated abdominal organ injuries
Barium swallow examination	Diagnosis of esophageal wounds
Peritoneal lavage	Diagnosis of transdiaphragmatic intra-abdominal injuries
Bronchoscopy	Diagnosis of tracheobronchial penetration

*These techniques should be done only in stable patients.

In patients with suspected diaphragmatic injury, *videothoracoscopy* has become a safe and reliable diagnostic technique. If an associated injury to an abdominal organ is suspected, laparoscopic examination or peritoneal lavage can also be done. If the trajectory of the missile is close to the airway or esophagus as documented by CT scanning, the patient may need a barium swallow examination or bronchoscopy to rule out a tracheobronchial or esophageal penetration.

These additional investigations are possible and indeed useful in *hemodynamically stable victims,* but patients in immediate danger of cardiac arrest may be better managed by an urgent operation without prior specific investigation.

MANAGEMENT OF THE PATIENT WITH PENETRATING CHEST INJURY

Possible Indications for Emergency Department Thoracotomy
(Table 12-14)

During the initial assessment period, all patients should have two large intravenous lines inserted, and blood should be sent for typing and crossmatching. Patients with severe respiratory difficulties and those in profound shock should be intubated and mechanically ventilated.

Emergency department thoracotomy (Table 12-14) is usually performed in moribund patients or in patients who have suffered a cardiac arrest shortly after arrival. The chest is opened anteriorly *through a left fourth interspace incision that can be extended across the sternum* if necessary. Effective open cardiac massage may then be instituted, the pericardium may be entered, and cardiorrhaphy may be performed. Lifesaving direct pressure can be applied to the site of major blood vessel penetration, and in cases of extensive lung injury, a vascular clamp can be placed across the entire pulmonary hilum. Midthoracic *aortic cross-clamping* for periods of 10 to 20 minutes may temporarily improve cerebral and coronary blood flow.

To be successful, emergency department thoracotomies must be performed by experienced teams operating in a well-equipped trauma center. Under such circumstances, survival is approximately 30% for patients with stab wounds and less than 10% for those with high-velocity bullet wounds. *A significant proportion of survivors will suffer from permanent neurologic sequelae.*

12

Chest Trauma

TABLE 12-14

POSSIBLE INDICATIONS FOR EMERGENCY DEPARTMENT THORACOTOMY IN PATIENTS WITH PENETRATING CHEST INJURIES

Postinjury cardiac arrest
Profound hypotension as a result of pericardial tamponade
Profound hypotension as a result of massive thoracic or thoracoabdominal bleeding

Possible Indications for Immediate Operating Room Thoracotomy
(Table 12-15)

Patients with severe hypotension but not in immediate danger of cardiac arrest should be given colloids initially followed by packed red cells as necessary. Open thoracic wounds should be covered by plastic sheets, and a large-bore thoracostomy tube should be inserted without waiting for radiologic confirmation of the presence of a hemothorax. Although there is no time for complex investigations, portable chest radiography and sometimes ultrasonography may be useful to document the likely cause of hypotension.

The next step is to decide whether the patient requires *immediate operating room thoracotomy.* A large amount of initial bleeding (>1500 mL) associated with an unstable blood pressure or a continuous high drainage (>250 to 300 mL/h) for 2 to 3 hours is generally considered an indication for emergency *operating room* exploration. This is particularly true if the penetration has occurred in cardiac proximity (cardiac box), which is defined as an anatomic territory bounded superiorly by the clavicles, inferiorly by the costal margins, and laterally by the midclavicular lines, or if the entrance wound is in the thoracic inlet or supraclavicular regions with possible great vessel injury. Immediate operating room surgery may also be indicated in unstable patients with a pericardial tamponade likely to be due to cardiac penetration.

A left anterior thoracotomy provides the most rapid exposure to the heart and allows excellent access to most of the cardiac surfaces, left hilum, and aorta. If the injury requires access to the right chest, the incision can be extended to the right across the sternum. The incision can also be *extended posteriorly* for access to the descending thoracic aorta. A median sternotomy can also be used for transmediastinal gunshot wounds, wounds to the right of the sternum, or injuries to vessels of the thoracic inlet (innominate, subclavian, and carotid arteries). Although *cardiopulmonary bypass is seldom required,* the surgical team should be ready to use it if necessary. Once the site of penetration has been identified (most commonly the right ventricle), digital pressure is applied until suture control can be accomplished.

TABLE 12-15

POSSIBLE INDICATIONS FOR IMMEDIATE OPERATING ROOM THORACOTOMY IN PATIENTS WITH PENETRATING THORACIC INJURIES

Severe and persistent hypotension unresponsive to fluid resuscitation

Severe hypotension and suspected major vascular injury (penetration in thoracic inlet)

Severe hypotension and suspected heart injury (penetration within cardiac box)

Initial thoracotomy tube blood loss > 1200-1500 mL or continued high drainage for 2-3 hours

Pericardial tamponade

Documented airway penetration

Management of the Stable Patient: Possible Indications for Early Operation

More than half the patients who are stable on admission or have become stable with fluid resuscitation will never require surgery. However, these patients should undergo *CT scan evaluation* as part of their trauma work-up, and if the wound is transmediastinal, they may also need angiography. Possible indications for surgery in such patients are listed in Table 12-16.

Penetration of the Chest Wall

Knife or low-velocity missile penetration of the chest wall may require surgery to control injuries to the *intercostal vascular bundle or internal mammary artery.* High-velocity missiles or shotgun blasts can also cause extensive loss of chest wall tissues, creating an open chest wound that must be completely débrided. The resulting defect is usually closed with a rotation muscle flap rather than with prosthetic meshes because these wounds are invariably contaminated.

Penetration of the Parietal Pleura

Most surgeons agree that if large amounts of blood clots are retained in the pleural space despite thoracostomy drainage, they should be evacuated usually through the use of *videothoracoscopy.* The evacuation of such clotted hemothoraces may *prevent* the occurrence of late empyemas or fibrothoraces.

Penetration of the Lung and Major Airway

In civilian practice, less than 5% of patients with penetrating chest trauma will require operative treatment of lung injuries, and in the majority of those cases, the indication is based on *hemorrhaging* from pulmonary blood vessels rather than on air leakage. Most lung injuries can be repaired by *direct suturing or by pulmonary tractotomy,* which involves dividing the parenchyma bridging the wound track and oversewing the

12

Chest Trauma

TABLE 12-16

POSSIBLE INDICATIONS FOR SURGERY IN THE STABLE PATIENT WITH PENETRATING THORACIC INJURIES

Injury	Surgical Indication
Chest wall injury	Control bleeding from intercostal or internal mammary arteries
	Repair of extensive loss of chest wall tissues
Retained hemothoraces	Evacuation to prevent late empyemas and fibrothoraces
Penetration of lung and major airway	Control bleeding from pulmonary blood vessels
	Repair of airway penetration
Penetration of the esophagus	Repair of site of injury
Penetration of the diaphragm	Repair of site of injury

bleeding sites. Extensive lung destruction may require lobectomy or pneumonectomy, but the latter procedure is associated with significant mortality rates.

Penetrating trauma to the airway is usually associated with other major mediastinal injuries. Once diagnosed, the site of injury should be primarily repaired during immediate operating room thoracotomy. Surprisingly, many of these patients will have stabilized both hemodynamically and from a respiratory point of view, and the lesion will have been discovered at bronchoscopy done for hemoptysis, subcutaneous emphysema, or stridor. This is because tracheobronchial injuries associated with penetrating trauma are *almost always partial ruptures* as opposed to the usually complete ruptures associated with blunt trauma. Low-velocity handgun bullets can cause minor tracheobronchial lacerations that can be treated conservatively.

Penetration of the Esophagus

Penetration of the esophagus is uncommon. The diagnosis is often made because the emergency department physician had a high index of suspicion and alertness in looking for such an injury. The diagnosis is confirmed by esophagography or CT scan, and *primary repair is always indicated*. Middle and upper third esophageal injuries are best approached through a right thoracotomy, and lower third injuries by a left thoracotomy.

Penetration of the Diaphragm

The incidence of diaphragmatic injury is high (40% to 50%) in patients with penetrating trauma to the left lower chest or in those with thoracoabdominal injuries. In the acute setting, these patients are often asymptomatic, and the peritoneal lavage will be negative in up to one third of cases. If there is still a high suspicion of diaphragmatic injury (penetrating trauma to the thoracoabdominal area), *video-assisted thoracoscopic surgery is useful to identify or to rule out such injuries.* Small lacerations can be repaired through this approach; larger defects may require conversion to open thoracotomy. It is agreed that diaphragmatic defects should be repaired as soon as possible because they can result in diaphragmatic herniation with potential for incarceration and strangulation of abdominal viscera.

Diaphragmatic penetration can also be assessed *laparoscopically* and by laparotomy. Both techniques have the advantage of including the evaluation of potentially associated intra-abdominal injuries that may not be clinically evident.

MANAGEMENT OF THE PATIENT WITH SYSTEMIC ARTERIAL AIR EMBOLISM

The physiology of pulmonary blood vessels and current techniques of mechanical ventilation are conducive to the formation of systemic air embolism in patients with penetrating injuries to the lung or major airways.

In such cases, a dynamic fistula is created between lung parenchyma and pulmonary venous circulation, with air potentially gaining access to the aorta and coronary arteries.

The clinical diagnosis of air embolism is difficult, but once it is made, the only possible treatment is to *interrupt the source of air* emboli by immediate clamping of the pulmonary hilum. Hyperbaric oxygen treatment should be considered in such patients because good results have been reported in patients with systemic air embolism from other causes.

CONCLUSION

During the past 25 to 40 years, urbanization and ready availability of firearms have resulted in a significant increase in the number of penetrating thoracic wounds. Successful management rests on basic knowledge of normal cardiopulmonary anatomy, rapid determination of the most likely trajectory of the penetration, and immediate resuscitation. On occasion, emergency department thoracotomy may be lifesaving.

12

Chest Trauma

SUGGESTED READINGS

Review Articles

Feliciano DV: The diagnostic and therapeutic approach to chest trauma. Semin Thorac Cardiovasc Surg 1992;4:156-162.

Pezzella AT, Silva WE, Lancey RA: Cardiothoracic trauma. Curr Probl Surg 1998;35:647-790.

Penetrating Trauma—Cardiovascular

Asensio JA, Berne JD, Demetriades D, et al: One hundred five penetrating cardiac injuries: a 2-year prospective evaluation. J Trauma 1998;44:1073-1082.

Hanpeter DE, Demetriades D, Asensio JA, et al: Helical computed tomographic scan in the evaluation of mediastinal gunshot wounds. J Trauma 2000;49:689-695.

Penetrating Trauma—Lung

Gasparri M, Karmy-Jones R, Kralovich KA, et al: Pulmonary tractotomy versus lung resection: viable options in penetrating lung injury. J Trauma 2001;51:1092-1097.

Penetrating Trauma—Diaphragm

Murray JA, Demetriades D, Cornwell EE III, et al: Penetrating left thoracoabdominal trauma: the incidence and clinical presentation of diaphragm injuries. J Trauma 1997;43:624-626.

Penetrating Trauma—Pediatric

Reinhorn M, Kaufman HL, Hirsch EF, Millham FH: Penetrating thoracic trauma in a pediatric population. Ann Thorac Surg 1996;61: 1501-1505.

Air Embolism

Estrera AS, Pass LJ, Platt MR: Systemic arterial air embolism in penetrating lung injury. Ann Thorac Surg 1990;50:257-261.

Indications for Thoracotomy

Demetriades D, Rabinowitz B, Markides N: Indications for thoracotomy in stab injuries of the chest: a prospective study of 543 patients. Br J Surg 1986;73:888-890.

Baxter BT, Moore EE, Moore JB, et al: Emergency department thoracotomy following injury: critical determinants for patient salvage. World J Surg 1988;12:671-675.

Thompson DA, Rowlands BJ, Walker WE, et al: Urgent thoracotomy for pulmonary or tracheobronchial injury. J Trauma 1988;28:276-280.

Branney SW, Moore EE, Feldhaus KM, Wolfe RE: Critical analysis of two decades of experience with postinjury emergency department thoracotomy in a regional trauma center. J Trauma 1998;45:87-95.

Demetriades D, Velmahos GC: Penetrating injuries of the chest: indications for operation. Scand J Surg 2002;91:41-45.

Videothoracoscopy and Penetrating Trauma

Lang-Lazdunski L, Mouroux J, Pons F, et al: Role of videothoracoscopy in chest trauma. Ann Thorac Surg 1997;63:327-333.

Freeman RK, Al-Dossari G, Hutcheson KA, et al: Indications for using video-assisted thoracoscopic surgery to diagnose diaphragmatic injuries after penetrating chest trauma. Ann Thorac Surg 2001;72:342-347.

Pons F, Lang-Lazdunski L, de Kerangal X, et al: The role of videothoracoscopy in management of precordial thoracic penetrating injuries. Eur J Cardiothorac Surg 2002;22:7-12.

Case Series

Mandal AK, Sanusi M: Penetrating chest wounds: 24 years experience. World J Surg 2001;25:1145-1149.

MANAGEMENT OF RIB FRACTURES AND FLAIL CHEST

The chest wall and its attached muscles and soft tissues are often injured during high-speed motor vehicle accidents or occupational trauma. Rib fractures, for instance, are the *most common of all blunt chest injuries* and occur in approximately 40% to 50% of patients sustaining chest trauma. Isolated rib fractures are uncommon, however, and many such patients will have concomitant trauma to the head or to intrathoracic structures. Indeed, the patient's outcome is often more dependent on the nature and severity of these associated injuries than on the rib fracture itself.

Because the main function of the chest wall is to participate in respiratory mechanics, any loss of its integrity is likely to bring about significant alterations in the respiratory function. These alterations are the result of chest wall pain, loss of integrity of both ribs and muscles of respiration, and associated pulmonary contusion.

RIB FRACTURES

Rib fractures are the most common form of thoracic injury due to nonpenetrating trauma. Although they can be documented in nearly 35% to 50% of all patients, their actual incidence is probably higher because they are notoriously difficult to detect on standard chest radiographs. *Pain control and maintenance of pulmonary function* are key treatment objectives, especially in the elderly and in patients with poor pulmonary reserve.

Mechanisms of Injury and Epidemiology

Motor vehicle accidents account for approximately 70% to 75% of all rib fractures, and in most cases, the injury is related to a *direct blow over the chest wall.* The number of ribs fractured, the number of fractured sites, and the degree of displacement of rib fragments are generally dependent on the *force of impact.* Indeed, the presence of three or more fractured ribs or the presence of a flail segment with chest wall instability is associated with increased pulmonary morbidity and overall mortality (see thoracic Abbreviated Injury Scale, Table 12-17). The fourth through the ninth ribs are the most commonly fractured ribs, and they usually break at the point of impact or at the posterior angle (Table 12-18).

Falls from a height, industrial and farm accidents, sport injuries, and assaults can also be associated with rib fractures. In children younger than 3 years, *child abuse* is a common cause of chest wall injury and rib fractures. In the elderly, rib fractures can result from *violent and sudden muscle pull during coughing* (spontaneous rib fracture).

Diagnosis

Simple rib fractures can be diagnosed by their clinical manifestations, such as pain often made worse by coughing or motion, *localized tenderness on palpation,* and muscle spasm. *Bone crepitus* can be felt if there is displacement of the bone fragments at the site of fracture.

TABLE 12-17

THORACIC ABBREVIATED INJURY SCALE (AIS)

AIS	Severity	Injury Description
1	Minor	Rib contusion, fracture, or both
		Sternal contusion
2	Moderate	2 or 3 rib fractures, stable chest
		Multiple fractures of a single rib
		Sternal fracture
3	Severe, not life-threatening	Rib fracture: open, displaced, comminuted
		Less than 3 rib fractures, stable chest
4	Severe, life-threatening	Flail chest (unstable chest wall)
5	Critical	Severe flail chest (requiring ventilatory support)

TABLE 12-18

SITE OF RIB FRACTURES

Incidence	Ribs	Comment
More common	Ribs 4-9	Break laterally at the point of impact or posteriorly (structural weakness)
Least common	Ribs 1-2	Protected by shoulder girdle
	Ribs 11-12	Mobile ribs (attached only posteriorly) Protected by muscles of abdominal wall

All patients with possible rib fractures should have an initial chest radiograph even if the site of fracture may be difficult to appreciate either because it is incomplete or because the fragments are undisplaced. Chest radiographs are also important *to diagnose or to rule out* associated conditions such as pneumothoraces, hemothoraces, and pulmonary contusions.

Complications (Table 12-19)

Isolated or multiple rib fractures even without chest wall instability often lead to complications, and this is the main reason why many patients, especially the elderly and the debilitated, require hospitalization. Whether each patient should be hospitalized is a question of clinical judgment, understanding that complications and ultimately mortality are proportional to the *number of fractured ribs, age of the patient, and presence or absence of comorbidities.*

Local Complications of Rib Injury

Most of these complications occur early and are related to rib fragments being driven inward at the time of impact. These fragments may cause *lung lacerations* with secondary pneumothoraces, hemothoraces, or both, or they may perforate intercostal blood vessels with resultant intrapleural bleeding (rare).

On occasion, subcutaneous emphysema may occur despite the absence of visible pneumothorax. This finding may be secondary to a

TABLE 12-19

POSSIBLE COMPLICATIONS OF RIB FRACTURES WITHOUT CHEST WALL INSTABILITY

Local complications of rib injury
    Pneumothorax
    Hemothorax
    Pneumohemothorax
    Surgical (subcutaneous) emphysema
    Pulmonary contusion (related to crushing impact)
Pulmonary complications related to inadequate pain control
    Atelectasis, pneumonia
    Respiratory failure

still undiagnosed airway injury or more commonly to a laceration of the lung in the presence of preexisting pleural symphysis. In such cases, *the air escapes directly into the subcutaneous tissues* at the site of laceration.

Pulmonary Complications Related to Inadequate Pain Control

Pulmonary complications related to inadequate pain control are the result of *ineffective cough and shallow breathing* leading to retained secretions and atelectasis, decreased ventilatory function, and impaired gas exchange. When these factors are associated with changes in chest wall mechanics and lung compliance (pulmonary contusion), they may ultimately cause frank respiratory failure.

Management

Management of patients with rib fractures includes pain control, pulmonary toilet, and treatment of associated conditions.

Pain Control (Table 12-20)

Analgesia should be tailored to every clinical situation with the objectives of pain control and prevention of pulmonary complications.

Most patients with isolated rib fractures can be treated with *oral opioids*. *Narcotics* must obviously be administered with caution, especially in elderly patients, because they can lead to hypoventilation and respiratory failure. *Nonsteroidal anti-inflammatory drugs* are reliable, but their use can be associated with gastrointestinal side effects.

Intercostal nerve blocks are of definite assistance. They are done with 1% lidocaine or 0.25% bupivacaine, and ideally one or two ribs above and one or two ribs below the site of fracture should be infiltrated. Unfortunately, the effect of intercostal nerve blocks wears off after 5 to 6 hours so that they have to be repeated. Transcutaneous electrical nerve stimulation is an alternative pain control method usually reserved for patients with *minor rib fractures*.

As the number of rib fractures increases, pain control becomes more of a problem. In this setting, *patient-controlled analgesia* in combination with intercostal nerve blocks may be useful. *Epidural analgesia* with narcotics, local anesthetics, or both is also effective; for many patients, it is the procedure of choice given the possibility of continuous administration of short-acting opioids such as fentanyl. *Intrapleural catheter analgesia* can be used, but its effectiveness depends on several factors including proper positioning of the catheter, thickness of the pleura, and presence or absence of an associated hemothorax.

Local measures, such as *adhesive chest strapping,* can be effective in young and otherwise healthy patients. They are contraindicated in older patients or in patients with preexisting chronic obstructive lung disease because their use prevents deep breathing, thus maximizing the dangers of secondary atelectasis, pneumonia, and respiratory acidosis.

TABLE 12-20

MOST COMMONLY USED PAIN CONTROL METHODS IN PATIENTS WITH RIB FRACTURES

Method	Description	Agent	Attributes	Disadvantages
Systemic (orally or parenterally)	Intermittent (q 3-4 h) administration	Narcotics	Adequate pain control	May lead to hypoventilation and respiratory failure
Nonsteroidal anti-inflammatory drugs	Intermittent	Ibuprofen Ketorolac	Adjunct to narcotics No respiratory depression	Gastrointestinal problems Risk of renal damage
Intercostal nerve blocks	Multiple injections of intercostal nerves	1% lidocaine 0.25% bupivacaine	Simple technique Efficient	Multiple injections q 4-6 h Risks of pneumothorax
Transcutaneous electrical nerve stimulation	Continuous through skin electrodes	Electrical energy across surface of skin	Safe, no toxicities	Technique not proven Effective only in minor rib fractures
Patient-controlled analgesia	IV narcotics self-administered	Narcotics	Immediate dosing for comfort Maximum dosing limits	Requires compliance of patient and staff May lead to hypoventilation Inefficient in multiple rib fractures
Epidural analgesia	Continuous or intermittent infusion	Local anesthetics, narcotics, or both	Best effectiveness for pain control Can be placed with chest tube	Side effects: pruritus, nausea, urinary retention
Intrapleural analgesia	Continuous or intermittent infusion	Local anesthetics	Minimal side effects	Variable success

Modified with permission from Mayberry JC, Trunkey DD: The fractured rib in chest wall trauma. Chest Surg Clin N Am 1997;7:239-261.

Pulmonary Toilet

Although adequate sedation may effectively alleviate the pain, patients may still have a reluctance or inability to cough. In such cases, nursing staff and physiotherapists can be helpful, particularly during the first few days after injury. *Support of the injured area* by the physiotherapist's hands, for instance, stabilizes the chest wall and helps patients to have a more effective cough. If the patient has retained secretions, more aggressive techniques, such as bedside *fiberoptic bronchoscopy,* should be carried out without hesitation (see Chapter 7, "Atelectasis and Pneumonia").

Treatment of Complications

When rib fractures are complicated by significant pneumothoraces, hemothoraces, or both, these must be drained promptly so that the lung can fully re-expand and the amount of bleeding can be monitored. Under such circumstances, insertion of a chest tube should *always be prioritized.*

Rib Fractures Under Special Circumstances

First and Second Rib Fractures

Fractures of the first two ribs and particularly of the first rib (Table 12-21) are *uncommon* because these ribs are *anatomically protected* by the clavicles, scapulas, and muscles of the upper chest. Such fractures result from a direct severe impact applied over the area or from indirect forces transmitted from adjacent anatomic regions to which the ribs are structurally related. In every patient with a first rib fracture, significant injuries to underlying structures, particularly to blood vessels, must be considered a possibility, and *these must be ruled out* by appropriate diagnostic techniques.

Fractures of the Lower Ribs

Fractures of the eleventh and twelfth ribs are uncommon because these ribs are attached only posteriorly (floating ribs) in addition to being protected by the large muscles of the abdominal wall. Fracture of lower ribs can be associated with injuries to the liver, spleen, and kidneys.

Fractures of the Costal Cartilages

Blunt injuries to the anterior chest wall can result in *fracture of one or more costal cartilages* or in complete separation of an anterior rib from its

12

Chest Trauma

TABLE 12-21

FACTS ABOUT FIRST RIB FRACTURES

They result from severe direct impact or from indirect forces transmitted from adjacent anatomic regions.

They are uncommon because the first rib is well protected.

Significant associated injuries are common and must be ruled out.

They can result in abnormal callus formation with chronic neurovascular syndromes of the thoracic outlet (post-traumatic thoracic outlet syndrome).

costal cartilage. These injuries are characterized by extreme local tenderness, which can in some cases last for long periods because of diminished blood supply and poor healing capacity of the cartilage. *A clicking sensation* is often present at the site of fracture.

Treatment is similar to that of rib fractures, but infiltration of local anesthetics is generally more efficient than it is with rib fractures.

Rib Fractures in Children (Table 12-22)

Most rib fractures seen in children are the result of motor vehicle accidents in which children are *pedestrian victims*. By contrast to adults, rib fractures are uncommon in children because bones are softer and more elastic and thus more able to absorb forceful impacts without breaking. Indeed, children with rib fractures are more likely to be severely injured (thoracic or multisystem), and they have a worse outcome than do children without rib fractures.

Rib Fractures in Elderly

The ribs of elderly individuals are brittle and osteoporotic and can be broken easily. In this population, a minor injury can result in several rib fractures. Apparently minor or isolated rib fractures also have the potential to become serious problems because older patients have an increased incidence of associated comorbidities as well as limited reserve.

Late Sequelae of Rib Fractures

Healing of rib fractures usually results in the formation of a callus, which can become palpable and, as its size increases, be misinterpreted as a chest wall tumor. The callus can also impinge on the adjacent intercostal bundle, resulting in chronic pain within the dermatome supplied by the involved intercostal nerve.

Malunion is not uncommon and usually results in local pain often increased by movement or cough. Symptomatic malunited fractures are best treated with local infiltration of long-lasting anesthetic agents mixed with corticosteroid preparations. On occasion, the site of malunion fracture will require resection for persistent symptoms, but this should only be done after prolonged periods of observation.

Fracture of the first rib may potentially narrow the interscalene triangle, and this narrowing may result in *mechanical compression of the brachial plexus and subclavian artery*. Management is similar to that of patients with thoracic outlet syndromes due to other causes.

TABLE 12-22

RIB FRACTURES IN CHILDREN

Most result from motor vehicle accidents (children are often pedestrian victims).

Rib fractures in infants or toddlers can result from abuse.

Children with rib fractures are more likely to be severely injured than are adults.

There is a direct relationship between number of broken ribs, severity of trauma, and final outcome.

Intercostal pulmonary hernias are rare and usually related to malunion or nonunion of several sites of rib fractures. Most are located *parasternally* or paravertebrally, and most are also small and relatively asymptomatic. Surgery can be considered for large and symptomatic hernias.

Post-traumatic chronic thoracic pain occurs in approximately 30% of victims of thoracic trauma and can last for months or even years. Patients typically complain of tingling sensation and swelling over the anterior chest and upper abdominal wall. Therapy can be *frustrating and generally benefits from a multidisciplinary approach* (see Chapter 11).

FLAIL CHEST

Flail chest is caused by *consecutive ribs being broken in at least two different sites*. As a result, the damaged segment is no longer in continuity with the remainder of the chest wall and becomes unstable and free moving. Flail chest can be observed in 10% to 15% of all patients with severe blunt chest trauma and is associated with significant mortality rates.

Definition and Terminology

Most flail chests are the result of forceful direct impact or compression of the thoracic cage suffered in a motor vehicle accident. The impact causes multiple fractures of consecutive ribs or multiple rib fractures associated with a sternal fracture. Four or more consecutive ribs need to be broken in at least two different sites to create a flail segment, and the *likelihood of instability increases with the number of fractured ribs*.

Three varieties of flail chest can be clinically recognized (Table 12-23). The *anterior flail* occurs when the ribs are separated at their costochondral junction or when the patient has unilateral or bilateral anterior rib fractures with or without sternal fracture. This type of flail chest is commonly associated with respiratory difficulties. The *lateral variety,* which is due to consecutive rib fractures over the lateral chest wall, is the most commonly observed. Posterior flail chests result from posterior rib fractures. They are not only the *least common variety* of flail chest but also the *least dangerous* because the posterior chest wall is strongly supported by muscles and scapula.

TABLE 12-23

TYPES OF FLAIL CHEST

Type	Comment
Anterior flail chest	Caused by anterior rib fractures with or without sternal fracture
	Most dangerous for respiratory complications
Lateral flail chest	Caused by fractures of at least 4 consecutive ribs at 2 or more sites over the lateral chest wall
	Most common variety of flail chest
Posterior flail chest	Related to fractures of posterior ribs
	Least common variety of flail chest and least dangerous for pulmonary complications

One of the most controversial aspects of thoracic traumatology is the *paradoxical motion* created by an unstable chest and its contribution to the pathogenesis of respiratory complications. In normal individuals, inspiration is characterized by an outward movement of the chest wall, and this movement produces a negative intrapleural pressure that draws air into the lungs. In patients with flail segments, the intact portion of the chest wall still moves outward during inspiration, but the flail segment, which is no longer in continuity with the rib cage, moves inward owing to the negative intrapleural pressure. This type of movement (which is contrary to normal respiratory movement) is called *paradoxical respiration*.

Diagnosis

The clinical diagnosis of a flail segment can often be made by *careful observation of the chest wall* during breathing. In some patients, the paradoxical movement *will be obvious;* in others, it *may not be* visible because associated chest wall swelling, contusion, or hematoma will obscure the paradox. In some patients, the flail segment may not be apparent initially (because of shallow breathing), but it will become obvious when breathing becomes more of an effort or when the intrapleural pressure becomes more negative because of atelectasis.

Although the initial chest radiograph may show multiple rib fractures and inward displacement of portions of the chest wall, CT is a better imaging technique to delineate the area of flail chest and to provide information about possible associated thoracic or intra-abdominal injuries.

Pathophysiology of Respiratory Failure in Patients with Flail Chest
(Table 12-24)

Because of the severe chest wall pain, changes in mechanical properties of both the rib cage and respiratory muscles, and underlying lung contusion, flail chests are likely to generate significant alterations in the normal physiology of respiration.

Acute Chest Wall Pain

Acute chest wall pain impairs deep breathing, cough, and expectoration of sputum. As a result, *respiration becomes shallow and labored,* secretions are retained, and atelectasis develops. Because reflex muscle spasm holds the chest in an expiratory pattern, the patient will generate small tidal volume at low resting lung volumes and at an increased rate. Together these factors will bring about major *alterations in the ventilation/perfusion (V̇/Q̇) relationship* with secondary hypoxemia.

In patients with preexisting chronic obstructive pulmonary disease and in elderly individuals, restriction of ventilation is also likely to result in alveolar hypoventilation and carbon dioxide retention.

Changes in Chest Wall Compliance

Muscle spasm, edema, and hematoma of the chest wall reduce chest wall compliance and may further increase the overall work of breathing. The loss of structural integrity of the thoracic cage with secondary flail and

TABLE 12-24

PATHOPHYSIOLOGY OF RESPIRATORY FAILURE IN PATIENTS
WITH FLAIL CHEST

Factor	Consequence	Result
Chest wall pain	Impairment in deep breathing, cough, expectoration	Shallow respiration
		Retention of secretions
		Atelectasis
		Alteration in $\dot{V}/\dot{Q}$ ratio and hypoxemia
		Carbon dioxide retention
Alteration in chest wall compliance	Increased work of breathing	Atelectasis
	Inadequate lung expansion	Hypoxemia
	Ineffective cough	Respiratory failure
Pulmonary contusion	Parenchymal hemorrhage and edema	$\dot{V}/\dot{Q}$ mismatch
		Hypoxemia
Pneumohemothorax	Collapsed lung	Hypoxemia
Cardiac contusion	Decreased cardiac output	Hypotension
		Post-traumatic shock

12

Chest Trauma

paradoxical respiration may also result in *inadequate lung expansion and inefficient cough,* and both factors can further aggravate the hypoxemia.

The pendelluft theory, whereby oxygen-depleted air is thought to move from the injured to the noninjured side because of the paradoxical movement of the rib cage, may exist but plays a minor part in the pathogenesis of respiratory complications due to flail chest.

Pulmonary Contusion

Direct damage to the underlying lung produces *hemorrhage and edema in the contused area*. As a result, there is a ventilation/perfusion mismatch throughout the area, and this derangement also aggravates the hypoxemia. The patient's efforts to correct these abnormalities result in increased work of breathing (due to increased oxygen demand) and muscle fatigue.

Other Factors

Other factors that may contribute to the physiologic derangements related to flail chest include associated hemopneumothoraces, concomitant injuries to other systems, and cardiac deficits due to cardiac contusion or tamponade of the heart by an anterior flail segment.

Management

Patients with minimal compromise can be adequately managed with pain control and aggressive pulmonary therapy. Patients with more significant respiratory compromise may require intubation and mechanical ventilation. Management of the flail segment by open surgical fixation remains controversial.

Treatment of Pain

In patients with flail chests, optimal analgesia is often difficult to achieve because the pain radiates over wide areas of the chest wall.

Epidural analgesia is currently *the standard of pain therapy* not only because it is effective but also because it avoids the problems associated with excessive parenteral narcotics. It should be maintained for approximately 3 to 5 days after trauma, especially if it provides efficient pain control.

Management of the Flail Segment

For advocates of the theory that chest wall instability contributes significantly to the pathophysiology of respiratory complications, operative stabilization of the flail segment is important because it may reduce the need for mechanical ventilation.

It is mostly indicated (Table 12-25) in patients with isolated chest injuries in which *chest wall disruption is severe and pulmonary contusion minimal.* Preferably, it should be done in younger patients with anterior or lateral flail chest when prolonged mechanical ventilation is expected. Surgical fixation can also be done in patients who require thoracotomy for some other reason, such as hemorrhage or bronchial trauma. If the operation is indicated to prevent prolonged mechanical ventilation, it should be done *within 2 to 4 days* of the injury because after that time, the respiratory derangements will have become established, and the patient will still require mechanical ventilation.

Management of Pulmonary Contusion

Many surgeons think that the chest wall injury is relatively unimportant and that the underlying lung contusion is totally responsible for the respiratory complications that may follow severe chest wall injuries and flail chest. In this context, Trinkle and associates were the first to emphasize the concept of *selective management of flail chest (Table 12-26).* They viewed the underlying lung contusion as the primary problem and showed that most patients do not require mechanical ventilation if supportive maneuvers

---

TABLE 12-25

POSSIBLE INDICATIONS AND CONTRAINDICATIONS FOR SURGICAL STABILIZATION OF FLAIL CHESTS

Indications
Deterioration of gas exchange in the absence of significant lung contusion
Isolated chest trauma (no injury to other systems)
Significant anterior or lateral flail chests
Best done in younger patients
Obvious need for prolonged mechanical ventilation
Patient seen within 2-4 days of the injury
Patient needs emergency thoracotomy for other reasons

Contraindications
Severe cerebral injury
Lung contusion requiring mechanical ventilation irrespective of the flail segment
Patient seen > 4 days after trauma
Better cosmetic result

including limitation of intravascular fluid volume, pain relief, and chest physiotherapy are applied. Although several of these recommendations have been modified over the years, Trinkle and colleagues clearly showed that *ventilatory assistance is not required* for most patients with flail chest. The use of broad-spectrum antibiotics is recommended only if the patient shows signs of a developing pneumonia.

In addition to the general indications already described in Chapter 7 ("Mechanical Ventilation for the Surgeon"), patients with flail chest who require intubation and mechanical ventilation are those in shock, those with closed head injury, and those with severe pulmonary contusion. By itself, paradoxical respiration is not considered to be an indication for mechanical ventilation. Mechanical ventilation provides *internal pneumatic stabilization of the unstable segment, reduces the work of breathing* and *discomfort*, and helps support the patient until pulmonary function has recovered.

Late Sequelae of Flail Chest

The most common sequelae of flail chest are persistent chest wall pain, chest wall deformity, and dyspnea on exertion. Dyspneic patients usually present with a *restrictive pattern* due to persistent pain, scarred chest wall, sequelae of contusion, and fibrothoraces. On occasion, struts that have been used for surgical stabilization may have to be removed because of chronic chest wall pain.

CONCLUSION

The physiologic alterations associated with rib fractures and flail chests may decrease ventilation of the ipsilateral lung and produce ventilation/perfusion mismatches leading to hypoxemia. In many patients, conservative efforts to correct these abnormalities will be successful and mechanical ventilation will be avoided. In certain cases, such as those associated with fractured sternum, there is a place for surgical stabilization.

12

Chest Trauma

TABLE 12-26

TRINKLE'S REGIMEN TO AVOID MECHANICAL VENTILATION IN PATIENTS WITH FLAIL CHEST

Intravenous fluids restricted to 1000 mL during resuscitation and 50 mL/h thereafter

Furosemide, 40 mg IV, given on admission and daily for 3 days

Methylprednisolone, 500 mg IV q 6 h, for 2-3 days

Salt-poor albumin, 25 g (100 mL), given daily

Blood loss replaced only with plasma or whole blood, not with crystalloid solutions

Frequent nasotracheal suction, blow bottles, and intermittent positive-pressure breathing

Pain control with morphine or intercostal nerve blocks

Supplemental oxygen as required

Mechanical ventilation only by indication

SUGGESTED READINGS

Review Articles

Kirsh MM, Sloan H: Blunt Chest Trauma. General Principles of Management. Boston, Little, Brown, 1977.

Todd TR: Flail Chest 1989. Proceedings of the University of Toronto Annual Postgraduate Course in Thoracic Surgery. Toronto, June 1989.

Mayberry JC, Trunkey DD: The fractured rib in chest wall trauma. Chest Surg Clin North Am 1997;7:239-261.

Rib Fracture

Kattan KR: What to look for in rib fractures and how. JAMA 1980;243:262-264.

Garcia VF, Gotschall CS, Eichelberger MR, Bowman LM: Rib fractures in children: a marker of severe trauma. J Trauma 1990;30:695-700.

Ziegler DW, Agarwal NN: The morbidity and mortality of rib fractures. J Trauma 1994;37:975-979.

Graham SGA, Schwartz RJ, Jacobs LM, et al: Clinical management of blunt trauma patients with unilateral rib fractures: a randomized trial. World J Surg 1995;19:388-393.

Easter A: Management of patients with multiple rib fractures. Am J Crit Care 2001;10:320-329.

Sirmali M, Türüt H, Topçu S, et al: A comprehensive analysis of traumatic rib fractures: morbidity, mortality and management. Eur J Cardiothorac Surg 2003;24:133-138.

Rib Fractures in Elderly

Bulger EM, Arneson MA, Mock CN, Jurkovich GJ: Rib fractures in the elderly. J Trauma 2000;48:1040-1047.

Albaugh G, Kann B, Puc MM, et al: Age-adjusted outcomes in traumatic flail chest injuries in the elderly. Am Surg 2000;66:978-981.

Bergeron E, Lavoie A, Clas D, et al: Elderly trauma patients with rib fractures are at greater risk of death and pneumonia. J Trauma 2003;54:478-485.

First Rib Fracture

Lazrove S, Harley DP, Grinnell VS, et al: Should all patients with first rib fracture undergo arteriography? J Thorac Cardiovasc Surg 1982;83:532-537.

Flail Chest

Trinkle JK, Richardson JD, Franz JL, et al: Management of flail chest without mechanical ventilation. Ann Thorac Surg 1975;19:355-363.

Clark GC, Schecter WP, Trunkey DD: Variables affecting outcome in blunt chest trauma: flail chest vs. pulmonary contusion. J Trauma 1988;28:298-304.

Freedland M, Wilson RF, Bender JS, Levison MA: The management of flail chest injury: factors affecting outcome. J Trauma 1990;30: 1460-1468.

Ahmed Z, Mohyuddin Z: Management of flail chest injury: internal fixation versus endotracheal intubation and ventilation. J Thorac Cardiovasc Surg 1995;110:1676-1680.

Tanaka H, Yukioka T, Yamaguti Y, et al: Surgical stabilization or internal pneumatic stabilization? A prospective randomized study of management of severe flail chest patients. J Trauma 2002;52: 727-732.

Athanassiadi K, Gerazounis M, Theakos N: Management of 150 flail chest injuries: analysis of risk factors affecting outcome. Eur J Cardiothorac Surg 2004;26:373-376.

Pain Control

Mackersie RC, Karagianes TG, Hoyt DB, Davis JW: Prospective evaluation of epidural and intravenous administration of fentanyl for pain control and restoration of ventilatory function following multiple rib fractures. J Trauma 1991;31:443-451.

Oncel M, Sencan S, Yildiz H, Kurt N: Transcutaneous electrical nerve stimulation for pain management in patients with uncomplicated minor rib fractures. Eur J Cardiothorac Surg 2002;22:13-17.

Operative Stabilization

Mouton W, Lardinois D, Furrer M, et al: Long-term follow-up of patients with operative stabilization of a flail chest. Thorac Cardiovasc Surg 1997;45:242-244.

Voggenreiter G, Neudeck F, Aufmkolk M, et al: Operative chest wall stabilization in flail chest—outcomes of patients with or without pulmonary contusion. J Am Coll Surg 1998;187:130-138.

MANAGEMENT OF THE PATIENT WITH AIRWAY TRAUMA

Tracheobronchial injuries have been recognized as a source of intrathoracic trauma for many years, but their true incidence is still unknown because many patients will die before reaching the hospital. There seems to have been, however, an increase in the number of reported cases in recent years, probably because of the larger number of traffic accidents, better on-site care of trauma victims, and development of specialized regional trauma units.

Although the estimated mortality of patients with tracheobronchial injuries is 30%, 90% of patients reaching the hospital alive can anticipate full recovery. Successful outcome depends on *early diagnosis, accurate assessment of the extent of injury,* and *appropriate treatment.*

12

Chest Trauma

LARYNGOTRACHEAL TRAUMA

Because of the protected position of the larynx and cervical trachea in the neck (mandible, sternum, spine), penetrating or nonpenetrating injuries to these structures are *uncommon*. If they are undiagnosed or improperly managed, however, they can be associated with *significant mortality* or serious *long-term morbidities*.

Injury

Mechanism of Injury (Table 12-27)

Most penetrating injuries of the larynx or upper trachea are due to knife or bullet wounds. Blunt injuries are produced by localized blows over the hyperextended neck often related to steering wheel or dashboard impacts. Indeed, the classic *dashboard airway injury* involves an unrestrained (no seat belt) driver or front seat passenger whose hyperextended neck strikes the dashboard during a head-on collision.

Another possible mechanism of blunt injury is strangulation. This can be due to a seat belt, which applies a compressive force to the neck during a head-on collision, or a rope. Another typical example of this type of injury is the *snowmobile or motorbike rider* who hits an unseen rope while traveling at high speed.

Type of Injuries

Fracture of the cricoid arch with cricotracheal separation results from a sharp transverse blow at the level of the cricoid cartilage. The cricoid arch may be fractured in one or more places, or the cricotracheal junction can be completely transected with distal retraction of the trachea. As discussed by Dr. F. G. Pearson, *both recurrent laryngeal nerves are usually avulsed* when the injury is complete. The injury may be associated with a vertical fracture of the posterior cricoid plate and a tear in the anterior wall of the esophagus, resulting in a tracheoesophageal fistula (see Chapter 11, "Management of the Adult Patient with a Tracheoesophageal Fistula").

Blunt injuries to the cervical trachea are usually due to a direct impact over the hyperextended neck. In such cases, retraction of the distal trachea in the mediastinum may occur, but surprisingly, the patency of the airway is *often maintained by a sleeve of areolar peritracheal tissue*.

Associated Injuries (Table 12-28)

Because of the many adjacent neck structures, penetrating cervical airway trauma is often associated with esophageal or vascular injuries, and these

TABLE 12-27

MECHANISM OF INJURY IN LARYNGOTRACHEAL TRAUMA

Type of Trauma	Mechanism of Injury
Penetrating	Knife or shotgun wound
Blunt	Localized blow over hyperextended neck
	Strangulation by direct compression (seat belt)
	Strangulation by rope

TABLE 12-28

INJURIES COMMONLY ASSOCIATED WITH LARYNGOTRACHEAL TRAUMA

Type of Injury	Commonly Associated Injuries
Penetrating	Esophageal, vascular structures
Blunt	Head, thoracic, cervical spine
	Esophageal, recurrent nerves

are important predictors of morbidity and mortality. Indeed, several series have shown that associated major injuries occur in 50% to 80% of cases.

In cases of blunt trauma, the magnitude of impact necessary to produce airway disruptions makes it likely that associated injuries *will also be common.* Cervical spine fractures or dislocations are particularly important to recognize because extending or flexing the neck to manage the airway of such patients would be dangerous.

Diagnosis

The diagnosis of laryngotracheal injuries often requires a high index of suspicion.

In the emergency department, the surgeon will be confronted with either a *conscious patient,* who can provide useful information about the accident and cooperate with examination, or an *unconscious patient,* who has an unsecured airway or one that has already been intubated or tracheostomized. In the conscious patient, the most common symptoms (Table 12-29) are those of respiratory difficulties and stridor (75% to 90% of patients), hemoptysis, change of voice, and neck pain. Physical findings include erosion of the neck with bruising, laceration, or edema and cervicomediastinal emphysema, which is present in 50% to 80% of cases.

If time is allowed, the most useful early diagnostic studies (Table 12-30) are chest and cervical spine radiographs. *Deep cervical emphysema* can be observed in 80% of patients with airway trauma, and the cervical spine radiographs may further show a *disruption of the tracheal air column* or spine fracture or dislocation. Once the patient has stabilized,

12

Chest Trauma

TABLE 12-29

MOST COMMON SYMPTOMS IN PATIENTS WITH LARYNGOTRACHEAL INJURY DUE TO BLUNT TRAUMA

Symptom	Characteristic
Respiratory difficulty (75%-90% of patients)	Most serious symptom
	May be absent early after the trauma
	Ranges from slight stridor to acute respiratory distress
Change in tone of voice (75%-90% of patients)	Slight dysphonia, hoarseness or aphonia
Hemoptysis	Rarely severe
Neck pain	Often during swallowing
	May indicate spine fracture

TABLE 12-30

DIAGNOSTIC STUDIES IN STABLE PATIENTS WITH POSSIBLE LARYNGOTRACHEAL TRAUMA*

Diagnostic Study	Purpose
Initial chest radiograph	May show associated injuries or deep cervical emphysema
Initial cervical spine radiograph	Necessary to rule out cervical spine fracture or dislocation
Upper chest CT scanning	May provide useful information about larynx, upper trachea, upper mediastinum, and upper ribs (1-2)
Thoracic CT scanning	Must be part of routine trauma work-up
Contrast esophagogram	To rule out associated esophageal injury
Angiography	To rule out associated vascular injury
Flexible laryngobronchoscopy	Most definitive diagnostic technique
	Should be done in operating room setting with ENT surgeon and anesthetist
	Examiner should be ready for possible emergency tracheostomy

*Should be done only in patients with stable airway.

the airway integrity can be further defined by CT scanning and associated injuries can also be ruled out by CT scanning, contrast esophagogram, or aortic angiography.

Flexible laryngotracheal examination should be attempted because it is the most definitive technique to assess airway injuries. Since the examination can sometimes precipitate complete airway obstruction or extend a partial rupture into a complete separation, it must be done in an operating room environment with the assistance of an ENT surgeon and experienced anesthetist. Rigid bronchoscopy is seldom indicated because the rigid bronchoscope can extend the airway injury in addition to being contraindicated in patients with suspected cervical spine injuries.

Management

Prompt recognition and management of patients with possible laryngotracheal trauma are keys to preventing fatal respiratory obstruction or difficult-to-manage long-term sequelae.

Initial Airway Management

Securing the airway is the most important initial step in managing such trauma victims. In patients with severe distress, orotracheal intubation can be attempted, but repeated attempts at intubation should be avoided. In many cases, intubation will be facilitated by the guidance of a flexible bronchoscope, which will direct the endotracheal tube past the area of trauma.

If any difficulties are encountered during bronchoscopy or in patients with severe maxillofacial trauma, an emergency tracheostomy with intubation of the distal segment may be required. If the distal segment has retracted in the mediastinum, it is best found by inserting a finger in the mediastinum, palpating the trachea, and grasping it with a clamp to bring it back out to the neck.

Stabilization of Associated Injuries

Once the airway is secure, the priority shifts to the *diagnosis of possible associated injuries* such as intra-abdominal bleeding and cardiovascular trauma and the sequencing of approaches to their management.

Definitive Management

Early surgical exploration, best achieved by a low cervical collar incision, and primary repair of most laryngotracheal injuries will provide the best results.

Any devitalized fragments of cartilage or segments of cartilage denuded of mucosa *should be removed;* care must also be taken to preserve as much viable airway as possible. In patients with extensive laryngeal injuries, it is possible to resect the cricoid arch with a primary anastomosis between the distal trachea and the thyroid cartilage. Because of possible bilateral vocal cord injury, it is recommended to leave either a *temporary Montgomery T tube or a tracheostomy cannula* after the primary repair. If there is an associated esophageal tear, the defect should be closed primarily and viable muscle interposed at the time of early repair.

When the cervical trachea has been transected transversely, a primary anastomosis is easily achieved, and a tracheostomy is usually not necessary.

Long-term Sequelae

Unrecognized injuries to the larynx or cervical trachea may result in late subglottic or tracheal strictures with progressive airway obstruction. In most such cases, *an emergency tracheostomy had been performed* at the time of initial trauma, and the laryngotracheal injury was overlooked until one tried to remove the tracheotomy cannula.

The management of these sequelae is difficult and requires the combined expertise of both the thoracic surgeon and the otorhinolaryngologist. As a rule, primary repair should only be attempted when the patient *no longer requires mechanical ventilation* and when all associated injuries have resolved. Preoperatively, the full extent of injury and possible involvement of adjacent structures such as the esophagus (see Chapter 11, "Management of the Adult Patient with a Tracheoesophageal Fistula") must be carefully evaluated, and the functional status of the larynx and especially of the vocal cords must also be assessed.

DISRUPTION OF THE INTRATHORACIC TRACHEA

Rupture of the intrathoracic trachea is the *least common* of airway injuries. The usual mechanism is a bursting disruption due to a sudden increase in intratracheal pressure against a closed glottis. Laceration of the

12

Chest Trauma

intrathoracic trachea can also result from difficult or forceful intubations. Although complete disruption may occur under such circumstances, it is much more common to have a vertical laceration in the membranous trachea.

The diagnosis of intrathoracic tracheal rupture can be suspected with the development of mediastinal emphysema, hemoptysis, and pneumothorax if there is air leakage into one or both pleural spaces. Definitive diagnosis is usually established at bronchoscopy.

Management requires the establishment of a safe airway, usually by orotracheal intubation, followed by prompt primary repair.

BRONCHIAL RUPTURE

Injury

Mechanism of Injury (Table 12-31)

Most bronchial tears are the result of severe crushing injury suffered in automobile accidents. Forceful *thoracic compression in the anteroposterior diameter,* such as may occur in a car accident, being run over by a vehicle, or being compressed behind a heavy object, produces lateral widening of the chest with distracting forces acting mostly at the relatively fixed carina. Rupture occurs when the elasticity of the tracheobronchial tree is exceeded.

If the glottis is closed moments before the impact, the crushing of the chest will result in *sudden increase of intrabronchial pressure,* producing a shearing or explosive force within the airway. Rapid deceleration may also generate shearing forces at points of fixation, causing bronchial disruption.

Type of Injuries

Eighty percent of all tears occur within 2.5 cm of the carina, and the lobar or segmental bronchi are seldom affected. The site of rupture is generally at bronchial bifurcations or at the union between membrane and cartilage. In most reports, the right main bronchus is disrupted *more often* than the left, possibly because of its shorter length and larger diameter or because the left main bronchus has more natural protection from surrounding mediastinal structures.

Larger bronchi rupture *more frequently than smaller ones* because the forces acting on the bronchial wall at any given time and intraluminal pressure are greater in large bronchi than in small ones (Laplace law). The type of injury ranges from small laceration to extensive linear tear and from

---

TABLE 12-31

MECHANISMS OF INJURY ASSOCIATED WITH BRONCHIAL RUPTURES

Forceful thoracic compression in anteroposterior axis produces lateral widening of chest

Sudden increase of intrabronchial pressure with closed glottis

Rapid deceleration may generate shearing forces

partial (rare) to complete transection (more common). Despite complete separation, *bronchial continuity and air entry* are often maintained by peribronchial tissues.

Associated Injuries

In patients reaching the hospital alive, there are no associated injuries in about half of cases. Diaphragmatic and aortic ruptures are uncommon, and pulmonary artery damage is almost never found. Upper rib fractures should always raise the possibility of a bronchial tear because both lesions share the same mechanism of injury.

Diagnosis (Table 12-32)

The presenting symptoms and radiographic signs of bronchial disruptions deserve emphasis because early diagnosis and repair are the keys to lung preservation and survival.

Clinical Presentation and Imaging

The clinical features depend on the degree of communication between the site of rupture and the free pleural space.

Free Communication with Pleural Space. With *free communication* between ruptured bronchus and pleural space, typical clinical features are those of *respiratory distress, subcutaneous emphysema,* and *hemoptysis.* The major clues to diagnosis are pneumothorax (on the side of rupture or bilateral), persistent lung collapse despite tube drainage, and large air leak through the chest tube. There is often *increased respiratory distress* or even suffocation when suction is applied to the chest tube because most of the inspired air will be sucked away from the functioning lung.

Early radiologic signs include a radiolucent shadow along the anterior aspect of the cervical spine (deep cervical emphysema) and obstruction in the course of an air-filled bronchus. CT scan may show mediastinal air, deviation of the airway, or the specific site of bronchial rupture. In patients with complete main bronchus rupture, the affected lung may fall over the diaphragm rather than collapse over the hilum as seen with standard pneumothoraces.

TABLE 12-32

CONDITIONS IN WHICH BRONCHIAL RUPTURE SHOULD BE SUSPECTED

Upper thoracic crushing injury (automobile accident)
Fracture of ribs 1-3
Respiratory distress, subcutaneous emphysema, hemoptysis
Pneumothorax (ipsilateral or bilateral)
Persistent lung collapse despite tube drainage
Large air leak
Increased distress when active suction is applied to chest tube
Mediastinal or deep cervical emphysema
Radiologic obstruction in air-filled bronchus

12

Chest Trauma

TABLE 12-33

BRONCHOSCOPY IN PATIENTS WITH POSSIBLE BRONCHIAL RUPTURE

Most useful procedure to confirm diagnosis
Should be done in operating room conditions
Flexible bronchoscopy is preferred to rigid bronchoscopy
Should be done under local anesthesia and light sedation
Most ruptures are clearly seen
Indirect signs include local bleeding, local edema, and air bubbling during respiration

---

Little or No Communication with Pleural Space. In this group, the site of disruption is *within the mediastinum*. The symptoms are *more subtle* because bronchial continuity is often maintained by apposition of peribronchial soft tissues, and the tear is sealed by fibrin or blood clot deposits. Pneumothorax may or may not be present, but in most cases, the lung expands readily with tube drainage.

Definitive Diagnosis

Bronchoscopy (Table 12-33) is the *most useful procedure to* confirm the diagnosis of bronchial rupture, to determine its location and extent, and to plan the repair. It should be done under operating room conditions in the event that the injury is aggravated by endobronchial manipulations. Although there is often an abundance of blood in the airway, we prefer the use of flexible bronchoscopy under local anesthesia and light sedation over rigid bronchoscopy.

The rupture can often clearly be seen, although the full extent of injury may not be apparent. If the disruption is not clearly visualized, indirect endoscopic signs, such as local bleeding, air bubbling, and local edema, may suggest the diagnosis.

Management

Resuscitation and Early Management (Table 12-34)

Contrary to what one might expect, the airway of patients with bronchial rupture is *seldom obstructed*. It is thus possible to manage most of these patients without intubation until such time as bronchoscopy and surgical repair can be carried out.

TABLE 12-34

EARLY MANAGEMENT OF PATIENTS WITH POSSIBLE BRONCHIAL RUPTURE

It is possible to manage most patients without ventilatory support.
Blind insertion of an endotracheal tube can be hazardous:
    It may extend the tracheobronchial laceration.
    Use of muscle relaxants may eliminate the respiratory drive that keeps the patient
    alive.
Emergency tracheotomy may be preferable to blind intubation.
Thoracostomy tubes connected to an underwater seal system should be inserted
    bilaterally.

TABLE 12-35

IMPORTANT RULES TO BE FOLLOWED BY ANESTHESIOLOGIST INDUCING A PATIENT WITH BRONCHIAL RUPTURE

Patient should be intubated while breathing spontaneously.

Patient should not be intubated until surgeon and operating room personnel are ready to perform immediate thoracotomy.

Chest tubes must remain under water seal system until chest is opened.

The primary and only objective is to gain control of the normal lung.

If intubation is deemed necessary, *blind insertion of an endotracheal tube can be extremely hazardous* and should probably be avoided if one is not ready to proceed immediately with bronchoscopy or thoracotomy. Under those circumstances, especially if the trauma victim is far from a specialized center, emergency tracheotomy may be preferred to blind orotracheal intubation. The most significant advantage of a tracheotomy is the easy access given to the airway for aspiration of blood while the patient is transported from a peripheral medical center to a major trauma unit. Tracheostomy also provides an opening by which trapped mediastinal air can be released, and it considerably reduces intratracheal pressures.

Thoracostomy tubes should be inserted *bilaterally and connected to underwater seal drainage systems* without suction.

Definitive Management

All major bronchial disruptions require immediate repair, and the procedure should be *carefully planned with the anesthesiologist* at the time of endoscopy. The important rules to be followed by the anesthesiologist inducing a patient with a bronchial rupture are listed in Table 12-35. We prefer intubation with a disposable double-lumen tube whose proper position can be verified with a flexible bronchoscope and that provides single-lung ventilation during the repair.

The main goal of surgery is the primary repair of the bronchial tear without sacrificing normal lung. In general, pulmonary resection is almost never required other than in ruptures involving smaller bronchi, where reconstruction may be difficult and parenchymal damage more

TABLE 12-36

SURGICAL PRINCIPLES INVOLVED IN THE REPAIR OF TORN BRONCHI

Thorough exploration with particular attention to possible undiagnosed tears of distal bronchial tree, pulmonary artery, or esophagus

Proper exposure of the site of injury and full assessment of extent of damage

Excision of all devitalized and necrotic tissues, mostly at bronchial edges

Primary end-to-end approximation with interrupted absorbable sutures

Use of pedicled flaps to protect site of reconstruction

Fiberoptic bronchoscopy performed at completion of procedure

TABLE 12-37	
LATE SEQUELAE OF UNDIAGNOSED BRONCHIAL RUPTURES	
Type of Rupture	Late Sequelae
Partial	Saccular bronchiectasis and irreversible lung damage
Complete	Atelectasis but no irreversible lung damage

difficult to assess. The principles involved (Table 12-36) are the same as in any other tracheobronchial reconstruction.

Conservative Management of Small Bronchial Tears

Most minor bronchial tears *can be managed conservatively* if the patient has few symptoms and the lung has fully expanded on radiographic examination. These lesions usually consist of a linear tear on the membranous portion of the bronchial wall or a local and limited separation between membrane and cartilage.

All of these patients should be examined by bronchoscopy at regular intervals until the laceration has healed perfectly.

Late Sequelae (Table 12-37)

If a partial bronchial rupture is undiagnosed at the time of injury or shortly thereafter, a *stricture* may develop at the site of rupture and lead within 4 to 6 weeks to saccular bronchiectasis and irreversible lung damage. In this event, pulmonary resection (lobectomy or pneumonectomy) is the only therapeutic alternative.

If the rupture was initially complete, each of the two stumps will separately heal by granulation, and the *distal lung* will fill with noninfected mucus. These patients can be asymptomatic for long periods or present with signs of arterial desaturation due to physiologic intrapulmonary shunting. In this situation, every effort should be made to preserve the distal lung. Bronchoplastic reconstruction should be attempted no matter how long it has been after the initial injury.

CONCLUSION

Tracheobronchial injuries usually result from crushing injuries to the neck or upper thorax. Their diagnosis is possible *through clinical features and judicious use of imaging and endoscopic modalities*. Although excellent results can be expected with early reconstruction, there must be an important coordination and cooperation among the surgeon operating, the anesthesiologist, and the operating room personnel. In cases of upper airway injuries, the otorhinolaryngologist must also be involved in the diagnostic and management processes.

SUGGESTED READINGS

Review Articles

Davies D, Hopkins JS: Patterns in traumatic rupture of the bronchus. Injury 1973;4:261-264.

Urschel HC, Razzuk MA: Management of acute traumatic injuries of tracheobronchial tree. Collective reviews. Surg Gynecol Obstet 1973;136:113-117.

Beesinger DE, Grover FL, Trinkle JK: Tracheobronchial injuries secondary to blunt thoracic trauma. Tex Med 1974;70:74-77.

Pearson FG: Acute Tracheal Trauma. Proceedings of the University of Toronto Annual Postgraduate Course in Thoracic Surgery. Toronto, June 1984.

Kelly JP, Webb WR, Moulder PV, et al: Management of airway trauma I: tracheobronchial injuries. Ann Thorac Surg 1985;40:551-555.

Schaefer SD, Close LG: Acute management of laryngeal trauma. Update. Ann Otol Rhinol Laryngol 1989;98:98-104.

Symbas PN, Justicz AG, Ricketts RR: Rupture of the airways from blunt trauma: treatment of complex injuries. Ann Thorac Surg 1992;54: 177-183.

Devitt JH, Boulanger BR: Lower airway injuries and anaesthesia. Can J Anaesth 1996;43:148-159.

Kiser AC, O'Brien SM, Detterbeck FC: Blunt tracheobronchial injuries: treatment and outcomes. Ann Thorac Surg 2001;71:2059-2065.

Chu CPW, Chen PP: Tracheobronchial injury secondary to blunt chest trauma: diagnosis and management. Anaesth Intensive Care 2002;30:145-152.

Trauma to Cervical Trachea and Larynx

Angood PB, Attia EL, Brown RA, Mulder DS: Extrinsic civilian trauma to the larynx and cervical trachea. Important predictors of long-term morbidity. J Trauma 1986;26:869-873.

Reece GP, Shatney CH: Blunt injuries of the cervical trachea: review of 51 patients. South Med J 1988;81:1542-1547.

Couraud L, Velly JF, Martigne C, N'Diaye M: Posttraumatic disruption of the laryngo-tracheal junction. Eur J Cardiothorac Surg 1989;3: 441-444.

Wu MH, Tsai YF, Lin MY, et al: Complete laryngotracheal disruption caused by blunt injury. Ann Thorac Surg 2004;77:1211-1215.

Case Series

Deslauriers J, Beaulieu M, Archambault G: Diagnosis and long-term follow-up of major bronchial disruptions due to non-penetrating trauma. Ann Thorac Surg 1982;33:32-39.

Fuhrman GM, Stieg FH III, Buerk CA: Blunt laryngeal trauma: classification and management protocol. J Trauma 1990;30:87-92.

Baumgartner F, Sheppard B, de Virgilio C, et al: Tracheal and main bronchial disruptions after blunt chest trauma: presentation and management. Ann Thorac Surg 1990;50:569-574.

Rossbach MM, Johnson SB, Gomez MA, et al: Management of major tracheobronchial injuries: a 28-year experience. Ann Thorac Surg 1998;65:182-186.

12

Chest Trauma

Cassada DC, Munyikwa MP, Moniz MP, et al: Acute injuries of the trachea and major bronchi: importance of early diagnosis. Ann Thorac Surg 2000;69:1563-1567.

Gabor S, Renner H, Pinter H, et al: Indications for surgery in tracheobronchial ruptures. Eur J Cardiothorac Surg 2001;20: 399-404.

Follow-up

Taskinen SO, Salo JA, Halttunen PEA, Sovijarvi ARA: Tracheobronchial rupture due to blunt chest trauma: a follow-up study. Ann Thorac Surg 1989;48:846-849.

Palliation for Lung and Esophageal Carcinoma

PALLIATION FOR LUNG CARCINOMA

The most important treatment objective in resectable lung cancer is the complete removal of the neoplasm. Unfortunately, 70% of patients newly diagnosed with lung cancer will have advanced disease that is too extensive for resection, or they will be found to be medically unfit for operation (inoperable disease). In addition, 60% of patients who have had prior complete resection will eventually have recurrence in the ipsilateral hemithorax or at distant sites. Thus, 80% to 85% of all patients with lung cancer are or will possibly become candidates for palliative therapy.

In such situations, management objectives are to palliate as quickly as possible the symptoms that are a cause of morbidity, to maintain the patient's quality of life, and to prolong, it is hoped, his or her life.

PALLIATION OF SYMPTOMS RELATED TO LOCOREGIONAL DISEASE

Tracheobronchial Obstruction

Tracheobronchial obstruction secondary to an endobronchial tumor or to extrinsic compression can be associated with significant *dyspnea, cough, and stridor*. Whether the cause of obstruction is intrinsic, extrinsic, or both, external beam radiation therapy is often considered the treatment of choice even if it relieves symptoms in only 25% of patients. Newer treatment options that may provide better palliation for patients with proximal airway obstruction include endobronchial tumor ablation, brachytherapy, and stent placement. For patients with distal obstruction, external beam radiotherapy is still the preferred method.

Endobronchial Obstructing Tumors

Endobronchial Tumor Ablation (Table 13-1). Attempts to debulk the tumor with a *rigid bronchoscope and large biopsy forceps* can be successful, but the procedure is associated with significant risks of hemorrhage from the tumor base. Because of such risks, *laser photocoagulation* with the neodymium: yttrium-aluminum-garnet (Nd:YAG) laser has now replaced biopsy forceps debulking. The procedure can be done with a rigid bronchoscope (general anesthesia) and a laser power of 40 to 60 watts or through a fiberoptic bronchoscope (topical anesthesia). Better results are obtained in patients where the length of the tumor is less than 4 cm.

Alternatives to laser ablation include *cryoablation* and *ablation with electrocautery probes*. These procedures are somewhat easier to perform, but they are not as precise as laser photocoagulation with respect to direction of energy and depth of tissue penetration. With electrocautery tumor ablation, relief of symptoms can be obtained in up to 75% of patients.

13

POSSIBLE AIRWAY INTERVENTIONS FOR ENDOBRONCHIAL TUMOR ABLATION

Tumor debulking with rigid bronchoscope and biopsy forceps
Nd:YAG laser photocoagulation
Cryoablation
Ablation with electrocautery probes
Brachytherapy
Photodynamic therapy

Endobronchial brachytherapy refers to a technique whereby *radiotherapy* is delivered through a radioactive source (commonly high-intensity iridium Ir 192) into or close to the endobronchial tumor. The main limitation of the technique is that the radiation field has only a 1.0- to 1.5-cm radius, so tumor cells beyond that radius are relatively unaffected by the treatment. Possible but uncommon complications include hemorrhage and bronchopleural fistulas. With high-dose radiation, the *entire treatment* can be completed in less than 5 minutes.

Photodynamic therapy is an alternative approach that uses a *photosensitive porphyrin agent* administered intravenously 48 hours before the procedure. The porphyrin disseminates to all cells of the body but is retained only in cancer cells (rapidly moves out of normal cells). When it is photoactivated by laser (red light), the porphyrin absorbs the light and initiates an intracellular photochemical reaction that *causes cell destruction* (oxidation of cellular biologic components). Advantages of photodynamic therapy over other methods include *technical ease, safety,* and *possibility of treating distal obstructions* less amenable to laser treatment. The main disadvantages are that patients must avoid exposure to sunlight for periods of 6 to 8 weeks after the injection of the porphyrin and that they require additional bronchoscopy to remove necrotic tissue. Another possible adverse effect is that the edema that sometimes develops within the tumor may temporarily increase the degree of obstruction.

Stent Implantation. Because airway obstruction often recurs after endobronchial tumor ablation, these procedures can be complemented by the insertion of airway stents (Tables 13-2 and 13-3). On the basis of the composing material, airway stents can be classified into silicone tubes and metal prostheses.

The main advantage of silicone tube stents is that they *are removable* and thus can be repositioned. Disadvantages are that they are *prone to migration* and are susceptible to granuloma formation and mucous plugging. Silicone stents also require insertion with a rigid bronchoscope. The most commonly used of such stents is the *Dumon stent,* which has external studs to prevent its migration.

TABLE 13-2

MOST COMMONLY USED BRONCHIAL STENTS

Type of Stent	Characteristics
Tube stents	
Dumon	Considered to be the "gold standard"
	Silicone tube with external studs to prevent migration
	Y-shaped and right main bronchus design available
Polyflex	Self-expandable stent made of polyester wire mesh with a thin layer of silicone
NovoStent	Silicone stent with small metallic hook of nitinol alloy and bands on the ends to prevent migration
Self-expandable metallic stents	
Gianturco	Stainless steel monofilament bent into a zigzag configuration to form a cylinder
	Fixation achieved by small hooks at proximal and distal extremities
	Reported high complication rates (stent disruption, hemoptysis)
Wallstent	Wire mesh made of cobalt-based alloy filaments and coated with silicone
	Uncovered metallic ends prevent migration
Ultraflex	Cylindrical wire mesh of nitinol

Modified from Lee P, Kupeli E, Mehta AC: Therapeutic bronchoscopy in lung cancer. Clin Chest Med 2002;23:241-256, with permission.

Metallic stents are easier to insert, and indeed the procedure can be done under local anesthesia with a fiberoptic bronchoscope. Self-expanding metallic stents, such as the Wallstent and Ultraflex stent, achieve proper bronchial configuration when they are released from their delivery catheter; but once they have been inserted, they *can be difficult* to reposition or to remove.

TABLE 13-3

ADVANTAGES AND DISADVANTAGES OF AIRWAY STENTS

Characteristic	Metal Stents	Silicone Stents
Internal lumen	Larger	Smaller
Insertion	Easier	Needs expertise (rigid bronchoscopy needed)
Repositioning, removal	Almost impossible	Possible and easy
Mucus stasis	More frequent	Less frequent
Displacement	Less frequent	More frequent
Granulation formation	More frequent	Less frequent
Cost	More	Less
Examples	Gianturco stent	Dumon stent
	Wallstent	

Modified from Kim H: Stenting therapy for stenosing airway disease. Respirology 1998;3:221-228, with permission.

Extrinsic Airway Obstruction

When airway obstruction is secondary to external compression, palliation is best achieved by *a combination* of airway stenting and external beam radiation therapy. Chemotherapy alone or in combination with radiotherapy may also play a role in the management of such patients.

Tracheobronchoesophageal Fistula

A malignant tracheobronchoesophageal fistula due to lung cancer is an uncommon but *devastating* complication. Symptoms include coughing while drinking or eating, fever, and recurrent pulmonary infection. Once a fistula has developed, the median survival is generally less than 2 months.

Treatment should therefore be strictly palliative and aim at preventing the flow of esophageal contents into the respiratory tract. Management options are discussed in Chapter 11 (see "Management of the Adult Patient with a Tracheoesophageal Fistula").

Malignant Effusions
Malignant Pleural Effusion

Recurrent malignant pleural effusions are common in lung cancer patients. They can be the cause of significant dyspnea, orthopnea, chest discomfort, and cough. Because 80% of such patients will die within 4 to 6 months of the occurrence of the effusion, *treatment must be expeditious and efficient.* A number of techniques, such as repeated thoracentesis, chemical pleurodesis, and indwelling catheter insertion, are available; their indications and results are discussed in Chapter 11 (see "Management of the Patient with Malignant Pleural Effusion").

Malignant Pericardial Effusion

Pericardial involvement by lung cancer (direct invasion or retrograde progression of disease through lymphatics) can result in *pericardial effusion, occasionally associated with tamponade.* The most common symptoms secondary to nontamponading effusions are dyspnea, cough, and chest pain; those of tamponade include increasing dyspnea and orthopnea or new arrhythmias, such as sinus tachycardia and atrial fibrillation. Diagnosis requires a *high index of suspicion* based on the tumor's location, evidence of increased cardiac size on chest radiograph, and ultimately echocardiography. Because a pleural effusion may also be present, the recognition of a pericardial effusion is often delayed.

Treatment objectives are to *palliate the symptoms, to release the tamponade,* and *to prevent recurrences.* This can be accomplished by simple pericardial drainage and chemical sclerosis or by the creation of a pericardial window through a thoracoscopic or more commonly a subxiphoid approach (Table 13-4). Both procedures allow adequate exploration of the pericardial cavity, with biopsy if necessary.

If it has been elected to proceed with sclerotherapy, a 9 Fr pigtail catheter is first inserted under ultrasound guidance. Once the fluid has

TABLE 13-4

TECHNIQUE OF SUBXIPHOID PERICARDIAL WINDOW

It is usually done under general anesthesia but can be done under local anesthesia.

A 4- to 6-cm vertical incision is made below the xiphoid.

The xiphoid is resected or bisected.

The dissection plane is developed posterior to sternum and anterior to pericardium.

The lower part of anterior pericardium is identified and incised.

The pericardial fluid is drained, and the pericardium is explored with the finger.

One or two chest tubes (separate incisions) are left in pericardial space for 4 or
5 days.

been evacuated, intrapericardial doxycycline can be used to stimulate sclerosis and prevent recurrences (success rate of 75% to 90%).

Superior Vena Cava Syndrome

In lung cancer patients, a superior vena cava syndrome nearly always reflects the presence of N2 disease causing an extrinsic compression of the vein. The syndrome can be recognized in 4% to 5% of patients, and characteristically, the obstruction and thus the symptoms slowly develop during a period of a few weeks.

Relief of superior vena cava obstruction is best achieved through *self-expanding endoprostheses* implanted percutaneously (see Chapter 11, "Management of the Patient with Superior Vena Cava Obstruction"). Because venous thrombosis may also contribute to the obstruction, thrombolysis is often part of endovascular stenting. Once the stent is in place, combined modality treatment approaches with chemoradiation therapy can be carried out.

Patients with *small cell lung cancer* and superior vena cava syndrome can be treated with chemotherapy alone or in combination with thoracic irradiation.

Palliation of Other Symptoms

Hemoptysis

Whereas hemoptysis occurs in up to 25% to 40% of lung cancer patients, it usually involves simple blood streaking of sputum rather than massive hemorrhage. In the majority of such cases, *external beam radiotherapy* will provide symptomatic relief. If the hemoptysis is massive, one can consider bronchial artery or even pulmonary artery embolization (see Chapter 11, "Management of the Patient with Massive Hemoptysis").

Cough

Although cough is a common symptom in smokers without lung cancer, it may become severe or even incapacitating in a significant proportion of lung cancer patients.

Immediate symptomatic relief is best achieved with *codeine-based antitussive medication.* In patients whose cough is secondary to endobronchial or extrinsic tumors causing bronchial irritation or distal atelectasis and pneumonia, external thoracic radiation may be useful.

13

Palliation for Lung and Esophageal Carcinoma

POSSIBLE CAUSES OF THORACIC PAIN IN LUNG CANCER PATIENTS

Parietal pleura contact

True invasion of ribs and chest wall muscles

Abutment or invasion of prevertebral fascia or thoracic spine by posteriorly
    located tumors

Invasion of upper ribs, cervicothoracic spine (C8-T1), and brachial plexus by
    superior sulcus tumors

Invasion of mediastinal pleura and phrenic nerve

Pleural or pericardial effusions

Chest Pain

Lung cancer can cause thoracic pain (Table 13-5) by *contacting* or
invading the parietal pleura or by *true invasion* of ribs and chest wall
muscles. Invasion of intercostal neurovascular bundles may also produce
radicular chest wall pain.

Patients with superior sulcus tumors (see Chapter 11) have *variable
combinations of shoulder and back pain* and radicular arm pain. These are
the result of direct invasion of the upper ribs (one to three), cervicothoracic
spine (C8-T1), chest wall muscles, or C8 and T1 nerve roots.

Direct invasion of the mediastinal pleura and of the phrenic nerve may
cause thoracic back pain often referred to the shoulder because of the
origin of the phrenic nerve from the C3, C4, and C5 nerve roots. Pain can
finally be related to the presence of a pleural or pericardial effusion.

Palliative management of thoracic pain due to locally advanced lung
tumors must begin with a comprehensive assessment to *determine the
most likely source of pain*. If, for instance, the pain is secondary to a
malignant pleural effusion, specific treatment should be that of the
effusion. If the pain is secondary to chest wall or thoracic spine invasion,
external beam radiotherapy is an effective means of palliation. Severe pain
associated with superior sulcus tumors can also be effectively controlled or
even completely relieved by radiation therapy.

Pain management must also include analgesic therapy, and numerous
guidelines for the management of cancer pain are available. Such guidelines
emphasize that therapy must achieve pain relief *within an acceptable time
frame* and *with minimal adverse or side effects* (Table 13-6). Commonly used

PRINCIPLES OF ANALGESIC DRUG THERAPY IN LUNG CANCER PATIENTS

Therapy must achieve adequate pain relief.

Therapy must be safe.

Pain relief must be achieved within an acceptable time frame.

Therapy must have minimal side effects.

Route of administration must be convenient to patient and physician
    (oral and transdermal routes are preferred).

Physician must understand tolerance and dependence.

TABLE 13-7

COMMONLY USED ANALGESICS

Nonopioid analgesics
Aspirin
Acetaminophen
Ibuprofen
Naproxen

Opioid analgesics
Codeine
Oxycodone
Morphine
Hydromorphone
Fentanyl

drugs include nonopioid analgesics, such as acetaminophen, aspirin, and other nonsteroidal anti-inflammatory drugs, and opioid drugs, such as codeine, oxycodone, morphine, and fentanyl (Table 13-7). Transdermal patches can provide pain relief for extended periods; compact portable pumps can deliver medications by both intravenous and subcutaneous infusions.

In selected patients with severe chest pain, *intermittent or continuous epidural infusion of either local anesthetics or opioid analgesics* can provide excellent palliation.

Role of Palliative Pulmonary Resection (Table 13-8)

The role of surgery for the palliation of symptoms in patients with unresectable tumors is highly controversial. There may be clinical situations, such as bronchial obstruction with distal infection, massive hemoptysis, and painful invasion of the chest wall, in which one may want to consider such an option. As a whole, however, palliative procedures are indicated only *when more conservative measures have failed* and when the patient and the patient's relatives clearly understand that operative morbidity and mortality are significantly higher than what is observed after more conventional operations.

PALLIATION OF METASTATIC DISEASE FROM LUNG CANCER

Brain Metastases

Brain metastases constitute nearly one third of all observed distant recurrences in patients with resected non–small cell lung cancer, and twice

TABLE 13-8

POSSIBLE INDICATIONS FOR PALLIATIVE RESECTIONAL
SURGERY OF THE LUNG

Lung abscesses distal to an obstructing tumor
Significant or massive hemoptysis
Excruciating chest wall or back pain due to invasion of thoracic bony structure

that incidence is found at autopsy of all patients dying with lung cancer. They can cause significant morbidity and are often accompanied by widespread metastatic disease.

Radiotherapy is the standard treatment for the palliation of symptomatic brain metastases. The recommended dose fractionation may vary, although in most cases, 30 Gy is given in 10 fractions during 2 weeks. Success rates in improving symptoms range from 50% to 75%. Symptomatic patients with peritumoral edema should also receive *dexamethasone (Decadron) initially given intravenously,* 4 mg four times a day, as well as anticonvulsant medications if they have seizures. Most patients, especially those with severe headaches, will improve within 48 to 72 hours of starting the dexamethasone.

Patients with a limited number of brain metastases can be treated by *stereotactic radiosurgery,* a technique that uses multiple convergent beams to concentrate high radiation doses to a treatment target.

Skeletal Metastases

Bone Metastases

Bone metastases occur in up to 25% of all lung cancer patients; the most common sites are the spine, the pelvis, the ribs, and the proximal ends of long bones. These metastases are primarily *osteolytic and produce localized pain* that is often activity related. Median survival of patients with bone metastases is less than 6 months.

Standard treatment is by radiation therapy (30 Gy given in 10 fractions during 2 weeks), which can attain symptomatic relief of pain in up to 80% of patients. If there is significant pain or high risk of pathologic fracture, patients can also be treated with a single fraction of 8 Gy. *Pain relief usually starts within 2 weeks of completion of the treatment,* and patients often continue to improve up to 3 months after radiotherapy.

In patients with long bone fractures and a life expectancy of more than 3 months, *operative internal fixation* is the most efficient method to control pain, restore function, and allow return to normal activities.

Spinal Cord Compression

Spinal cord compression is secondary to vertebral body metastases. It is a significant clinical problem because if left untreated, it may rapidly lead to complete paraplegia. Treatment (Table 13-9) is initially with dexamethasone followed by radiation therapy to decompress the spinal cord and nerve roots. Provided patients have a life expectancy of more than

---

TABLE 13-9

TREATMENT OF SPINAL CORD COMPRESSION BY METASTATIC DISEASE FROM LUNG CANCER

Dexamethasone, loading dose of 8 mg IV followed by 4 mg q 6 h

Radiotherapy if no or minimal symptoms

Surgery if progression of symptoms or spinal instability

2 or 3 months, surgery may be indicated when there is spinal instability or progression of neurologic symptoms.

PALLIATION OF SYMPTOMS RELATED TO PARANEOPLASTIC SYNDROMES

Paraneoplastic syndromes associated with lung cancer are relatively uncommon. Primary treatment *is that of the underlying neoplasm,* and if the cancer can be completely resected, all symptoms will disappear, often within hours of the operation. Unfortunately, the majority of paraneoplastic syndromes occur in patients with small cell lung cancer or in those who have unresectable disease so that treatment objectives become strictly palliative.

Hypertrophic Pulmonary Osteoarthropathy

Hypertrophic pulmonary osteoarthropathy is characterized by a proliferating periostitis of tubular bones (tibia, fibula, radius), leading to tenderness and swelling, and by digital clubbing. On occasion, these symptoms will become debilitating, especially if they are associated with acute migrating polyarthritis.

Excellent and often dramatic palliation can be achieved with *aspirin or other nonsteroidal anti-inflammatory agents.* Ipsilateral vagotomy proximal to the hilum has been reported to be of some benefit but is no longer done.

Metabolic Syndromes

Hypercalcemia

Although 10% of patients with lung cancer will develop hypercalcemia, only a minority will be symptomatic. In the majority of cases (85%), hypercalcemia is due to *metastatic bone disease,* in which there is bone destruction and release of calcium, or it is *mediated through ectopic parathormone production.* When it becomes symptomatic, hypercalcemia causes general symptoms, such as fatigue and dehydration, as well as neurologic symptoms, such as lethargy, confusion, and muscle weakness (Table 13-10).

Patients with severe (serum calcium concentration ≥ 12 mg/dL) or symptomatic hypercalcemia should be treated by intravenous hydration, especially if they have been vomiting, and infusion of bisphosphonates (pamidronate, 60 to 90 mg during 24 hours). These drugs inhibit calcium release from the bones and will lower the serum calcium concentration in approximately 75% of patients during 24 to 48 hours. In the longer term, pamidronate can be given at a dose of 60 to 90 mg intravenously (infused during 2 to 4 hours) every 7 to 14 days.

TABLE 13-10

SYMPTOMS THAT CAN BE ASSOCIATED WITH HYPERCALCEMIA

General symptoms: fatigue, dehydration, weight loss
Neurologic symptoms: lethargy, muscle weakness, confusion
Gastrointestinal symptoms: nausea, vomiting

TABLE 13-11

CHARACTERISTICS OF THE SYNDROME OF INAPPROPRIATE ANTIDIURETIC HORMONE SECRETION

Early symptoms: fatigue, anorexia, headaches, nausea, vomiting
Late symptoms: confusion, lethargy, seizures
Hyponatremia
Decreased serum osmolarity (<275 mOsm/kg)
Inappropriately high urine osmolarity
Urine osmolarity $>$ serum osmolarity

Syndrome of Inappropriate Antidiuretic Hormone Secretion

The syndrome of inappropriate antidiuretic hormone secretion is due to an *abnormal production of antidiuretic hormone or antidiuretic hormone–like substances by the cancer.* Secretion of large quantities of antidiuretic hormone leads to hyponatremia (water intoxication); symptoms of anorexia, nausea, and vomiting; and symptoms of central nervous system toxicity, such as confusion, lethargy, and seizures (Table 13-11). The diagnosis is made by demonstration of serum hyponatremia, low serum osmolarity, and inappropriately high urine osmolarity.

Because the syndrome of inappropriate antidiuretic hormone secretion is often associated with small cell lung cancer, primary treatment is chemoradiation. Supportive measures include treatment of the hyponatremia with fluid restriction.

CONCLUSION

Although resectional surgery is the treatment of choice in lung cancer, only a small number of patients can be submitted to such operations. For most other patients, the primary objective of management is palliation. Under such circumstances, effective palliation can be of benefit through relief of symptoms, maintenance of quality of life, psychological support, and prolonged survival.

SUGGESTED READINGS

Review Articles

Pizzo PA: Management of fever in patients with cancer and treatment-induced neutropenia (Review article). N Engl J Med 1993;328: 1323-1332.

Ashburn MA, Lipman AG: Management of pain in the cancer patient. Anesth Analg 1993;76:402-416.

Kanner R: Recent advances in cancer pain management. Cancer Invest 1993;11:80-87.

Tchekmedyian NS: Clinical approaches to nutritional support in cancer. Curr Opin Oncol 1993;5:633-638.

Shepherd FA: Treatment of advanced non–small cell lung cancer. Semin Oncol 1994;21:7-18.

Feld R: Recent advances in supportive care in patients with lung cancer. Lung Cancer 1994;11(suppl 3):S101-S110.

American Society of Clinical Oncology: Clinical practice guidelines for the treatment of unresectable non–small-cell lung cancer [special article]. J Clin Oncol 1997;15:2996-3018.

Lee P, Kupeli E, Mehta AC: Therapeutic bronchoscopy in lung cancer. Laser therapy, electrocautery, brachytherapy, stents, and photodynamic therapy. Clin Chest Med 2002;23:241-256.

Wood DE: Management of malignant tracheobronchial obstruction. Surg Clin North Am 2002;82:621-642.

Wood DE, Liu YH, Vallières E, et al: Airway stenting for malignant and benign tracheobronchial stenosis. Ann Thorac Surg 2003;76:167-174.

Bezjak A: Palliative therapy for lung cancer. Semin Surg Oncol 2003;21:138-147.

Potter J, Higginson IJ: Pain experienced by lung cancer patients: a review of prevalence, causes, and pathophysiology. Lung Cancer 2004;43:247-257.

Endobronchial Therapy

de Souza AC, Keal R, Hudson NM, et al: Use of expandable wire stents for malignant airway obstruction. Ann Thorac Surg 1994;57:1573-1578.

Tojo T, Iioka S, Kitamura S, et al: Management of malignant tracheo-bronchial stenosis with metal stents and Dumon stents. Ann Thorac Surg 1996;61:1074-1078.

Monnier P, Mudry A, Stanzel F, et al: The use of the covered Wallstent for the palliative treatment of inoperable tracheobronchial cancers. A prospective multicenter study. Chest 1996;110:1161-1168.

Wasserman K, Eckel HE, Michel O, Müller RP: Emergency stenting of malignant obstruction of the upper airways: long-term follow-up with two types of silicone prosthesis. J Thorac Cardiovasc Surg 1996;112:859-866.

Sutedja TG, van Boxem TJ, Schramel FM, et al: Endobronchial electrocautery is an excellent alternative for Nd:YAG laser to treat airway tumors. J Bronchology 1997;4:101-105.

Kim H: Stenting therapy for stenosing airway disease. Respirology 1998;3:221-228.

Moghissi K, Dixon K, Stringer T, et al: The place of bronchoscopic photody-namic therapy in advanced unresectable lung cancer: experience of 100 cases. Eur J Cardiothorac Surg 1999;15:1-6.

Maiwand MO: The role of cryosurgery in palliation of tracheobronchial carcinoma. Eur J Cardiothorac Surg 1999;15:764-768.

Simoff MJ: Endobronchial management of advanced lung cancer. Cancer Control 2001;8:337-343.

Wood DE: Airway stenting. Chest Surg Clin North Am 2001;11:841-860.

Madden BP, Datta S, Charokopos N: Experience with Ultraflex expandable metallic stents in the management of endobronchial pathology. Ann Thorac Surg 2002;73:938-944.

13

Palliation for Lung and Esophageal Carcinoma

Morris CD, Budde JM, Godette KD, et al: Palliative management of malignant airway obstruction. Ann Thorac Surg 2002;74:1928-1933.

Maziak DE, Markman BR, Mackay JA, Evans WK, and the Cancer Care Ontario Practice Guidelines Initiative Lung Cancer Disease Site Group: Photodynamic therapy in nonsmall cell lung cancer: a systematic review. Ann Thorac Surg 2004;77:1484-1491.

Freitag L: Interventional endoscopic treatment. Lung Cancer 2004;45(suppl):s235-s238.

Radiotherapy

Baldini EH: Palliative radiation therapy for non–small cell lung cancer. Hematol Oncol Clin North Am 1997;11:303-319.

Budach W, Belka C: Palliative percutaneous radiotherapy in non–small-cell lung cancer. Lung Cancer 2004;45(suppl):s239-s245.

Effusions

Palatianos GM, Thurer RJ, Pompeo MQ, Kaiser GA: Clinical experience with subxiphoid drainage of pericardial effusions. Ann Thorac Surg 1989;48:381-385.

Liu G, Crump M, Goss PE, et al: Prospective comparison of the sclerosing agents doxycycline and bleomycin for the primary management of malignant pericardial effusion and cardiac tamponade. J Clin Oncol 1996;14:3141-3147.

Girardi LN, Ginsberg RJ, Burt ME: Pericardiocentesis and intrapericardial sclerosis: effective therapy for malignant pericardial effusions. Ann Thorac Surg 1997;64:1422-1428.

Cardillo G, Facciolo F, Carbone L, et al: Long-term follow-up of video-assisted talc pleurodesis in malignant recurrent pleural effusions. Eur J Cardiothorac Surg 2002;21:302-306.

Superior Vena Cava Syndrome

Gross CM, Krämer J, Waigand J, et al: Stent implantation in patients with superior vena cava syndrome. AJR Am J Roentgenol 1997;169:429-432.

Tracheoesophageal Fistula

Burt M: Management of malignant esophagorespiratory fistula. Chest Surg Clin North Am 1996;6:765-776.

Brain Metastases

Taimur S, Edelman MJ: Treatment options for brain metastases in patients with non–small-cell lung cancer. Curr Oncol Rep 2003;5:342-346.

Zabel A, Debus J: Treatment of brain metastases from non–small-cell lung cancer (NSCLC): radiotherapy. Lung Cancer 2004;45(suppl):s247-s252.

Hypercalcemia

Bilezikian JP: Management of acute hypercalcemia [review article]. N Engl J Med 1992;326:1196-1203.

Hall TG, Burns Schaiff RA: Update on the medical treatment of hypercalcemia of malignancy [therapy update]. Clin Pharm 1993;12:117-125.

PALLIATION FOR ESOPHAGEAL CARCINOMA

Patients with unresectable esophageal carcinoma often require palliation of local symptoms. For individuals with *esophageal obstruction,* the objectives of therapy are to restore the esophageal lumen, to relieve dysphagia, and to improve nutrition. For those with airway fistulization, the primary goal is to occlude the fistulous track.

To achieve those objectives, numerous forms of interventions are available, including chemoradiation, insertion of stents, photodynamic therapy, laser photocoagulation therapy, and in selected cases, surgical bypass of the obstructed esophagus. Because the median survival of such patients is less than 6 months, these interventions must carry *low morbidity and mortality* as well as have high *short-term* success rates.

SYMPTOMS REQUIRING PALLIATION

Symptoms Related to Esophageal Obstruction (Table 13-12)

The most common presenting symptom in patients with esophageal obstruction is dysphagia, *initially for solids and later for liquids* as the obstruction progresses and becomes more complete. Eventually, patients become unable to swallow even their own saliva, and indeed, esophageal obstruction is often associated with *reflex hypersalivation.* Patients with high-grade obstruction may also have regurgitations, often worse at night when they are lying supine; these regurgitations can lead to coughing, aspiration, and pulmonary suppuration.

Odynophagia (retrosternal pain associated with swallowing) is not uncommon. When the tumor has spread beyond the esophageal wall into the posterior mediastinum, patients may also have *persistent back pain.*

Symptoms Related to Airway Fistulization

As the tumor enlarges, fistulization between the esophageal lumen and the tracheobronchial tree can occur. The clinical consequences of such fistulization are related to the *spillage of esophageal contents* such as saliva and food into the airway with secondary bronchial obstruction, refractory pneumonia, and respiratory distress. The severity of symptoms requiring palliation is generally proportional to the width and length of the fistula.

13

Palliation for Lung and Esophageal Carcinoma

| TABLE 13-12 |

SPECTRUM OF SYMPTOMS ASSOCIATED WITH ESOPHAGEAL OBSTRUCTION

Dysphagia
Odynophagia (retrosternal pain associated with swallowing)
Hypersalivation
Regurgitation, aspiration, cough
Chronic pulmonary suppuration

TABLE 13-13

TECHNIQUES THAT CAN BE USED TO PALLIATE SYMPTOMS DUE TO ESOPHAGEAL OBSTRUCTION

Tumor dilatation
Chemoradiation therapy (external beam) or radiotherapy alone
Endoscopic interventions
    Laser ablation
    Photodynamic therapy
    Brachytherapy
    Electrocautery excision
Esophageal stenting
Surgical bypass

Other Symptoms That May Require Palliation

Other symptoms that may need to be palliated include *chronic anemia* secondary to low-grade blood loss from the tumor, pain (whether or not related to swallowing), and *chronic malnutrition*. Palliation of symptoms related to metastatic disease is similar to what has already been outlined in the palliation of lung cancer (see "Palliation of Lung Cancer").

PALLIATION OF ESOPHAGEAL OBSTRUCTION

Techniques that may be used to relieve esophageal obstruction and to improve dysphagia (Table 13-13) include tumor dilatation; chemoradiation therapy; endoscopic interventions, such as laser ablation, photodynamic therapy, electrocautery excision, and brachytherapy; use of esophageal stents; and on occasion, esophageal bypass.

Tumor Dilatation and External Beam Radiotherapy With or Without Chemotherapy (Tables 13-14 and 13-15)

Tumor dilatation can be accomplished with mercury bougies, but the procedure is associated with *significant risks* of perforating the esophagus or creating airway fistulization. Because relief of dysphagia is short-lived, tumor dilatation is *seldom used* as a solitary procedure.

    External beam radiation therapy (Table 13-15) is well tolerated and relieves symptoms of esophageal obstruction in more than 50% of patients. The response can be short-lived, however, and dysphagia will often persist because the tumor may have been replaced by fibrous tissue. Radiation therapy requires *prolonged treatment courses* (30 days), and it can be associated with *significant complications* such as airway fistulization. Concurrent chemoradiation does not appear to result in improved palliation.

TABLE 13-14

ADVANTAGES AND DISADVANTAGES OF TUMOR DILATATION

Advantage	May be necessary in preparation for other palliative measures
Disadvantages	Short-lived relief of dysphagia
	Dangers of perforation or fistulization
Comment	Almost never used for palliation of esophageal cancer

TABLE 13-15

ADVANTAGES AND DISADVANTAGES OF EXTERNAL BEAM RADIOTHERAPY

Advantages
Well tolerated by patients
Causes significant tumor shrinkage and improvement
   in symptoms in 50% of patients

Disadvantages
Treatment course is prolonged
Complications are common (one third of cases)
Tumor may be replaced by fibrous tissue, and dysphagia may
   persist (stricture formation)
Patients often unable to complete treatment

13

Chemotherapy alone is almost never used because the *toxicity can be significant* in the setting of debilitated patients with poor performance status.

Endoscopic Interventions (Table 13-16)

Endoscopic interventions can be quite useful if the indications are respected and the patients well selected.

Laser photocoagulation (Nd:YAG laser) is the most popular of these techniques because it is easy to use (flexible esophagoscope) and the laser beam has excellent coagulating and tissue penetration properties. It is *ideally suited* for endoluminal fungating tumors located in the midportion of the esophagus. Potential drawbacks include significant perforation rates (depth of penetration unpredictable) and the fact that most patients will require repeated treatments.

With photodynamic therapy, selective endoscopic delivery of light (specific wavelength) activates a photosensitizing agent that results in tumor cell death. Despite its potential advantages (see Table 13-16), the technique is seldom used not only because it requires *specialized equipment* but also because the photosensitizing agent is expensive, and there is a high incidence of patients requiring re-treatment. In the short-term, photodynamic therapy relieves dysphagia in more than 80% of patients.

Brachytherapy involves the intraluminal delivery of high-dose radiotherapy, usually given in two or more fractions 1 week apart. Improvement in dysphagia occurs in more than 50% of patients; the level of improvement depends on *tumor size* (i.e., better results with smaller tumors). Complications such as strictures and fistulization are common.

The BICAP tumor probe delivers bipolar electrocoagulation energy to the tumor. Although it is seldom used, the technique can help quickly relieve dysphagia. It has a low incidence of complications.

Palliation for Lung and Esophageal Carcinoma

TABLE 13-16

ADVANTAGES AND DISADVANTAGES OF TECHNIQUES
OF ENDOSCOPIC INTERVENTION

Technique	Advantages	Disadvantages	Comment
Laser ablation (Nd:YAG)	Ease of use (flexible endoscope) Excellent tissue penetration Excellent coagulation properties (control of bleeding) Provides immediate relief of dysphagia	Complications in 5%-10% of cases Repeated treatment often necessary (>50%)	Ideally suited for fungating tumor in midportion of esophagus Less popular since advent of metallic self-expandable stents Requires experienced endoscopist
Photodynamic therapy (photosensitizing agents)	Improvement in dysphagia in majority of patients (>80%) Improvement within days of treatment Low perforation rate	Skin photosensitivity for 4-6 weeks High costs of specialized equipment and photosensitizing agent Re-treatment often necessary	Ideal candidates have primarily endoluminal disease with minimal extrinsic compression Seldom used technique except in specialized centers
Brachytherapy (intraluminal radiation)	Improvement in dysphagia in 40%-80% of cases Short treatment time (few minutes) Rapid improvement in dysphagia	Most patients require at least 2 fractions Requires highly specialized radiation equipment and experienced radiotherapist Often associated with strictures (25%) and tracheoesophageal fistula Inefficient in large tumors	Seldom used technique

Esophageal Stents

The best method currently available to relieve dysphagia is the *intubation of the obstructed esophagus* with prosthetic tubes. Indeed, the biggest advantage of intubation techniques is that they provide immediate relief of obstruction.

Plastic and Self-Expandable Metallic Stents (Table 13-17)

Over the years, various prostheses have been developed. These can generally be classified into plastic tubes and self-expandable metallic stents.

TABLE 13-17

COMPARISON OF EXPANDABLE STENTS AND PLASTIC TUBES

	Expandable Stents	Plastic Tubes
Deployment	Easy	More difficult
Dilation	Minimal or unnecessary	Necessary
Complications	Seldom	Common
Lengthening of the device	Possible	Not possible
Removability	No	Yes
Tumor ingrowth	Seldom/often	Seldom
Migration of device	Seldom/often	Often

From Frenken M: Best palliation in esophageal cancer: surgery, stenting, radiation, or what? Dis Esophagus 2001;14:120-123, with permission.

13

Plastic tubes (Celestin tube, Atkinson tube) are rigid and feature a *distal flange,* which helps prevent their migration, and a *proximal funnel* to help guide ingested food through the lumen of the prosthesis. They are notoriously difficult to deploy, and their use is associated with *significant complication rates.* Since the advent of self-expandable metallic stents, the indications for plastic tubes have decreased significantly.

Self-expanding metal stents are designed to be placed in narrow areas *where they exert an outward radial force during their deployment.* Two models of self-expanding metallic stents are currently popular. The Ultraflex stent* is made of nitinol and available in coated (silicone) and uncoated versions. The stent itself is bound to an introducer, which is manipulated into position by a combination of endoscopic and fluoroscopic techniques. It is deployed by simply pulling on a string, which results in the release of the stent (Fig. 13-1). The Wallstent is made of a woven stainless steel mesh, and it also comes in covered and uncovered versions.

Metal stents are effective in relieving obstruction, and both the Ultraflex and the Wallstent are associated with low incidence of esophageal perforation (<1%). Potential drawbacks include the fact that they can be very difficult to remove once they have been deployed and that tumor ingrowth might occur through the mesh (especially if the stent is uncovered) and reocclude the esophageal lumen.

Stent Insertion According to the Location of the Obstruction

Before an esophageal prosthesis is deployed, an important issue to consider is the *location of the obstruction* (Table 13-18). For high cervical or cricopharyngeal obstructions, the foreign body sensation may be difficult to tolerate and metallic stents should be avoided. Indeed, patients with tumors in those locations are perhaps better managed with *repeated dilatations or electrocautery probe debulking* of the tumor. On occasion, softer and thinner salivary tubes (Montgomery-Hood) will also work well under such circumstances.

*Microinvasive, Boston Scientific, Watertown, Mass.

Palliation for Lung and Esophageal Carcinoma

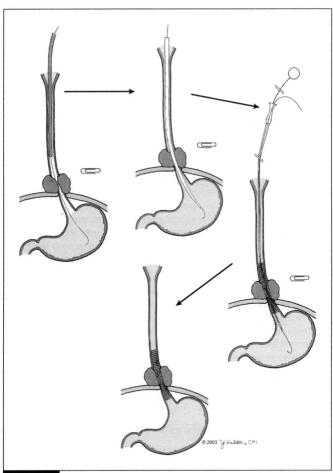

FIG. 13-1

Technique of insertion of a self-expandable metallic stent of the Ultraflex variety. Once the holding catheter and stent have been manipulated into precise position, the operator pulls on the holding thread, which results in the deployment of the stent. The paper clip is used as a reference on fluoroscopy of the proximal extent of the tumor.

For lesions at the gastroesophageal junction, passage of a tube into the stomach may generate significant reflux. To decrease the consequences of such a problem, patients can be managed by elevating the head of the bed and by long-term antacid therapy. In patients with severe reflux, the prosthesis may have to be completely removed.

TABLE 13-18

CONSIDERATIONS IN STENT PLACEMENT ACCORDING TO THE LOCATION
OF THE OBSTRUCTION

Location of Obstruction	Comment
Proximity to cricopharyngeal muscle or high cervical	Foreign body sensation may be difficult to tolerate. Avoid hard metallic prosthesis. Soft and thin salivary tubes may be useful.
Mid esophageal lesions	4 cm of prosthesis should protrude beyond the tumor in either direction.
Gastroesophageal junction	Significant gastroesophageal reflux may occur. Stents are more likely to migrate.

Management of Stent Failure

The insertion of an endoesophageal stent is usually associated with
immediate relief of dysphagia. Because of such relief, patients may
become enthusiastic toward eating, and this enthusiasm can *generate food
impaction* within the prosthesis. To prevent this problem, patients should
be advised to cut their food in small pieces ($1\ cm^3$) and to drink carbonated
fluids while eating (this will increase food migration across the prosthesis).

Another potential source of stent failure is the development of a stricture
over the uncovered portion of the stent. This is usually due to *tumor
ingrowth* but can also be secondary to ingrowth of normal mucosa through
the meshing of the prosthesis. The best way to avoid such a problem is to
use covered stents. If the problem still occurs, treatment consists of tissue
debulking with the Nd:YAG laser or large biopsy forceps.

Esophageal Bypass

Palliative esophageal bypass procedures are *seldom indicated* because they
are associated with significant morbidity and mortality rates and often result
in worsening of the patient's quality of life. As a rule, these operations
should be proposed only to well-selected younger patients in otherwise
relatively good health.

Practice Guidelines

Dysphagia can be a significant problem in patients with unresectable
tumors of the esophagus or in patients with local recurrences after
esophagectomy. Because the surgeon may not be familiar with the entire
spectrum of palliative techniques, it is important that she or he works
within *a multidisciplinary group* so that patients can be offered the most
appropriate method of palliation.

In general, external beam radiotherapy has little role in palliation of
dysphagia because it requires several weeks before an effect can be noted.
If external beam radiotherapy is given concurrently with chemotherapy, it
probably has better palliative effects, but the treatment can be associated
with *life-threatening toxicities*.

13

Palliation for Lung and Esophageal Carcinoma

Photocoagulated laser therapy may be indicated for tumors that are relatively short in length, especially those located in the *mid or distal esophagus*. Laser therapy provides immediate relief of dysphagia, but often the procedure must be repeated. Laser therapy is contraindicated in patients with dysphagia secondary to extrinsic compression of the esophagus.

Endoluminal plastic stents are seldom used because they must be positioned under general anesthesia and they are associated with high complication rates (25%), including perforation, tube migration, and airway fistulization. *Self-expanding metal stents* are safer and can be used in nearly all patients, even those with external compression of the esophageal lumen. Most patients will note significant improvement early after the procedure, and the incidence of complications is low. Tumor ingrowth through the stent with secondary obstruction is possible, but this complication can be prevented by use of coated stents.

Bypass surgery is almost never indicated in debilitated patients or in patients whose median survival is expected to be less than 6 months.

For patients with a reasonably good performance status, one can *combine modality regimens* so that survival can be prolonged in addition to the palliation of dysphagia. Stents may, for instance, be deployed before radiotherapy or chemotherapy. In other patients, laser photocoagulation can be followed by intubation, which is then followed by external beam radiotherapy.

PALLIATION OF AIRWAY FISTULIZATION

Airway fistulization arises from tumor necrosis with secondary erosion in the membranous portion of the airway. This process will occasionally have been enhanced by radiation therapy. For most patients, treatment should strictly be palliative, and the options are limited to esophageal intubation and supportive care (see Chapter 11, "Management of the Adult Patient with a Tracheoesophageal Fistula"). *Covered self-expandable metallic stents are particularly well suited for treatment of such patients.* Despite effective palliation, few patients will survive more than a few months after the diagnosis of airway fistulization.

PALLIATION OF SYMPTOMS RELATED TO CHRONIC BLOOD LOSS

Patients with unresectable esophageal carcinomas will often have symptoms related to anemia that is due to chronic blood loss from the tumor bed. This is seldom a significant clinical problem and can be managed by laser photocoagulation followed by external beam endotherapy.

CONCLUSION

Palliation of esophageal carcinoma is *best achieved* through the use of self-expandable metallic stents. Improved stents that are silicone covered can provide longer palliation by preventing recurrent obstruction due to tumor ingrowth. In patients with good performance status, chemoradiation can be added in the hope of prolonging survival.

SUGGESTED READINGS

Review Articles

Lerut TE, de Leyn P, Coosemans W, et al: Advanced esophageal carcinoma. World J Surg 1994;18:379-387.

Ell C, May A: Self-expanding metal stents for palliation of stenosing tumors of the esophagus and cardia: a critical review. Endoscopy 1997;29:392-398.

Siersema PD, Dees J, Van Blankenstein M: Palliation of malignant dysphagia from oesophageal cancer. Scand J Gastroenterol Suppl 1998;33(suppl 225):75-84.

Wong R, Malthaner R: Esophageal cancer: a systematic review. Curr Probl Cancer 2000;24:297-373.

Frenken M: Best palliation in esophageal cancer: surgery, stenting, radiation, or what? Dis Esophagus 2001;14:120-123.

Weigel TL, Frumiento C, Gaumintz E: Endoluminal palliation for dysphagia secondary to esophageal carcinoma. Surg Clin North Am 2002;82:747-761.

Specific Therapy—Photodynamic Therapy

Saidi RF, Marcon NE: Nonthermal ablation of malignant esophageal strictures. Photodynamic therapy, endoscopic intratumoral injections, and novel modalities. Gastrointest Endosc Clin North Am 1998;8:465-491.

Maier A, Tomaselli F, Gebhard F, et al: Palliation of advanced esophageal carcinoma by photodynamic therapy and irradiation. Ann Thorac Surg 2000;69:1006-1009.

Litle VR, Luketich JD, Christie NA, et al: Photodynamic therapy as palliation for esophageal cancer: experience in 215 patients. Ann Thorac Surg 2003;76:1687-1693.

Specific Therapy—Brachytherapy

Jager J, Langendijk H, Pannebakker M, et al: A single session of intraluminal brachytherapy in palliation of esophageal cancer. Radiother Oncol 1995;37:237-240.

Sur RK, Donde B, Levin VC, Mannell A: Fractionated high dose rate intraluminal brachytherapy in palliation of advanced esophageal cancer. Int J Radiat Oncol Biol Phys 1998;40:447-453.

Sharma V, Mahantshetty U, Dinshaw KA, et al: Palliation of advanced/recurrent esophageal carcinoma with high-dose-rate brachytherapy. Int J Radiat Oncol Biol Phys 2002;52:310-315.

Specific Therapy—Laser

Norberto L, Ranzato R, Marino S, et al: Endoscopic palliation of esophageal and cardial cancer: neodymium-yttrium aluminum garnet laser therapy. Dis Esophagus 1999;12:294-296.

Specific Therapy—Esophageal Bypass and Palliative Resection

Mannell A, Becker PJ, Nissenbaum M: Bypass surgery for unresectable esophageal cancer: early and late results in 124 cases. Br J Surg 1988;75:283-286.

13

Palliation for Lung and Esophageal Carcinoma

Mitani M, Kuwabara Y, Shinoda N, et al: The effectiveness of palliative resection for advanced esophageal carcinoma: analysis of 24 consecutive cases. Surg Today 2002;32:784-788.

Specific Therapy—Stents

Knyrim K, Wagner HJ, Bethge N, et al: A controlled trial of an expansile metal stent for palliation of esophageal obstruction due to inoperable cancer. N Engl J Med 1993;329:1302-1307.

Mehran R, Duranceau A: The use of endoprosthesis in the palliation of esophageal carcinoma. Chest Surg Clin North Am 1994;4:331-346.

Dittler HJ, Pfister KGM: Palliation of esophageal cancer: stents and tubes. Dis Esophagus 1996;9:105-116.

Acunas B, Rozanes I, Akpinar S, et al: Palliation of malignant esophageal strictures with self-expanding nitinol stents: drawbacks and complications. Radiology 1996;199:648-652.

Moores DWO, Ilves R: Treatment of esophageal obstruction with covered, self-expanding esophageal Wallstents. Ann Thorac Surg 1996;62: 963-967.

Maier A, Pinter H, Frieas GB, et al: Self-expandable coated stent after intraluminal treatment of esophageal cancer: a risky procedure? Ann Thorac Surg 1999;67:781-784.

Christie NA, Buenaventura PO, Fernando HC, et al: Results of expandable metal stents for malignant esophageal obstruction in 100 patients: short-term and long-term follow-up. Ann Thorac Surg 2001;71: 1797-1802.

O'Donnell CA, Fullarton GM, Watt E, et al: Randomized clinical trial comparing self-expanding metallic stents with plastic endoprostheses in the palliation of oesophageal cancer. Br J Surg 2002;89:985-992.

Specific Therapy—Radiotherapy

Hayter CRR, Huff-Winters C, Paszat L, et al: A prospective trial of short-course radiotherapy plus chemotherapy for palliation of dysphagia from advanced esophageal cancer. Radiother Oncol 2000;56;329-333.

Comparison Between Treatments

Low DE, Pagliero KM: Prospective randomized clinical trial comparing brachytherapy and laser photoablation for palliation of esophageal cancer. J Thorac Cardiovasc Surg 1992;104:173-179.

Lightdale CJ, Heier SK, Marcon NE, et al: Photodynamic therapy with porfimer sodium versus thermal ablation therapy with Nd:YAG laser for palliation of esophageal cancer: a multicenter randomized trial. Gastrointest Endosc 1995;42:507-512.

Cwikiel M, Cwikiel W, Albertsson M: Palliation of dysphagia in patients with malignant esophageal strictures. Acta Oncol 1996;35:75-79.

Aoki T, Osaka Y, Takagi Y, et al: Comparative study of self-expandable metallic stent and bypass surgery for inoperable esophageal cancer. Dis Esophagus 2001;14:208-211.

Malignant Tracheoesophageal Fistula

Mohammed S, Moss J: Palliation of malignant tracheo-oesophageal fistula using covered metal stents. Clin Radiol 1996;51:42-46.

Low DE, Kozarek RA: Comparison of conventional and wire mesh expandable prostheses and surgical bypass in patients with malignant esophagorespiratory fistulas. Ann Thorac Surg 1998;65:919-923.

Appendices

APPENDIX 1: WEANING PROTOCOL

Guidelines

1. Communication between all bedside caregivers is key to the successful care of the patient.
2. All ventilator changes must be communicated to and coordinated with the attendant nurse in charge of the patient.
3. Decisions to place patients on protocol or to take patients off protocol and changes in the patient's status must be communicated by the physician to the nursing and respiratory care personnel.
4. Failure to progress through the protocol or worsening of clinical status must be communicated from respiratory care personnel and nurses to physicians.
5. All changes in ventilator settings and patient's status must be completely documented.
6. Extubation requires physician's consent.
7. Protocol-directed screening for extubation will take place only between 0500 and 1600.

Protocol Entry Criteria

1. Written physician order to enter into the protocol.
2. ABG on entry, with $Pao_2/Fio_2 \geq 200$.
3. Entry static compliance ≥ 25 mL/cm H_2O.
4. Entry minute volume ($\dot{V}E$) ≤ 15 mL/min.
5. No failure of ventilator discontinuation in past 24 hours.

Oxygenation/Ventilation Weaning

1. Initial settings: SIMV to deliver 6-12 mL/kg, rate high enough to support at most 80% of patient's minute volume; PS to deliver tidal volume of 5-7 mL/kg; PEEP, 0-15 cm H_2O; Fio_2 to maintain sat $\geq 92\%$; and $Pao_2 \geq 60$ mm Hg.
2. In conjunction with nursing personnel, ensure that the following are within acceptable limits for the patient: hemodynamics, temperature, blood pressure, pain control, heart rhythm, mental status, blood loss, patient's cooperation, electrolytes, reversal of anesthetic agents.
3. Obtain an ABG within 1 hour of ICU arrival and ensure acceptable correlation with monitors. Subsequent ABGs as indicated.
4. Incrementally decrease ventilator support as follows, with **no less than 30 minutes and no more than 1 hour** between changes:
   a. Decrease Fio_2 to ≤ 0.50 (increments of 0.10).
   b. Decrease PEEP to ≤ 6 cm H_2O.
   c. Decrease IMV rate to ≤ 6 bpm (increments of 2 bpm).
   d. Decrease PS to ≤ 8 cm H_2O.
   e. Alternate oxygenation changes (a or b) with ventilation changes (c or d).

    f. Perform above to maintain $Sao_2 \geq 92\%$, spontaneous RR $\leq$ 30, $V_T \geq 5$ mL/kg, normal respiratory drive, and $Petco_2 \leq 45$ mm Hg.

5. If the above changes are not tolerated, reverse the most recent change. If not improved by 10 minutes, **notify physician** and hold weaning protocol.

6. Once the above target values (IMV $\leq$ 6, PS $\leq$ 8, $Fio_2 \leq 0.50$, PEEP $\leq$ 6) are met, the patient will be screened for **Extubation Criteria.** Screening times are between the hours of 0600 and 1600.

Extubation Criteria

1. Changes to PS ventilation (IMV zero) and flow-by; with tolerance of target values (above) for Fio_2, PEEP, and PS; for 30 minutes. *Observe:*
   a. O_2 sat $\geq$ 92%.
   b. Respiratory rate < 30 bpm.
   c. Spontaneous tidal volume > 5 mL/kg body weight.
   d. No respiratory distress, agitation, or clinical signs of increased work of breathing.
   e. Hemodynamic changes < 20% of baseline.
   f. $Petco_2 \leq 45$ mm Hg.

If the above is observed for 30 minutes, then:

2. Patient must have GCS score $\geq$ 10 or tracheostomy.
3. Patient must have MAP $\geq$ 60 mm Hg, no pressors (except dopamine at ≤ 5 μg/kg/min).
4. Patient must have good cough not limited by pain.
5. Patient must be able to clear airway of secretions.
6. Respiratory rate/tidal volume $\leq$ 105 br/min/L.
7. NIF $\geq$ 25 cm H_2O.
8. $\dot{V}_E \leq 12$ L/min.
9. Hours between 0600 and 1600.
10. ABG obtained.
11. Physician notification and approval for extubation.

Extubation

1. Physician consent obtained and documented.
2. Extubation to nasal cannula or aerosol determined by physician before extubation.
3. Incentive spirometry every 15 minutes $\times$ 2 hours, then every 1 hour after extubation.
4. Obtain ABG $\frac{1}{2}$ hour after extubation.

ABG, arterial blood gas; GCS, Glasgow Coma Scale; ICU, intensive care unit; IMV, intermittent mandatory ventilation; MAP, mean arterial pressure; NIF, negative inspiratory force; PEEP, positive end-expiratory pressure; PS, pressure support; SIMV, synchronized intermittent mandatory ventilation.

WEANING PROTOCOL FROM RESPIRATOR

Parameter	Threshold
Gas exchange	
Pao_2/Fio_2	>200 mm Hg
Pao_2 ($Fio_2 = 0.21$)	>50 mm Hg
Pao_2 ($Fio_2 = 1.0$)	>350 mm Hg
Ventilatory	
Respiratory rate (f)	<30/min
Tidal volume (V_T)	>5 mL/kg
Vital capacity (VC)	>10 mL/kg
Minute ventilation ($\dot{V}_E$)	<10 L/min
Negative inspiratory force	< −20 to −30 cm H_2O
Breathing pattern	
Respiratory alternans	Absent

Appendices

APPENDIX 2: STAGING OF LUNG CANCER

THE INTERNATIONAL TNM STAGING SYSTEM FOR THE STAGING OF LUNG CANCER

PRIMARY TUMOR (T)

TX	Primary tumor cannot be assessed, or the tumor proven by the presence of malignant cells in sputum or bronchial washings but not visualized by imaging or bronchoscopy
T0	No evidence of primary tumor
Tis	Carcinoma in situ
T1	Tumor <3 cm in greatest dimension, surrounded by lung or visceral pleura, without bronchoscopic evidence of invasion more proximal than the lobar bronchus* (i.e., not in the main bronchus)
T2	Tumor with any of the following features of size or extent: >3 cm in greatest dimension Involves main bronchus, ≥2 cm distal to the carina Invades the visceral pleura Associated with atelectasis or obstructive pneumonia that extends to the hilar region but does not involve the entire lung
T3	Tumor of any size that directly invades any of the following: Chest wall (including superior sulcus tumors), diaphragm, mediastinal pleura, or parietal pericardium; or Tumor in the main bronchus <2 cm distal to the carina but without involvement of the carina; or Associated atelectasis or obstructive pneumonitis of the entire lung
T4	Tumor of any size that invades any of the following: Mediastinum, heart, great vessels, trachea, esophagus, vertebral body, or carina; or Tumor with a malignant pleural or pericardial effusion†; or Tumor with satellite tumor nodule(s) within the ipsilateral primary-tumor lobe of the lung

Continued

THE INTERNATIONAL TNM STAGING SYSTEM FOR THE STAGING OF LUNG CANCER—cont'd

REGIONAL LYMPH NODES (N)

NX	Regional lymph nodes cannot be assessed
N0	No regional lymph node metastasis
N1	Metastasis to ipsilateral peribronchial or ipsilateral hilar lymph nodes and intrapulmonary nodes involved by direct extension of the primary tumor
N2	Metastasis to ipsilateral mediastinal or subcarinal lymph node(s)
N3	Metastasis to contralateral mediastinal, contralateral hilar, ipsilateral or contralateral scalene, or supraclavicular lymph node(s)

DISTANT METASTASIS (M)

MX	Presence of distant metastasis cannot be assessed
M0	No distant metastases detected
M1	Distant metastasis present‡

*The uncommon superficial tumor of any size with its invasive component limited to the bronchial wall, which may extend proximal to the main bronchus, is also classified T1.

†Most pleural effusions associated with lung cancer are due to tumor. However, there are a few patients in whom multiple cytopathologic examinations of pleura fluid show no tumor. In these cases, the fluid is nonbloody and is not an exudate. When these elements and clinical judgment indicate that the effusion is not related to the tumor, the effusion should be excluded as a staging element and the patient's disease should be staged T1, T2, or T3. Pericardial effusion is classified according to the same rules.

‡Separate metastatic tumor nodule(s) in the ipsilateral nonprimary-tumor lobe(s) of the lung are also classified M1.

STAGE GROUPING OF TNM SUBSETS*

Stage 0	Tis	Carcinoma in situ	
Stage IA	T1	N0	M0
Stage IB	T2	N0	M0
Stage IIA	T1	N1	M0
Stage IIB	T2	N1	M0
	T3	N0	M0
Stage IIIA	T3	N1	M0
	T1-3	N2	M0
Stage IIIB	T4	Any N	M0
	Any T	N3	M0
Stage IV	Any T	Any N	M1

*Staging is not relevant for occult carcinoma, designated TXN0M0.

Reprinted from Mountain CF: Revisions in the International System for Staging Lung Cancer. Chest 1997;111:1710-1717.

APPENDIX 3: NODAL MAPPING OF LUNG CANCER
MEDIASTINAL LYMPH NODE MAP DEFINITIONS* (FIG. A-1)

Nodal Station	Anatomic Location
N2 nodes: All N2 nodes lie within the mediastinal pleural envelope.	
1 Highest mediastinal nodes	Nodes lying above a horizontal line at the upper rim of the brachiocephalic vein where it ascends to the left, crossing in front of the trachea at its midline
2 Upper paratracheal nodes	Nodes lying above a horizontal line drawn tangential to the upper margin of the aortic arch and below the inferior boundary of 1 nodes
3 Pretracheal and retrotracheal nodes	Pretracheal and retrotracheal nodes may be designated 3a and 3p; midline nodes are considered to be ipsilateral
4 Lower paratracheal nodes	The lower paratracheal nodes on the right lie to the right of the midline of the trachea between a horizontal line drawn tangential to the upper margin of the aortic arch and a line extending across the right main bronchus at the upper margin of the upper lobe bronchus and are contained within the mediastinal pleural envelope.
	The lower paratracheal nodes on the left lie to the left of the midline of the trachea between a horizontal line drawn tangential to the upper margin of the aortic arch and a line extending across the left main bronchus at the level of the upper margin of the left upper lobe bronchus, medial to the ligamentum arteriosum, and are contained within the mediastinal pleural envelope.
	The lower paratracheal nodes may be classified into 4s (superior) and 4i (inferior) subsets. The 4s nodes may be defined by a horizontal line extending across the trachea and drawn tangential to the cephalic border of the azygos vein. The 4i nodes may be defined by the lower boundary of 4s and the lower boundary of 4, as described above.
5 Subaortic (A-P window)	Subaortic nodes are lateral to the ligamentum arteriosum or the aorta or left pulmonary artery and proximal to the first branch of the left pulmonary artery and lie within the mediastinal pleural envelope
6 Para-aortic nodes (ascending aorta or phrenic)	Nodes lying anterior and lateral to the ascending aorta and the aortic arch or the innominate artery, beneath a line tangential to the upper margin of the aortic arch
7 Subcarinal nodes	Nodes lying caudal to the carina of the trachea, but not associated with the lower lobe bronchi or arteries within the lung
8 Paraesophageal nodes (below carina)	Nodes lying adjacent to the wall of the esophagus and to the right or left of the midline, excluding subcarinal nodes
9 Pulmonary ligament nodes	Nodes lying within the pulmonary ligament, including those in the posterior wall and lower part of the inferior pulmonary vein

Appendices

Continued

MEDIASTINAL LYMPH NODE MAP DEFINITIONS* (FIG. A-1)—cont'd

Nodal Station	Anatomic Location
N1 nodes: All N1 nodes lie distal to the mediastinal pleural reflection (takeoff of the upper lobe bronchi) and within the visceral pleura.	
10 Hilar nodes	The proximal lobar nodes, distal to the mediastinal pleural reflection and the nodes adjacent to the bronchus intermedius on the right
	Radiographically, the hilar shadow may be created by enlargement of both hilar and interlobar nodes.
11 Interlobar nodes	Nodes lying between the lobar bronchi
12 Lobar nodes	Nodes adjacent to the distal lobar bronchi
13 Segmental nodes	Nodes adjacent to the segmental bronchi
14 Subsegmental nodes	Nodes around the subsegmental bronchi

*According to the combined staging system of the American Joint Committee on Cancer (AJCC) and the Union Internationale Contre le Cancer (UICC).

From Mountain CF, Dresler CM: Regional lymph node classification for lung cancer staging. Chest 1997;111:1718-1723.

NOTE FROM THE EDITOR

Regional Lymph Node Classification

The lymph node–bearing regions of the thorax have been classified for the last 15 years according to two different staging systems, the one used by the American Joint Committee on Cancer (AJCC) and the other used by the Union Internationale Contre le Cancer (UICC). The AJCC staging is based on the map proposed by the American Thoracic Society[1] (Fig. A-2); the one used by the UICC is based on the original description of Naruke[2] (Fig. A-3). The first map is principally used in North America, whereas the second is mainly used in Europe and Asia. The unification of these two maps led to the combined map as described by Mountain and Dresler. However, this map is still not used universally. Since the two original maps are still in use, it is important to continue to mention them and to understand their dissimilarities. The main differences affect the definition of the lymph node territories 1, 3, and 10.

In the AJCC system, level 1 lymph nodes are supraclavicular. The UICC system includes also the lymph nodes in the upper third of the thorax above the level of the left innominate vein.

Level 3 lymph nodes in the AJCC system are either 3a, anterior to the superior vena cava, or 3p, around the esophagus. The AJCC system has

---

[1]American Thoracic Society: Clinical staging of lung cancer. Am Rev Respir Dis 1983;127:659-664.

[2]Naruke T, Suemasu K, Ishikawa S: Lymph node mapping and curability at various levels of metastasis in resected lung cancer. J Thorac Cardiovasc Surg 1978;76:832-839.

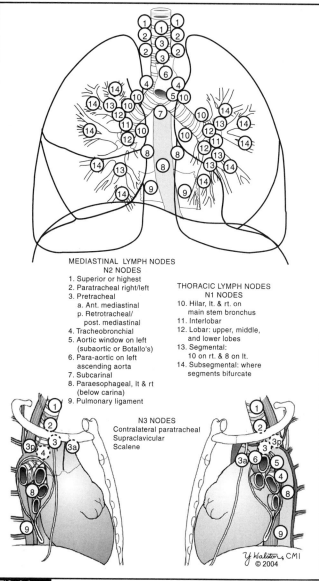

MEDIASTINAL LYMPH NODES
N2 NODES
1. Superior or highest
2. Paratracheal right/left
3. Pretracheal
   a. Ant. mediastinal
   p. Retrotracheal/
      post. mediastinal
4. Tracheobronchial
5. Aortic window on left
   (subaortic or Botallo's)
6. Para-aortic on left
   ascending aorta
7. Subcarinal
8. Paraesophageal, lt & rt
   (below carina)
9. Pulmonary ligament

THORACIC LYMPH NODES
N1 NODES
10. Hilar, lt. & rt. on
    main stem bronchus
11. Interlobar
12. Lobar: upper, middle,
    and lower lobes
13. Segmental:
    10 on rt. & 8 on lt.
14. Subsegmental: where
    segments bifurcate

N3 NODES
Contralateral paratracheal
Supraclavicular
Scalene

Y. Walston, CMI
© 2004

FIG. A-1

Mediastinal lymph node map, combined staging system of the American Joint
Committee on Cancer and the Union Internationale Contre le Cancer.

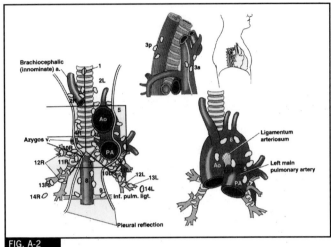

Regional lymph node map, staging classification of the American Joint Committee on Cancer.

no description for pretracheal lymph nodes; these lymph nodes are labeled 3 in the UICC system.

The anatomic landmarks for station 10 are not clear in either system. Level 10 lymph nodes are hilar lymph nodes. For the AJCC system, these lymph nodes are situated at the takeoff of the upper lobar bronchi. In the UICC system, level 10 lymph nodes involve also lymph nodes found around the main stem bronchi.

The differences in the definition of the lymph node–bearing territories of the chest can lead to confusion in the interpretation of research data. Obviously, a unified system was necessary to combine the information obtained by both staging systems. This led to the creation of a revised system proposed by Mountain in 1997. The new system presented here should be the system used in clinical settings worldwide.

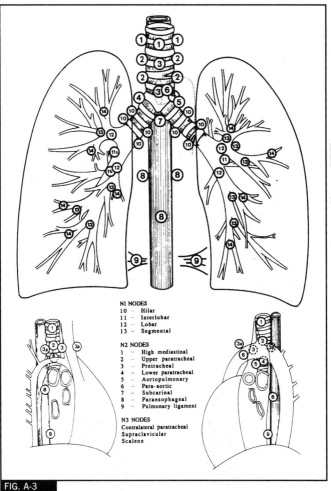

FIG. A-3

Regional lymph node map, staging classification of the Union Internationale Contre le Cancer.

APPENDIX 4: STAGING OF ESOPHAGEAL CANCER
TNM STAGING OF ESOPHAGEAL CARCINOMA
T: PRIMARY TUMOR

TX	Tumor cannot be moved
T0	No evidence of tumor
Tis	High-grade dysplasia
T1	Tumor invades the lamina propria, muscularis mucosa or submucosa; does not breach the submucosa
T2	Tumor invades into but not beyond the muscularis propria
T3	Tumor invades the paraesophageal tissue but does not invade adjacent structures
T4	Tumor invades adjacent structures

N: REGIONAL LYMPH NODES

NX	Regional lymph nodes cannot be assessed
N0	No regional lymph node metastases
N1	Regional lymph node metastases

M: DISTANT METASTASES

MX	Distant metastases cannot be assessed
M1a	Upper thoracic esophagus metastatic to cervical lymph nodes
	Lower thoracic esophagus metastatic to celiac lymph nodes
M1b	Upper thoracic esophagus metastatic to other nonregional lymph nodes or other distant sites
	Midthoracic esophagus metastatic to either nonregional lymph nodes or other distant sites
	Lower thoracic esophagus metastatic to other nonregional lymph nodes or other distant sites

STAGE GROUPINGS	T	N	M
Stage 0	T in situ	N0	M0
Stage I	T1	N0	M0
Stage IIA	T2	N0	M0
	T3	N0	M0
Stage IIB	T1	N1	M0
	T2	N1	M0
Stage III	T3	N1	M0
	T4	Any N	M0
Stage IVA	Any T	Any N	M1a
Stage IVB	Any T	Any N	M1b

APPENDIX 5: STAGING OF THYMOMA
MASAOKA STAGING SYSTEM FOR THYMOMA

Stage	Definition
I	Macroscopically—completely encapsulated
	Microscopically—no capsular invasion
II	Macroscopic invasion into surrounding fatty tissue or mediastinal pleura
	Microscopic invasion into capsule
III	Macroscopic invasion into neighboring organ (i.e., pericardium, great vessels, or lung)
IVA	Pleural or pericardial dissemination
IVB	Lymphogenous or hematogenous metastasis

From Masaoka A, Monden Y, Nakahara K, Tanioka T: Follow-up study of thymomas with special reference to their clinical stages. Cancer 1981;48:2485-2492.

APPENDIX 6: STAGING OF MALIGNANT MESOTHELIOMA

IMIG STAGING SYSTEM FOR DIFFUSE MALIGNANT PLEURAL MESOTHELIOMA

T—Tumor

T1	T1a	Tumor limited to the ipsilateral parietal ± mediastinal ± diaphragmatic pleura
		No involvement of the visceral pleura
	T1b	Tumor involving the ipsilateral parietal ± mediastinal ± diaphragmatic pleura
		Tumor also involving the visceral pleura

T2   Tumor involving each of the ipsilateral pleural surfaces (parietal, mediastinal, diaphragmatic, and visceral pleurae) with at least one of the following features:

Involvement of diaphragmatic muscle

Extension of tumor from visceral pleura into the underlying pulmonary parenchyma

T3   Describes locally advanced but *potentially resectable* tumor

Tumor involving all of the ipsilateral pleural surfaces (parietal, mediastinal, diaphragmatic, and visceral pleurae) with at least one of the following features:

Involvement of the endothoracic fascia

Extension into the mediastinal fat

Solitary, completely resectable focus of tumor extending into the soft tissues of the chest wall

Nontransmural involvement of the pericardium

T4   Describes locally advanced *technically unresectable* tumor

Tumor involving all of the ipsilateral pleural surfaces (parietal, mediastinal, diaphragmatic, and visceral pleurae) with at least one of the following features:

Diffuse extension or multifocal masses of tumor in the chest wall, with or without associated rib destruction

Direct transdiaphragmatic extension of tumor to the peritoneum

Direct extension of tumor to the contralateral pleura

Direct extension of tumor to mediastinal organs

Direct extension of tumor into the spine

Tumor extending through to the internal surface of the pericardium with or without a pericardial effusion; or tumor involving the myocardium

N—LYMPH NODES

NX	Regional lymph nodes cannot be assessed
N0	No regional lymph node metastases
N1	Metastases in the ipsilateral bronchopulmonary or hilar lymph nodes
N2	Metastases in the subcarinal or the ipsilateral mediastinal lymph nodes including the ipsilateral internal mammary nodes
N3	Metastases in the contralateral mediastinal, contralateral internal mammary, ipsilateral, or contralateral supraclavicular lymph nodes

M—METASTASES

MX	Presence of distant metastases cannot be assessed
M0	No distant metastasis
M1	Distant metastasis present

Continued

Appendices

IMIG STAGING SYSTEM FOR DIFFUSE MALIGNANT PLEURAL MESOTHELIOMA—cont'd

Staging

Stage			
Stage I			
Ia	T1a	N0	M0
Ib	T1b	N0	M0
Stage II	T2	N0	M0
Stage III	Any T3	Any N1	M0
		Any N2	
Stage IV	Any T4	Any N3	Any M1

From Rusch VW: A proposed new international TNM staging system for malignant pleural mesothelioma. From the International Mesothelioma Interest Group. Chest 1995; 108:1122-1128.

Index

Page numbers followed by *f* indicate figures; those followed by
t indicate tables.